DICTIONARY OF
MEDICAL
BIOGRAPHY

EDITORIAL BOARD

DICTIONARY OF MEDICAL BIOGRAPHY

Volume 2, C–G

Edited by

W. F. Bynum *and* Helen Bynum

GREENWOOD PRESS
Westport, Connecticut • London

Library of Congress Cataloging-in-Publication Data

Dictonary of medical biography / edited by W. F. Bynum and Helen Bynum.
     p.   cm.
    Includes bibliographical references and index.
    ISBN 0–313–32877–3 (set : alk. paper) — ISBN 0–313–32878–1 (v. 1 : alk. paper) —
    ISBN 0–313–32879–X (v. 2 : alk. paper) — ISBN 0–313–32880–3 (v. 3 : alk. paper) —
    ISBN 0–313–32881–1 (v. 4 : alk. paper) — ISBN 0–313–32882–X (v. 5 : alk. paper)
  1. Medicine—Biography. 2. Healers—Biography. I. Bynum, W. F. (William F.), 1943– . II. Bynum, Helen.
R134.D57   2007
610—dc22   2006022953

British Library Cataloguing in Publication Data is available.

Library of Congress Catalog Card Number: 2006022953
ISBN: 0–313–32877–3 (set)
         0–313–32878–1 (vol. 1)
         0–313–32879–X (vol. 2)
         0–313–32880–3 (vol. 3)
         0–313–32881–1 (vol. 4)
         0–313–32882–X (vol. 5)

First published in 2007

Greenwood Press, 88 Post Road West, Westport, CT 06881
An imprint of Greenwood Publishing Group, Inc.
www.greenwood.com

Printed in the United States of America

The paper used in this book complies with the
Permanent Paper Standard issued by the National
Information Standards Organization (Z39.48–1984).

10   9   8   7   6   5   4   3   2   1

CONTENTS

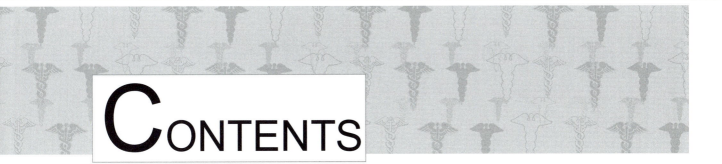

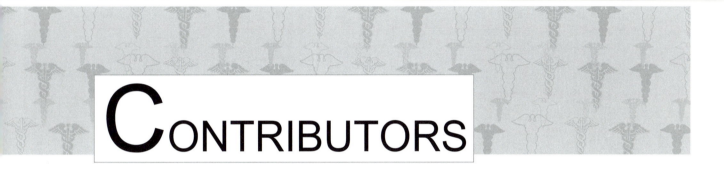

CONTRIBUTORS

Göran Åkerström
Academic Hospital, Uppsala, Sweden
Sandström

Seema Alavi
Jamia Millia University, New Delhi, India
Aziz

Angelo Albrizio
Institut d'Histoire de la Médecine et de la Santé,
Geneva, Switzerland
De Giovanni

W. R. Albury
University of New South Wales, Sydney,
Australia
Bichat, Broussais, Corvisart des Marets, Magendie

Marta de Almeida
Museu de Astronomia e Ciências Afins,
Rio de Janeiro, Brazil
Ribas

Cristina Álvarez Millán
UNED, Madrid, Spain
*Ibn Buṭlān, Al-Majūsī, Ibn al-Nafīs, Al-Rāzī, Ibn Rushd,
Ibn Zuhr*

Stuart Anderson
LSHTM, London, England
Beecham, Holloway, Squibb

Warwick Anderson
University of Wisconsin–Madison, Madison, WI,
USA
Burnet, Cleland

Jon Arrizabalaga
CSIC, Barcelona, Spain
Laguna, Sanches, Torrella

S. N. Arseculeratne
University of Peradeniya, Peradeniya,
Sri Lanka
M. Paul, Wickramarachchi

Mikel Astrain
Universidad de Granada, Granada, Spain
Lardizábal Dubois

Guy Attewell
Wellcome Trust Centre for the History of Medicine
at UCL, London, England
*Medical Traditions in South Asia, Abd ul-Hamīd,
M. Ajmal Khān, M. A'zam Khān, Saīd*

Nara Azevedo
Casa de Oswaldo Cruz, Fundação Oswaldo Cruz,
Rio de Janeiro, Brazil
Cruz

Søren Bak-Jensen
Medical Museion, Copenhagen, Denmark
*Fibiger, Friderichsen, Gram, Hagedorn,
Pindborg, Salomonsen*

Martha Baldwin
Stonehill College, Easton, MA, USA
Dionis

Marta Aleksandra Balinska
Institut national du cancer, Paris, France
Hirszfeld, Rajchman, Śniadecki

Rosa Ballester
Universidad Miguel Hernández, Alicante-Valencia, Spain
Martínez Vargas

Scott Bamber
UNICEF, Bangkok, Thailand
Jivaka

Richard Barnett
Wellcome Trust Centre for the History of Medicine
at UCL, London, England
Godlee, Knox, Long, W. Morton, Read, Simpson, Wakley

Josep Lluís Barona
Universidad de Valencia Blasco, Valencia, Spain
Ramón y Cajal, Trueta i Raspall

Penelope Barrett
Wellcome Trust Centre for the History of Medicine
at UCL, London, England
Li Shizhen

Alexander R. Bay
Chapman University, Orange Campus, CA, USA
Takaki

Elaine Beale
Cherhill, Wiltshire, England
Ingen Housz

Norman Beale
Cherhill, Wiltshire, England
Ingen Housz

Denise Best
California State University, Fresno, CA, USA
Pokrovskaia

Anne-Emanuelle Birn
University of Toronto, Toronto, ON, Canada
Morquio

Carla Bittel
Loyola Marymount University, Los Angeles, CA, USA
Baker, A. Jacobi, M. P. Jacobi, Van Hoosen

Johanna Bleker
ZHGB, Institut für Geschichte der Medizin,
Berlin, Germany
Henle, Schoenlein

Michael Bliss
University of Toronto, Toronto, ON, Canada
Cushing, Dandy

Hans Blom
Erasmus Universiteit, Rotterdam, the Netherlands
Mandeville

Michel Bonduelle
University of Paris, Paris, France
Duchenne de Boulogne, Guillain

Christopher Booth
Wellcome Trust Centre for the History of Medicine
at UCL, London, England
Haygarth, Hurst, Lettsom, Sherlock

Cornelius Borck
McGill University, Montreal, QC, Canada
Berger

Mineke Bosch
Universiteit Maastricht, Maastricht,
the Netherlands
Jacobs

David Bradley
LSHTM, London, England
Macdonald

Gunnar Broberg
University of Lund, Lund, Sweden
Linnaeus

Alejandra Bronfman
University of British Columbia, Vancouver,
BC, Canada
Finlay y Barres, Guiteras Gener

Linda Bryder
University of Auckland, Auckland, New Zealand
Gordon, King, Liley

Chris Burton
University of Lethbridge, Lethbridge, AB,
Canada
Burdenko, Fedorov, Semashko, Solev'ev

Helen Bynum
Shadingfield, Suffolk, England
Halsted, Harinasuta, Rogers, Snow, Steptoe

Ricardo Campos
CSIC, Madrid, Spain
Rubio Gali

Franco Carnevale
Azienda Sanitaria di Firenze, Florence, Italy
Devoto, Ramazzini

Ana María Carrillo
UNAM, Mexico City, Mexico
Montoya Lafragua

Ian Carter
University of Auckland, Auckland, New Zealand
M. Bell

Ramón Castejón-Bolea
Universidad Miguel Hernández, Alicante, Spain
Azúa y Suárez

Rafael Chabrán
Whittier College, Whittier, CA, USA
Hernández

Iain Chalmers
The James Lind Initiative, Oxford, England
Cochrane

Joël Chandelier
Ecole française de Rome, Rome, Italy
Gentile da Foligno

Rethy Chhem
University of Western Ontario, London, ON,
Canada
Yajnavaraha

Indira Chowdhury
Tata Institute of Fundamental Research,
Mumbai, India
*Chopra, Dharmendra, Mukerji, Pandit,
Ramalingaswami, P. Sen, Vakil*

Charlotte Christensen-Nugues
University of Lund, Lund, Sweden
Harpestreng

Amy Eisen Cislo
Washington University, St Louis, MO, USA
Gilbert the Englishman

Catherine S. Coleborne
Waikato University, Hamilton, New Zealand
Manning

Andrea Contini
University of Paris XII, Paris, France
Basaglia

Roger Cooter
Wellcome Trust Centre for the History of Medicine
at UCL, London, England
Braid, Charnley, Gall, R. Jones, Treves, Wells

Anne Cottebrune
Ruprecht-Karls-Universität Heidelberg,
Heidelberg, Germany
Fischer, Wagner

Christopher Crenner
KUMC, Kansas City, KS, USA
*Bowditch, Codman, Edsall, J. Jackson, Jarvis,
Minot*

Anna Crozier
University of Edinburgh, Edinburgh, Scotland
Atiman, Cook, Kasili, Spoerry, C. Williams

Ivan Crozier
University of Edinburgh, Edinburgh, Scotland
*Dickinson, Ellis, Haire, Hirschfeld, C. Mosher,
E. Mosher, Reich, Sanger, Stopes*

Marcos Cueto
Universidad Peruana Cayetano Heredia,
Lima, Peru
*Balmis, Candau, Horwitz Barak, Houssay,
Monge Medrano, Núñez Butrón, Paz Soldán,
Soper*

Michael Z. David
University of Chicago, Chicago, IL, USA
Pavlovskii, Sklifosovskii

Rosalie David
University of Manchester, Manchester,
England
Imhotep

Annemarie de Knecht-van Eekelen
CITO International, Arnhem, the Netherlands
De Lange

Ana Cecilia Rodríguez de Romo
Universidad Nacional Autónoma de México,
Mexico City, Mexico
*Arias de Benavides, Bernard, Bustamante
Vasconcelos, Chávez Sánchez, Izquierdo
Raudón, Liceaga, Martínez Báez, Montaña
Carranco*

Michelle DenBeste
California State University, Fresno, CA, USA
Pokrovskaia

Michael Denham
Wellcome Trust Centre for the History of Medicine
at UCL, London, England
M. Warren

Sven Dierig
Max-Planck-Institut, Berlin, Germany
Brücke, Ludwig

Derek A. Dow
University of Auckland, Auckland, New
Zealand
Buck, Gillies, Hercus, G. Robb, Scott

Alex Dracobly
University of Oregon, Eugene, OR, USA
Fournier, Ricord

Jean-Jacques Dreifuss
Centre Médical Universitaire, Geneva,
Switzerland
Coindet, Prevost

Ariane Dröscher
University of Bologna, Bologna, Italy
*Bassini, Bizzozero, Cotugno, Lombroso, Perroncito,
Rasori, Rizzoli*

Jacalyn Duffin
Queen's University, Kingston, ON, Canada
Laennec

Marguerite Dupree
University of Glasgow, Glasgow, Scotland
Anderson, Blackwell, Jex-Blake

Achintya Kumar Dutta
University of Burdwan, West Bengal, India
Brahmachari

William Eamon
New Mexico State University, Las Cruces, NM, USA
Nicholas of Poland

Myron Echenberg
McGill University, Montreal, QC, Canada
Brazil, Girard, A. Gregory, Jamot, Simond, Yersin

Wolfgang U. Eckart
Ruprecht-Karls-Universität Heidelberg,
Heidelberg, Germany
*Büchner, Dietl, Domagk, Sachs, Sauerbruch, Schwalbe,
Sennert, Skoda, Wundt, Zeiss*

Flávio Coelho Edler
Casa de Oswaldo Cruz, Fundação Oswaldo Cruz,
Rio de Janeiro, Brazil
Wucherer

Martin Edwards
Wellcome Trust Centre for the History of Medicine
at UCL, London, England
Balint

Kristen Ann Ehrenberger
University of Illinois, Urbana-Champaign, IL, USA
Drake

Antoinette Emch-Dériaz
University of Florida, Gainsville, FL, USA
Tissot

Eric J. Engstrom
ZHGB, Berlin, Germany
Kraepelin

Gunnar Eriksson
Uppsala Universitet, Uppsala, Sweden
Rudbeck

Bernardino Fantini
Institut d'Histoire de la Médecine et de la Santé,
Geneva, Switzerland
*Baglivi, Bovet, Celli, Dubini, Fabrizi da Acquapendente,
Golgi, Grassi, Lancisi, Pacini, Puccinotti, Redi, Sanarelli*

F. N. Fastier
University of Otago, Dunedin, New Zealand
Smirk

Morten Fink-Jensen
University of Copenhagen, Copenhagen, Denmark
Bartholin

Michael A. Flannery
University of Alabama at Birmingham,
Maylene, AL, USA
*J. Jones, Lloyd, McDowell, Newton, Nott, E. Warren,
D. Williams*

Yajaira Freites
IVIC, Caracas, Venezuela
Balmis, Beauperthuy, Gabaldón, Razetti

Charlotte Furth
University of Southern California, Los Angeles,
CA, USA
Zhu Zhenheng

Namrata R. Ganneri
Independent scholar, Mumbai, India
Joshi, Rakhmabai, Scudder

Michelle Garceau
Princeton University, Princeton, NJ, USA
Chauliac, William of Saliceto

Amy Gardiner
LSHTM, London, England
Burkitt

Nina Rattner Gelbart
Occidental College, Los Angeles, CA, USA
Du Coudray

Toby Gelfand
University of Ottawa, Ottawa, ON, Canada
Bayle, Bernheim, Bourneville, Charcot, Desault, Hayem,
Lapeyronie, Lasègeu, Péan, Petit, Sée

Jacques Gélis
University of Paris, Paris, France
Baudelocque

Dario Generali
Edizione Nazionale delle Opere di Antonio Vallisneri,
Milan, Italy
Vallisneri

Norman Gevitz
Ohio University, Athens, OH, USA
A. Still

James Gillespie
University of Sydney, Sydney, Australia
Argyle, Cilento

Florence Eliza Glaze
Coastal Carolina University, Conway, SC, USA
Constantine the African, Gariopontus

Christopher Goetz
Rush University Medical Center, Chicago, IL,
USA
Déjerine, Marie

Asaf Goldschmidt
Tel Aviv University, Tel Aviv, Israel
Li Gao, Liu Wansu, Qian Yi, Wang Weiyi,
Xu Shuwei

Christoph Gradmann
University of Oslo, Oslo, Norway
Klebs, Koch, Pettenkofer, Rabinowitsch-Kempner

John L. Graner
Mayo Clinic, Rochester, MN, USA
C. Mayo, W. Mayo

Joanna Grant
London, England
Wang Ji

Monica H. Green
Arizona State University, Tempe, AZ, USA
Trota

Samuel H. Greenblatt
Brown University, Pawtucket, RI, USA
Broca

David Greenwood
University of Nottingham, Nottingham,
England
Florey

Alberto Alonso Guardo
Universidad de Vallodolid, Vallodolid, Spain
Bernard of Gordon

Patrizia Guarnieri
Università degli Studi de Firenze, Florence, Italy
Bufalini, Cerletti, Chiarugi, Concetti, De Sanctis,
Morselli, Mya

Annick Guénel
LASEMA, Villejuif, France
Tùng Tôn Thất

Anita Guerrini
University of California, Santa Barbara, CA,
USA
G. Cheyne

Anne Y. Guillou
L'Université de Haute-Bretagne, Rennes, France
Pen

Bert Hall
University of Toronto, Toronto, ON, Canada
Guido da Vigevano

June Hannam
University of the West of England, Bristol, England
R. Paget

Caroline Hannaway
NIH History, Bethesda, MD, USA
Alibert, Cruveilhier, Dunglison, Dupuytren, Louis, Parran

Signe Lindskov Hansen
Copenhagen, Denmark
Finsen

Marta E. Hanson
Johns Hopkins University, Baltimore, MD, USA
Wu Youxing, Ye Gui, Zhang Jiebin

Susan Hardy
University of New South Wales, Sydney, Australia
Gillbee

Mark Harrison
Wellcome Unit for the History of Medicine, University of Oxford, Oxford, England
Carter, Christophers, Fayrer, Martin, Parkes, Ross

Joy Harvey
Independent scholar, Somerville, MA, USA
Bert, Bertillon, Brès, Edwards-Pilliet, Littré, Rayer, Tardieu, Trousseau, Vulpian

Mike Hawkins
Wellcome Trust Centre for the History of Medicine at UCL/Imperial College, London, England
Willis

E. A. Heaman
McGill University, Montreal, QC, Canada
Fleming, Sanderson, Wright

R. van Hee
Universiteit Antwerpen, Antwerp, Belgium
Depage, Vesalius

Jürgen Helm
Martin Luther Universität, Halle-Wittenberg, Halle, Germany
Brunfels, Erxleben, Frank, Gersdorff, Hoffmann, Stahl

John Henry
University of Edinburgh, Edinburgh, Scotland
Caius, Dubois, Fernel, Harvey, Linacre, Lower, Turquet, Winsløw

Volker Hess
ZHGB, Berlin, Germany
Behring, Frerichs, Kraus, Leyden, Traube, Wunderlich

Martha Hildreth
University of Nevada, Reno, NV, USA
Brouardel, Grancher

Caroline Hillard
Washington University, St Louis, MO, USA
Del Garbo, Mondino de' Liuzzi

Gilberto Hochman
Casa de Oswaldo Cruz, Fundação Oswaldo Cruz, Rio de Janeiro, Brazil
Barros Barreto, Chagas, Cruz, Fraga, Penna, Pinotti, Ribas, Wucherer

Hans-Georg Hofer
University of Manchester, Manchester, England
Krafft-Ebing, Wagner-Jauregg

Eddy Houwaart
Vrije Universiteit Medisch Centrum, Amsterdam, the Netherlands
Ali Cohen

Joel D. Howell
University of Michigan, Ann Arbor, MI, USA
Elliotson, Flick, Gerhard, Heberden, Herrick, Lewis

Elisabeth Hsu
University of Oxford, Oxford, England
Chunyu Yi

Christian Huber
Sigmund Freud-Privatstiftung, Vienna, Austria
Breuer, Jung

Rafael Huertas
CSIC, Madrid, Spain
Orfila i Rotger, Rodríguez Lafora

Teresa Huguet-Termes
Universitat Autònoma de Barcelona, Barcelona, Spain
Cardenal Fernández

Frank Huisman
University Medical Center, Utrecht/Universiteit Maastricht, Maastricht, the Netherlands
Einthoven, Hijmans van den Bergh, Loghem, Sylvius

Marion Hulverscheidt
Ruprecht-Karls-Universität Heidelberg,
Heidelberg, Germany
Basedow, Hegar

J. Willis Hurst
Emory University, Atlanta, GA, USA
White

Erik Ingebrigsten
Norwegian University of Science and Technology,
Trondheim, Norway
Holst

Lorentz M. Irgens
University of Bergen, Bergen, Norway
Hansen

Mark Jackson
University of Exeter, Exeter, England
Blackley, Down, Floyer, Freeman, Seguin, Tredgold

Bengt Jangfeldt
Center for the History of Science, Royal Academy of
Science, Stockholm, Sweden
Munthe

Mark Jenner
University of York, York, England
*Chamberlen, Clowes, Glisson, D. Turner, Wiseman,
Woodall*

William Johnston
Wesleyan University, Middletown, CT, USA
*Gotō Konzan, Hanaoka, Manse, Sugita, Yamawaki,
Yoshimasu*

Peter Jones
King's College Library, Cambridge, England
Arderne, Yperman

Eric Jorink
Constantijn Huygens Instituut, the Hague,
the Netherlands
*J. Heurnius, O. Heurnius, Lemnius, Piso,
Swammerdam*

Robert Jütte
Robert Bosch Stiftung, Stuttgart, Germany
*Auenbrugger, Hahnemann, Hirsch, Hufeland, Kaposi,
Rolfink, Rubner*

Oliver Kahl
University of Manchester, Manchester, England
Ibn at-Tilmīdh

Harmke Kamminga
University of Cambridge, Cambridge, England
Eijkman

Amalie M. Kass
Harvard Medical School, Boston, MA, USA
Cabot, Channing, Churchill, Dameshek, Kelly, Sims

Matthew Howard Kaufman
University of Edinburgh, Edinburgh, Scotland
Ballingall, C. Bell, Brodie, Guthrie, Liston, McGrigor

Amy Kemp
Indiana University, Bloomington, IN, USA
Souza

Helen King
University of Reading, Reading, England
*Agnodice, Archagathus, Hippocrates, Machaon,
Podalirius*

Stephanie Kirby
University of the West of England, Bristol, England
Nightingale

Rina Knoeff
Universiteit Maastricht, Maastricht,
the Netherlands
G. Bidloo, Boerhaave

Carl Henrik Koch
University of Copenhagen, Copenhagen,
Denmark
Stensen

Peter Koehler
Wever Hospital, Heerlen, the Netherlands
Babinski, Brown-Séquard, Winkler

Luuc Kooijmans
Universiteit van Amsterdam, Amsterdam,
the Netherlands
Ruysch

Maria Korasidou
Panteion University of Athens, Athens, Greece
Geroulanos, Goudas, Papanicolaou, Vouros, Zinnis

Jan K. van der Korst
Loosdrecht, the Netherlands
Camper, Swieten

Samuel Kottek
Hebrew University, Jerusalem, Israel
Astruc

Simone Petraglia Kropf
Casa de Oswaldo Cruz, Fundação Oswaldo
Cruz, Rio de Janeiro, Brazil
Chagas

Howard I. Kushner
Emory University, Atlanta, GA, USA
Gilles de la Tourette

Ann F. La Berge
Virginia Tech, Blacksburg, VA, USA
Parent-Duchâtelet, Villermé

Paul A. L. Lancaster
University of Sydney, New South Wales, Australia
Gregg

Øivind Larsen
University of Oslo, Oslo, Norway
Schiøtz

Christopher Lawrence
Wellcome Trust Centre for the History of
Medicine at UCL, London, England
*Cheselden, Culpeper, Lind, Mead, Pott, Pringle,
Salk, Sydenham, Trotter*

Sean Hsiang-lin Lei
National Tsing-hua University, Hsinchu, Taiwan
Yu Yan

Efraim Lev
University of Haifa, Haifa, Israel
Asaph

Milton James Lewis
University of Sydney, Sydney,
Australia
Cumpston

Shang-Jen Li
Institute of History and Philology, Academia
Sinica, Taipei, Taiwan
*Bruce, Hobson, Leishman, Lockhart, Manson,
Parker*

Kai Khiun Liew
Wellcome Trust Centre for the History of Medicine
at UCL, London, England
Chen Su Lan

Vivienne Lo
Wellcome Trust Centre for the History of Medicine
at UCL, London, England
Medicine in China

Stephen Lock
Aldeburgh, Suffolk, England
*The Western Medical Tradition, Beecher, Cooper,
Crile, Dale, Doll, Ferrier, Fishbein, Gull, Hart,
Hastings, G. Holmes, Keynes, Mitchell,
Pappworth, Pickles, Ryle, Saunders, Trudeau*

Winifred Logan
Glasgow, Scotland
Stephenson

Brigitte Lohff
Medizinische Hochschule Hannover,
Hannover, Germany
Autenrieth, Baer, Blumenbach, Müller, Oken, Reil

Jorge Lossio
University of Manchester, Manchester, England
Carrión, Espejo, Unanue

Ilana Löwy
CERMES, Villejuif, France
Aleksandrowicz, Bieganski, Biernacki, Korczak

Kenneth M. Ludmerer
Washington University, St Louis, MO, USA
Flexner

Joan E. Lynaugh
University of Pennsylvania Nursing School,
Philadelphia, PA, USA
L. Dock, L. Richards, I. Robb

Kan-Wen Ma
Wellcome Trust Centre for the History of Medicine
at UCL, London, England
Bian Que

Helen MacDonald
University of Melbourne, Carlton, Victoria,
Australia
W. MacKenzie

Andreas-Holger Maehle
University of Durham, Durham/Wolfson Research
Institute, Stockton, England
Moll

Susanne Malchau
Aarhus Universitet, Aarhus, Denmark
Mannerheim, Reimann

John Manton
University of Oxford, Oxford, England
Johnson, Lambo, Schweitzer

Predrag J. Markovic
Institute for Contemporary History, Belgrade, Serbia
Batut, Djordjević, Lazarević, Kostić, Nešić, Štampar,
Subbotić

Shula Marks
SOAS, London, England
Gale, Gear, Gillman, Gluckman, Kark, Waterston

José Martínez-Pérez
Universidad de Castilla-La Mancha, Albacete, Spain
Calandre Ibáñez, Jiménez Díaz, Marañón Posadillo

Àlvar Martínez-Vidal
Universidad Autónoma de Barcelona, Barcelona,
Spain
Gimbernat i Arbós, Giovannini

Romana Martorelli Vico
Università di Pisa, Pisa, Italy
Lanfranc, Ugo Benzi

J. Rosser Matthews
Williamsburg, VA, USA
Biggs, Bouchard, Bouchardat, Chapin, Greenwood, Hill

Janet McCalman
University of Melbourne, Melbourne, Australia
Balls-Headley, Bryce, Campbell, Macnamara,
Scantlebury Brown

Louella McCarthy
University of Sydney, Sydney, New South Wales,
Australia
D'Arcy

Laurence B. McCullough
Baylor College of Medicine, Houston, TX, USA
Hooker, Rush

Susan McGann
RCN Archives, Edinburgh, Scotland
Fenwick

James McGeachie
University of Ulster, Newtownabbey, Northern Ireland
Corrigan, Graves, W. Jenner, M. Mackenzie, Stokes, Wilde

Alessandro Medico
Washington University, St Louis, MO, USA
Peter of Abano

Rosa María Medina-Doménech
Universidad de Granada, Granada, Spain
Goyanes Capdevilla, Guilera Molas

Alfredo Menéndez
Universidad de Granada, Granada, Spain
Casal Julián

Sharon Messenger
Wellcome Trust Centre for the History of Medicine
at UCL, London, England
Livingstone

Alexandre Métraux
Dossenheim, Germany
S. Freud, Goldstein

Dmitry Mikhel
Saratov State University, Saratov, Russia
Botkin, Erisman, Manassein, Molleson, Ostroumov, Zakhar'in

Bridie Andrews Minehan
Bentley College, Waltham, MA, USA
Ding Fubao, Yen

Consuelo Miqueo
Universidad de Zaragoza, Zaragoza, Spain
Piquer Arrufat

Néstor Miranda Canal
Universidad El Bosque y de la Universidad de Los Andes,
Bogotá, Colombia
Vargas Reyes

Jorge Molero-Mesa
Universidad Autònoma de Barcelona, Barcelona, Spain
Sayé i Sempere

Laurence Monnais
Université de Montréal, Montreal, QC, Canada
Medical Traditions in Southeast Asia: From Syncretism to
Pluralism

Maria Teresa Monti
CSPF-CNR, Milan, Italy
Spallanzani

Francisco Moreno de Carvalho
Independent scholar, São Paulo, Brazil
Amatus Lusitanus, Orta

Edward T. Morman
Baltimore, MD, USA
Bartlett, H. Bigelow, J. Bigelow, Billings, Da Costa, Pepper,
Thayer, Welch

Barbara Mortimer
Edinburgh, Scotland
Sharp

Anne Marie Moulin
CNRS-CEDEJ, Cairo, Egypt
Bordet, Davaine, Laveran, Netter, Roux, Widal

Wolf-Dieter Müller-Jahncke
Hermann-Schelenz-Institut für Pharmazie und
Kulturgeschichte, Heidelberg, Germany
Paracelsus

Jock Murray
Dalhousie University, Halifax, Nova Scotia, Canada
*Abbott, Banting, Bethune, Gowers, Grenfell, Huggins,
J. H. Jackson, Macphail, Osler, Parkinson, Penfield, Selye*

Takeshi Nagashima
Keio University, Tokyo, Japan
Gotō Shinpei, Kitasato, Miyairi, Nagayo, Noguchi, Shiga

Michael J. Neuss
Columbia University, New York, NY, USA
Al-Anṭākī

Michael Neve
Wellcome Trust Centre for the History of Medicine
at UCL, London, England
Beddoes, Gully, Head, Prichard, Rivers, Winslow

Malcolm Nicolson
University of Glasgow, Glasgow, Scotland
Alison, Baillie, Donald, J. Hunter, W. Hunter, Lister, Smellie

Ingemar Nilsson
University of Gothenburg, Gothenburg, Sweden
Acrel

Sherwin Nuland
Yale University, New Haven, CT, USA
Beaumont, Bloodgood, Kubler-Ross, McBurney, Mott, Murphy

Eva Nyström
University of Uppsala, Uppsala, Sweden
Rosén von Rosenstein

Ynez Violé O'Neill
UCLA, Los Angeles, CA, USA
Paré

Diana Obregón
Universidad Nacional de Colombia Edificio Manuel
Ancizar, Bogotá, Colombia
Carrasquilla, García-Medina

Ambeth R. Ocampo
National Historical Institute, Manila, Philippines
Rizal

Guillermo Olagüe de Ros
Universidad de Granada, Granada, Spain
García Solá, Nóvoa Santos, Urrutia Guerezta

Jan Eric Olsén
University of Lund, Lund, Sweden
Gullstrand, Holmgren

Todd M. Olszewski
Yale University, New Haven, CT, USA
Cannon, D. Dock

Willie T. Ong
Makati Medical Center, Makati, Philippines
Acosta-Sison

Giuseppe Ongaro
Ospedale di Padova, Padova, Italy
*Aranzio, Aselli, Bellini, Benivieni, Berengario da Carpi,
Borelli, Cardano, Cesalpino, Colombo, Cornaro,
Da Monte, Eustachi, Falloppia, Malpighi, Mattioli,
Mercuriale, Morgagni, Santorio, Scarpa, Severino,
Tagliacozzi, Valsalva, Zacchia*

Ooi Keat Gin
Universiti Sains Malaysia, Penang, Malaysia
Danaraj, Lim Boon Keng, Wu Lien-Teh

Teresa Ortiz-Gómez
Universidad de Granada, Granada, Spain
Arroyo Villaverde, Soriano Fischer

Abena Dove Osseo-Asare
University of California, Berkeley, CA, USA
Ampofo, Barnor, De Graft-Johnson, C. Easmon

Nelly Oudshoorn
Universiteit Twente, Enschede,
the Netherlands
Laqueur

Caroline Overy
Wellcome Trust Centre for the History of
Medicine at UCL, London, England
Livingstone

Steven Palmer
University of Windsor, Windsor, Ontario,
Canada
*Calderón Guardia, Durán Cartín,
Fernández y Hernández*

José Pardo-Tomás
CSIC, Barcelona, Spain
Monardes

Lawrence Charles Parish
Jefferson Medical College, Philadelphia, PA, USA
Bateman, Duhring, Gross, Hutchinson, Shippen, Willan

Eldryd Parry
Tropical Health and Education Trust, London, England
Burkitt

Adell Patton Jr.
University of Missouri, St Louis, MO, USA
Boyle, J. Easmon, Odeku, Togba

Harry W. Paul
University of Florida, Gainesville, FL, USA
Pasteur, Rothschild

John Pearn
University of Queensland, Brisbane, Australia
*Bancroft, Beaney, Coppleson, Fairley, Halford,
MacGregor*

Steven J. Peitzman
Drexel University College of Medicine,
Philadelphia, PA, USA
Addis, Bright, A. Richards, Scribner

Kim Pelis
National Institutes of Health, Bethesda, MD, USA
*Barker, Councilman, Gorgas, Hammond, Nicolle, Reed,
T. Smith*

Concetta Pennuto
Université de Genève, Geneva, Switzerland
Ficino, Fracastoro

José Morgado Pereira
Universidade de Coimbra, Coimbra, Portugal
Egas Moniz

Jacques Philippon
Salpêtrière-Pitié Hospital, Paris, France
Mondor

Howard Phillips
University of Cape Town, Rondebosch, South Africa
Abdurahman, Barnard, Barry, Naidoo, Orenstein, Xuma

Jean-François Picard
CNRS, Paris, France
Debré, Delay, Hamburger, Leriche, Roussy, Vincent

Mikhail Poddubnyi
Voenno-meditsinskii Zhurnal, Moscow, Russia
*N. Bidloo, Buial'skii, Dobroslavin, Gaaz, Inozemtsev,
Pirogov, Pletnev*

Hans Pols
University of Sydney, Sydney, Australia
*Beard, Beers, Bowlby, Burton-Bradley, Grinker, Klein,
Laing, Stillé*

María-Isabel Porras-Gallo
University of Castilla-La Mancha, Madrid, Spain
Obrador Alcalde

Patricia E. Prestwich
University of Alberta, Edmonton, AB, Canada
Magnan, Moreau de Tours, Morel

Lawrence M. Principe
Johns Hopkins University, Baltimore, MD, USA
Helmont

Armin Prinz
Medizinische Universität Wien, Vienna, Austria
Wenckebach

Cay-Ruediger Pruell
Albert-Ludwigs-Universität, Freiburg, Germany
Aschoff, Cohnheim, Conti, Ehrlich, Rokitansky, Virchow

Constance Putnam
Independent scholar, Concord, MA, USA
*Balassa, Bene, Duka, O. W. Holmes, Korányi,
Markusovszky, Meigs, Morgan, Semmelweis, G. Shattuck,
N. Smith, J. Warren*

Emilio Quevedo
Universidad Nacional de Colombia, Bogotá, Colombia
Franco

Sean Quinlan
University of Idaho, Moscow, ID, USA
A. Louis, Quesnay

Camilo Quintero
University of Wisconsin–Madison, Madison, WI, USA
Mutis y Bosio

Roger Qvarsell
University of Linköping, Linköping, Sweden
Huss

Karina Ramacciotti
Universidad de Buenos Aires, Buenos Aires, Argentina
Carrillo, Mazza, Rawson

Mridula Ramanna
SIES College, University of Mumbai, Mumbai, India
*Bentley, Choksy, Jhirad, Khanolkar, Lad, Morehead,
J. Turner*

Matthew Ramsey
Vanderbilt University, Nashville, TN, USA
Civiale, Desgenettes, Fourcroy, Portal, Richerand, Velpeau, Vicq d'Azyr

Ismail Rashid
Vassar College, Poughkeepsie, NY, USA
Fanon, Horton

Carole Reeves
Wellcome Trust Centre for the History of Medicine
at UCL, London, England
Abt, Battey, Buchan, Budd, Cole, Darwin, Holt, Keen, Lane, S. Morton, Prout, Rock, Sabin, Scharlieb, Seacole, Spock, Tait

C. Joan Richardson
University of Texas Medical Branch, Galveston, TX, USA
Barton

Philip Rieder
Université de Genève, Geneva, Switzerland
Bonet, De La Rive, Le Clerc, Odier, Reverdin, Tronchin

Ortrun Riha
Universität Leipzig, Leipzig, Germany
Isaac Israeli

Julius Rocca
University of Birmingham, Birmingham, England
Aëtius, Aretaeus, Aristotle, Asclepiades, Caelius Aurelianus, Celsus, Dioscorides, Empedocles, Erasistratus, Herophilos, Pliny, Scribonius Largus, Soranus, Whytt

Julia Rodriguez
University of New Hampshire, Durham, NH, USA
Aráoz Alfaro, Coni, Grierson, Ingenieros

Esteban Rodríguez-Ocaña
Universidad de Granada, Granada, Spain
Ferrán y Clúa, Pittaluga Fattorini

Volker Roelcke
Justus-Liebig Universität, Giessen, Germany
Alzheimer, Bleuler, Kretschmer, Mitscherlich, Rüdin

Hugo Röling
Universiteit van Amsterdam, Amsterdam, the Netherlands
Rutgers

Naomi Rogers
Yale University, New Haven, CT, USA
Kenny

Anastasio Rojo
University of Valladolid, Valladolid, Spain
Bravo de Sobremonte, Mercado, Valles

Nils Rosdahl
Medical Museion, Copenhagen Denmark
Madsen

Barbara Gutmann Rosenkrantz
Harvard University, Cambridge, MA, USA
Hardy, L. Shattuck

Leonard D. Rosenman
UCSF, San Francisco, CA, USA
Frugard

Fred Rosner
Mount Sinai School of Medicine, New York, NY, USA
Maimonides

Lisa Rosner
Richard Stockton College, Pomona, NJ, USA
Bennett, Brown, Christison, Cullen, Ferriar, J. Gregory, Laycock, Monro, Percival, Withering

Frederic Roy
Université de Montréal, Montreal, QC, Canada
Suvannavong

Marion Maria Ruisinger
Friedrich-Alexander-Universität, Erlangen-Nuremberg, Germany
Heister

Han van Ruler
Erasmus Universiteit, Rotterdam, the Netherlands
Blankaart, Bontekoe, Graaf

Andrea Rusnock
University of Rhode Island, Kingston, RI, USA
Arbuthnot, Bond, Boylston, E. Jenner, Jurin, Sutton, Waterhouse

Fernando Salmón
Universidad de Cantabria, Santander, Spain
Arnald, López Albo

Lutz D. H. Sauerteig
University of Durham, Durham/Wolfson Research Institute, Stockton, England
Blaschko

Walton O. Schalick III
Washington University, St Louis, MO, USA
Gilles de Corbeil, Henry of Mondeville, John of Gaddesden, John of Saint-Amand, Peter of Abano, Peter of Spain, Richard the Englishman, Taddeo, William of Brescia

Volker Scheid
University of Westminster, London, England
Ding Ganren, Fei Boxiong, Yun Tieqiao

Aina Schiøtz
Universitetet i Bergen, Bergen, Norway
Evang

William Schneider
Indiana University, Indianapolis, IN, USA
Hirszfeld, Pinard, Richet, Tzanck

Heinz Schott
Rheinische Friedrich-Wilhelms-Universität, Bonn, Germany
Mesmer

Andrew Scull
University of California San Diego, San Diego, CA, USA
Brigham, Cotton, Dix, Earle, Haslam, Meyer, Ray, Tuke

Nikolaj Serikoff
The Wellcome Library, London, England
The Islamic Medical Tradition, Aḥmad, Ibn al-Bayṭār, Al-Bīrūnī, Clot Bey, Foley, Ḥaddād, Ibn al-Haytham, Mahfouz, Ibn al-Māsawayh, Meyerhof, Ibn Sīnā, Sournia, Van Dyck, Waldmeier, Al-Zahrāwī

Jole Shackelford
University of Minnesota, Minneapolis, MN, USA
Severinus

Sonu Shamdasani
Wellcome Trust Centre for the History of Medicine at UCL, London, England
Adler, Forel, A. Freud, Gesell, Janet, Menninger, Putnam, Sullivan

Patrick Henry Shea
Rockefeller Archive Center, Sleepy Hollow, NY, USA
Carrel

Sally Sheard
University of Liverpool, Liverpool, England
Bevan, Beveridge, Chadwick, Farr, Newman, Newsholme, Shuttleworth, T. S. Smith

Dongwon Shin
Korean Advanced Institute of Science and Technology, Taejon, Korea
Choe Han'gi, Heo, Sejong, Yi Jema

Barry David Silverman
Northside Hospital, Atlanta, GA, USA
Taussig

Mark E. Silverman
Emory University, Atlanta, GA, USA
Flint, Hope, J. Mackenzie

Jelena Jovanovic Simic
Zemun, Serbia
Batut, Djordjević, Lazarević, Kostić, Nešić, Štampar, Subbotić

P. N. Singer
London, England
Galen

Kavita Sivaramakrishnan
Public Health Foundation of India, New Delhi, India
G. Sen, P. Sharma, T. Sharma, Shukla, Vaid, Varier

Morten A. Skydsgaard
University of Aarhus, Aarhus, Denmark
Panum

Jean Louis De Sloover
Erpent (Namur), Belgium
Dodonaeus

David F. Smith
University of Aberdeen, Aberdeen, Scotland
Orr

F. B. Smith
Australian National University, Canberra, Australia
W. Thomson

Thomas Söderqvist
Medical Museion, Copenhagen, Denmark
Jerne

Marina Sorokina
Russian Academy of Sciences, Moscow, Russia
Al'tshuller, Briukhonenko, Haffkine, Ilizarov, Iudin, Negovskii, Semenovskii

David Sowell
Juniata College, Huntingdon, PA, USA
Perdomo Neira

Eduard A. van Staeyen
Leiden, the Netherlands
Guislain

Frank W. Stahnisch
Johannes Gutenberg-Universität, Mainz, Germany
Graefe, Griesinger, His, C. Vogt, O. Vogt, Warburg,
Wassermann

Ida H. Stamhuis
Vrije Universiteit Amsterdam, Amsterdam,
the Netherlands
Quetelet

Darwin H. Stapleton
Rockefeller Archive Center, Sleepy Hollow, NY, USA
Hackett

Jane Starfield
University of Johannesburg, Bertsham, South Africa
Molema, Moroka

Martin S. Staum
University of Calgary, Calgary, AB, Canada
Cabanis

Hubert Steinke
University of Bern, Bern, Switzerland
Haller

Oddvar Stokke
National Hospital, Oslo, Norway
Følling, Refsum

Michael Stolberg
Universität Würzburg, Würzburg, Germany
Bartisch, Fabricius, Fuchs, Platter, Rösslin, Scultetus

Marvin J. Stone
Baylor University Medical Center, Dallas, TX, USA
Coley, Ewing, Farber, E. Graham, Hodgkin, Wintrobe

Hindrik Strandberg
Helsinki, Finland
Willebrand, Ylppö

Karin Stukenbrock
Martin-Luther-Universität Halle-Wittenberg,
Halle, Germany
Brunfels, Erxleben, Frank, Gersdorff, Hoffmann,
Stahl

Charles Suradji
Jakarta, Indonesia
Soedarmo

Akihito Suzuki
Keio University, Yokohama, Japan
Medicine, State, and Society in Japan, 500–2000,
Asada, Baelz, Conolly, Hata, Mori, Ogata, Pompe van
Meerdervoort, Siebold, Yamagiwa

Mika Suzuki
Shizuoka University, Shizuoka, Japan
Ogino, Yoshioka

Victoria Sweet
UCSF, San Francisco, CA, USA
Hildegard of Bingen

Simon Szreter
University of Cambridge, Cambridge,
England
McKeown

Cecilia Taiana
Carleton University, Ottawa, ON, Canada
Lacan

Ian Tait
Aldeburgh, Suffolk, England
Browne

Jennifer Tappan
Columbia University, New York, NY, USA
Trowell

Robert Tattersall
University of Nottingham, Nottingham,
England
Abel, Addison, Albright, Doniach, Hench, Horsley,
Joslin, Minkowski, Starling

Kim Taylor
Kaimu Productions, Shanghai, China
Hatem, Zhu Lian

Manuela Tecusan
University of Cambridge, Cambridge, England
Alcmaeon, Anaximander, Andreas, Democedes,
Democritus, Diocles, Diogenes, Oribasius, Paul
of Aegina, Philistion, Plato, Praxagoras, Rufus

Bert Theunissen
Universiteit Utrecht, Utrecht, the Netherlands
Donders

Michel Thiery
Stichting Jan Palfyn en Museum voor
Geschiedenis van de Geneeskunde, Ghent, Belgium
Palfyn

C. Michele Thompson
Southern Connecticut State University,
New Haven, CT, USA
Lán Ông, Tuệ Tĩnh

Carsten Timmermann
University of Manchester, Manchester, England
*Bauer, Grotjahn, McMichael, Pickering, D. Richards,
Rosenbach*

Tom Treasure
St George's Hospital Medical School, London,
England
*Beck, Blalock, C. E. Drew, C. R. Drew, Favaloro, Gibbon,
Hufnagel*

Ulrich Tröhler
University of Bern, Bern, Switzerland
*Bergmann, Billroth, Kocher, Langenbeck,
Mikulicz-Radecki, Nissen, Quervain*

Arleen Marcia Tuchman
Vanderbilt University, Nashville, TN, USA
Zakrzewska

Marius Turda
Oxford Brookes University, Oxford, England
Babeş, Cantacuzino, Ciucă, Marinescu

Trevor Turner
Homerton University Hospital, London, England
Maudsley

Peter J. Tyler
Edgecliffe, New South Wales, Australia
*W. Armstrong, Bland, Fiaschi, Mackellar, Skirving,
Stuart, Thompson*

Michael Tyquin
Making History, Darlington, New South Wales,
Australia
Dunlop

Tatiana Ul'iankina
Institute of the History of Science and Technology,
Moscow, Russia
Mechnikov, Sechenov

G. van der Waa
Rotterdam, the Netherlands
Gaubius

Lia van Gemert
Universiteit Utrecht, Utrecht, the Netherlands
Beverwijck

Maria Vassiliou
University of Oxford, Oxford, England
Belios, Livadas

Jan Peter Verhave
UMCN, Nijmegen, the Netherlands
Swellengrebel

Joost Vijselaar
Trimbos-Instituut, Utrecht, the Netherlands
Schroeder van der Kolk

Jurjen Vis
Amsterdam, the Netherlands
Foreest

An Vleugels
National University of Singapore, Singapore
Kerr

Hans de Waardt
Vrije Universiteit Amsterdam, Amsterdam,
the Netherlands
Wier

Keir Waddington
Cardiff University, Cardiff, Wales
*Abernethy, Brunton, Garrod, Gee, Lawrence,
J. Paget*

Lisa K. Walker
University of California, Berkeley, CA, USA
Khlopin, Teziakov

John Walker-Smith
Wellcome Trust Centre for the History of
Medicine at UCL, London, England
G. Armstrong, G. Still, Underwood, West

Paul Weindling
Oxford Brookes University, Oxford, England
Verschuer

Dora B. Weiner
UCLA, Los Angeles, CA, USA
Esquirol, Larrey, Percy, Pinel, Tenon

Kathleen Wellman
Southern Methodist University, Dallas, TX, USA
La Mettrie, Patin, Renaudot

Ann Westmore
The University of Melbourne, Parkville, Victoria,
Australia
Cade

James Whorton
University of Washington, Tacoma, WA, USA
Eddy, S. Graham, Kellogg, Lust, B. Palmer, D. Palmer,
S. Thomson, Trall

Ann Wickham
Dublin City University, Dublin, Ireland
A. Jones

Elizabeth A. Williams
Oklahoma State University, Stillwater, OK, USA
Boissier de la Croix de Sauvages, Bordeu

Sabine Wilms
Paradigm Publications, Taos, NM, USA
Ge Hong, Sun Simiao, Tao Hongjing

Warren Winkelstein, Jr.
University of California, Berkeley, CA, USA
Emerson, Frost, Goldberger, Hamilton, Kinyoun,
Lane-Claypon, Park, Paul, Wynder

Michael Worboys
University of Manchester, Manchester, England
Allbutt, Bristowe, W. W. Cheyne, Moynihan, Simon, Syme

Jill Wrapson
University of Auckland, Auckland,
New Zealand
Barnett

Marcia Wright
Columbia University, New York, NY, USA
Park Ross

Rex Wright-St Clair (deceased)
Huntingdon, Hamilton, New Zealand
A. Thomson

Henrik R. Wulff
Medical Museion, Copenhagen, Denmark
Hirschsprung

Ronit Yoeli-Tlalim
Warburg Institute, London, England
Sangye Gyatso, Yuthog Yontan

William H. York
Portland State University, Portland, OR,
USA
Despars, Valesco of Tarenta

Benjamin Zajicek
University of Chicago, Chicago, IL, USA
Bekhterev, Korsakov, Pavlov

Soledad Zárate
Universidad de Chile, Santiago, Chile
Cruz-Coke Lassabe

Alfons Zarzoso
Museu d'Història de la Medicina de Catalunya,
Barcelona, Spain
Pedro-Pons, Puigvert Gorro

Franz Zehentmayr
Salzburg, Austria
Zhang Yuansu

Barbara Zipser
Wellcome Trust Centre for the History of Medicine
at UCL, London, England
Al-Mawṣilī

Patrick Zylberman
CERMES, Villejuif, France
Sand

ABBREVIATIONS

AMA	American Medical Association
ANB	*American National Biography*
BA	Bachelor of Arts
BCE	Before Common Era
BCG	Bacillus Calmette-Guérin (tuberculosis vaccination)
BM	Bachelor of Medicine
BMA	British Medical Association
BMJ	*British Medical Journal*
CBE	Commander, The Most Excellent Order of the British Empire
CE	Common Era
ChB	Bachelor of Surgery
ChD	Doctor of Surgery
ChM	Master of Surgery
CIE	Companion, The Most Eminent Order of the Indian Empire
KCIE	Knight Commander, The Most Eminent Order of the Indian Empire
CM	Master of Surgery
CMB	Combat Medical Badge (U.S. Army)
CMG	Companion, The Most Distinguished Order of St Michael and St George
CMO	Chief Medical Officer
CMS	Church Missionary Society
CSI	Companion, The Most Exalted Order of the Star of India
CSIRO	Commonwealth Scientific and Industrial Research Organization (Australia)
DAMB	*Dictionary of American Medical Biography*
DAuB	*Dictionary of Australian Biography* (available online)
DBE	Dame of the British Empire
DBI	*Dizionario Biografico degli Italiani*
DGMS	Director General Medical Service (military)

DMed	Doctor of Medicine
DNZB	*Dictionary of New Zealand Biography* (available online)
DPM	Diploma of Psychological Medicine
DSB	*Dictionary of Scientific Biography*
DSO	Distinguished Service Order (military British)
ECT	Electo-convulsive Therapy
EEG	Electroencephalogram
FAO	Food and Agriculture Organization (United Nations)
FRCP	Fellow Royal College of Physicians
FRCPEdin/FRCPEd	Fellow Royal College of Physicians Edinburgh
FRCS	Fellow of the Royal College of Surgeons
FRCSEdin/FRCSEd	Fellow Royal College of Surgeons Edinburgh
FRS	Fellow of the Royal Society
FRSEdin/FRSEd	Fellow of the Royal Society of Edinburgh
GBH	General Board of Health (England and Wales)
GMC	General Medical Council (UK)
GP	General Practitioner
ICN	International Council of Nursing
ICS	Indian Civil Service
IHB	International Health Board (Rockefeller Foundation)
IMS	Indian Medical Service
IOC	Institute Oswaldo Cruz
JAMA	*Journal of the American Medical Association*
KCSI	Knight Commander, The Most Exalted Order of the Star of India
LLD	Doctor of Laws
LMS	Licentiate in Medicine and Surgery
LRCP	Licentiate of the Royal College of Physicians
LRCPEdin/LRCPEd	Licentiate of the Royal College of Physicians Edinburgh
LRCSEdin/LRCSEd	Licentiate of the Royal College of Surgeons Edinburgh
LRFPS	Licentiate of the Royal Faculty of Physicians and Surgeons of Glasgow
LSA	Licentiate of the Society of Apothecaries
LSHTM	London School of Hygiene and Tropical Medicine
LSMW	London School of Medicine for Women
MA	Master of Arts
MB	Bachelor of Medicine
MBCM	Bachelor of Medicine Master of Surgery
MC	Military Cross
MD	Doctor of Medicine
mg	milligram
MMed	Master of Medicine
MO	Medical Officer
MoH	Medical Officer of Health
MRC	Medical Research Council
MRCNZ	Medical Research Council of New Zealand
MRCOG	Member of the Royal College of Gynaecologists
MRCP	Member of the Royal College of Physicians
MRCS	Member of the Royal College of Surgeons
MS	Multiple Sclerosis
NHMRC	National Health and Medical Research Council (Australia)
NSDAP	National Socialist Party (Nazi Germany)
NSW	New South Wales (Australia)
OAS	Organization of American States
OBE	Officer, The Most Excellent Order of the British Empire
Oxford DNB	*Oxford Dictionary of National Biography* (UK)
PASB	Pan American Sanitary Bureau

PhD	Doctor of Philosophy
QVJIN	Queen Victoria Jubilee Institute of Nursing
RACP	Royal Australasian College of Physicians
RACS	Royal Australasian College of Surgeons
RAMC	Royal Army Medical Corps (UK)
RBNA	Royal British Nurses Association
RCP	Royal College of Physicians
RCPEdin	Royal College of Physicians of Edinburgh
RCS	Royal College of Surgeons
RCSEdin	Royal College of Surgeons of Edinburgh
RMO	Resident Medical Officer
RSTMH	Royal Society of Tropical Medicine and Hygiene
SA	Sturm Abteilung [Storm Section] (Nazi Germany)
SLSAA	Surf Lifesaving Association of Australia
SS	Schutzstaffel [Protective Squadron] (Nazi Germany)
STD	Sexually Transmitted Diseases
UCH	University College Hospital (London, England)
UCL	University College London (England)
UNICEF	United Nations Children's Fund
UNRRA	United Nations Relief and Rehabilitation Administration
WHO	World Health Organization
YMCA	Young Men's Christian Association

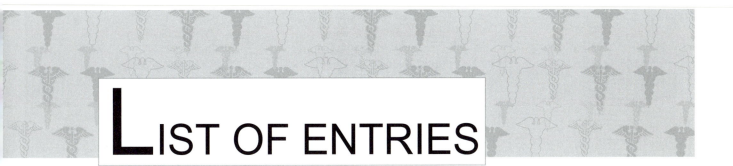

LIST OF ENTRIES

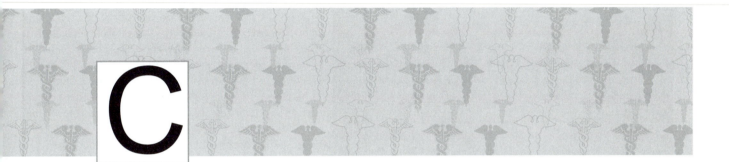

C

CABANIS, PIERRE-JEAN-GEORGES (b. Cosnac, France, 5 June 1757, d. Rueil-Seraincourt, France, 5 May 1808), *medicine, psychophysiology, clinical theory.*

Cabanis was the son of an upper bourgeois seigneurial court judge, Jean-Baptiste Cabanis, and a noblewoman, Marie-Hélène d'Escarolle de Souleyrac. He studied at the Paris Faculty of Medicine from 1780 to 1783 but took his degree at the less demanding Faculty of Reims in 1784.

In his two major works on method in medicine, *On the Degree of Certainty in Medicine* (written 1788, published 1798) and *Sketch of the Revolutions of Medical Science and Views Relating to Its Reform* (written 1795, published 1804), Cabanis demonstrated how the empiricist philosophy of Condillac, including methods of 'analysis', could be adapted to a science of precise neo-Hippocratic clinical observation of symptom patterns and therapeutic adjustments to the individual. The first essay argued that physicians could attain only highly probable truths, but that large numbers of observations would justify belief in empirical regularities and disease classifications. The full discussion of analytic method in the second work was more characteristic of the 'old clinic', in Foucault's formulation, rather than of the new pathological anatomy.

Cabanis also published *Observations on Hospitals* (1790), which favored small hospices for better ventilation, cleanliness, and more individualized treatment. However, in a 1798 speech to the Council of 500 (lower house of the legislature), he recognized that large hospitals would provide the data for sound clinical treatments.

In 1795, colleagues in the new French National Institute elected Cabanis a member of the 'analysis of sensations and ideas' section of the new Class of Moral and Political Sciences. With Destutt de Tracy, he led the Idéologue circle of physicians and philosophers aspiring to construct a 'science of man'. He also held three appointments at the new Paris School of Medicine from 1796 to 1803 but does not appear to have done much teaching.

From 1796 he read in the Institute the series of memoirs that would ensure his lasting reputation, *On the Relations between the Physical and Moral Aspects of Man.* His most original contribution was his argument that empiricist philosophers' notions of conscious sensations ignored internal impressions from subcenters of sensitivity or from the nervous system that might affect ideas and passions. A physician aware of these relationships could use climate (travel or, at the social level, land reclamation) or regimen (diet, exercise, stimulants, change of occupation) to act on these impressions. Modification of innate individual temperament by hygiene and physical habits could make the individual more sanguine, sensitive, or sociable and thus provide great assistance to the moralist or legislator. Cabanis never correlated temperaments with social class, but his assertion of an indelibly sensitive female temperament assigned women to traditional social roles.

Aside from Enlightenment materialism, the influence of Montpellier school vitalism (Bordeu and Barthez) convinced Cabanis to see sensitivity as a physiological unknown, despite his notorious comparison of digesting impressions to digesting food. His posthumous *Letter on First Causes* (1806–07, published in 1824) reveals more of a monist or pantheist metaphysic than mechanical materialism.

Cabanis never completed a proposed treatise on human perfectibility. However, contemporary physicians Bichat, Pinel, Richerand, and Alibert, and their successors Broussais and Magendie, all paid tribute to his work on physical-mental relations. Physiological Ideology also provided a favorable cultural context for the diffusion of Gall's phrenology.

Bibliography

Primary: 1956. Lehec, Claude and Jean Cazeneuve, eds. *Oeuvres philosophiques* (Paris); 1806. *Sketch of the Revolutions of Medical Science, and Views Relating to Its Reform* [1804], (London) (reprint 1975, Ann Arbor); 1981. Mora, George, ed. *On the Relations between the Physical and Moral Aspects of Man* [1802] (Baltimore).

Secondary: Rôle, André, 1994. *Georges Cabanis, le médecin de Brumaire* (Paris); Staum, Martin, 1980. *Cabanis: Enlightenment and Medical Philosophy in the French Revolution* (Princeton); Moravia, Sergio, 1974. *Il pensiero degli Idéologues: Scienza e filosofia in Francia 1780–1815* (Florence).

Martin S. Staum

CABOT, RICHARD CLARKE   (b. Brookline, Massachusetts, USA, 21 May 1868; d. Cambridge, Massachusetts, USA, 8 May 1939), *medicine.*

Cabot was the son of James and Elizabeth (Dwight) Cabot, members of a prominent family that played a leading role in Boston's intellectual, civic, and business life for several generations. He graduated from Harvard College, summa cum laude, in 1889 and from Harvard Medical School in 1892.

Cabot's professional life was a reflection of the Progressive Era with its emphasis on social reform and his personal belief that medicine offered an opportunity to serve as an agent of moral as well as scientific progress. He interned at the Massachusetts General Hospital (MGH) where he remained on staff until his retirement in 1920 as Clinical Professor of Medicine and Chief of the Medical Staff. Initially committed to laboratory research, he soon discovered that he preferred clinical practice, 'the looking after bodies with souls in them rather than bodies without'. (letter to Ella Lyman, 27 June 1893, quoted in Dodds, 1993, p. 3). He maintained a large private practice in addition to his hospital duties and teaching responsibilities.

Cabot's reputation rests on his development of the scientific diagnosis of disease, resulting in *Physical Diagnosis*, the standard textbook for many years, and creation of the Clinico-Pathological Conference at the MGH, where cases were presented in which diagnosis of disease was correlated with autopsy results. Accounts of these conferences were so popular that, starting in 1924, they were routinely published by the *Boston Medical and Surgical Journal* and continue to the present in its successor, the *New England Journal of Medicine and Surgery.*

He is also remembered for his commitment to the social aspects of medicine, for example, by the importance he gave to the hospital's outpatient clinic, where the health of most patients often reflected the social conditions in which they lived. He created a department of medical social work at the MGH (1905) and, unlike most of his colleagues, was an early advocate of group practice and prepaid medical care. His humanistic approach to medicine and his concern for the patient rather than the disease mark him as a forerunner to contemporary critics of bio-medicine.

Cabot was also a serious medical ethicist. He wrote and taught extensively on the subject, was professor of social ethics (1920–34) at Harvard University, and was professor of natural theology at Andover-Newton Theological School (1935–39). His interest in the relationship of religion to medical therapy and his early recognition of the work of Freud and other psychiatrists placed him outside mainstream American medicine.

In addition to his work at MGH, where he maintained a part-time relationship after his formal retirement, he was a consultant to the New England Hospital for Women and Children, although many people still questioned the propriety of the women physicians. He was also a consultant to Westboro School for Boys and Lancaster School for Girls, both reform schools for wayward youth. He served on the hospital ship *Bay State* during the Spanish American War and at an army hospital in France during World War I.

Cabot married Ella Lyman (1866–1934) in 1894. There were no children.

Bibliography

Primary: 1905–41. *Physical Diagnosis* [12 edns.] (New York and Baltimore); 1909. *Social Service and the Art of Healing* (New York); 1936. (with Dicks, Russell R.) *The Art of Ministering to the Sick* (New York).

Secondary: Crenner, Christopher, 2005. *Private Practice in the Early Twentieth-Century Office of Dr. Richard Cabot* (Baltimore); Crenner, Christopher, 2002. 'Diagnosis and Authority in the Early Twentieth-Century Practice of Richard C. Cabot.' *Bulletin of the History of Medicine* 76: 30–55; Dodds, T. Andrew, 1993. 'Richard Cabot, Medical Reformer during the Progressive Era.' *Annals of Internal Medicine* 119: 417–422; Williams, Thomas Franklin, 1950. 'Cabot, Peabody and the Care of the Patient.' *Bulletin of the History of Medicine* 24: 462–481; White, Paul Dudley, 1939. 'Richard Clarke Cabot.' *New England Journal of Medicine* 222: 1049–1052; *DAMB.*

Amalie M. Kass

CADE, JOHN FREDERICK JOSEPH ('JACK')   (b. Horsham, Victoria, Australia, 18 January 1912; d. Melbourne, Victoria, 16 November 1980), *psychiatry.*

Cade, the eldest of three sons of David Duncan Cade, a pillar of the British Empire, war veteran, and mental diseases specialist, and Ellen Edwards, a sports-loving nursing matron, lived on the grounds of several mental hospitals during his childhood and youth, mixing with the sorts of troubled people whose treatment he would later revolutionize. He attended Scotch College (1925–28) and Melbourne University (1929–34) and then, as a resident at Melbourne's Children's Hospital (1936), met his future wife Estana ('Jean') Charles, a triple-certificate nursing sister assigned to nurse him through a severe bout of pneumonia. He joined the Victorian Mental Hygiene Department in September 1936, undertaking basic psychiatric training at Royal Park Mental Hospital before marrying and continuing on-the-job training in government mental hospitals.

His decision to combine research with psychiatric practice was encouraged by Dr John Catarinich, a close friend of his father. Catarinich became head of Victoria's mental health service (1937–51) and supported Cade's research ambitions, which he demonstrated early by coauthoring with Frank Macfarlane Burnet a novel study of subclinical influenza infection (1940).

In 1941 Cade, nicknamed the 'Mad Major', was posted to Malaysia as a senior company commander in the 2nd/9th Field Ambulance, 8th Division, Australian Imperial Force. Captured by the Japanese at Singapore the following year, he was incarcerated in the Changi POW Camp, one of only two sites noted for conducting medical research in the official history of Australia's wartime participation, in this case on treatments for omnipresent nutritional deficiency diseases. On leaving Singapore in August 1945, Cade wrote home that the long period of captivity had crystallized his notions of psychiatry, 'and I'm just bursting to put them to the test'.

Cade was a founding member of the Australasian Association of Psychiatrists (1946) but soon became a self-described 'lone wolf researcher' testing the theory that a metabolite in excess and demonstrable in the urine caused particular forms of mental illness. This led to studies of the anticonvulsant properties of creatinine (1947) and the discovery that lithium could quell episodes of acute and chronic mania (1949). The finding led him to speculate on the possible etiological significance of lithium in mania and the concept of specific psychopharmaceuticals. It provided the first hard evidence supporting chemical imbalance as an explanation for mental disorder.

When concerns about lithium's life-threatening toxicity in manic patients emerged (1950), Cade asked his colleagues to discuss any adverse effects with him. Simultaneously, pharmacological research on lithium commenced in Melbourne, resulting in modified lithium regimens to reduce toxicity problems (1951, 1955).

Lithium's striking effect in mania attracted little initial attention from American and British psychiatrists, but galvanized numerous studies in France. Danish psychiatrist Mogens Schou and colleagues confirmed the efficacy of lithium in psychiatry's first controlled clinical trial (1954), later demonstrating that it could also prevent recurrences of bipolar disorder (1973). Although Cade retained a strong interest in lithium, he did not publish any new findings after 1949, instead studying the effects on mental illnesses of other alkali metals and nutritional factors. Schou's numerous lithium publications consolidated its acceptance, and in 1974 he and Cade were jointly awarded the International Kittay Award, then the world's richest prize in psychiatry.

Throughout his career Cade, a devout Catholic and trenchant critic of Freudian psychotherapy, stressed the importance of research by psychiatrists of all theoretical persuasions in advancing understanding of mental illness and its causes. He required strong persuasion to mention Freud in his postretirement project, a pocket-sized book on twentieth-century psychiatry (1979) and, in a chapter on lithium, modestly consigned to a footnote his own landmark contribution.

Bibliography

Primary: 1949. 'Lithium Salts in the Treatment of Psychotic Excitement.' *Medical Journal of Australia* 36: 349–352.

Secondary: 1998–2004. Interviews with Jean Cade, Eric Cunningham Dax, Ed Chiu; Healy, David, 1997. *The Antidepressant Era* (Cambridge, MA); Johnson, F. Neil, 1984. *The History of Lithium Therapy* (London); Ayd, F. J., and B. Blackwell, 1970. *Discoveries in Biological Psychiatry* (Philadelphia).

Ann Westmore

CAELIUS AURELIANUS (b. Sicca Veneria [now Le Kef, Tunisia]; fl. late fourth or early fifth century), *gynecology, nosology, medicine, rehabilitative medicine, surgery.*

Caelius Aurelianus was born in Sicca Veneria, in the province of Africa Proconsularis. Little else is known of him. His dating to the late fourth century is based principally on comparative philological analysis with the African medical writer Cassius Felix (c. 450 BCE). That Caelius was a practicing physician is probable, and that he worked in Rome is tenable. It is thanks to Caelius that we possess a Latin version of two important works by the great second-century Methodist doctor, Soranus of Ephesus: *Celeres Passiones* [Acute Diseases] in three books and *Tardae Passiones* [Chronic Diseases] in five books. The Greek originals are lost. There are also parts of two other works by Soranus that Caelius Latinized. The first was *Medicinales Responsiones* [Medical Responses], an erotematic (question-and-answer) compendium of the rules of health (*salutaria praecepta*). Strictly speaking, this work should be regarded as that of Caelius, albeit utilizing Soranian material. The second comprised parts of his *Genecia* [Gynecology]. A comparison of this Latin fragment with Soranus's original indicates that Caelius was a careful translator. Caelius also prepared versions of other works by Soranus, which like the originals, are now lost. The chief features of *Acute and Chronic Diseases* were the organizational layout and attention to detail. The volumes constituted a practical manual, concerned with the description of diseases and their treatment in accord with the Methodist doctrine that theoretical considerations have no place in medical treatment. Methodism laid great stress on the use of those features of a disease that were manifest; these could be amenable to treatment, whereas hidden causes could not, and therefore such speculation was useless for medical practice. This did not prevent Caelius from discussing apparent hidden causes, the physiological role of pneuma being one such example, because speculation of its existence did not necessarily hinder treatment. A few examples suffice to give a flavor of the work. The signs and symptoms of sciatica were accurately described, and where Caelius linked it to what is now regarded as osseous tuberculosis, this nevertheless allows a window into the nature of tuberculosis in antiquity. Caelius's range of treatment for sciatica was a good illustration of the holistic nature of Methodism. Here treatment began with massage, bed rest, the application of heat, and passive exercise and progressed to the application of leeches and venesection in refractory cases. The treatment regimen in cases of paresis, stressing early rehabilitation, showed remarkable foresight. Caelius's views on the treatment of mania were also enlightened, condemning the usual harsh treatments employed. He also discussed migraine (*hemicrania*) and the use of catheterization in cases of paralysis or hemorrhage from the urinary tract, as well as for the application of medical preparations.

Caelius's work survived the depredations of North Africa by the Vandals, Byzantine Empire, and Muslim conquest and eventually made its way to south Italy. The first edition of *Chronic Diseases*, based on a manuscript in the former Benedictine Abbey of Lorsch in Hesse, was published in Basel in 1529. *Acute Diseases* was published in Paris in 1533, and the first entire edition was published in Lyons in 1566.

The degree of fidelity of Caelius's work to the Soranian original, as well as to Soranus's Methodism, is a subject of continuing debate. It is perhaps best to view these texts as capturing the spirit of Soranus and illustrating Caelius's own accomplishments as a doctor, redactor, and compiler. And although Soranus in his *Gynecology* provided what he regarded as necessary correctives to deviations from earlier Methodist teaching, Caelius, in his discussions of causal explanations and definitions, for example, perhaps offered further evidence of Methodist adaptability. Whether these were representative of wider Methodist teaching cannot be determined. Be that as it may, Caelius Aurelianus should not be viewed simply as the Latinizer of Soranus's work, but as a learned and insightful medical writer in his own right.

Bibliography

Primary: 1950. Drabkin, Israel, ed. and trans., *Caelius Aurelianus, On Acute and Chronic Diseases* (Chicago); 1990–93. Bendz, Gerhard, ed., Pape, Ingeborg, trans. *Caelii Aureliani Celerum Passionum libri III, Tardanum Passionum libri V*, CML VI, 1 (Berlin).

Secondary: Van der Eijk, Philip, 2005. 'The Methodism of Caelius Aurelianus: Some Epistemological Issues' in Van der Eijk, Philip, ed., *Medicine and Philosophy in Classical Antiquity* (Cambridge) pp. 299–327; Nutton, Vivian, 1998. 'To Kill or Not to Kill? Caelius Aurelianus on Contagion' in Fischer, Klaus-Dietrich, Diethard Nickel, and Paul Potter, eds., *Text and Tradition. Studies in Ancient Medicine and Its Transmission* (Leiden) pp. 233–242.

Julius Rocca

CAIUS, JOHN (b. Norwich, England, 6 October 1510; d. London, England, 29 July 1573), *medicine, classical scholarship, zoology.*

The son of Robert and Alice Keys or Kees, Caius is the Latinized version of John's name but is always pronounced as 'keys'. He entered Gonville Hall, Cambridge, in September 1529 as a student of theology but seems to have found some of the changes wrought by the Reformation as uncongenial to his conservative nature. He graduated in 1533 and was elected a fellow of Gonville that same year. He then seems to have decided to focus on medicine, and in 1539 he continued his studies at Padua, the leading medical school in Europe. Although well acquainted with Andreas Vesalius (1514–64) at just the time he was compiling the anatomical studies for his *De humani corporis fabrica* (1543) (they even shared a house in Padua together for eight months), Caius was much more profoundly influenced by the celebrated medical humanist, Giovanni Battista Da Monte (aka Montano, Montanus 1489–1551). Caius became convinced by Montanus that current problems with medicine could be solved by returning to Galen in the original Greek, thus avoiding the errors introduced by inadequate translations. He refused throughout his life to countenance criticisms of Galen, regarding them as stemming from an inadequate understanding of the ancient physician. Caius himself, by contrast, expended great efforts to establish scholarly editions of Galen's works. After taking his MD from Padua in 1541, he toured Italian libraries, collecting and copying Greek manuscripts. He published seven Galenic texts at Basel in 1544, *Galeni libri aliquot graeci*, on his way back home to England.

He resigned his fellowship in 1545 and set up a practice in London. From 1546 to 1563 he lectured on anatomy to the Company of Barbers and Surgeons, who were granted the bodies of four executed criminals annually by statute. He was elected fellow of the College of Physicians in 1547, serving on the Council from 1551 and as President from 1555 to 1560 and again in 1562, 1563, and 1571. He was also a generous benefactor of the College, being wealthy from his practice and a confirmed bachelor with no family. He paid for the refurbishment of the tomb of the College's founder, Thomas Linacre (1460?–1524). Caius also lavished donations on his old Cambridge college, enabling it to expand in size and personnel. In September 1557 Gonville Hall was refounded by royal Charter as Gonville and Caius College, and in January 1559 Caius was elected Master.

Caius's conservatism hampered his Mastership. Students protested against his autocratic rule, and the religious conservatism of the College, in an increasingly Calvinist Cambridge, began to attract criticism. Although very short (just over five feet tall) and possessed of a weak voice, Caius evidently had a domineering personality, and this, together with some eccentricities (Dr Caius in Shakespeare's *Merry Wives of Windsor* is said to be modeled on him), exacerbated feeling against him. He refused to hand over the medieval treasures and relics of the College to the university authorities, and in 1572, at the instigation of the precisionist Archbishop of York, Edwin Sandys (1519–88), his rooms were ransacked and much of his property destroyed. Caius returned to London, resigning the Mastership in June of the following year, shortly before his death. He bequeathed virtually all his wealth to the College.

Although primarily devoted to scholarship, Caius was evidently a highly successful practitioner. This may have been due not only to the intimate knowledge of Hippocrates and Galen but also to his own careful observations, as displayed, for example, in his description of the sweating sickness, *Counseil . . . againste . . . the Sweate* (1552). Considerable observational skills were also manifested in his studies of exotic animals, mostly North African, and his detailed study of British dogs (*De canibus Britannicis*, 1570), which he undertook for his friend, the famed naturalist, Conrad Gesner (1516–65), whom he had met on his journey back from Padua. Although, even here, on one occasion Gesner had to correct Caius's assumption that a report of an elk in Caesar's *Gallic War* disproved a contradictory modern report.

Bibliography

Primary: 1556. *Opera aliquot et versiones* (Louvain); 1912. Roberts, E. S. ed. *The works of John Caius, M.D., second founder of Gonville and Caius College and Master of the College, 1559–1573, with a memoir of his life by John Venn.* (Cambridge).

Secondary: Nutton, Vivian, 1987. *John Caius and the Manuscripts of Galen* (Cambridge); O'Malley, C. D., 1965. *English Medical Humanists: Thomas Linacre and John Caius* (Lawrence, KS); Clarke, G., and A. M. Cooke, 1964. *A History of the Royal College of Physicians of London* (Oxford); Raven, Charles E., 1947. *English Naturalists from Neckham to Ray* (Cambridge); *DSB*; *Oxford DNB*.

John Henry

CALANDRE IBÁÑEZ, LUIS (b. Cartagena, Spain, 26 March 1890; d. Madrid, Spain, 29 September 1961), *medicine, histology, cardiology.*

Calandre was the son of a doctor who broke with the family tradition of being in business. He was educated at the Faculty of Medicine in Madrid (1906–11), where he was influenced by various teachers interested in developing research, such as Ramón y Cajal (1852-1934), Juan Madinaveitia (1861–1938), and Nicolás Achúcarro (1880–1918). After obtaining a grant, he went to Germany in 1912 to work in histology with G. F. Nicolai (1864–1964). When he returned to Spain in 1914, he continued his work in the Histology Laboratory of the Board for Advanced Studies and Scientific Research—*Junta de Ampliación de Estudios*—which helped him be noticed by Cajal as one of the young men who would continue consolidating the Spanish school of histology.

At this time he began to work for Juan Madinaveitia in his internal medicine department, taking increasing interest in cardiology. In 1920 he founded, along with Gustavo Pittaluga, the journal *Archivos de Cardiología y Hematología*. He then dedicated much time speaking, teaching, and writing on cardiology. In 1925 the Royal Academy of Medicine awarded him a prize for his work on the influence of the recent histological and physiological discoveries of the myocardium on the interpretation of cardiac pathology. All this led to his appointment as a consultant in heart disease at the Central Hospital of the Spanish Red Cross (1925), and he soon went on to be appointed staff physician (1927).

His resignation as a member of the *Laboratorio de Histología* in 1931 seems to suggest that he was concentrating his efforts on cardiology. A series of appointments came his way at this time, including assistant manager of the previously mentioned hospital in 1932 and vice-chairman of the Central Committee of the Spanish Red Cross in 1933. These illustrate his decision to devote his time to health care management.

The Civil War (1936–39) brought this period to an abrupt end. He received his last public appointment during the war, as head of a provisional hospital in Madrid. He undertook no other public appointment from 1939, dedicating his time to private medicine. The end of the war meant prison for him, and after an initial acquittal in 1940, he was sentenced to six years, which he never served, as he was granted probation in 1942. Earlier, in 1941, he was sanctioned by the College of Physicians and banned from practicing medicine in Madrid for five years.

Calandre is therefore an example of the Civil War's repercussions on the careers of some Spanish scientists whom the new totalitarian government considered political enemies. Until the Civil War he stood out in the group of doctors that Laín called, after their best renowned member, 'the Marañón Generation', which advocated modern medicine in Spain, where clinical medicine was based on research. Calandre thus pioneered the development of cardiology as a specialist area in Spain via original work on anatomy, histology, and cardiac physiology in addition to further research on heart diseases. After the war, at a time when he was professionally removed from the centers of scientific production and health care management, he was limited to private practice and he wrote only three manuals: *Electrocardiografía* (1942), *Tratamiento de las enfermedades del corazón* (1942), and *Electrocardiografía práctica* (1955).

Bibliography

Primary: 1942. *Electrocardiografía,* (Madrid) [2nd edn. 1945, 3rd edn. 1952]; 1947. *Calandre: Historia familiar* (Madrid); 1962. *Luis Calandre Ibáñez: MDCCCXC–MCMLXI* (Madrid).

Secondary: Laín Entralgo, Pedro, 1991. 'Medicina', in López Piñero, José María, ed., *España-Ciencia,* (Madrid) pp. 333–352; Ramón y Cajal, Santiago, 1981. *Recuerdos de mi vida: Historia de mi labor científica* (Madrid).

José Martínez-Pérez

CALDERÓN GUARDIA, RAFAEL ÁNGEL (b. San José, Costa Rica, 10 March 1900; d. San José, 9 June 1970), *medicine, social security.*

One of the most important figures in Costa Rican history, Calderón Guardia was the son of an influential and popular San José physician, Rafael Calderón Muñoz, and Ana María Guardia Mora, a member of an important oligarchic family. Despite this privileged background, he grew up at a time when the patrician families still lived in the heart of the city and daily intermingled with the laboring classes. Calderón Guardia later recalled how, as a child, he had witnessed his father's medical work with the poor, and he attributed the birth of his social conscience to these experiences. His parents were actively involved in Catholic charity organizations, and his father, a congressional deputy, was part of a group seeking to organize a Catholic political arm. His childhood and youth coincided with a tumultuous time in the political and economic history of the small Central American republic. The growth of a manufacturing sector in the capital city, San José, was accompanied by the rise of labor organizations that forced the social question onto the political agenda. Competitive electoral politics expanded considerably only to enter a crisis when the social reform government of President Alfredo González Flores (1914–17) met with elite opposition in the context of an economic crisis provoked by the shrinking of world markets during World War I and was overthrown in a coup. The brief military dictatorship that followed was itself toppled in 1919 by a civic coalition that succeeded in mobilizing the San José masses and restoring political democracy.

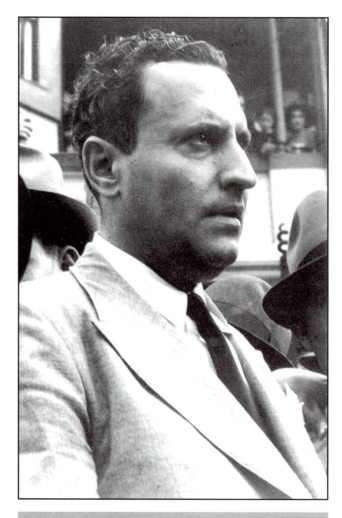

Rafael Ángel Calderón Guardia, probably speaking at a political rally, *c.* 1940. Courtesy Archivo Nacional de Costa Rica.

A Catholic Route into Medicine and Politics

In the early 1920s, Calderón Guardia went to Belgium to pursue university studies (Costa Rica was still without a university or a medical school), dividing his medical training between the Free University of Brussels and the Catholic University of Louvain. While in Belgium he was strongly influenced by the teachings of Cardinal Desiré Joseph Mercier, a reformist theologian trying to formulate a neo-Thomist spiritual doctrine of social reconciliation that could overcome the two competing materialist creeds of the age, Marxism and laissez-faire liberalism. In 1927, Calderón Guardia returned to Costa Rica to practice medicine. He was part of a wave of young physicians who had studied abroad after World War I and who would rejuvenate the profession in Costa Rica over the next two decades.

Following in his father's footsteps, he established a general practice in San José and developed a reputation as a caring, devoted, and charitable doctor in the working-class neighborhoods of the city. This took place in a milieu of increasing unemployment, poverty, and suffering as Costa Rica's export-based economy was hit hard by the Great Depression. In 1934 Calderón Guardia was elected to congress and enjoyed a mercurial rise to the top of the political pyramid. The ascent was paralleled by a rise in his stature as a medical professional, as he was named head of surgery at the country's principal hospital, the Hospital San Juan de Dios, and president of the country's medical association. A leading figure in the Catholic wing of the dominant National Republican Party, he was selected to run as the party's presidential candidate in the elections of 1939 and was victorious, receiving an extraordinary 82.5 percent of the popular vote.

Social Security and the Foundations of the Welfare State

Calderón Guardia is remembered for the great social reform he initiated during his four years in office (1940–44), which laid the foundations of the welfare state. He created the University of Costa Rica, enshrined social guarantees in the constitution, and established a labor code. Most notable, however, was his audacious creation of a social security program in 1941. The social security reform was very much mandated from above by Calderón Guardia and a small group of political confidants (among them physicians, including his father and the former minister of public health, Solón Núñez). Nevertheless, it came at a time when Costa Rica's institutions of state medicine had reached a significant level of development, with the government having assumed control over hospital budgets and having developed a system of health units in towns and cities that was national in scope. Modeled on the Chilean system, the *Caja Costarricense de Seguro Social* (the Costa Rican Social Security Institute) guaranteed medical and maternity benefits to the insured. Beneficiaries were initially concentrated among the salaried labor force of the public sector and large companies, but within two years the system offered coverage to 20 percent of economically active Costa Ricans. In Central American terms, the implementation of social security with medical benefits was quite precocious, predating other countries in the isthmus by many years. *La Caja*, as Costa Ricans call it, continued to expand its reach and currently approaches universal coverage of the population. The institution remains at the heart of the symbolic and real orders of Costa Rican life.

Medical Populism

Calderón Guardia is a good example of a figure peculiar to Latin America: the medical populist. Although physicians have not played significant leadership roles in Anglo-American politics, twentieth-century Latin America has propelled a number of charismatic physicians with populist appeal to the heights of public life: Ramón Grau San Martín in Cuba, Juscelino Kubitschek in Brazil, Arnulfo Arias in Panama, and Salvador Allende in Chile (one is tempted to include Ernest 'Ché' Guevara as well). Calderón Guardia's populist credentials and charismatic style were attributable in essential ways to his work as a doctor, and he justified his political program on the basis of his experiences in medicine and his privileged knowledge of the suffering of the poor. His popular appeal was enhanced by the way he represented himself as a blend of three different types of healer: the Catholic doctor who saw healing as integral to the spiritual health of the community, and spirituality as integral to healing; the good general practitioner who worked among the people; and the modern professional at home in the institutions of biomedicine. His social security reform was likewise billed as a synthesis of all three domains and so must be considered as much the projection of popular medical practices and beliefs as the creation of a biomedical institutional array.

Civil War

In 1942–43, as his reformist agenda expanded and he was confronted by an increasingly hostile and largely conservative establishment, Calderón Guardia forged an alliance with the Communist Party (less controversial at the time because of the wartime alliance between the United States and the USSR) and progressive sectors of the Catholic Church. Although constitutionally barred from re-election, he remained powerful during the subsequent government of a hand-picked political ally, and ran for the presidency again in 1948. Calderón Guardia's nepotism and authoritarian tendencies, as well as an alliance with the Communists that was now taboo because of the Cold War, led the opposition increasingly to advocate violence to keep him from power again. A polarized country descended into a short, sharp civil war following the disputed and fraud-ridden elections of 1948, and Calderón Guardia and his allies were defeated and sent into exile. His subsequent efforts to recapture the presidency were unsuccessful, but his social reforms have remained the touchstone of modern Costa Rican politics.

Bibliography

Primary: 1942. *El gobernante y el hombre frente al problema social costarricense* (San José); 1942. 'Páginas autobiográficas del Dr. Calderón Guardia, presidente de la república' *Revista de los Archivos Nacionales* 6: 11–12, 561–576.

Secondary: Palmer, Steven, 2004. 'A Governor and a Man Faces the Social Problem' in Palmer, Steven, and Iván Molina eds., *The Costa Rica Reader: History, Culture, Politics* (Durham, NC) pp. 135–138; Palmer, Steven, 2003. *From Popular Medicine to Medical Populism: Doctors, Healers and Public Power in Costa Rica, 1800–1940* (Durham, NC); Rosenberg, Mark, 1983. *Las luchas por el seguro social en Costa Rica* (San José); Rosenberg, Mark, 1981. 'Social Reform in Costa Rica: Social Security and the Presidency of Rafael Angel Calderón Guardia.' *Hispanic American Historical Review* 61(2): 279–296.

Steven Palmer

CAMPBELL, KATE ISOBEL (b. Hawthorn, Victoria, Australia, 22 April 1899; d. Camberwell, Victoria, 12 July 1986), *pediatrics*.

Campbell was the third of four children of a Scottish-born clerk, Donald Campbell, and his New Zealand-born wife, Janet Duncan, née Mill, a former schoolteacher. The family had limited means, and the first two sons left school early despite their parents' reverence for education. (Her youngest brother, Donald Campbell QC, was a distinguished and witty barrister who defended Frank Hardy in the *Power without Glory* trial.) Kate shone at Manningtree Road primary school and won a junior government scholarship in the same year as (Sir) Frank Macfarlane Burnet, which enabled her to attend the nearby Methodist Ladies' College. In 1917, supported by a Senior Government Scholarship, she proceeded to the University of Melbourne Medical School; she graduated from there in the stellar year of 1922 alongside Burnet; (Dame) Jean Macnamara (also destined to work in child health); the distinguished hematologist Lucy Bryce; (Sir) Rupert Willis, described by some as the father of modern tumor pathology; and obstetrician and gynecologist George Simpson.

Even as a student, Campbell distinguished herself with her powers of clinical observation and sympathy with patients. (Of almost three thousand home deliveries recorded by medical students at the Melbourne Women's Hospital between 1921 and 1937, her 1922 records were the only ones to note and monitor signs of fetal distress.) Having graduated within the top twelve, she and Jean Macnamara were grudgingly admitted to residencies at the Melbourne hospital, where women residents were habitually restricted to the less interesting cases and excluded from Casualty.

On completion, she chose private general practice but believed she needed more experience in child and maternal health. The Children's Hospital, however, after taking women residents during World War I, was again claiming it lacked the toilet facilities to accommodate female doctors. Sir William Upjohn pleaded the special cases of Drs Campbell and Macnamara with the hospital's board, and in later years would boast that when he got to heaven and Saint Peter asked him what he had done on earth to deserve entry, he need only say 'I got Jean Macnamara and Kate Campbell on at the Children's.' It was while holding the hand of a two-year-old girl at the hospital that she suddenly decided she would specialize in children.

Her time at the Children's was followed by a happier residency at the Women's Hospital. In 1923 and 1924 she began working closely with Dr Vera Scantlebury Brown as they both studied for their MD, and in 1927, when Brown was touring New Zealand to investigate the infant care methods of Dr Truby King, Kate Campbell took over the training school for infant welfare nurses. Thus began a lifelong association with the Victorian Baby Health Centres Association, for which she acted as medical officer until 1965. She visited centers throughout Victoria, 'seeing all the difficult babies', lectured to nurses, and acted as exam-

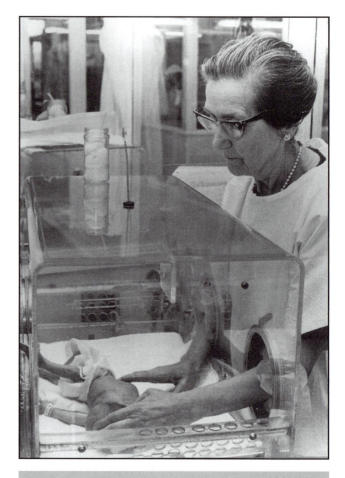

Dame Kate Campbell examines a premature baby in an isolette. Photograph, 1974. Medical History Museum, University of Melbourne.

iner for the State Infant Welfare certificate. With Vera Scantlebury Brown she wrote *A Guide to the Care of the Young Child* (1929), which remained the standard textbook for infant welfare sisters for decades.

She began in general practice in Essendon in 1927, but in 1937 she moved to specialist pediatric practice in Collins Street and into a familiar routine that saw her conducting her hospital visits in the small hours and many of her consultations in the evening. In 1926 she was appointed honorary pediatrician to the Queen Victoria Hospital, where she began her work on newborn babies, an appointment she held until 1965. She was also honorary pediatrician at the Royal Women's Hospital from 1944 until 1965, when she was made consultant pediatrician. In 1929 she began her teaching career in the University of Melbourne after Professor Marshall Allan saw her lecture at an Australian Medical Association meeting. It was an inspired appointment, and she trained generations of doctors in the intricate medicine of the newborn and in tiny babies' 'vocabulary', hilariously imitating their squeaks, snuffles, and grimaces—all of which told her what the baby was feeling. Through her private practice, her consultant positions at the Women's and Queen Victoria hospitals, and her inimitable university teaching, she established an outstanding reputation as a diagnostician. She was remembered for spending hours late at night simply observing babies in special care wards. She developed her own tests for newborns' reflexes and neurological function long before such procedures were discovered by others and disseminated in the literature, and she chatted away to tiny pre-term babies as fascinating fellow human beings.

This habit of clinical observation was the foundation of her most important contributions to neonatal pediatrics. As Dr Elizabeth Turner observed, 'long before neonatology had become a sub-specialty of paediatrics, Kate Campbell was collecting and storing information concerning the reactions of new-born infants to various perinatal stresses, and relating maternal antenatal illness and disease to intra-uterine health and development of the foetus.' This unusual blend of clinical sensitivity, epidemiological curiosity, and meticulousness translated into pioneering work on neonatal intensive care and a range of significant advances in the medicine of the newborn.

Her neonatal care work included infection control, neonatal feeding, jaundice in the premature infant, electrolyte and fluid tolerance in the newborn, and the effects of trauma in delivery. She also collaborated with medical scientists, in particular in the pioneering work conducted in Melbourne by Lucy Bryce and Rachel Jakobowicz of the Red Cross Blood Bank into Rh incompatibility of mother and child, the treatment of consequent hemolytic disease of the newborn, and the development of exchange blood transfusion. At the end of her career, she was publishing on sudden infant death syndrome.

Her most outstanding contribution was the clinical research that established that it was excess therapeutic oxygen that lay behind acquired retrolental fibroplasia in the newborn, first published in 1951. For this work she shared the inaugural Britannica Australia Award for medical research in 1964. She published widely for her generation of researcher clinicians, and in 1965 she became the first woman president of the Australian Paediatric Association.

She irritated some colleagues with her almost uncanny gift of diagnosis and her tenacity in debate, but she was revered by most for her combination of wisdom, diffidence, courtesy, and sense of fun. Nursing staff respected her for being one of the few senior doctors to treat nurses in special care wards as colleagues. She derived enormous pleasure from the human comedy, especially at the rougher end of public medicine. She was also of a generation of women doctors who dressed impeccably and was rarely seen without a hat. She brought both diagnostic brilliance and clinical rigor to neonatal medicine in Australia, but she also championed the virtues of maternal bonding and humane flexibility in an era beset by fads and lingering Puritanism. She had a 'magic touch' with the most distressed of babies, who often found her as fascinating as she did them. She introduced unrestricted visiting in children's wards in 1947 and typically later reviewed the policy, with her colleagues at the Queen Victoria Hospital, Marion Ievers and Mona Blanch, for *Lancet*. Her singularity of character bordered on the eccentric. Her fellow university exhibitioner of 1922–23, Sir Macfarlane Burnet, commented on her seventy-fifth birthday: 'It was interesting to see how, with fame and authority, she changed only by becoming more true to her own individuality.' She never married, but her private life was well organized by a devoted housekeeper-companion.

She was awarded the OBE in 1954, and created a Dame in 1971. In 1966, Kate Campbell and her contemporary and friend, Dame Jean Macnamara, were the first women made honorary doctors of law by the University of Melbourne. It was an indication of their stature that recipients of this honor since 1960 had included three Australian Nobel Prize Winners—Sir Frank Burnett, Lord Florey, and Sir John Eccles.

Dame Kate Campbell remains Australia's most highly regarded pediatrician and probably achieved more than any other female practitioner in establishing women's equality in Australian medicine, and Melbourne owes its continuing high standing in neonatology to her inspiration.

Bibliography

Primary: 1945. (with Brown, Vera Scantlebury) *A Guide to the Care of the Young Child* (Melbourne) [revised edition]; 1949. (with Bryce, Lucy M., J. J. Graydon, Rachel Jakobowicz, and Lorna Kiel) 'The Effect of Heterospecific Pregnancies on the Haemoglobin and Red Cells Levels of the Newborn Infant.' *Medical Journal of Australia* ii: 337–342; 1951. 'Intensive Oxygen Therapy as a Possible Cause of Retrolental Fibroplasia: A Clinical Approach.' *Medical Journal of Australia* ii: 48–50; 1954. 'Care of the Premature Baby.' *Medical Journal of Australia* ii: 404–410.

Secondary: Campbell, Kate, 1982. 'A Medical Life: An Interview with Dame Kate Campbell' in Grimshaw, Patricia, and Lynne Strahan, eds., *The Half-open Door: Sixteen Modern Australian Women Look at Life and Achievement* (Sydney), pp. 154–171; Turner, Elizabeth (guest editor), 1974. *Australian Paediatric Journal* 10(2): 48–54 (Special edition in honor of Dame Kate Campbell's 75th birthday).

Janet McCalman

CAMPER, PETRUS (b. Leiden, the Netherlands, 11 May 1722; d. The Hague, the Netherlands, 7 April 1789), *obstetrics, surgery, anatomy, physical anthropology.*

Camper was the son of Florentinus Camper and Sara Geertruida Ketting. His father was a minister of the Dutch Reformed Church in Batavia in the Dutch East Indies (now Djakarta in Indonesia), where he met his wife, who was born there to a Dutch family. At the time of Camper's birth his parents were living in prosperous conditions in the town of Leiden. His father actively took part in the cultural and scientific life of this small university town. Among the frequent visitors to his parental house was Herman Boerhaave, who was a friend of the family. At the age of twelve (1734), Camper was matriculated at Leiden University, a privilege for all pupils of the local Latin school. However, he started his academic studies some years later. Newtonian empiricists such as W. J. 's Gravesande and P. van Musschenbroek were among his teachers. He completed his studies on 14 October 1746, obtaining a doctorate in Arts as well as in Medicine. Both theses concerned an ophthalmologic subject. In the meantime Camper was trained in practical obstetrics as a pupil of the obstetrician Trioen. Soon after obtaining his doctorate, he settled as medical practitioner in his hometown. Apparently, medical practice did not give him enough satisfaction because after two years he traveled to London, mainly to attend a course in obstetrics given by William Smellie. He stayed in England for about six months, meeting people such as Richard Mead, John Pringle, and Sir Hans Sloane. In the summer of 1749 he left England for Paris, visiting, among others, the Comte du Buffon, Félix Vicq d'Azyr, and Antoine Louis.

Franeker and Amsterdam

While he continued his voyage through France, Switzerland, and Germany, Camper received word that he was appointed professor of philosophy at the University of Franeker in the northern Dutch province of Friesland. Back in Leiden, he became seriously ill, which prevented him from starting his lectures before the spring of 1750. Very soon, his assignment was extended; henceforth, it included the chair of medicine and surgery as well. Notwithstanding his academic obligations, he visited London again in 1752, where he contributed some drawings to the obstetric atlas of Smellie. In the meantime a severe conflict about priority arose between Camper and the only other professor in the medical faculty of Franeker, Tiberius Lambergen. The affair ended only when the provincial court of justice fined Camper twenty gold guilders, to be paid to his opponent.

Both contestants left Franeker soon afterward: whereas Lambergen went to the University of Groningen in 1753, Camper accepted a municipal professorship in Amsterdam in 1755; he was expected to teach anatomy and surgery to members of the surgeon's guild. Three years later he also received a professorship in medicine at the Amsterdam Athenaeum. In April 1756, Camper married Johanna Bourboom, the wealthy widow of one of his former patients in Franeker. From this marriage three sons were born. In 1761, Camper resigned from his Amsterdam appointments to retreat to a rural estate belonging to his wife: Klein Lankum in the neighborhood of Franeker.

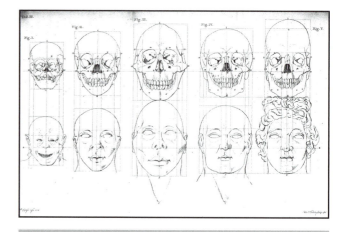

Comparative human skulls and physiognomy of ethnic and historical groups. Engraving from *Dissertation physique de M. Pierre Camper . . .* Utrecht, 1791. Rare Books, Wellcome Library, London.

First Interlude

It was two years before Camper accepted an academic appointment again. In 1763, he was appointed professor of medicine, surgery, anatomy, and botany at the University of Groningen. In the meantime, he spent several productive years in the Frisian countryside, publishing on a variety of surgical and obstetrical subjects. Two problems occupied him in particular: the 'jammed head' and the surgery of bladder stones. With regard to the latter he advocated—to no avail—an operation in two sessions: first incise the bladder and a few days later remove the stone(s). Concerning the rather frequent problem of a discrepancy between the size of the fetal head and the diameter of the pelvic inlet, Camper proposed to perform a symphyseotomy in the last resort, based on experiments he had performed on pigs and human cadavers. His request to perform this intervention on a young woman who had been sentenced to death was rejected by the stadtholder William V. This operation was performed only a very few times before it fell into oblivion. Camper preferred practical skill to theory, and he experimented with obstetric instruments of his own design. He was one of the most fervent advocates of variolation in the Netherlands, belittling the risks involved. During this period, in which he lived in Friesland, he became involved in provincial politics, being chosen as representative of one of the thirty 'grietenijen' (rural districts) to the Diet of Friesland.

Groningen

In 1764, Camper began his professorial duties in Groningen by delivering an inaugural address concerning the remarkable analogy between plants and animals. Although his assignment clearly stated medicine as one of the subjects to be taught, he confined his lectures to obstetrics, surgery, and anatomical demonstrations. When students asked for a course in materia medica, Camper refused, arguing that all that was known about drugs could be told in one afternoon. During his years in Groningen Camper became involved in the struggle against rinderpest, a disease that repeatedly decimated the livestock in the countryside of Groningen and elsewhere. Based on an assumed analogy between human smallpox and rinderpest, Camper and his colleague, Professor Wouter van Doeveren, studied the effects of inoculation in diverse variations but without any effect. When Camper later tried to continue his inoculation experiments in Friesland, local farmers revolted, causing Camper to stop his veterinarian escapade.

Early in his life Camper took lessons in drawing and painting from the Leiden painter Carel de Moor and his son. He showed a remarkable talent and produced beautiful anatomical and pathological illustrations to his own work as well as to that of Smellie, as mentioned earlier. In 1770, he held a lecture at the Amsterdam drawing academy on the physiognomy of people from various regions and of different age groups. Among other things, he argued that one of the features that separated Negroes from Caucasians was the so-called facial angle, which measures the relative flatness versus the forward extension of the face. He also noted that this angle changed during life. Although Camper claimed that the facial angle was not an inborn racial characteristic—but largely depended on a variety of external factors—the concept was misused in the nineteenth century as an identifying mark of the black race.

Retirement

In 1770, one of Camper's former teachers, Professor B. S. Albinus, died. Camper seems to have had aspirations for this chair at the University of Leiden. The curators of Groningen University did their utmost to keep him. They were successful but not for long; in 1773 Camper left Groningen, to retire once again to his country estate Klein Lankum. It has been suggested that his wife became homesick for her Friesland. However, she was not granted much time to enjoy her native country; she died in 1776 of breast cancer. After his wife's death, Camper took up traveling. He traveled through Belgium and Germany and went to Paris to lecture on—amongst other topics—physiognomy. In 1779, 1780, and 1782, he traveled through Germany, visiting many scientists. In 1780 he was accompanied by his youngest son Adrian Gilles. Frederick the Great of Prussia granted him an audience. In 1785 he visited London, this time accompanied by one of his other sons, Jacques. Two years later his last trip brought him to Paris once again.

After taking leave from the University of Groningen, Camper's interest in practical medicine declined, and he showed a growing interest in comparative anatomy and paleontology. He dissected a variety of exotic animals, such as the orangutan and the deer. He gathered a large collection of animal bones and fossils in his natural history cabinet. Shortly before his death he bought a collection of remnants of a mastodon found on the borders of the Mississippi. He maintained a large international correspondence on these subjects.

During his second stay at Klein Lankum, Camper became more and more involved in Frisian politics. During the 1780s, the Dutch Republic was moving steadily to its chaotic end; it became the battle scene of various political factions, such as the Orangists, the 'democrats', and the regents. Camper became a very outspoken member of the faction of Frisian Orangists. As a protégé of stadtholder William V, he was appointed mayor of the small town of Workum, member of the executive committee of the Estates of Friesland, and councilor of the admiralty. In 1787, he even became a member—and later president—of the Council of State of the Dutch Republic, making it necessary for him to move to The Hague. The same year, a group of radical democrats occupied Franeker, where they formed a revolutionary government. Camper moved most of his precious natural history collection to Amsterdam and The Hague.

Evaluation

Petrus Camper was an ambitious and energetic man who divided his attention between various fields of interest: anatomy, surgery, obstetrics, anthropology, zoology, paleontology, drawing, and politics. Although a medical doctor by training, he had little regard for the scientific medicine of his time. Being a faithful Newtonian, he rejected the speculative character of contemporary medical theory. In his inaugural address *De certo in medicina* [On certainty in medicine] (1758), he advocated an empirical approach to medicine, whereby diseases are defined by their symptoms, disregarding etiology. He was a keen observer, both as an anatomist and as a zoologist. Combining practice and theory, he successfully engaged in comparative anatomy and anthropology. Although one can hardly point to a concrete and lasting contribution to medicine by Camper, through his publications, lectures, and his vast correspondence he certainly contributed to the emancipation of surgery and obstetrics.

Bibliography

Primary: 1760. *Demonstrationum anatomico-pathologicarum liber primus, continens brachii humani fabricam et morbos* (Amsterdam); 1762. *Demonstrationum anatomico-pathologicarum liber secundus, continens pelvis humanae fabricam et morbos* (Amsterdam); 1801. *Vermischte Schriften, die Arzney-, Wundarzney- und Entbindungskunst betreffend* (Lingen); 2002. Bots, H., and R. Visser, eds., *La correspondance, 1785–1787, de Petrus Camper (1722–1789) et son fils Adriaan-Gilles Camper (1759–1820)* (Amsterdam).

Secondary: Sluis, Jacob van, 2003. 'Camper, Petrus' in Bunge, Wiep van et al., eds., *The Dictionary of Seventeenth and Eighteenth-Century*

Dutch Philosophers 2 vols. (Bristol) pp. 196–199; Meijer, Miriam Claude, 1999. *Race and Aesthetics in the Anthropology of Petrus Camper (1722–1789)* (Amsterdam and Atlanta); Gould, Stephen Jay, 1991. *Bully for Brontosaurus* (New York and London) esp. 229–240; Schuller tot Peursum-Meijer, J., and W. R. H. Koops, 1989. *Petrus Camper (1722–1789). Onderzoeker van nature* (Groningen); Visser, R. P. W., 1985. *The Zoological Work of Petrus Camper (1722–1789)* (Amsterdam); *DSB.*

Jan K. van der Korst

CANDAU, MARCOLINO GOMEZ (b. Rio de Janeiro, Brazil, 30 May 1911; d. Geneva, Switzerland, 23 January 1983), *international health.*

Born in Rio de Janeiro, then the capital of Brazil, Candau completed his medical training at Rio's Medical School in 1933. In his first job, as head of a provincial local health unit in São João Marcos, in the state of Rio de Janeiro, he demonstrated administrative skill and devotion to his duties and was promoted to assistant to the Director of the State's Department of Health. In 1938, Fred L. Soper, the representative of the Rockefeller Foundation in Brazil, asked Candau to work under his direction in a major eradication campaign against a malaria outbreak spread by the *Anopheles gambiae.* Thereafter he pursued graduate studies in public health at Johns Hopkins University. Upon his return from the United States in the early 1940s, he worked with the Special Service of Public Health (SESP in Portuguese), an organization created thanks to U.S. bilateral assistance to organize health campaigns and construct public health infrastructure. By 1947 Candau was superintendent, namely, SESP's Brazilian head of this organization.

In 1950 Candau was called to the World Health Organization's headquarters in Geneva to head the Division of Organization of Health Services. Within a year he was promoted to Assistant Director General in charge of Advisory Services. During 1952 he returned briefly to the Americas as second in command of the Pan American Health Organization, under the directorship of his old boss Soper. During the first months of the next year he was elected and ratified by a WHO Assembly as the successor of the first Director General, Canadian Brock Chisholm.

Candau was WHO's Director-General for over twenty years (1953–1973), being re-elected to four successive terms. Under his command, WHO enhanced its membership, infrastructure, staff, and prestige. In 1953, WHO had a membership of eighty-one countries, a staff of 1,500, and a budget of U.S. $9 million. Twenty years later, WHO included 138 nations, its staff was almost 4,000, and its budget was over U.S. $106 million. In addition, it had a splendid building in Geneva and a regional organizational scheme with five main continental field offices. It had also signed agreements with other multilateral agencies, such as UNICEF and PASB, and with U.S. bilateral agencies. The latter was important during a political period that combined the Cold War between the superpowers and the decolonization movements in many Third World nations. His diplomatic personality, sound judgment, wit, and power of persuasion had an easy way with heads of state, politicians, and medical leaders.

Candau was a strong advocate of malaria eradication when it was launched in a World Health Assembly held in Mexico City in 1955 (another theme he championed was the medical use of atomic energy). He strongly believed, along with many experts, that indoor spraying of residual insecticides and new drugs would eliminate malaria from developing countries. He also eventually believed that all major infectious diseases would surrender to new scientific tools. However, the goal was never achieved. The worldwide malaria burden was only temporarily reduced. The campaign was a learning experience for WHO regarding the limitations of vertical programs, and from the 1960s WHO emphasized the development of basic health services.

Candau supported WHO in a renewed smallpox eradication campaign launched in 1967 (that achieved its target in 1978). He also played a crucial role in the fight against onchocerciasis, combining the efforts of the World Bank and FAO. Candau standardized the advice of scientists with the formation of an Advisory Committee on Medical Research. The WHO Committee included Nobel Prize laureates and provided fellowships for young researchers.

Upon his retirement Candau became WHO's Director-General Emeritus, participated in WHO meetings, and declined to become Health Minister of President Goulart's government. Among the prizes he received was the Geraldo de Paula de Souza Medal from the Public Health Association of Sao Paulo and the Leon Bernard Medal and Prize from WHO.

Bibliography

Primary: 1954. 'WHO and the Modern Concept of Public Health.' *Journal of the Indian Medical Association* 24(7): 272–274; 1971. 'La Salud en el Segundo Decenio para el Desarrollo' *Crónica de la Organización Mundial de la Salud* 25(1): 3–8; 1973. 'International Public Health: Some Reflections after 25 Years.' *WHO Chronicle* 26(6): 225–235.

Secondary: 1983. 'In Memory of Dr. M. G. Candau.' *WHO Chronicle* 37(4): 144–147; 1982. 'Marcolino Gomez Candau' *Revista de Malariologia e Doenças Tropicais* 34: 119–22; 1973. 'Retirement of Dr. M.G. Candau.' *Lancet* ii(7821): 138.

Marcos Cueto

CANNON, WALTER BRADFORD (b. Prairie du Chien, Wisconsin, USA, 19 October 1871; d. Franklin, New Hampshire, USA, 1 October 1945), *physiology.*

Cannon was the only son of Colbert Hanchett Cannon, a railroad worker, and Sarah Wilma Denio, a schoolteacher. He was born in Prairie du Chien, Wisconsin, site of Fort

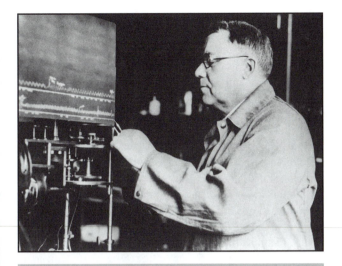

Walter Bradford Cannon. Photograph, Iconographic Collection, Wellcome Library, London.

Crawford, where William Beaumont carried out his gastric experiments on Alexis St Martin in the 1820s. Cannon attended public schools in Milwaukee, Wisconsin, and St Paul, Minnesota. When he was fourteen, his father put him to work in a railroad office for two years. In 1888 Cannon entered St Paul High School and graduated in three years, subsequently taking a postgraduate year to prepare for college examinations. May Newsom, an English literature teacher at St Paul High School, encouraged Cannon to apply to Harvard College and helped him secure financial aid.

In 1892 Cannon entered Harvard College. While at Harvard, he studied the biological sciences but took no mathematics. He studied biology and zoology under George H. Parker and Charles B. Davenport and became interested in neurology and psychology. He wrote his first research paper, 'On the Determination of the Direction and Rate of Movement of Organisms by Light', with Davenport. Cannon graduated *summa cum laude* in 1896. After a letter to Dean William H. Welch of the Johns Hopkins Medical School went unanswered, he enrolled in medical school at Harvard in the fall of 1896.

Cannon immediately sought out opportunities to conduct research at Harvard. At the suggestion of Henry Bowditch, professor of physiology, Cannon and second-year student Albert Moser tested the mechanics of swallowing by using the newly discovered x-ray. Cannon and Moser observed the phenomena in the frog and goose by watching the passage of gelatin capsules filled with bismuth subnitrate. At the December 1896 meeting of the American Physiological Society in Boston, Cannon made the first public demonstration of the mechanics of digestion in a goose by means of x-rays. Cannon's gastric research yielded his first individual publication, 'The Movements of the Stomach Studied by Means of the Röntgen Rays', which was printed in the first issue of the *American Journal of Physiology* in January 1898.

As a medical student, Cannon was innovative not only in the laboratory but also in the classroom. He grew envious of the interactive educational methods employed by Christopher Langdell at the Harvard Law School. Cannon adapted the case system for medical education, utilizing case histories gathered from various hospitals. Several departments at the Harvard Medical School later adopted Cannon's case system methodology.

Sometime during the winter of 1900, while teaching comparative vertebrate anatomy, Cannon accepted an instructorship in physiology for the following year. On 25 June 1901 Cannon married Cornelia James, a Radcliffe student whom he had met as a senior at Harvard. They would later have five children. In 1902 he was promoted to assistant professor. Upon Bowditch's retirement in 1906, Cannon became the George Higginson Professor of Physiology as well as chair of the physiology department, a position he held until his own retirement in 1942. As he gained administrative responsibilities, he continued his research on the digestive system, examining the nature of swallowing, gastrointestinal motility, gastric peristalsis, and the time it took for foodstuffs to pass out of the stomach into the duodenum. He summarized his research in a 1911 text, *The Mechanical Factors of Digestion.*

In 1908 the American Medical Association appointed Cannon as chair of the AMA's Council on the Defense of Medical Research. The AMA established the Council in response to vociferous antivivisectionist attacks on the Rockefeller Institute. Cannon sought to defend animal experimentation. He devised a model code of laboratory regulations that was circulated to medical schools and research institutions across the country. Cannon resigned his position in 1926 but continued in an advisory capacity.

During his investigations of digestion, Cannon noticed how emotions impacted the digestive process. He realized that when experimental animals were emotionally excited, the movement of the stomach and intestines ceased. These observations led Cannon to investigate the sympathetic nervous system. In the early 1910s, he developed the concept of the emergency function of the sympathetic nervous system, otherwise known as the 'fight or flight' mechanism.

World War I interrupted Cannon's research. In the fall of 1916, the National Research Council named him a member of a committee on traumatic shock. He joined the Harvard University Hospital Unit and traveled to France, where he served as director of a surgical research laboratory in Dijon. In 1923 he recapitulated his wartime experiences in *Traumatic Shock.*

In 1917 Western Reserve University physiologists George N. Stewart and Julius M. Rogoff severely criticized Cannon's research on the sympathetic nervous system. Stewart and Rogoff challenged Cannon's contention that secretion of the adrenal medulla increased during emergency situations; they insisted that adrenal secretion was continuous. Surprised, although not dissuaded, Cannon responded to such criticism by developing a new line of research. With the aid of Harold F. Price, a Harvard graduate student, Cannon adopted the denervated cat heart preparation. The removal of the stellate ganglia from the cat's heart eliminated any influence the thyroid had upon the cat and made the heart an indicator of adrenalin levels in the blood. This methodology enabled Cannon to confirm his earlier investigations of the sympathetic control of adrenal secretion.

Cannon then turned to investigating the autonomic nervous system and determining how the body maintained a state of internal equilibrium. Building on French physiologist Claude Bernard's notion of the *milieu interieur*, Cannon coined the term 'homeostasis'. Cannon first presented the concept in a 1924 article in the *American Journal of Physiology*, suggesting that an organism responds to external disturbances by making autonomic adjustments. At a meeting of the Congress of American Physicians in 1925, Cannon expanded further on how the body maintained a steady state of equilibrium. Cannon, however, did not introduce the term 'homeostasis' until 1926, in a paper entitled 'Physiological Regulation of Normal States: Some Tentative Postulates Concerning Biological Homeostatics'.

Cannon believed that the scientific and medical communities had certain social obligations to uphold. The international scientific community found itself increasingly threatened by fascist governments in the 1930s and 1940s. His scientific and political views coalesced during these tumultuous years. Cannon believed that a productive scientist also had to be a good citizen. Cannon became very politically involved and he helped organize the Medical Bureau to Aid Spanish Democracy, served as president of the American-Soviet Medical Society, and participated in the American Bureau for Medical Aid to China and the United China Relief. Cannon also developed a close friendship with Russian physiologist Ivan Pavlov. In 1923 Pavlov visited the United States at Cannon's suggestion, returning again in 1929 for the International Physiological Congress in Boston. Cannon returned the favor, visiting Moscow in 1935 to attend the fifteenth International Physiological Congress. Just as Cannon believed that a productive scientist had an obligation to be a good citizen, he also insisted that the lay public have access to accurate medical knowledge. At his suggestion, the AMA began publishing *Hygeia*, a family health magazine, in 1923.

Throughout the 1930s Cannon collaborated with Arturo Rosenblueth, a Mexican physician and physiologist. Rosenblueth was Cannon's most favored collaborator, with whom he worked until his death. The Cannon-Rosenblueth collaboration marked the second phase of research on the chemical mediation of nerve impulses for Cannon. In 1921 Cannon and Joseph Uridil demonstrated that stimulation of the hepatic nerve brought about acceleration of the denervated heart, hinting at the plausibility of neurochemical transmission of nerve impulses. In 1933 Cannon and Rosenblueth proposed that two sympathins, one excitatory and the other inhibitory, directed chemical mediation of nerve impulses. Ulf von Euler later demonstrated that Cannon and Rosenblueth's hypothetical sympathins were epinephrine and norepinephrine.

During World War II, Cannon revisited the problem of shock as chair of the National Research Council's Committee on Shock and Transfusion. Occupying a primarily administrative role, Cannon watched as Edwin J. Cohn refined methods of blood procurement in order to assist in the prevention and treatment of soldiers suffering from shock. Cannon retired from Harvard in 1942, although he served as visiting professor at the New York University Medical School in 1944 and continued his collaboration with Rosenblueth. Throughout his career, Cannon maintained numerous professional obligations. Elected to the American Physiological Society in 1900, Cannon served as treasurer from 1905 until 1912 and as president from 1914 until 1916. Cannon also served as president of the American Association for the Advancement of Science in 1939.

Later in life, Cannon suffered from radiation damage caused by overexposure to x-rays during his early years of research. In 1931 he was diagnosed with mycosis fungoides, a lymphoma of the skin. He later developed several other cancerous conditions, eventually succumbing in October 1945. Although Cannon performed little research on homeostasis after publishing *The Wisdom of the Body* in 1932, his closing statement in a 1929 *Physiological Reviews* article best summarizes his impact on physiology in the twentieth century. Cannon remarked that 'regulation in the organism is the central problem of physiology'. Cannon's legacy was multifold, as he tackled an array of research topics: the mechanics of digestion, the autonomic and sympathetic nervous systems, traumatic shock, homeostasis and hormonal regulation, and the neurochemical transmission of nerve impulses.

Bibliography

Primary: 1911. *The Mechanical Factors in Digestion* (London); 1932. *The Wisdom of the Body* (New York); 1945. *The Way of an Investigator: A Scientist's Experiences in Medical Research* (New York).

Secondary: Wolfe, Elin, A. Clifford Barger, and Saul Benison, 2000. *Walter B. Cannon, Science and Society* (Cambridge, MA); Benison, Saul, 1991. 'Walter B. Cannon and the Politics of Medical Science, 1920–1940.' *Bulletin of the History of Medicine* 65: 234–251; Benison, Saul, A. Clifford Barger, and Elin Wolfe, 1987. *Walter B. Cannon: The Life and Times of a Young Scientist* (Cambridge, MA); Brooks, Chandler McC., Kiyomi Koizumi, and James O. Pinkston, eds., 1975. *The Life and Contributions of Walter Bradford Cannon, 1871–1945* (Albany, NY); *DSB*; *DAMB*.

Todd M. Olszewski

CANTACUZINO, IOAN   (b. Bucharest, Romania, 13 November 1863; d. Bucharest, Romania, 14 January 1934), *microbiology.*

Cantacuzino was the son of Ion Cantacuzino, a former minister of Prince Alexandru Ioan Cuza (r. 1859–66), and Maria Cantacuzino, née Mavros, the daughter of General Mavros, secretary to Pavel Kiseleff, the governor of the Danubian Principalities (1830–34). He was tutored at home and then continued his education at the lyceum 'Louis le Grand' in Paris. In 1882 Cantacuzino obtained his baccalaureate and enrolled at the Faculty of Philosophy and the Faculty of Natural Sciences from which he graduated in 1885 and 1891, respectively. Between 1890 and 1892 he worked as an assistant at several hospitals in Paris. It was during this period that he published his first medical research on hysteria syndrome, which simulated sclerosis in the cell plates.

Between 1892 and 1893 Cantacuzino was a student of the Russian immunologist and embryologist Elie Mechnikov (1845–1916). In 1894 he obtained his doctorate in medicine from the Faculty of Medicine in Paris, with a thesis on *Recherches sur le mode de destruction du vibrion cholérique dans l'organisme. Contribution à l'étude du probléme de l'immunité.* In the same year he was appointed professor of animal morphology at the Faculty of Natural Sciences in Iai (eastern Romania). In 1896 he returned to Paris and worked with Mechnikov at the Pasteur Institute. In 1901 he was appointed professor at the Faculty of Medicine in Bucharest and became the director of the newly founded Laboratory of Experimental Medicine. Between 1908 and 1910 he was the director of the Sanitary Service in Romania. During the Balkan Wars (1912–13) Cantacuzino supervised the study of the cholera epidemic in Bulgaria and organized several vaccination campaigns among the Romanian troops known as 'the great Romanian experiment of 1913'. His campaigns against cholera, typhus, and exanthemas fever continued during World War I. In 1921 Cantacuzino founded 'The Institute of Serums and Vaccines' (today the 'Institute of Microbiology, Parasitology and Epidemiology Dr. I. Cantacuzino'), which specialized in the preparation of serums, vaccines, and other biological products necessary for the diagnosis, prophylaxis, and treatment of infectious diseases.

Cantacuzino expanded Mechnikov's research on the phagocytes and the problem of immunity in invertebrates. Cholera and the defense mechanisms used by organisms against cholera vibrios, in particular, were given constant consideration. Cantacuzino combined the existing theories of Mechnikov, Behring, and Koch with his own research and suggested that the organism defends itself against cholera by destroying cholera vibrios. There was, Cantacuzino believed, a correlation between the intensity of leucocytes and phagocytes, on the one hand, and the elimination of vibrios on the other hand. In 1912 he discovered in a species of invertebrates, *Eupagurus prideauxii,* a type of natu-

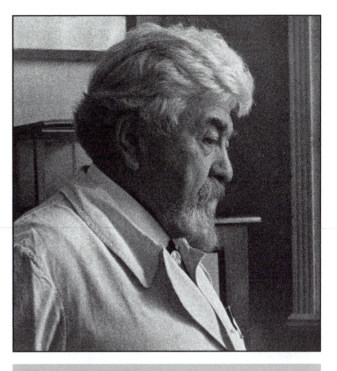

Ioan Cantacuzino. Photograph, Iconographic Collection, Wellcome Library, London.

ral antibody. Cantacuzino also worked extensively on the anticholera vaccine; for example, he invented a method of antimalaria vaccination (the 'Cantacuzino Method'), which is still used today. Connected to his research of cholera was the research on scarlet fever. After researching various manifestations of scarlet fever and streptococcus infections, Cantacuzino discovered the phenomenon of 'transmissible agglutination' of the streptococcus, which contributed to a better understanding of the etiology of scarlet fever.

Moreover, Cantacuzino was interested in tuberculosis, as illustrated by his first experimental clinical and epidemiological study (1928) of over 3,000 children, whom he vaccinated successfully. Due to Cantacuzino's efforts, Romania was the second country in the world, after France, to introduce the BCG vaccine ('Bacillus Calmette-Guérin'). Cantacuzino was the recipient of several honorary titles, such as *Doctor honoris causa* of the University of Lyon (1922), Montpellier (1930), Athens (1932), and Bordeaux (1934), and a member of numerous scientific organizations, including the Hygiene Committee of the League of Nations (1923), the Romanian Academy, and the Society of Exotic Pathology in Paris. Much of Cantacuzino's research on the immunity of invertebrates was re-discovered by the American scientist F. B. Bang who presented it in *Nature* in 1962.

Bibliography

Primary: 1965. *Opere alese* (Bucharest); 1905. 'Recherches sur la maladie expérimentale provoquée par l'inoculation de bacilles tuberculeux dégraissés' *Ann. Inst. Pasteur*, 1929. 'Sur l'étiologie de la scarlatine' *Rapport, XXe Congrès Français Médicine*, 1932. 'Vaccination par le B.C.G. en Roumanie'. *Ann. Inst. Pasteur.*

Secondary: Bacaloglu, C., Stella Litarczek, V. Baroni, Valeriu Bologa, A. Boivin, A. Besredka, A. Boquet, et al., eds., 1934. *Hommage à la mémoire du professeur Jean Cantacuzène* (Paris).

Marius Turda

CARDANO, GIROLAMO (b. Pavia, Italy, 24 September 1501; d. Rome, Italy, 20 September 1576), *medicine, mathematics, physics, philosophy.*

Cardano, the illegitimate son of Fazio Cardano, jurist and mathematician, and Chiara Micheri, had an unhappy childhood. He began his medical studies in 1520 at the University of Pavia; in 1524 he transferred to the University of Padua, and in June 1524 he obtained his degree in arts at the Venetian College of Physicians. At Padua in 1525 he was elected rector of the University of Arts and Medicine, and on 13 August 1526 he graduated in medicine. Almost immediately he began to practice medicine in Piove di Sacco, a small town near Padua, where he spent nearly six years. In 1534 Cardano became a teacher of mathematics in the Piattine schools of Milan. In 1543 he accepted the first chair of theoretical medicine at the University of Pavia, where he taught until 1562, with an interruption from 1552 to 1559. In 1547 he was asked, through Andreas Vesalius (1514–64), to become personal physician to King Christian III of Denmark, but he refused. Instead he went to Scotland in 1552 at the request of John Hamilton, archbishop of St Andrews, to cure his allergic asthma.

In 1560 his elder son was executed for having poisoned his wife. Cardano left Pavia and in 1562 he was offered the first chair of theoretical medicine at the University of Bologna. But in 1570 he was accused of heresy and thrown into prison. Upon his release a few months later Cardano went south to Rome, where in 1573 Pope Gregory XIII granted him a pension. He dedicated the last year of his life to writing *De vita propria liber*, an autobiography published posthumously (1643) that is the principal source for his biography.

Cardano wrote more than 200 works on medicine, mathematics, physics, philosophy, astrology, religion, and music. His *De subtilitate* (1550) and *De rerum varietate* (1557) are expressions of his encyclopedic talent.

Cardano's fame rests mostly on his contributions to mathematics. In this field his greatest work was the *Ars magna* (1545), which gave rise to a well-known priority dispute with Nicolò Tartaglia concerning the procedure for solving third-degree equations. Many new ideas in algebra were presented, including Cardano's rule for solving reduced third-degree equations, and the solution of the quartic equation. In a later edition of the *Ars magna* (1570) he also tackled the 'irreducible case' of the cubic equation. Cardano also made important contributions in various

fields of physics. He is credited with the invention of the so-called Cardano's suspension and of the Cardano's (or universal) joint. He also sustained the impossibility of perpetual motion.

Cardano was a renowned physician. His copious medical production has yet to be suitably and systematically studied. His medical works included Hippocratic commentaries and treatises on therapeutics and various aspects of medical practice and on debated issues in medicine, such as plague, venereal diseases, saliva, consultations, etc., in which he never failed to demonstrate his extraordinary capacity for observation. He was also very interested in anatomy and enjoyed excellent relations with Vesalius, who he considered the foremost anatomist of his time. In 1536 Cardano first described typhus fever while differentiating measles from typhus, which he called *morbus pulicaris* (fleabite disease) due to the likeness between the rash and fleabites. He maintained that the seeds of disease were in fact living organisms.

Cardano was also a forerunner in the fields of psychiatry and criminal anthropology. In 1550 he proposed a device for teaching the blind to read and write by sense of touch; he was also convinced of the possibility of teaching deaf mutes by the visual pathway.

Bibliography

Primary: 1663. *Opera omnia* 10 vols. (Spon, Charles, ed.) (Lyons); 1658. *Metaposcopia* (Paris) (omitted by Spon in the *Opera omnia*).

Secondary: Baldi, Marialuisa, and Guido Canziani, eds., 1999. *Girolamo Cardano. Le opere, le fonti, la vita* (Milan); Siraisi, Nancy G., 1997. *The Clock and the Mirror: Girolamo Cardano and Renaissance Medicine* (Princeton); Simili, Alessandro, 1969. *Gerolamo Cardano lettore e medico a Bologna* (Bologna); Eckman, James, 1946. 'Jerome Cardan.' *Bulletin of the History of Medicine, Supplement, 7; DSB*.

Giuseppe Ongaro

CARDENAL FERNÁNDEZ, SALVADOR (b. Valencia, Spain, 1 September 1852; d. Barcelona, Spain, 24 April 1927), *surgery.*

The son of an engineer, Cardenal spent most of his childhood in Urgell, a Catalan provincial town. After he recovered from a purulent pleurisy, he became interested in surgery. He attended the Faculty of Medicine of the University of Barcelona, and upon graduation in 1872 he worked with José de Letamendi. Together with him he spent some time in Brussels, where he started to publish on anesthesia. Soon after his return to Spain he became attached to the Faculty of Medicine of the University of Madrid and obtained his PhD there in 1877 on the subject of septicemias. He was appointed anatomic demonstrator at the Faculty of Medicine of Barcelona (1877–84) and entered the *Casa de la Caritat*, a Poor Law shelter institution, to serve as a physician. At the same time, he worked as orthopedist for an industrial firm, Girona Brothers.

During the years 1875–79 he spent much time abroad, training in major European surgical centers. In Vienna he learned about stomach surgery with Theodor Billroth and became acquainted with goiter techniques under Emil Kocher in Bern. In 1879 he became director of a newly founded charity institution, the *Sagrat Cor* (Holy Heart) Hospital of Barcelona, which was to be the theatre for the deployment of his surgical skills and new knowledge, together with his privately owned *Clinicum*. But during his visits to England between 1880 and 1887, he became especially interested in the role of microbes in wound sepsis and in mastering antiseptic methods, thanks to the guidance of Joseph Lister. His earlier training in France, Switzerland, and Austria had given him a preliminary knowledge of Louis Pasteur's and Robert Koch's microbiology. The first two editions (1880, 1887) of his handbook on surgery, which contained the explanation of antiseptic methods, were quickly sold out and won for him a reputation as the leader of what has been known as the modern Catalan school of surgery.

Despite earlier attempts by people such as Juan Giné y Partagás, it was Cardenal's achievement to introduce and popularize antiseptic surgical practice in Spain. He devoted himself to practicing and teaching Listerian doctrines, experimenting with products brought with him from his travels, which he reassumed in 1889. Particularly, he introduced several antiseptic products, such as rubber gloves and impregnated bandages, in the surgical theatre.

In 1887 he became physician in chief of the *Casa de la Caritat* and obtained the appointment as head of the surgical department at the *Sacrat Cor* Hospital. In 1890 he became an Honorary Fellow of the Royal College of Surgeons of England, and he was President of the Academy and Laboratory of Medical Sciences of Barcelona from 1893 to 1895. By the time of the third edition (1896) of his handbook, antiseptic methods were commonplace; but, needless to say, as with most of the early Listerians, he moved on toward aseptic surgery. He also presided over the Royal Academy of Medicine (1901–10), and upon retirement he was awarded an Honorary Professorship at the Faculty of Medicine of Barcelona (1922). Among his contributions to medical journalism was his coeditorship, with Santiago Ramón y Cajal, of the *Revista de Medicina y Cirugía* (1898–1920).

Bibliography

Primary: *c.* 1880. *Guía práctico para la cura de las heridas y la aplicación del método antiséptico. (Lecciones dadas en la Academia y Laboratorio de Ciencias Médicas de Cataluña)* (Barcelona); 1887. *Manual práctico de cirugía antiséptica* [2nd edn. (Barcelona), 3rd edn. 1896 (Barcelona)].

Secondary: Vázquez de Quevedo, Francisco, 2003. *Dos escuelas de cirugía: Madrid y Barcelona. Ribera i Sans y Salvador Cardenal* (Santander); Danon, Josep, 1996. 'De la antisepsia a la asepsia en la obra de Salvador Cardenal.' *Medicina e Historia*, n. 61, Tercera época; Calbet, Josep M., and Jacint Corbella, 1981. *Diccionari biogràfic de metges catalans.* (Barcelona); Corachán García, Manuel, 1928. 'El Dr. Cardenal cirujano.' *Anales de la Real Academia de Cirugía y Medicina de Barcelona* 10: 3–9.

Teresa Huguet-Termes

CARRASQUILLA, JUAN DE DIOS   (b. Bogotá, Colombia, 1 March 1833, d. Bogotá, 14 July 1908), *bacteriology*.

Carrasquilla, son of Juan Manuel Carrasquilla, a farmer and importer of European animals and agricultural machinery, attended the Universidad Central in Bogotá, graduating MD in 1852. During most of his life he was interested in scientific agriculture and natural sciences, and he published on meteorology, geology, and paleontology. As his father did before him, Carrasquilla imported cattle, seeds, and machinery and taught scientific methods applied to agriculture. Partly thanks to his agricultural experience and interest, he learned a great deal about Darwinism and in 1888 presented to a meeting of the Society of Medicine and Natural Sciences of Bogotá what is considered the first solid defense of Darwinism in Colombia, then a devoted Catholic country unwilling to accept 'foreign', unreligious ideas. As to medicine, Carrasquilla stood out as an introducer of the new microbiological theories of Robert Koch and Louis Pasteur and as an innovator of therapies based on these bacteriological methods. He was one of the first doctors ready to develop and apply medical laboratory science and to intermingle medicine and natural sciences. In nineteenth-century rural Colombia, such a mixing of occupations and interests was not common.

Carrasquilla studied the etiology of infectious diseases such as leprosy and malaria. In his work he supported the specificity of these diseases by taking a reductionist standpoint, claiming that germs were the only source of disease causation. He was also strongly committed to naturalistic interpretations of illnesses. Using Darwinian arguments, he opposed the hereditary theory of leprosy transmission. He contended that accidental or intentional changes of the individual reproducer were unable to be transmitted hereditarily. Therefore, according to Carrasquilla, leprosy could not be transmitted from parents to offspring; Hansen's bacillus was the unique cause of leprosy. In the last years of his life he modified this radical reductionism, and emphasized hygiene and public health, arguing that poverty and social misery explained the rapid spread of leprosy and other infectious diseases in Colombia.

Inspired by Richet's antisyphilitic serum, Carrasquilla developed a serum to treat leprosy that was widely used in Colombia and several Latin American countries, as well as in Algeria and South Africa. Although some patients under serotherapy seemed to have improved, the First International Leprosy Congress held in Berlin (1897) and the

Colombian National Academy of Medicine in 1899 judged that Carrasquilla's serum was not an effective treatment. Nonetheless, Carrasquilla's research contributed to current debates on immunity and to the founding of Colombia's applied scientific medicine.

Given that all attempts at inoculating Hansen's bacillus in animals and humans had failed, and that leprosy transmission was still unknown, Carrasquilla focused on studying fleas as a possible vector of leprosy. Using laborious methods, he found the leprosy bacillus in fleas' intestines and presented his theory of the transmission of leprosy by fleas at the Third Latin American Scientific Congress held in Rio de Janeiro in 1905. This hypothesis was still being debated in the early 1940s, when researchers tried to prove it, but some years later it was shown to be erroneous.

Carrasquilla's interest in leprosy went beyond research. He strongly disagreed with the official policy of mandatory segregation of leprosy patients sanctioned by the Berlin congress. He complained that the sick were treated as criminals based on the erroneous belief that leprosy was highly contagious. He advocated the creation of urban hospitals, as opposed to isolated leper colonies. These city hospitals were to be devoted to the study of the disease, good medical treatment, and research.

Bibliography

Primary: 1889. 'Disertación sobre la etiología y el contagio de la lepra.' *Revista Médica* 13(137): 441–484; 1897. 'Memoria sobre la Lepra Griega en Colombia.' *Mittheilungen und Verhandlungen der internationalen wissenschaftlichen Lepra-Conferenz zu Berlin im October 1897* vol. 1 (Berlin) pp. 122–124.

Secondary: Rico, Edmundo, 1925. 'Doctor Juan de Dios Carrasquilla.' *Repertorio de Medicina y Cirugía* 16–17(187): 304–313.

Diana Obregón

CARREL, ALEXIS (b. Sainte-Foy-Les-Lyon, near Lyon, France, 28 June 1873; d. Paris, France, 5 November 1944), *surgery, tissue culture.*

Carrel was the eldest child of devout Catholics Alexis Carrel-Billiard and Anne-Marie Ricard. He received a Jesuit education at the St Joseph's Day School in Lyon and received the degrees of LB (1890) and MD (1900) from the University of Lyon and an ScB from the University of Dijon (1891). As an intern he demonstrated remarkable skill and dexterity in operative surgery and spent two years teaching anatomy and experimental surgery while preparing to take his surgical exams. In 1901 he completed his doctoral thesis on cancer of the thyroid, but his most promising work concerned techniques for suturing blood vessels.

A few medical pioneers, including some of Carrel's teachers, experimented with suturing the walls of blood vessels but had difficulty manually stitching a small thin-walled structure while preventing blood clots and bacterial infections. Carrel developed several techniques to

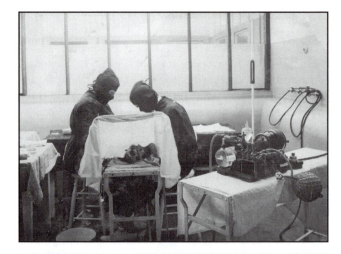

Alexis Carrel (left) and colleague operating on a dog at the Rockefeller Institute. They are wearing the black gowns and masks that Carrel favored for laboratory experiments. Courtesy of Rockefeller Archive Center.

overcome these problems. He took embroidery lessons to improve his dexterity and used exceptionally fine needles and thread coated in paraffin jelly to prevent clotting. He then conceived a method of uniting vessels end-to-end without exposing circulating blood to anything but the smooth lining of the vessel. To prevent infections, Carrel adhered to scrupulous aseptic methods, which often meant not allowing any visitors into his lab. Indeed, Carrel was quickly annoyed by interruptions and could be blunt when he felt individuals were wasting his time or contaminating his lab.

In the summer of 1903, Carrel was invited to serve as a physician on a 'sick train' making a pilgrimage to the Catholic shrine in Lourdes, France. He relished the opportunity to make objective observations on mystical occurrences but was unprepared for what he witnessed. On the train, Carrel tended to a young girl he believed to be on the verge of death. Moments after her arrival at Lourdes, however, Carrel watched as all of the girl's symptoms diminished until she was completely cured. Forever moved by what he saw, Carrel returned to Lourdes nearly every year for the rest of his life.

Upon returning to Lyon, Carrel reported the inexplicable cure to his colleagues. He stopped short of calling it a miracle but declared there were still many mental and physical processes not fully understood by the medical profession. Carrel's mystical perspective was not well received by his colleagues and his credibility was irreversibly damaged within Lyon's conservative medical community. One of Carrel's colleagues advised him not to bother trying to pass his surgical examinations, which were needed to secure a coveted hospital appointment, because he would never pass. This advice would prove prophetic.

New Beginnings in North America

After failing his surgical examination for a third and final time, Carrel left France for a fresh start in Montreal, Canada (1904). Shortly after arriving, he delivered a paper at the Second Medical Congress of the French Language of North America on blood vessel surgery. His paper was an immediate success, and within weeks Carrel was fielding job offers from several American universities.

He accepted a position at the University of Chicago, where he collaborated with Charles Guthrie, a promising young physiologist. During the twenty-two months Carrel and Guthrie worked together, they performed many groundbreaking experiments in vascular medicine and jointly wrote twenty-one papers. One of the first things they did was to perfect Carrel's triangulation technique of vascular suture, which revolutionized what was considered surgically possible. With his new suturing technique, Carrel explored the viability of reattaching body parts such as limbs, kidneys, thyroids, intestines, hearts, and lungs. Carrel succeeded in restoring blood flow to these transplanted organs in cats and dogs, but they were not always transplanted into their true anatomical position, and in most cases the animals died from infections that followed.

Carrel's growing reputation for surgical skill and daring experimentation drew the attention of several distinguished scientists, most notably Simon Flexner, director of the recently established Rockefeller Institute for Medical Research in New York City. Within weeks of their first meeting, Carrel accepted an offer from Flexner as a fellow in experimental surgery at the institute. The Rockefeller Institute provided Carrel with an ideal environment to conduct research, as he received substantial financial support and was free to run his lab without any interference.

In New York, Carrel continued his previous experiments and tested his suturing techniques on human subjects. In one procedure, Carrel gave a direct blood transfusion to a baby by attaching the child's femoral vein to the radial artery of the child's father. Experiments such as this caught the attention of journalists, who were quick to report on Carrel's seemingly bizarre experiments.

Carrel's work with tissue culture also became the subject of several sensationalized news stories that dwelled on Carrel's mystical inquiry into the immortality of organs. In 1912 he took tissue from the heart of a chicken embryo and reportedly kept it alive in a medium of chicken plasma for over three decades. The experiment was inaccurately described in the press as a growing, beating heart and was considered a monstrosity by some.

Undeniably eccentric, Carrel was also aware of the importance of a germ-free atmosphere in his lab and strongly discouraged colleagues from dropping in for casual visits. Those who did found themselves surrounded by assistants clad in black gowns and masks, who worked in rooms painted black. Dark colors were used to reduce glare in the laboratory, but some people decided it was evidence that Carrel was involved with the occult.

The Medical Celebrity

Application of Carrel's methods for human organ transplants must have seemed close at hand, because in 1912 he was awarded the Nobel Prize in Physiology or Medicine. At thirty-nine, Carrel was the youngest Nobel laureate in history and had the distinction of being the first person to be awarded the prize for research conducted in America.

While Carrel was on his annual vacation to France in the late summer of 1914, Germany declared war on France, and Carrel, still a French citizen, received mobilization orders. He was posted to a hospital in Lyon to treat war wounds, but found that there were no effective techniques for treating the massive infections found in the wounds of injured soldiers. Carrel received funding to open a hospital in Compiegne, just eight miles from the front lines, but no funds were allocated for research. Undaunted, Carrel secured a grant from the Rockefeller Foundation to fund the hospital's research laboratories and recruited the English biochemist, Henry Dakin, to develop an antiseptic solution for wound irrigation. Carrel then created a method to apply Dakin's solution, and by 1915 the Carrel-Dakin technique of wound management was in full use.

Before the war ended, Carrel returned to New York and set up a War Demonstration Hospital at the Rockefeller Institute to demonstrate battlefield surgical techniques. Nearing fifty years of age, Carrel sought a new orientation for his medical research. Surgical experiments required precise dexterity, good vision, and physical endurance, which Carrel was losing with age. Instead, he devoted his time to growing tissue cultures. Just as Carrel's suturing techniques were used by future surgeons to transplant human limbs and organs, his innovative work with tissue culture paved the way for scientists to grow viruses *in vitro* and ultimately develop vaccines. Carrel used his tissue culture techniques to grow human sarcoma cells outside of the body. For this, he was awarded the Nordhoff-Jung Cancer Prize (1931).

At the request of Charles Lindbergh, Carrel explored the possibility of creating an artificial heart. Lindbergh's sister-in-law was in dire need of heart surgery, but doctors were unable to perform the operation because it was impossible to stop the heart long enough for the operation to be completed. Lindbergh worked with Carrel to solve this problem and together they designed a glass perfusion pump that could circulate nutrient fluid around an organ. By 1935, the pump was able to keep the thyroid gland of a cat alive for eighteen days, but it was not an artificial heart as was reported in the press.

The Controversial Scientist

Carrel's experiments were frequently reported to the public with a great deal of embellishment. Stories of beating hearts in jars and whole organs grown in labs both flattered and annoyed Carrel. To set the record straight, he published *Man, the Unknown* (1935), which summarized his knowledge of both biology and humanity. The book expressed Carrel's belief that in spite of scientific and technological progress, man was still largely unknown. Carrel touched on mystical matters in the book, covering topics such as clairvoyance, mental telepathy, and faith healing. He also optimistically asserted that through selective reproduction, and rule by a spiritually minded aristocracy, mankind could banish disease, prolong life, improve the race, and reach new spiritual heights.

The book created an immediate sensation. It was translated into nineteen languages and became an international best seller. Critical readers, however, noted many unsupported generalizations and dogmatic statements that exposed Carrel's chauvinistic, racist, and elitist sentiments. The book came under increased attacks during World War II, when passages on eugenics were offered as evidence of Carrel's Nazi sympathies.

Carrel's opinions alienated many of his colleagues at the Rockefeller Institute. One such colleague was Herbert Gasser, who in 1935 replaced Carrel's friend and mentor, Simon Flexner, as the director of the institute. One of Gasser's first acts was to institute a mandatory retirement age of sixty-five for all employees. In July 1939 Carrel officially retired and his lab was closed.

Returning to France in the opening days of World War II, Carrel immediately set to work on one of his long-held ambitions, creating a think tank of experts that could formulate a science of man. Chartered by the Vichy regime in 1941, the French Foundation for the Study of Human Problems brought together biologists, physicians, philosophers, anthropologists, lawyers, architects, and economists to expound on the ideas found in *Man, the Unknown*. Although the foundation did explore aspects of eugenics and parapsychology, the primary focus of the institute was on more traditional forms of public health.

As head of the foundation, Carrel frequently dealt with the Vichy government as well as with German occupation officials. These actions, coupled with his open distrust of democracy, caused many of his contemporaries to label Carrel a Nazi collaborationist. This claim, however, has not withstood historical scrutiny. Throughout the war Carrel wrote to friends and colleagues on the flawed vision of National Socialism and frequently condemned it. He was undoubtedly an elitist who strongly believed in a well-disciplined society but was opposed to both genocide and anti-Semitism. He vehemently denied rumors that he was a Nazi collaborator or apologist, but news did not freely travel out of occupied France and his reputation never recovered.

In August 1943 Carrel suffered the first of two heart attacks that would eventually lead to his death. The second episode occurred one year later and left Carrel bedridden in his Paris apartment as France was being liberated. The new French government placed Carrel under house arrest, where, severely depressed, he died on 5 November 1944 from heart failure.

Although Carrel's politics have not stood the test of time, he was revered throughout his life as a scientist. He was honored by memberships of learned societies all over the world and received honorary doctorates from numerous universities. He was a Commander in the Legion of Honor of France and the recipient of other decorations from Spain, Serbia, Great Britain, Belgium, Sweden, and the Holy See.

Bibliography

Primary: 1935. *Man, the Unknown* (New York); 1936. (with Lindbergh, Charles A.) *The Culture of Organs* (New York); 1950. *The Voyage to Lourdes* (New York); 1953. *Reflections on Life* (Portland).

Secondary: Le Voy, David, 1996. *The Perfectibility of Man* (Rockville, MD); Malinin, Theodore, 1979. *Surgery and Life: The Extraordinary Career of Alexis Carrel* (New York); Edwards, Peter D., and Charles Lindbergh, 1974. *Alexis Carrel: Visionary Surgeon* (Springfield, IL); Durkin, Joseph T., 1965. *Hope for Our Time: Alexis Carrel on Man and Society* (New York); *DSB*; *DAMB*.

Patrick Henry Shea

CARRILLO, RAMÓN (b. Santiago del Estero, Argentina, 7 March 1906; d. Belém do Pará, Brazil, 20 December 1956), *neurosurgery, public health*.

Educational Background

Carrillo was the oldest son of journalist and later conservative representative Ramón Carrillo and his wife, María Salomé Gómez Carrillo. He attended elementary and secondary school in his home province and then moved to Buenos Aires to study at the School of Medical Sciences of the University of Buenos Aires. He began his medical coursework in 1924.

Under the supervision of Manuel Balado, Carrillo used iodized oil injections to detect brain lesions during his last years of graduate study. Thanks to this work he established the 'Carrillo sign', a diagnostic method to establish deviations of the aqueduct of Sylvius in tumors of the cerebellopontine angle. This study was the basis of his 1937 doctoral thesis, which received the prestigious Medical School's Award and an honorable mention at the National Science Award competition, organized by the National Science Academy.

Between 1927 and 1929, while he was still a medical student, Carrillo published a series of articles on neurological and political issues in *Revista del Círculo Médico Argentino y Centro de Estudiantes de Medicina*. The medical magazine published research conducted by advanced students and political commentaries on sociomedical issues. Carrillo's role, first as a contributor and later as magazine editor (from 1930), is evidence on the one hand, of his interest in transmitting knowledge and, on the other, of his desire to gain legitimacy among his peers.

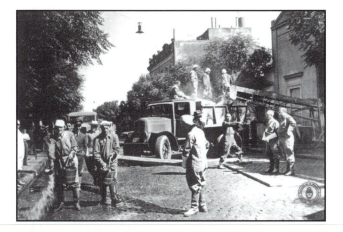

Ramón Carrillo (far right) supervising the disinfection crew of the Argentinian Public Heath Secretariat, December, 1946. Photograph, courtesy Departamento Documentos Fotográficos, Archivo General de la Nación, Argentina.

In 1930 the young Carrillo won a scholarship for top-score students from the University of Buenos Aires to pursue postgraduate studies in Europe. For two years, he was an assistant at the Brain Anatomy Laboratory and at the Histology Laboratory at Amsterdam University. In 1932 he was the Argentine representative at the First International Congress on Neurology, which took place in Bern, Switzerland. Throughout 1933 he continued his training first in Berlin, at the *Hirnforschung Institut*, and then in Paris, where he visited several research centers. During that period, he devoted his attention to a series of issues such as the examination of brain sclerosis, experimental polyneuritis, and histological staining methods in neurology.

Upon returning to Buenos Aires in 1933, Carrillo was appointed head of the Neuropathology Laboratory at the Instituto de Clínica Quirúrgica, sponsored by the Hospital de Clínicas. In 1939 he received a proposal from the Ministry of War to organize the Army's Neurosurgery Service at Hospital Militar Central. Carrillo noticed the appalling sanitary conditions of the young men joining the military service. He also elaborated a proposal focused on the need to improve the health of Argentineans, considering it a *sine qua non* for economic and military development. Carrillo expressed these concerns in a paper presented at the First Population Congress, held in Buenos Aires in 1940.

Until 1942 Carrillo was the assistant professor of the chair of Neurosurgery at the School of Medical Sciences at the University of Buenos Aires. In that year he won the contest for the position of associate professor of the chair and later, after the death of the incumbent, Manuel Balado, he was appointed to a prestigious full-professorship position. From October to December 1945, he was interim president of the School of Medical Sciences at the University of Buenos Aires. Short as his term of office was, it allowed him to strengthen his bonds with rising nationalistic political sectors at the university. Carrillo's liaison with both the military and nationalistic political groups at the university led him to collaborate in Colonel Juan Domingo Perón's electoral campaign.

Experience in Public Health

In February 1946 Perón was elected president of Argentina. In 1951 he was re-elected, and he kept his post until 1955, when he was overthrown by a military coup. Many of the health transformations seen in Argentina during those years were orchestrated by Ramón Carrillo. In May 1946 President-elect Perón appointed Carrillo to the newly created Public Health Secretariat, reporting directly to the president. The new organization replaced the National Public Health Board, an organization under the supervision of the Ministry of the Interior. The newly appointed Secretary held his position until March 1949, when he managed to have the Secretariat promoted to the Ministry of Public Health. In sum, Carrillo was the head—a powerful head—of the Argentinean health system between 1946 and 1954. The changes in the institutional fabric of the state that he led produced more autonomy, more staff, and increased budgets for national public services.

One of the main achievements of Carrillo's outstanding administration was increasing the number of beds available in hospitals and creating new health centers (he doubled the health care services in Argentina). This outcome benefited mainly the low-income sectors of society. As head of the Argentinean health system, Carrillo organized the 'First Sanitary Caravan', made up of sixty war trucks that departed from Buenos Aires and visited major provinces in the country carrying supplies to inaugurate new hospitals.

Most important among Carrillo's accomplishments was the creation of general hospitals, which offered care for several ailments and also featured maternity wards and pediatric services. Additionally, hospitals for specific conditions or that specialized in different stages of disease were built, and ambulatory health centers and frontier checkpoints were created.

According to Carrillo, hospitals were supposed to provide not only medical attention but also sanitary information to the community. Thus, free books were distributed, and short films, advertisements, and radio announcements were broadcast from medical establishments. Educational materials were also distributed in factories, schools, and military units. Medical doctors were in charge of the distribution and use of these materials. Additionally, campaigns were organized to control endemic diseases, such as the one against malaria that took place between 1947 and 1949 and was led by Carlos Alvarado, who with a combination of several techniques, succeeded in controlling the disease. A key technological innovation, DDT, was instrumental in achieving the control of malaria in only two years. Another important campaign was the Comprehensive Cleanup of the Patagonia, a remote region in Southern Argentina that had been formerly neglected by the state. The campaign aimed at preventing smallpox, diphtheria, typhoid fever, and goiter. In addition, rural dwellings were disinfected in the year 1948.

Another important preventive measure taken during Carrillo's administration was disseminating 'good advice' on nutrition practices. Carrillo thought it was essential for families to include more milk, fruit, and vegetables in their diets. According to him, a lack of these elements contributed to the decay of a people's biological potential. Thus, Carrillo increased school food subsidies and supported broadcast radio messages that carried healthy nourishing recipes. Those measures gave rise to some protests, such as one by the Argentine Women's Association, a pro-communism group, which pointed out that the advice was useless given the constant price increases of staple diet products.

Another goal of the government was to supply locally produced medicines and x-ray film. For penicillin-derived medicines, official authorization was granted to the American laboratories *Squibb and Sons* to produce them locally. For other frequently used medicines, the State Medical Specialties agency (EMESTA in Spanish), under the supervision of the health sector, was created. Furthermore, the Buenos Aires-based Malbrán Bacteriological Institute increased and diversified its production of serums, vaccines, drugs, and medicines. A board was appointed to study the country's technical capability to produce x-ray films. However, local production was not possible because of budgetary problems.

An important development in Argentina during the first four decades of the twentieth century was that major political and social players insisted on the need for more up-to-date statistical health records and an improved civil registration system. They thought that the state needed to update old practices in these areas by the systematic study of the role played by both public health interventions and disease in population growth. In 1947 Carrillo set up an agency in the Health Secretariat to deal with these issues. As a result, a leprosy census in Buenos Aires and other population activities took place. In addition, inspired by these activities, Argentina's first Health Census was conducted some years later (1954). This valuable quantitative record provided crucial information on population and medical resources in both the capital city and the provinces.

It is important to underscore that although health services increased and several health indicators improved in Argentina under Carrillo's leadership, those changes were not uniform across the country because many provinces lagged behind the capital city. As well, an uneven distribution of doctors and nurses, which concentrated their numbers in Buenos Aires, and insufficient sophisticated technical resources, especially unavailable in the provinces, made it difficult to take good care of complex or chronic cases. This was apparent during the poliomyelitis outbreak in the 1950s because medical care required long and difficult treatments based on modern technology not available then in Argentina.

By the early 1950s the health budget began to be cut. One of the reasons for this reduction was a shift in the political priorities and economic policy of the Peronist administration, which abandoned a redistributive policy to embrace economic adjustment policies and administrative rationalization. Furthermore, the Eva Perón Foundation's attempt to monopolize and set priorities in terms of health projects had an impact on the slowdown of investments by the Health Ministry.

As a result of the dispute over limited economic resources, in July 1954 Carrillo resigned. Formally his reasons for leaving the post included his poor health (he was afflicted by malignant hypertension) and the radicalization of the political conflict between Perón and the Catholic sectors. Always a conservative and a follower of the Catholic Church, Carrillo expressed his discontent with certain governmental proposals leading to the undermining of the power of the Church in some areas of Argentina.

In October 1954 Carrillo traveled to New York, where he visited research centers, sought treatment for his disease, and kept up to date regarding Argentine events (in 1955 Perón was overthrown). Unable to return to his home country due to the political persecution of anyone considered a follower of the deposed president, Carrillo obtained a job as a doctor in an American mining company located in the Brazilian city of Belém Do Pará. In this location, he combined his medical practice with lecturing. He died of a stroke on 28 November 1956.

In sum, thanks to Carrillo's remarkable leadership and contributions, Argentina's health policy experienced a substantial improvement from 1946 to 1954. Free health care, the infrastructure of public medical establishments, and broad educational health campaigns in the community were enhanced, and concern over population care issues deepened, benefiting a greater number of people who previously had only intermittent contact with health systems. In addition, Carrillo established resources for food control, improved nutrition and the local production and pricing of medicines and artificial milk. Consequently, Ramón Carrillo is remembered in Argentina as a national symbol of active state intervention in health issues.

Bibliography

Primary: 1937. *Yodoventriculografía* (Buenos Aires); 1951. *Contribuciones al conocimiento sanitario* (Buenos Aires); 1974. *Teoría del hospital* (Buenos Aires); 1975. *Planes de salud pública, 1952–1958 de Ramón Carrillo* (Buenos Aires).

Secondary: Ramacciotti, Karina, 2004. 'Las tensiones en la política sanitaria de Ramón Carrillo' in Berrotarán, Patricia, et al., eds., *Sueños de Bienestar en la nueva Argentina: estado y política pública durante el peronismo, 1946–1955.* (Buenos Aires) pp. 229–268; Torre, Juan Carlos, and Elisa Partoriza, 2002. 'La democratización del bienestar' in Juan Carlos Torre, ed., *Los años Peronistas, 1943–1955* (Buenos Aires) pp. 257–313; Ramacciotti, Karina, and Alfredo Kohn Loncarica, 2001. 'Una aproximación a las conexiones ideológicas del primer Ministro de salud de la Argentina (1929–1946)' *Horizontes* 21: 63–75.

Karina Ramacciotti

CARRIÓN, DANIEL ALCIDES   (b. Cerro de Pasco, Peru, 13 August 1857; d. Lima, Peru, 5 October 1885), *self-experimentation, verruga peruana.*

Carrión, son of the physician Baltazar Carrión and Dolores García, attended the prestigious school of Nuestra Señora de Guadalupe, the Faculty of Natural Sciences and the Faculty of Medicine of the University of San Marcos in Lima. Carrión's medical studies occurred during the War of the Pacific between Peru, Bolivia, and Chile (1879–83). This war led to Chilean military occupation of an important part of the Peruvian territory, including the country's capital, Lima, where Carrión lived. During the military occupation the medical community was mobilized for war emergencies and the Medical Faculty premises transformed into military barracks.

Immediately after the war, between 1883 and 1885, Carrión devoted himself to the clinical study of *verruga peruana*, a disease known since pre-Hispanic times, considered unique to the Peruvian Andean valleys, which was recognized by the protuberant warts that appeared on the skin. When Carrión initiated his studies, several aspects of the etiology of *verruga peruana* were still unknown. There was also debate about the relationship between this disease and Oroya fever. The latter was an illness that caused the death of hundreds of railway workers during the construction of the Lima–La Oroya Andean railway in 1870. Carrión's studies were partly motivated by nationalism (after the country's defeat in the War of the Pacific). For instance, he was aware of the studies on *verruga peruana* being performed by the Chilean physician Vicente Izquierdo.

In 1885 the Academia Libre de Medicina (a professional medical society formed by a group of physicians from San Marcos University who resisted the attempts made by the government to interfere with the autonomy of the Medical School) called for a contest to distinguish the best work on the etiology, pathology, and geographical distribution of *verruga peruana*. Carrión decided to enter the contest. In order to better understand the clinical aspects of the disease, Carrión also decided to 'self-experiment' with the disease. He admitted himself into Dos de Mayo Hospital and, with the assistance of a local practitioner, was inoculated with the blood of a hospital patient (27 August 1885). He also started a diary detailing his pre-eruptive symptoms. Carrión's case is also interesting because we find in his work a combination of ideas on miasmatic emanation and bacteriology. Although he was convinced that the experiment would follow a benign development, he died forty days after the inoculation. Before his death, however, he claimed that *verruga peruana* and Oroya fever had the same etiological origin. Carrión also demonstrated that the disease could be inoculated and transmitted from one person to another. Carrión's was the first case of self-experimentation in Peru.

Initially, authorities of the Medical Faculty of San Marcos University denounced self-experimentation as an unscientific

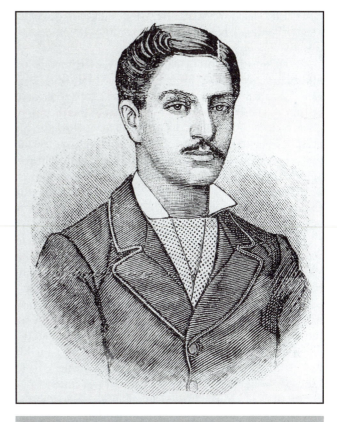

Daniel Carrión, a student at Lima, who died while studying Oroya fever in Peru and had Carrión's disease named after him. Engraving, Wellcome Library, London.

procedure, portrayed Carrión as a naïve student, and condemned his death as a disgrace to the medical community. However, his fellow students and the members of the Academia Libre de Medicina praised the courage of the medical student and launched a vigorous campaign portraying Carrión as a heroic scientist. Carrión's death date (5 October 1885) was established as the national medical day, and *verruga peruana* and the Oroya fever were unified in a single entity, renamed Carrión's disease. Carrión's experience helped legitimate the emergent Peruvian medical culture. In 1909 the Peruvian Alberto Barton discovered the causal agent of the disease afterward named *Bartonella bacilliformis*. In the 1920s Hideyo Noguchi confirmed the finding and validated Carrión's self experiment.

Bibliography

Primary: 1886. *La verruga peruana y Daniel A. Carrión* (Lima) (published posthumously).

Secondary: Cueto, Marcos, 1996. 'Tropical Medicine and Bacteriology in Boston and Peru: Studies of Carrión's Disease in the early Twentieth Century' *Medical History* 40(3): 344–364; Odriozola, Ernesto, 1898. *La maladie de Carrion; ou, la verruga péruvienne* (Paris).

Jorge Lossio

CARTER, HENRY VANDYKE (b. Hull, England, 22 May 1831; d. Scarborough, England, 4 May 1897), *pathology, epidemiology, leprology.*

Carter was the son of Henry Barlow Carter; there is no information regarding his mother. His brother, Joseph Newington Carter, followed in his father's footsteps as an artist, and Henry also showed some talent in this direction, assisting in the illustration of Gray's *Anatomy.* However, his passion from an early age was for science and, after leaving grammar school in Hull, he went on to study medicine at St George's Hospital, London. In 1852 Carter was admitted MRCS and LSA; four years later he graduated MD from the University of London and joined the Indian Medical Service (IMS) as an assistant surgeon in 1858.

Carter took the opportunity of service in India to actively pursue his scientific interests and he was soon appointed professor of anatomy and physiology at Grant Medical College, Bombay, of which he later became principal. From 1876 to 1880 he was engaged in research into 'famine' or 'spirillum fever', a disease common among those who fled famine in the Deccan. Carter found that the organism was similar to that causing relapsing fever and his work won him the BMA's Stewart Pathological Prize in 1882. The other disease with which Carter was closely associated was leprosy. His interest in the disease began in the 1860s, shortly after his arrival in India. His clinical and post-mortem observations at the Native Hospital in Bombay were stimulated by the work of Daniel C. Danielssen (1815–94) and Wilhelm Boeck (1808–75) in Norway, who had examined the anatomical characteristics of the disease. The results of his study of more than one hundred patients were published in the *Transactions of the Medical and Physical Society of Bombay* (1863).

His work on leprosy and his distinction as a scientist made Carter the obvious candidate for a fact-finding visit to Norway, which he conducted in 1873 at the behest of the government of India. The aim of the visit was to ascertain whether Norwegian leprosy was the same as that in India. Carter concluded that the disease was the same and, in his book *On Leprosy and Elephantiasis* (1874), he suggested that leprosy could be controlled in India through the establishment of leper asylums like those in Norway. At this point, Carter believed that leprosy was primarily a hereditary disease and that it could be extinguished only through segregation of the sexes in institutions.

But Carter was soon to change his mind about the cause of leprosy. The gradual acceptance of Norwegian G. H. A. Hansen's (1841–1912) claim to have discovered the bacterium causing leprosy (1873) led Carter to emphasize the role of contagion over that of heredity. This served only to strengthen Carter's commitment to asylums as a means of preventing the spread of leprosy and, in league with other Europeans and Indians, he also persuaded the Bombay government to pass by-laws to prevent the congregation of lepers begging for alms.

Carter's role as a scientist and public health activist led to his being promoted to the rank of deputy surgeon-general in the IMS. He was also appointed honorary surgeon to Queen Victoria. After leaving India, he retired to the East Riding of Yorkshire, where he lived in some comfort until his death.

Bibliography

Primary: 1863. 'On the symptoms and morbid anatomy of leprosy, with remarks.' *Transactions of the Medical and Physical Society of Bombay* 8: 1–105; 1874. *On Leprosy and Elephantiasis* (London).

Secondary: Robertson, Jo, 2003. 'Leprosy and the Elusive *M. leprae*: Colonial and Imperial Medical Exchanges in the Nineteenth Century.' *Manguinhos* 10(1): 13–40; Buckingham, Jane, 2002. *Leprosy in Colonial South India: Medicine and Confinement* (Basingstoke); Kakar, Sanjiv, 1996. 'Leprosy in British India, 1860–1940: Colonial Politics and Missionary Medicine.' *Medical History* 40: 215–230; [Obituary], 1897. *British Medical Journal* i: 1256–1257; *Oxford DNB.*

Mark Harrison

CASAL JULIÁN, GASPAR (b. Gerona, Spain, 31 December 1680; d. Madrid, Spain, 10 August 1759), *medicine, natural history.*

Casal is a fine example of the accomplishments of the revival of the Hippocratic tradition and clinical empiricism in late seventeenth- and eighteenth-century Spain. He successfully practiced medicine in different regions of Spain, particularly in Asturia in northern Spain, and in Madrid. He contributed to medical geography with a natural and medical history of Asturia and to nosography with the first documented clinical description of pellagra (1735).

The son of Federico Casal y Dajón, a Second Lieutenant of the Cavalry of probable Italian origin and Magdalena Julián from Utrilla in Castile, Casal spent the first third of his life in various places in the center and north of Castile. Between 1706 and 1712, he learned natural history, botany, and chemistry in apprenticeship to and in collaboration with Juan Manuel Rodríguez de Luna, former apothecary of Pope Innocent XI. In 1709 he entered the University of Sigüenza, a minor Spanish university, where he earned his BA (1713). He likely completed his studies of medicine at this university but there is no documentary evidence as to where he gained his MD and PhD.

Casal moved to Madrid in 1713, where he practiced until he left for Oviedo, Asturia, in 1717. Although he complained of difficulties in adapting to the Madrid climate, his leaving may have been prompted by accusations laid by the Inquisition against his first wife, María Ruiz, which ended in her conviction and the public declaration of her 'infamy'. His protector, the Duke of Parque, secured his appointment as physician of the city of Oviedo (1720), and from 1729 to 1751 he served as physician of the Oviedo Cathedral Council. Casal had four children by his first marriage, and after he was widowed he married (1730) María Rodríguez Fernández, with whom he also had four children.

In 1751, probably thanks to the influence of his friend Benito Jerónimo Feijóo, professor at the University of Oviedo and one of the most prestigious Spanish intellectuals of his time, Casal was called to Madrid to attend to the wife of King Ferdinand VI. In August of the same year he was named Royal Physician and in 1752 was designated member of the Royal Academy of Medicine of Madrid and member of the Castilian Tribunal of the *Protomedicato*, which controlled access to the medical profession.

All of his writings during his time in Asturia were compiled and posthumously published by his friend and Royal Physician Juan José García Sevillano in 1762 with the title of 'Medical and Natural History of the Principality of Asturia'. Among the texts, written in Spanish and Latin, stand out a conventional medical topography of Asturia (*Historia phisico-médica . . .*), a series of case reports that bear witness to his rigorous adherence to clinical empiricism (*Brevissimo tratado . . .*), and various writings on 'epidemic constitutions'. Also included is a clinical description of diseases endemic to the region (*Historia affectionum . . .*) including pellagra, called *mal de la rosa* in Asturia after the characteristic pink skin lesion. Consistent with his environmental approach, Casal attributed the origin of this disease of Asturian peasants to the quality of their food and to particular atmospheric influences in the area.

Part of his international recognition stems from his friendship with the French physician François Thiéry, whom he met in Madrid in 1755. Thiéry underlined the primary role of Casal in the description of pellagra in two widely read reports (1755 and 1791).

Bibliography

Primary: 1762. *Historia Natural y Medica del Principado de Asturias* (Madrid).

Secondary: García Guerra, Delfín, and Víctor Álvarez Antuña, 1993. *Lepra Asturiensis. La contribución asturiana en la historia de la pelagra (siglos XVIII-XIX)* (Madrid); López Piñero, José M. et al., 1983. *Diccionario histórico de la Ciencia moderna en España* (Barcelona); Major, Ralph, 1944. 'Don Gaspar Casal, François Thiéry and Pellagra.' *Bulletin of the History of Medicine* 16: 351–361.

Alfredo Menéndez

CELLI, ANGELO (b. Cagli, Italy, 25 March 1857; d. Monza, Italy, 2 November 1914), *medicine, parasitology, hygiene, social medicine.*

Born in the small town of Cagli, near Urbino, the son of Cristoforo, a farmer, and Teresa Amatori, Celli studied medicine at the University of Rome, receiving his MD in 1883. Immediately after his degree, Celli started collaborating with Ettore Marchiafava (1847–1916) on the parasites of the blood in intermittent fevers. Alphonse Laveran's observations of the parasitic forms in malarial cases (1880–81) were received with skepticism, and the French physician went to Rome to show his findings to Marchiafava and Celli. The Italian pathologists, after an initial period of skepticism and thanks to their powerful oil immersion microscopes, confirmed Laveran's ideas, observing in 1883 the active amoeboid ring in unstained blood and giving to the parasites the name *Plasmodium*. Over the same period, Marchiafava and Celli discovered the etiology of cerebrospinal meningitis, isolating the causal microorganism (*Micrococcus meningitides*) later isolated also by A. Weichselbaum (1887).

In 1886 Celli obtained his qualification (*libero docente*) and was named extraordinary professor of hygiene at the University of Palermo, where he founded an anti-rabies institute. However, a year later he was called back to Rome to the chair of experimental hygiene. In 1889 he founded a new journal, *Annali di igiene*.

In this period Celli extended his research on malaria, with epidemiological and environmental analyses, producing regular reports that in the following years became the main source of information about malaria in Italy. He studied other hygienic problems, such as the transmission of infectious diseases by insects, the quality of water, and the sanitation of houses. He became particularly interested in Texas fever, the malaria of cattle (babesiasis). He established an experimental field station in the Roman Campagna, and he was able to confirm Theobald Smith (1859–1934) and F. L. Kilborne's (1858–1936) discovery that the disease was spread by ticks and showed how to prevent the disease by keeping cattle inside and dipping them in chemical solutions to kill the ticks.

In 1892 he was elected to the Italian Parliament, and until his death he combined scientific research with social and political action. Convinced of the relevance of education to hygiene, with his wife Anna Frantzel and other Italian intellectuals he created rural schools in the Roman Campagna. As a deputy he proposed new laws against children's work and for an amelioration of working conditions, especially to prevent accidents. Together with the deputies Giustino Fortunato and Leopoldo Franchetti, Celli created the Italian Society for the Study of Malaria in 1898, which played a fundamental role in the approval of legislation for the distribution of quinine against malaria (*Chinino di Stato*) in the following years. The first law was approved in 1900, and the final version of 1904 provided for the free distribution of quinine in the whole national territory.

The years that followed Ronald Ross and Giovanni Battista Grassi's demonstration that Anopheles mosquitoes transmitted malaria saw the development of intense research on malaria epidemiology and prevention. Many different methods were proposed for the 'war on malaria' (Celli, 1906). Celli established in 1899 an experimental station at the Cervelletta, an estate near Rome, getting excellent results with mechanical protection and the use of quinine. However, he became convinced that 'with so many extensive marshes and so much intensive culture, one cannot succeed, save in exceptional cases and by long and assiduous work, in destroying malaria by means of the destruction of mosquitoes' (1908). He suggested, therefore, the extensive use of prophylactic quinine. According to him, 'with malaria, prevention was better than suppression; and the remedy itself, was easy to handle . . . the daily use of quinine' (1912).

Celli did not consider malaria merely a medical problem and its control a technological challenge. He saw malaria as closely linked to underdevelopment and emphasized the long-term need for improved living standards for the population. In his posthumous *History of Malaria in the Roman Campaign* (1925) he showed with detailed epidemiological and socioeconomic analyses the historical connection between malaria and underdevelopment.

Bibliography

Primary: 1883. (with Marchiafava, E.) 'Sulle alterazioni dei globuli rossi nella infezione della malaria e sulla genesi della melanemia.' *Mem. R. Acad. Lincei* 18: 381–401 (English trans, 1888); 1889. (with Guarnieri, G.) 'Sull'etiologia dell'infezione malarica' *Ann. Ig. Sperim.* 1: 109–134; 1899. *La malaria secondo le nuove ricerche* (Rome) (English trans. 1900. *Malaria according to the new researches* (London) with a preface by P. Manson); 1903. *La società per gli studi della malaria e la campagna antimalarica in Italia (1898–1902)* (Rome); 1913. 'The restriction of Malaria in Italy' in *Transactions of the XVth International Congress on Hygiene and Demography* (Washington, DC, September 23–28, 1912) (Washington, DC) pp. 1–15; 1925. *Storia della malaria nell'Agro Romano* (Rome) [English trans. 1933. *The History of Malaria in the Roman Campagna from Ancient Times* (London)].

Secondary: Snowdon, F., 2006. *The Conquest of Malaria: Italy, 1900–1962* (New Haven and London); Orazi, S., 1993. *Angelo Celli* (Rome); Berlinguer, G., 1957. 'L'opera medica e sociale di Angelo Celli nel centenario della nascita (1857–1914).' *Difesa sociale* 2: 3–32; D'Urso, G., 1925. *La lotta contro la malaria. L'opera di Angelo Celli* (Melfi); Marchiafava, E., 1915. 'La vita e l'opera di Angelo Celli.' *Nuova Antologia* 50: 3–16.

Bernardino Fantini

CELSUS, AULUS CORNELIUS (fl. *c.* 14–37), *history of medicine, medicine, surgery.*

There is little biographical information on Celsus, and his dates are not known, but he was active in the time of Tiberius. It is unlikely that he was a doctor; such an occupation would not have been considered fitting for a freeborn Roman of his class. Pliny the Elder did not refer to him as a *medicus*, although this by itself is not convincing. The first-century rhetorician Quintillian praised Celsus for his knowledge of agriculture, medicine, rhetoric, and warfare. There was nothing to prevent an educated Roman from compiling useful medical data; such information was a matter of practical concern.

De Medicina [On Medicine] is all that survives of a sixpart work that discussed agriculture, military matters, philosophy, rhetoric, and jurisprudence. It began with an introductory preface, in which Celsus provided an account of the history of medicine. Celsus noted that, while medicine did not originate in Greece, it was cultivated more assiduously there than in other nations. The medical art was complex (*multiplex*), made so by the practices of indolence and luxury, an affliction that first appeared in Greece. Celsus thus reflected a Roman mindset, albeit one not as dismissive as that of Pliny the Elder. Celsus praised Hippocrates, stating that it was he who separated medicine from natural philosophy. After him, Diocles of Carystus, Praxagoras, Chrysippus, Herophilus, and Erasistratus furthered the medical art. It was during this period, according to Celsus, that medicine was divided into healing by diet, drugs, and surgery. Further divisions resulted in the establishment of medical sects such as the Dogmatists, Empiricists, and Methodists. Celsus is also a key source on the practice of human dissection and vivisection performed by Herophilus and Erasistratus in third-century BCE Alexandria.

De Medicina consisted of eight books. Book I discussed matters that may keep a person in health (*sanus homo*), comprising an individual's constitution, diet, exercise, bathing, purgation, and the effects of the environment. The account of the seasons and their effects was continued in Book II, which also discussed the symptoms and signs of disease in general and specific terms. Acute and chronic diseases that affect the entire body were examined in Book III, and those that affect specific parts were dealt with in Book IV, which also provided an anatomical survey of the body before the diseases of specific organs and regions were discussed. Among others, Celsus gave accounts of what are recognized as facial neuralgia, tetanus, the effects of renal calculi, osteoarthritis of the hip, asthma, pneumonia, and the common cold. Book V listed over 300 pharmaceuticals and some of their applications in treating the body as a whole. The treatment of specific parts of the body was the subject of Book VI, while Books VII and VIII offered one of the most impressive accounts of the instruments and techniques of surgical practice (including orthopedics) that have survived from antiquity. Some of the treatments, especially concerning wound repair of defects, amputation, and cataract, still impress.

It has been said that what Cicero did for philosophy Celsus rendered in the service of medicine, earning him the epithet *Cicero medicus*. Apart from its medical and surgical content, Celsus's work is an important source for otherwise lost medical authors and practices. From 1478, when *De Medicina* was recovered and published, Celsus has had an admirable reputation and may be appreciated on many levels, not the least of which are the elegance of his prose and the insights he provides into the materials and practices of medicine in early imperial Rome.

Bibliography

Primary: Marx, Friderick, 1915. *A. Cornelii Celsi quae supersunt.* Corpus Medicorum Latinorum 1 (Leipzig and Berlin); Spencer, Walter, 1935–38. *Celsus. De Medicina*, with an English translation, 3 vols. (London and Cambridge, MA).

Secondary: Von Staden, Heinrich, 1999. 'Celsus as Historian?' in van der Eijk, Philip, ed., *Ancient Histories of Medicine. Essays in Medical Doxography and Historiography in Classical Antiquity* (Leiden) pp. 251–294; Spivack, Betty, 1991. 'A.C. Celsus: Roman Medicus.' *Journal of the History of Medicine and Allied Sciences* 46: 143–157; *DSB*.

Julius Rocca

CERLETTI, UGO   (b. Conegliano Veneto, Treviso, Italy, 26 September 1877; d. Rome, Italy, 25 July 1963), *psychiatry, neurology.*

The son of a vintner, Cerletti enrolled in the Faculty of Medicine of Turin University in 1896, transferring in 1898 to Rome to work as a clinical clerk in the Psychiatric Clinic. He graduated in 1901 with a thesis on cerebral lesions. As a student, he traveled to Germany and there became convinced of the importance of close links between clinical practice and neuropathological research at the laboratory bench. In Heidelberg, under the guidance of Franz Nissl, he studied the pathological anatomy of neurosyphilis ('progressive paralysis'). Several years later, in 1905–07, he published the findings of his research, distancing himself from Nissl's interpretation and arguing correctly that the cause of the disorder was infectious. He worked briefly in the laboratory of Giovanni Mingazzini and then became an assistant in the Psychiatric Clinic directed by the neurologist Ezio Sciamanna. Here Cerletti founded the laboratory of the pathology of the nervous system that he directed until 1919. In these years he often traveled to Heidelberg, then to Munich, to work in the clinic of Emil Kraepelin, in collaboration with Nissl and Alois Alzheimer. In 1906 Augusto Tamburini became professor of psychiatry in Rome, and Cerletti worked closely with both Sciamanna and Tamburini. Together with colleagues Paolo Pini and Gaetano Perusini, Cerletti also founded an institute for neuropathological research linked to the Mombello psychiatric hospital near Milan; he directed this from the end of World War I until becoming professor in 1925 at the University of Bari and founder of the Clinic of Nervous and Mental Diseases there. In 1928 he transferred to the University of Genoa, where he succeeded Enrico Morselli, devoting himself to the study of epilepsy. Finally, in 1935 he was called to Rome as director of the Psychiatric Clinic ('Clinic of Nervous and Mental Diseases').

Cerletti became interested in the new insulin and metrazol (pentamethylenetetrazole) shock therapies being intro-duced in the 1930s by Manfred Sakel and Ladislaus von Meduna. He set to work with his keen young assistants (who had already visited Sakel in Vienna): Ferdinando Accornero, who studied insulin coma; Lamberto Longhi, who was assigned to metrazol; and Lucio Bini, whose task was to determine if the canine experiments with electric current that Cerletti had conducted in Genoa could be applied in medical therapeutics as a more efficient way of inducing convulsions than metrazol. At a conference organized by Max Müller in 1937 at the Swiss cantonal psychiatric hospital in Münsingen on new treatments in schizophrenia, Bini presented a paper on the group's canine experiments, mentioning that the technique might also be applied to humans: the proposal elicited no reaction.

After learning that electric shocks were used at the municipal slaughterhouse in Rome to obtund the pigs before dispatching them, Cerletti and his assistants decided to proceed to clinical trials of 'electroshock' at the Clinic. The first patient was treated on 18 April 1938, a thirty-nine-year-old man from Milan, who was found wandering about the railway station in Rome hallucinating. After approximately eleven electroshock (ECT) treatments in one month, the patient was discharged in good condition and enthusiastic about his recovery, returning home to work—three months later his wife complained that his symptoms were recurring. ECT was not a cure for schizophrenia or melancholic depression, although it did relieve these and other disorders. Cerletti considered it superior to insulin coma and cardiazol (metrazol) convulsions, because it was more humane (the patients were immediately unconscious), because it did not cause cardiovascular side effects, and because it could be more economically administered. Thus in May 1938 he presented ECT at the Academy of Medicine in Rome. Cerletti rejected Sakel's and Meduna's explanations of the mechanism of action, and proposed convulsive therapy as a less invasive alternative to 'prefrontal leucotomy' (lobotomy) introduced by Egas Moniz and practiced at various Italian sites. Cerletti believed that electroshock opened new avenues in the understanding of psychiatric illness. Yet many of his research projects collided with the difficult conditions of scientific research in Italy, aggravated by the war.

In 1950 Cerletti participated in the World Congress of Psychiatry in Paris, the first of such congresses, where he gave voice to the hope that ECT might be surpassed by a pharmacological treatment based on the same cerebral effects. In his long activity as a psychiatrist and neurologist, he published 113 original papers on a range of subjects from the pathology of senile plaques in Alzheimer's disease to the structure of neuroglia, the blood-brain barrier, and neurosyphilis. In September 1953 he received the gold medal in recognition of his contributions to public health. The Cerletti papers have been deposited at the Kansas State Historical Society in Topeka, Kansas.

Bibliography

Primary: 1940. 'L'elettroshock.' *Rivista sperimentale di freniatria* 18: 209–310; 1954. 'Electroshock Therapy.' *Journal of Clinical and Experimental Psychopathology* 15: 191–217.

Secondary: Shorter, Edward, and David Healy, 2006. *A History of Shock Therapy* (forthcoming); Passione, Roberta, 2004. 'Italian Psychiatry in International Context: Ugo Cerletti and the Case of Electroshock.' *History of Psychiatry* 15: 83–104.

Patrizia Guarnieri

CESALPINO, ANDREA (b. Arezzo, Italy, *c.* 1524–1525; d. Rome, Italy, 15 March 1603), *medicine, botany.*

Andrea Cesalpino was the first-born son of Giovanni Cesalpino, a mason originally from Lombardy, and Giovanna de Bianchi. He began his education in Arezzo, and then in about 1544, he went to Pisa to study medicine. Among his teachers were the anatomist Realdo Colombo (*c.* 1510–59), the botanist Luca Ghini (*c.* 1490–1556), and the physician Guido Guidi (1509–69), and Simone Porzio tutored him in Peripatetic philosophy; moreover it seems that while he was at Pisa he attended the anatomical demonstrations and lectures held by Andreas Vesalius (1514–64) in January and February 1544. After being awarded his degree in medicine on 20 March 1551 Cesalpino stayed in Pisa, where in 1555 he was nominated prefect of the botanical garden and lecturer in the simples (medicinal herbs), soon gaining renown not only as a scholar of botany and the simples but also as a much sought-after and highly esteemed physician. At Pisa his students included the gifted botanist Michele Mercati (1541–93) and probably Galileo Galilei (1564–1642) himself. In 1569, following a rather uncertain period in his biography from 1558–63 (when, it is said he was forced to emigrate to Germany following an alleged crime) he obtained the first chair of practical medicine, which he occupied without interruption until 1592. The distinctive features of his scientific activity that clearly distinguished him from the other physicians and naturalists of his time were a decisive experimental vocation that did not clash with his explicit loyalty to the Peripatetic tradition, the sense of a full and total unity in the cosmic order, and an interest in logical instruments and methods that allowed one to go from the particular data of the experience to the formulation of general principles and rules.

During his sojourn in Pisa, Cesalpino published some of his most important works, such as his *Quaestiones peripateticae* (1571), *Daemonum investigatio peripatetica* (1583), and *De plantis* (1583). His teaching—which attracted many students from all over Italy and Europe—won him special renown. The reasons for abandoning the chair at Pisa in 1592 are not at all clear. Perhaps it had something to do with the many disagreements and arguments with the Platonic philosopher Francesco de Vieri, which were especially bitter between 1589 and 1590, and the accusations of heresy made against him by some of his own colleagues. It is

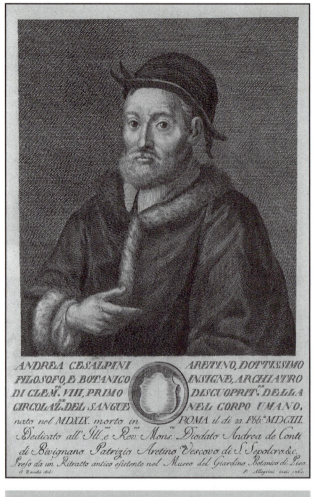

Andrea Cesalpino. Line engraving by F. Allegrini after Giuseppe Zocchi. Iconographic Collection, Wellcome Library, London.

more probable that Cesalpino's pride was wounded when Girolamo Mercuriale (1530–1606) was invited to the university, on an amazingly generous salary, which ensured him a special pre-eminence. With the help of his former student Mercati, Cesalpino tried to find another position, and in September 1592 was called to Rome by Pope Clement VIII as lecturer in medicine at the Sapienza and papal archiater. In Rome, where he passed the remaining eleven years of his life, Cesalpino dedicated himself above all to the publication of works of a more medical character: *Quaestiones medicae* (1593); *De metallis* (1596); *Praxis universa artis medicae* (1602–03), republished several times later with the title *Katoptron, sive speculum artis medicae hippocraticum*; and an *Appendix ad libros de plantis et quaestiones peripateticas* (1603).

De plantis libri XVI (1583), the first true textbook of botany, was the fruit of his meticulous and painstaking botanical research carried out in Tuscany and various parts of Italy. The first book, where Cesalpino presented the principles of botany and grouped a wealth of careful observations under broad categories, is of outstanding historical importance. It was he who first attempted a methodical classification of plants, inspired by the principle of a hierarchy of characteristics, founded on an a priori conception of the nature of the plant—an essentially Aristotelian inspiration. He tried to discover in the plant the fundamental elements of the animal organization, of which the plant would be a simplified reproduction. The root represented the head inserted in the ground—the equivalent of the mouth; thus the root was the organ of nutrition and the stem, the organ of fructification. Cesalpino considered the portion of the plant between roots and stem—which he called the 'heart' (cor)—to be the seat of the soul of plants. The fruit was the most important part of the plant. The nourishment, drawn up through the roots, was taken up through the stem, reaching the fruits, just as in animals the veins went to the heart. The flower corresponded to the membrane, which in animals enfolded the fetus. Cesalpino denied sexuality in plants; his completely artificial classification was based on the characteristics of the fruit.

Like Aristotle, Cesalpino divided plants into two groups, those with a persistent stem (arbores and frutices, i.e., trees and shrubs) and those with a non-persistent stem (suffrutices and herbae, i.e., shrubby herbs and herbs). Trees possessed a single stem or trunk, whereas shrubs were composed of many thin stems. Shrubby herbs lived for many years and often bore fruit, but herbs died after the formation of the seeds. Cesalpino believed that the distinction among species should be made only according to similarity and dissimilarity of forms. The remaining fifteen books of De plantis were devoted to the classification and description of plants. His description of tendrils on the shoots and leaves, the climbing petioles of Clematis, the anchoring roots of Hedera, the secretion of nectar from flowers, and many other phenomena testified to his extraordinary skill in observation.

Cesalpino was the first to elaborate a system of plants based on a unified and coherent group of notions. Not content to confine himself to describing plants, he also set forth the basic elements of general botany. By paying scant attention to the medicinal uses of plants—which were of crucial importance to his contemporaries—he raised botany to the level of an independent science. The genus Caesalpinia of the Mimosaceae family was named by Linnaeus in his honor. In his work De metallis (1596) he tried to establish a new classification of minerals.

For medicine, Cesalpino's views on the circulation of blood have attracted the most attention, giving rise to many heated debates and arguments about his priority over William Harvey (1578–1657). Cesalpino, follower of Aristotle and the Peripatetic tradition, claimed, contrary to Galen, that the heart and not the liver was the true center of the blood, and consequently of the arteries and veins, providing, moreover, unquestionably important indications for the circulation of the blood, the heart, and the blood vessels.

His views and observations appear in many of his works. The first indications regarding the circulation of the blood can be found in the first edition of the Quaestiones peripateticae published in 1571 but actually written earlier, before mid-1566. In this work Cesalpino actually used the term 'circulation' for the first time, claiming that there was a continuous movement of blood from the veins into the heart, and from the heart into the arteries. Moreover, he affirmed that the blood passed constantly from the arteries to the veins in all parts of the body by means of capillary anastomoses (capillamenta), namely, the finest branches into which the arteries—after having penetrated into the organs—resolved to give origin to the veins. He also dealt with cardiac valves, suggesting that their presence prevented the passage of blood from the heart to the vena cava. In De plantis (1583) he further developed his doctrine of the blood's perpetual movement from the veins to the right heart, from this to the lungs, from there to the left heart, and from the left heart to the arteries, which distributed it to all parts of the body. In another work, the Quaestiones medicae (1593), he provided experimental proof confirming his doctrine of circulation, being the first to use ligature of the veins to demonstrate the blood's centripetal course. The veins swell peripherally not centrally to the site of a ligature, as would have been the case according to Galen's doctrine; phlebotomists know this by experience and apply ligatures centrally to the site of incision, not peripherally; the veins swell peripherally, not centrally, between their capillary origins and the ligature. In another experiment, in order to demonstrate the continuity existing between arteries and veins by means of capillary anastomoses, Cesalpino exposed a vein in a living animal, ligated it, made an incision under the ligature (i.e., toward the periphery), and observed that the first blood to come out was dark, i.e., venous, whereas later it was lighter, i.e., arterial. Finally, Cesalpino was the first to identify and distinguish the structure of an 'artery' as the pulsating vessel that emerged from the right ventricle, then called the vena arteriosa (i.e., pulmonary artery), from the structure of a 'vein', the non-pulsating vessel, then called arteria venosa (i.e., pulmonary veins). His views on the continuous flow of blood into and from the heart were reiterated in his last work Praxis universae artis medicae, first published in 1602, one year before his death, and reprinted on several occasions thereafter. However, Cesalpino did not realize the importance of his studies for the development of scientific thought and failed to synthesize his ideas, as he might have done, in a work expressly dedicated to the circulation of the blood.

Bibliography

Primary: 1571. *Peripateticarum questionum libri V* (Venice) [2nd edn., 1593]; 1583. *Daemonum investigatio peripatetica* (Florence) [2nd edn., 1593 (Venice)]; 1583. *De plantis libri XVI* (Florence); 1593. *Quaestionum medicarum libri II* (Venice); 1596. *De metallis libri III* (Rome).

Secondary: Mägdefrau, Karl, 1973. *Geschichte der Botanik* (Stuttgart) pp. 37–38, 41–43; Pagel, Walter, 1967. *William Harvey's Biological Ideas. Selected Aspects and Historical Background* (Basel and New York) pp. 169–209; Arcieri, Giovanni P., 1939. *La circolazione del sangue scoperta da Andrea Cesalpino d'Arezzo* (Milan); Viviani, Ugo, 1922. *Vita e opere di Andrea Cesalpino* (Arezzo); *DSB.*

Giuseppe Ongaro

CHADWICK, EDWIN (b. Longsight, near Manchester, England, 24 January 1800; d. East Sheen, Surrey, England, 6 July 1890), *public health.*

After his early education in Longsight and Stockport, Chadwick moved with his widowed father, a radical journalist, to London in 1810, where he was taught by private tutors. He began a clerking apprenticeship in an attorney's office and then studied at the Inner Temple before being called to the Bar on 26 November 1830. He funded some of his legal education by writing articles for newspapers and for the *Westminster Review.* His article in the *London Review* (1829) on 'Preventive Police' gained him the attention of the philosopher Jeremy Bentham (1748–1832), with whom he subsequently lived and worked as an assistant until Bentham's death. He never resumed his legal career but moved instead through a series of civil service positions, which reflected his philosophical views on the socio-economic structure of Britain. He firmly believed that significant social problems, such as crime, poverty and disease, could be addressed with technical and administrative solutions.

By the mid-1820s Chadwick was already well associated with leading social reformers, including the doctors Neil Arnott (1788–1874) and Thomas Southwood Smith (1788–1861), and the political economists John Stuart Mill (1806–73) and Nassau Senior (1790–1864). He developed a 'sanitary idea', based on his personal observations of fever dens in the east end of London. He was able to exploit this knowledge when he was appointed as an assistant commissioner (through the intervention of Senior) on the new Poor Law Commission (1832) to investigate the rising levels of poverty in Britain, which the old (Elizabethan) Poor Law could no longer cope with. He was promoted to a full commissioner (1833) and in the same year served on the Royal Commission to investigate the conditions of factory children, which eventually led to the Ten Hours Act (1847) and the establishment of employers' liability for workplace health and safety. This established the concept of 'inspectors' as part of state bureaucracy—a role that Chadwick himself personified.

With the creation of the New Poor Law (1834), Chadwick was disappointed not to be made one of its commissioners, possibly because his social stature was not felt to be high enough. Instead, he was appointed as Secretary (chief executive officer). He exploited his position to develop a solution to the increasing demands of poverty on the British public through the introduction of workhouses based on the principle of 'less eligibility'—to deter dependency on the state by making relief so repellent. However, despite this feature, the new poor Law provoked considerable debate and discontent in Britain, especially because it was financed through a pro rata charge on property owners.

Chadwick was faced in the years after the New Poor Law with increasing political and public pressure because expenditure on poor relief had not fallen as he had predicted. Indeed, the new service required the creation of workhouse infirmaries—one of the earliest forms of state medicine in Britain—an additional expense for the public to bear. He thus began to search for statistical evidence to substantiate a relatively new theory that he was developing with the aid of other investigators (such as Dr William Henry Duncan in Liverpool) that much poverty was related to the ill health of the working classes. He used his considerable authority within Whitehall in the 1830s to push for the creation of a system of registration for births, marriages, and deaths (1838) (most importantly the *causes* of deaths), and the appointment of William Farr (1807–83) to a key position in the Registrar General's office. He was also influential in the creation of the first Sanitary Commission (1839), on which he found work for Neil Arnott, Thomas Southwood Smith, and James Kay Shuttleworth (1807–77), who worked as an assistant on the Poor Law Commission.

Of this triumvirate, Arnott has been least remembered. Born in Scotland on 15 May 1788, he qualified in medicine at Aberdeen before establishing a successful private practice in London's Hunter Street in 1811. His 1827 publication, *Elements of Physics: or natural philosophy, general and medical* was very influential in Britain and abroad. He was responsible for introducing Chadwick to his mentor Jeremy Bentham in the 1820s—thus establishing one of the most significant philosophical groupings to affect the health of the population. Arnott's investigations, particularly that of the typhoid epidemic at Croydon in 1852, were colored by his unwavering belief in the miasmatic theory of disease transmission, to which he held even in the face of strong statistical evidence from John Snow in 1854 that cholera was a water-born disease. He died on 2 March 1874.

The Sanitary Commission effectively marked the transition from Chadwick's Poor Law career to his fifteen years as a sanitary reformer. His monumental *Report on the Sanitary Condition of the Labouring Population of Great Britain*, published in 1842, provided the statistical evidence on the association between disease and poverty, which was needed to stimulate further investigations.

In 1844 he was instrumental in the creation of the Royal Commission on the Health of Towns, which he used to solicit evidence throughout Britain on the links between poverty, poor environment, and ill health. These investigations eventually resulted in the 1848 Public Health Act. This was a significant step toward sanitary reform, although

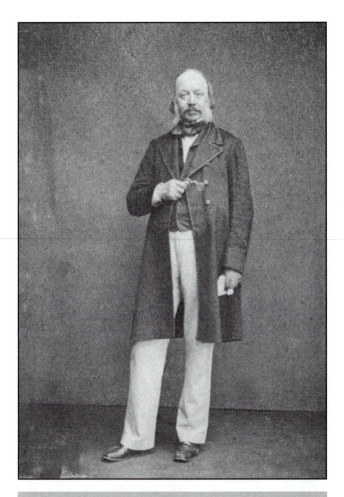

Sir Edwin Chadwick. Photograph by John & Charles Watkins. Iconographic Collection, Wellcome Library, London.

Chadwick's dogmatic approach to centralization stymied its full potential—the Act was only passed on condition that it was permissive rather than compulsory, and many towns were slow to adopt its recommendations, which included the municipalization of water supplies and the appointment of medical officers of health.

This first national public health legislation enabled Chadwick to propound his environmental policies of sanitary reform and preventive medicine based on the miasmatic theory, which held that disease was generated by breathing in poisonous gases produced by rotting matter. This broad theory was used to justify Chadwick's obsession with the design and installation of new egg-shaped sewer systems into urban areas, which would reduce the production of miasmas. He insisted on emulating the best designs of nature in his quest for a healthy environment, particularly the concept of the city as a natural system. He drew on arteriovenous theories to push for fully integrated sanitary systems, in which water was used to flush the sewage out of the urban area to surrounding farms where it was to be spread as fertilizer, thus producing more food for the urban population. However, the early sewers and associated water

provisions were often installed first in wealthy parts of towns (reflecting ratepayer pressure on councils) and not in the areas with the poorest housing conditions experiencing the highest rates of 'filth-related' disease. Chadwick also investigated the issue of urban burial as part of his sanitary enquiries, producing a supplementary *Interment Report* in 1843. He advocated that overcrowded urban cemeteries be closed as a measure to protect the public health and that new public burial grounds be provided by the local authorities, away from residential areas. These proposals, along with his plans to municipalize the water companies, were opposed by the government, local Poor Law organizations, and businesses.

Chadwick remained convinced throughout his life, and in spite of new scientific evidence, that 'all smell is disease'. Although he was appointed as one of the commissioners (the only salaried one) on the General Board of Health operating between 1848 and 1854, after its premature dissolution (caused in part by Chadwick's domineering attitude) he held no further public office.

Despite his social and political isolation after 1854, he continued to comment on a wide variety of national issues, including sanitary engineering, agricultural drainage, and the maintenance of a railway system as a public service. He attempted to begin a political career by standing at Parliamentary by-elections in 1859 and 1868 but was unsuccessful. He continued to be active in the Social Science Association and was president of the congress of the Sanitary Institute in 1878. Through his friendship with Florence Nightingale (1820–1910) he was able to continue to launch bitter attacks on new government personnel, such as John Simon (1816–1904), who had rejected the Chadwickian model of sanitary reform in favor of strategies recognizing that diseases such as cholera were waterborne rather than generated by miasmatic air.

Chadwick married Rachel Kennedy, the daughter of a textile manufacturer, in 1839 and had a son, Osbert, a civil engineer, and a daughter, Marion, who was active in the women's movement. The Kennedy money financed a relatively prosperous lifestyle, which his civil service salary would not have afforded, and they moved in 1869 to a self-designed cottage near Richmond Park, Surrey, with state of the art heating and ventilation. His public service was belatedly recognized when he was knighted in 1889.

Bibliography

Primary: 1842. *Report on the Sanitary Condition of the Labouring Population of Great Britain* (London); 1889. (Richardson, B. W., ed.) *The Health of Nations: A Review of the Works of Edwin Chadwick* 2 vols. (London).

Secondary: Hamlin, Christopher, 1998. *Public Health and Social Justice in the Age of Chadwick* (Cambridge); Brundage, Anthony, 1988. *England's 'Prussian Minister': Edwin Chadwick and the Politics of Government Growth, 1832–1854* (University Park, PA);

Finer, Samuel E., 1952. *The Life and Times of Sir Edwin Chadwick* (London); Lewis, Richard A., 1952. *Edwin Chadwick and the Public Health Movement* (London); *Oxford DNB*.

Sally Sheard

CHAGAS, CARLOS RIBEIRO JUSTINIANO (b. Oliveira, Brazil, 9 July 1879; d. Rio de Janeiro, Brazil, 8 November 1934), *parasitology, tropical medicine, public health.*

Early Years

Chagas was born on a farm near the city of Oliveira, Minas Gerais. His family, of Portuguese descent, raised coffee, then the mainstay of the Brazilian economy. He studied at Catholic schools and then moved to Rio de Janeiro to enter the School of Medicine in 1897. Upon reaching what was then the nation's capital and main seaport, Chagas encountered a city grappling with precarious sanitary conditions. Frequent epidemics (especially of yellow fever) jeopardized immigration and foreign trade. Urban sanitation was a major government concern.

Chagas studied medicine at a time when microbiology and tropical medicine were undergoing a process of institutionalization around the world. In tune with these changes in biomedical sciences, some professors at Rio's School of Medicine defended the idea that the precepts and practices of experimental medicine should be incorporated into teaching. Chagas was deeply influenced by two of these teachers: Miguel Couto was a prominent general practitioner who held that clinical practice should keep step with advances in medical science; Francisco Fajardo, a pioneer in Brazilian microbiology, introduced the young student to the experimental study of tropical diseases, especially malaria.

In 1902 Chagas began researching his MD thesis at the Federal Serum Therapy Institute, located at the Manguinhos farm on the outskirts of Rio de Janeiro and founded two years earlier to produce serum and vaccine against bubonic plague. The director, Oswaldo Cruz, was a prestigious physician who had specialized in microbiology at the Pasteur Institute. Cruz served as adviser to Chagas, who chose to investigate the hematological aspects of malaria. This was his first contact both with the institute that would become an integral part of his professional life and with the master to whom he would become heir. Renamed the Oswaldo Cruz Institute (IOC) in 1908, the establishment evolved into one of Brazil's leading centers of microbiology and tropical medicine.

After receiving his medical degree in 1903, Chagas turned down an invitation by Cruz to join the still small team of researchers at Manguinhos, opting instead to practice medicine. In 1904, he was appointed physician at the General Directorship of Public Health, headed since the previous year by Cruz, and began working at an isolation hospital. That same year, he set up a private practice in Rio

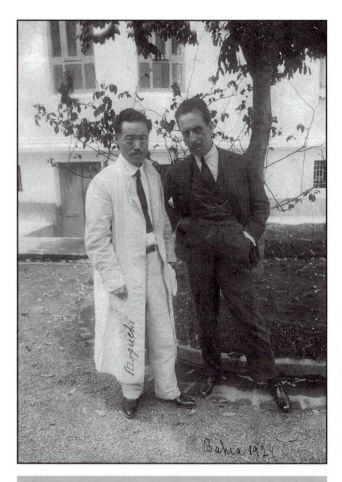

Hideyo Noguchi (see biographical entry) and Carlos Chagas, State of Bahia, Brazil, 1924. Photograph, Oswaldo Cruz Foundation Historical Archives.

de Janeiro and married Íris Lobo, daughter of a federal senator. Their sons Evandro Chagas (1905–1940) and Carlos Chagas Filho (1910–2000) both achieved distinguished scientific careers.

The Discovery of American Trypanosomiasis

In 1905 Cruz assigned Chagas to combat a malaria epidemic that had halted work on a hydroelectric power plant that was to serve the port of Santos, São Paulo. In 1907 he led another attack on malaria, this time in the vicinity of Rio de Janeiro to keep work going on the federal capital's water system. Directly connected to the modernization of the Brazilian economy, these prophylactic campaigns took place at a time of great world enthusiasm about the prospect of combating contagious diseases by controlling and even eliminating their vectors. In Rio this outlook had been evinced in Cruz's initiatives against the transmitters of yellow fever since 1903.

Chagas argued that malaria was transmitted chiefly inside the home. He therefore contended that preventive measures should not be limited to larval control alone but

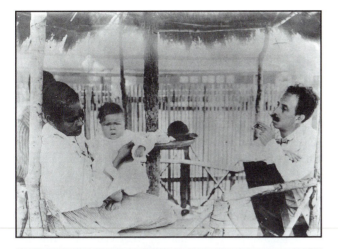

Carlos Chagas (far right) examines a little girl, one of the first acute cases of American trypanosomiasis, City of Lassance, State of Minas Gerais, *c.* 1910. Photograph, Oswaldo Cruz Foundation Historical Archives.

should focus on attacking adult mosquitoes in these environments through use of such insecticides as pyrethrum. Chagas's theory of intradomiciliary transmission of malaria and its related prophylactic method, which he used successfully in the 1905–07 campaigns, would later be recognized as pioneer contributions to malariology and to the widespread use of synthetic insecticides such as DDT.

Work with malaria took Chagas to the region where he made the scientific discovery that brought him international renown. In 1907 he was sent by Cruz to northern Minas Gerais to combat a malaria epidemic among workers on the Brazilian Central Railway, the main channel for the export of agricultural production, which was being extended from Rio de Janeiro to northern Brazil. In the small town of Lassance, located on the banks of the Rio das Velhas, he set up a laboratory inside a train car and devoted himself not only to the question of malaria but also to investigating the region's wild animals and insects.

A railroad engineer called Chagas's attention to a blood-sucking triatomine bug that infested the cracks of mud-walled huts, typical of poor rural housing in Brazil. This insect was known as a *barbeiro* ('barber' bug or, in English, the kissing or conenose bug) because rural folk still often relied on barber-surgeons who practiced blood-letting and because the insect tends to bite people on the face. Examining the bug's intestine, Chagas identified a protozoan as a possible intermediary form of a monkey trypanosome (*Trypanosoma minasense*) he had previously discovered at Lassance or of another vertebrate hemo-flagellate. He sent some specimens of *barbeiros* to Cruz, where they could feed on infection-free primates. When Chagas was informed that these same flagellates had been detected in the blood on one of those animals that became ill, he returned to Rio and in December 1908 described the parasite as a new spe-

cies of trypanosome, which he named *Trypanosoma cruzi* in honor of Cruz.

Suspecting *T. cruzi* could be pathogenic to man, Chagas then returned to Lassance in search of other vertebrate hosts. After discovering an infected cat, which confirmed the existence of household reservoirs, in April 1909 he detected the parasite in the blood of a feverish two-year-old girl named Berenice. Hers was considered the first case of the new disease that was named 'American trypanosomiasis', or Chagas' disease.

The scientific reasoning that guided Chagas reflected his adherence to the parasite-vector model, heart of the tropical medicine paradigm defined by the British physician Patrick Manson in the 1890s. This model applied to a set of diseases caused by protozoans or more complex organisms (usually parasites), whose transmission depended on completion of their life cycle inside a vector under geographical conditions typical of the tropics. The disease identified in Lassance thus contributed to affirmation of this model, as had the description (a few years earlier) of African trypanosomiasis, which had been causing colonizing nations on that continent much concern. Chagas's discovery displays certain singularities. First, it was made by a local doctor with no direct ties to colonialist interests. Furthermore, within a few months the same researcher identified the infectious agent, the insect vector, and human disease, a feat many cite as the only such instance in the history of medicine. The order of these events deviated from the normal sequence of such discoveries, where clinical description of the disease usually precedes the determination of its pathogen and mode of transmission. This served as further proof of the power of the parasite-vector model.

The new parasitic disease was identified at a moment when Cruz was investing heavily to transform the IOC into a center for the study of tropical diseases that would combine scientific research, manufacturing of biological products, and teaching of microbiology, much like the Pasteur Institute. In the realm of research, he endeavored to tighten the institute's relations with scientific institutions abroad, especially German institutes of tropical medicine. Because Chagas had produced original knowledge in a country lying outside the major scientific centers, the episode constituted a milestone in the consolidation of Cruz's project and in the institutionalization of Brazilian biomedical science itself.

On 15 April 1909, in Lassance, Chagas wrote a preliminary note announcing his discovery and sent it to *Brazil-Medico*, then one of the country's more important medical periodicals. The publication date (22 April) coincided with Cruz's formal notification of the finding to the National Academy of Medicine, Brazil's most prestigious medical association, which sent a commission to Lassance to verify Chagas's accomplishment; Miguel Couto took this opportunity to propose that the new malady be called 'Chagas' disease'.

The international scientific community learned of the discovery through papers published by Chagas in *Bulletin de la Société de Pathologie Exotique* and *Archiv für Schiffs- und Tropen-Hygiene*. In August 1909 the first volume of the IOC's journal *Memórias do Instituto Oswaldo Cruz* included a detailed study of *Trypanosoma cruzi* by Chagas.

Chagas was a member of the IOC research staff from March 1908. Thanks to his growing prestige, in 1910 he rose to second in the institute's hierarchy. That same year, the National Academy of Medicine made him a full member. Worldwide recognition was not long in coming, and at the International Hygiene Exposition, which took place in Dresden in 1911, Chagas' disease was the centerpiece of the Brazilian pavilion. One year later (1912) Chagas received the Schaudinn Award, bestowed every four years by the Hamburg Institute for Tropical Medicine for the best work in protozoology.

Throughout the rest of his life, Chagas earned various honors, titles, and decorations. He was the first Brazilian to be conferred an honorary degree from Harvard University (1921), a tribute he later received from the University of Paris as well (1926). He was a member of many medical and scientific institutions in Brazil and abroad, including the Brazilian Academy of Science, Argentina Medical Association, Pan-American Medical Association, Société de Pathologie Exotique, Royal Society of Tropical Medicine and Hygiene, Société Royale des Sciences Medicales et Naturelles de Bruxelas, and academies of medicine in Paris, Madrid, Rome, and New York. He was nominated for the 1913 and 1921 Nobel Prizes.

Studies and Controversies Surrounding the New Disease

The discovery of American trypanosomiasis helped reinforce protozoology as one of the Oswaldo Cruz Institute's main areas of investigation. The main research site for American trypanosomiasis was the municipality of Lassance, where Cruz had a small hospital built for the study of clinical cases of the disease. Likewise with the objective of supporting investigation into the subject at the IOC, in 1912 Cruz began to build a hospital for tropical diseases at Manguinhos (inaugurated in 1918), where cases from Lassance could be clinically studied.

Under Chagas's leadership, a number of IOC researchers began exploring different aspects of the new trypanosomiasis, including the biological characteristics of the vector, the parasite, and its life cycle; clinical presentation of the infection; means of transmission; and diagnostic techniques.

Between 1909 and the early 1920s, Chagas conducted his key studies on the disease's clinical, anatomical-pathological, and pathogenic characteristics. In 1910, he stated that it presents itself in two modalities: acute and chronic stages. During the acute phase, diagnosed directly from the presence of the parasite in the patient's blood, Chagas noted that the main symptom was fever, accompanied by a generalized edema and ganglionic hypertrophy and by splenomegally and hepatomegally (increase in size of the spleen and liver). Although most acute cases evolve into the chronic state, Chagas pointed out that more serious first-stage infections could involve cerebral manifestations that were usually fatal. Chronic infection—where clinical manifestations reflected changes to organs and tissues caused by *T. cruzi*—comprised the following types, according to Chagas's first formulation: nervous, myxedematous, pseudo-myxedematous, cardiac, and chronic with acute exacerbations. In chronic cases, indirect methods of diagnosis are required because the parasite disappears from the patient's blood.

In 1916 Chagas systematized information on the disease's clinical presentation, revising his earlier classification. He indicated that acute infection involved not only cases of serious meningoencephalitis but might also lead to cardiac disturbances, which generally evolved into the chronic state. He raised the hypothesis that dysphagia, or 'swallow disease' (recognized since the nineteenth century), might be a clinical manifestation of American trypanosomiasis. In the chronic modality, he maintained the nervous and cardiac forms but eliminated the chronic form with acute exacerbations and replaced the myxedematous and pseudo-myxedematous forms, respectively, with the hypothyroid and indeterminate forms. While affirming that the disease evolved progressively, Chagas observed that many cases could remain asymptomatic for a long time. For him, the infection was responsible for endocrine disturbances, as *T. cruzi* acted on a number of glands, mainly the thyroid. He thus defended the notion that endemic goiter—an ailment that jeopardized physical and mental development and was especially prevalent in rural Minas Gerais—was actually a clinical manifestation of Chagas' disease.

Later research did not confirm Chagas's statements regarding the nervous form of the disease nor its glandular manifestations, particularly endemic goiter. Yet his formulations of the cardiac form—which he viewed as one of the main clinical manifestations during the chronic stage—were widely confirmed and expanded. In his studies of how *T. cruzi* affects the myocardium, Chagas employed electrocardiography techniques (albeit depending on rudimentary equipment), and for this he is considered a pioneer in the use of electrocardiography in Brazil. Although he did not further explore his hypothesis regarding digestive system disturbances, this was another postulate proven after his death.

Chagas also produced important information about the parasite's natural reservoirs and the disease's epidemiological characteristics and its means of transmission. His hypothesis that trypanosomes were transmitted by bug bite was not confirmed; rather, it was shown that infection follows contamination by the bug's feces. Although research focused on the region of Lassance, from his earliest studies on, Chagas argued that this pathology affected vast areas of Brazil and the American continent, constituting an important social problem that public health authorities should address by combating the *barbeiro* and improving housing. In the 1910s, representatives of the public health movement spread this idea far and wide, especially through the IOC expeditions into rural Brazil; they called attention to how rural endemic diseases were immensely damaging to the country's development.

Chagas's scientific prestige in Brazil and abroad notwithstanding, and despite the political role the disease played within the public health movement's discourse, some of his ideas on the clinical characterization of American trypanosomiasis and its epidemiological importance were questioned by the medical field. During a medical conference in the Argentinean capital, held in 1916, the director of the Buenos Aires Bacteriological Institute, the Austrian researcher Rudolf Kraus, cast doubts on the Chagasic etiology of endemic goiter and on the thesis that the disease was widely distributed across the American continent. The issue he raised was that in spite of the large number of infected *barbeiros*, he had been unable to identify human cases of the disease in some regions of Argentina. Chagas's explanation was that the parasite had probably not yet adapted to human hosts in those areas.

In 1922 some physicians who nurtured political resentments over Chagas's appointment as director of the IOC and of the National Department of Public Health brought the questions raised by Kraus back to the table, within the forum of the National Academy of Medicine. Following a period of heated debates and much publicity, the Academy appointed a committee to evaluate the dispute. In November 1923 it acknowledged the scientific value of Chagas's work but declared that the link with goiter and the disease's epidemiological dimensions were still open questions. The doubts introduced during this polemic hampered research progress as well as the dissemination of information on American trypanosomiasis in Brazil and especially abroad. This state of affairs was finally reversed in the first years after Chagas's death, thanks to the work of Argentinean researchers and some of his disciples at Manguinhos, including his oldest son, Evandro Chagas.

Head of the Oswaldo Cruz Institute (1917–34)

In February 1917, three days after Cruz died, the president of Brazil appointed Chagas director of the IOC. In the climate of growing public health demands and economic modernization that followed World War I, Chagas's administration—which would last until his death—worked to expand research, production, and teaching activities.

Research remained centered on diseases endemic to Brazil and, to a lesser extent, on animal diseases. Chagas shaped the institute's work areas into a more formal framework, creating scientific divisions by field of knowledge, such as applied chemistry, mycology, bacteriology and immunity, medical zoology, pathological anatomy, protozoology, and physiology. Taught since 1908 by IOC researchers—including Chagas himself—the Applied Course program, which offered specialization in microbiology and medical zoology, was expanded. For Chagas, a doctor's learning should not be restricted to clinical practice but should go hand in hand with both the theory and practice of scientific investigation. Furthermore, he believed that students should be prepared to treat and prevent not just the common illnesses encountered in their urban offices but also—indeed, primarily—'Brazil's diseases', as he used to say, i.e., those endemic to rural areas. Thanks to a government educational reform in 1925, Chagas had the opportunity to put these guidelines into practice. The following year, he set up a chair in tropical medicine at the Rio de Janeiro School of Medicine, whose program was overseen by the IOC director; Chagas himself was appointed the course's first professor. He also deepened the institute's involvement in teaching activities at Rio's medical school by creating a Specialization Course in Hygiene and Public Health at that same time.

Chagas diversified the IOC's production of medications and biological products and promoted their marketing to boost the institute's income; from its earliest days, the IOC had been guaranteed a certain degree of autonomy from the federal budget. He maintained Cruz's polemic order that part of the profits from the sale of any products developed and patented by staff researchers must revert to these individuals. In 1918 Chagas created the Official Medication Service, which manufactured quinine and other products and supplied them to rural prevention posts, state governments, the Armed Forces, and public and private companies. In 1920 the IOC was made responsible for quality control of the biological preparations used in immunization that were manufactured or imported by Brazilian laboratories; it also absorbed the Municipal Vaccinogen Institute, which produced smallpox vaccine.

Throughout the 1920s the institute suffered the impacts of financial and political instability, intensified by the international crisis of 1929 and the first years of the Getúlio Vargas administration (1930–45). Chagas nonetheless managed to strengthen and enrich the model put in place by Cruz, fostering tight bonds between biomedical science, public health, and national interests. At the age of fifty-five (1934), he died suddenly from heart problems.

Public Health

After the trips to combat malaria in the early years of his career, Chagas came into further contact with issues in Brazilian nosology when he was assigned to an expedition to the Amazon River valley (October 1912–March 1913). The trip was planned by the federal government, which was concerned over the crisis in rubber production and its impact on the country's trade balance. Chagas evaluated

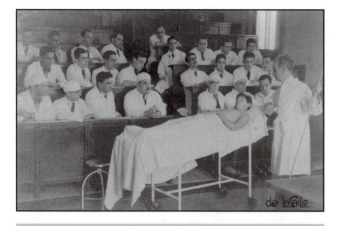

Carlos Chagas examines a malaria patient during a class at the Tropical Diseases Pavilion, School of Medicine of Rio de Janeiro, at São Francisco de Assis Hospital. Perhaps the last image of Chagas before his death. Rio de Janeiro, 1934. Photograph, Oswaldo Cruz Foundation Historical Archives.

the living and sanitary conditions of riverside dwellers and people working on rubber extraction and also conducted scientific investigations into the region's main diseases, such as malaria, all while working out of an improvised laboratory on the boat. In his final report, he drew attention to the medical and social neglect of the Amazon's inhabitants and urged immediate enforcement of sanitation measures that would allow the region to achieve economic development.

Reports by other IOC researchers who likewise took part in expeditions into the Brazilian hinterlands during the 1910s caused a stir among the public; they portrayed the living conditions of the country's rural inhabitants (which represented the majority of the population) and disseminated the view that Brazil was backward when compared to so-called civilized nations not because of its tropical climate or miscegenation but because endemic diseases impaired productivity in the countryside. This diagnosis became the banner of a political movement comprising scientists and intellectuals (among them Chagas himself) that favored increased government responsibility in public health.

When the Spanish flu reached Brazil and ravaged the federal capital (1918), the public health movement extended its grievances. Appointed by the federal government to coordinate relief efforts, Chagas set up hospitals and emergency posts around the city. His wholehearted commitment to battling the epidemic earned him the stature of hero in the pages of the press at the time.

Elected in 1919, President Epitácio Pessoa vowed to place reform of federal sanitary services at the top of his agenda, entrusting leadership of the process to Chagas. Following fierce debates in Congress, the National Department of Public Health was created in January 1920, and Chagas was appointed director. Like Cruz, he adminis-

trated the federal sanitary services while simultaneously serving as head of the IOC.

The new agency endowed the federal government with greater power to intervene in public health matters, in contrast with the decentralized state-based model previously in force. Chagas was author of an extensive Sanitary Code that organized and modernized Brazilian public health law. Up to then focused on urban areas, public health initiatives moved into the countryside, especially through the opening of health posts to combat rural endemic diseases. In these efforts, Chagas enjoyed the decisive collaboration of the Rockefeller Foundation, which since 1916 had worked in Brazil to prevent ancylostomiasis and yellow fever. Specialized agencies and institutions were also established to meet the specific needs of pregnant mothers and children, provide hospital assistance, and combat tuberculosis, syphilis, and leprosy.

Another vital aspect of Chagas's administration was investment in the training of specialized professionals. In collaboration with the Rockefeller Foundation, in 1923 he founded Brazil's first school of nursing in Rio de Janeiro: Escola de Enfermagem Anna Nery. Three years later, at the Rio de Janeiro School of Medicine, he organized the Specialization Course in Hygiene and Public Health, which was offered by Manguinhos research staff under the guidance of the IOC's director. The first of its kind in Brazil, this course guaranteed that its graduates would have direct access to positions within the federal sanitary services; it was a milestone in the institutionalization and professionalization of the career of sanitarians in this country.

Chagas's ideas and projects in the public health field reached an international audience through his role as the Brazilian representative to the League of Nations' Health Committee from 1922 until his death.

Chagas left his position as head of the National Department of Public Health in 1926 at the close of President Arthur Bernardes's administration. During Chagas's term of office, the department modernized, professionalized, and broadened the federal government's roles and responsibilities in public health, especially in rural Brazil.

Still revered today, Carlos Chagas stands as a symbol of how biomedical science can achieve successful institutionalization and produce innovations under difficult local condition, based on paradigms in microbiology and tropical medicine developed in so-called central nations. Both for his work as a scientist and for his active participation in civic life, Chagas represents a brand of science that forged its organizational framework and acquired legitimacy through commitment to the interests of society and to the formulation of a national project.

Bibliography

Primary: 1909. 'Nova especie morbida do homem, produzida por um Trypanozoma (*Trypanozoma cruzi*): Nota prévia.' *Brazil-Medico* 23: 161; 1909. 'Nova tripanozomiase humana: Estudos sobre a morfolojia e o ciclo evolutivo do Schizotrypanum cruzi n. gen., n. sp., ajente etiolojico de nova entidade morbida do homem.' *Memorias do Instituto Oswaldo Cruz* 1: 159–218; 1910. 'Nova entidade morbida do homem.' *Brazil-Medico* 24: 423–428, 433–437, 443–447; 1916. 'Processos patojenicos da tripanozomiase americana.' *Memorias do Instituto Oswaldo Cruz* 8: 5–35; 1922. 'The Discovery of *Trypanosoma cruzi* and of American Trypanosomiasis. Historic Retrospect.' *Memorias do Instituto Oswaldo Cruz* 15: 3–11.

Secondary: Kropf, Simone, Nara Azevedo, and Luiz Otávio Ferreira, 2003. 'Biomedical Research and Public Health in Brazil: The Case of Chagas' Disease (1909–1950).' *Social History of Medicine* 16: 111–129; Prata, Aluízio, 1999. 'Evolution of the Clinical and Epidemiological Knowledge about Chagas Disease 90 Years after Its Discovery.' *Memórias do Instituto Oswaldo Cruz* 94: 81–88, suppl. I; Coutinho, Marilia, Olival Freire Jr., João Dias, and Carlos Pinto, 1999. 'The Nobel Enigma: Chagas' Nominations for the Nobel Prize' *Memórias do Instituto Oswaldo Cruz* 94: 123–129, suppl. I; Hochman, Gilberto, 1998. *A era do saneamento. As bases da política de Saúde Pública no Brasil* (São Paulo); Perleth, Matthias, 1997. *Historical Aspects of American Trypanosomiasis (Chagas' Disease)* (Berlin); Chagas Filho, Carlos, 1993. *Meu pai* (Rio de Janeiro); Benchimol, Jaime Larry (coord.), 1990. *Manguinhos do sonho à vida. A ciência na belle époque* (Rio de Janeiro); *DSB*.

Simone Petraglia Kropf and
Gilberto Hochman

CHAMBERLEN, HUGH (THE ELDER) (b. London, England, 1630–34, d. Netherlands, after 1720), *medicine, midwifery.*

Chamberlen was born into the famous family of medical and man-midwifery practitioners of that name in London between 1630 and 1634. His father was Peter Chamberlen and his mother, Jane, was the daughter of Sir Hugh Myddelton, the London goldsmith who brought the New River water supply to London under James VI and I. His grandfather was Peter Chamberlen the Younger.

His education, training, and grounds for his claim to be a Doctor of Medicine remain obscure. By the early 1660s he was practicing in London, being sufficiently secure to marry in 1663. He was familiar with the obstetrical secret (probably a form of forceps) that members of the family used since earlier in the century. In 1670 he traveled to Paris, where he seems to have sought to sell the secret, but his demonstration of it at the Hôtel Dieu was unsuccessful. Three years later, he was appointed physician-in-ordinary to Charles II, and he also published a translation of a treatise of the French physician, François Mauriceau. In the preface he described how in cases of obstructed births he, his father, and brothers could deliver babies 'without prejudice' to mother or child because they did not use hooks.

Although this reference was tantalizing and omitted all details, it was the first step in a long drawn-out process by which the obstetrical forceps entered wider medical practice. The family sought to control the diffusion of their innovation and to profit from it. However, a proposal in 1678 that the secret should be passed to selected practitioners in each county came to nothing. Nor did Hugh's medical career progress smoothly. In 1682 he lost his position at court, possibly because of his Non-Conformist religion and Whig politics. In 1685 he joined the Earl of Monmouth's rebellion against King James II, being lucky to receive a pardon the next year. In 1687 Hugh tried unsuccessfully to obtain a patent for midwifery from the College of Physicians and found himself prosecuted for malpractice the following year. In 1692 he attended a delivery of the future Queen Anne but thereafter seems to have spent less time in medical practice, moving to Scotland by 1699; six years later he moved on to the Netherlands, where he died at some point after 1720.

His plans to institutionalize and control midwifery practice using the Chamberlen family secret paralleled other proposals for social and economic reform that he advanced during his life. Like his midwifery proposals, these often combined the language of public benefit with opportunities for personal profit. They overlapped with the ideas of contemporary advocates of political arithmetic and Baconian reform such as Thomas Houghton, who proposed him to the Royal Society, when he was elected to it in 1681. He remained in London through the plague of 1665, and in that and the following year submitted proposals to the Privy Council recommending a range of precautionary measures designed to prevent and avert the infection, including the raising of taxes in order to pay for their cost. In 1689 he drew up proposals for Parliament to initiate a complete reform and restructuring of medicine. In subsequent years he wrote several pamphlets that advocated a form of land bank, a penny post scheme, and other public works.

Bibliography

Primary: 1673. (Chamberlen, H., ed. and trans.) F. Mauriceau's *The Accomplisht Midwife* (London).

Secondary: Wilson, A., 1995. *The Making of Man-midwifery: Childbirth in England, 1660–1770* (London); Hunter, M., 1982. *The Royal Society and Its Fellows: The Morphology of an Early Scientific Institution* (Chalfont St. Giles); Gibbons, P., 1969. 'The Medical Projectors, 1640–1720.' *Journal of the History of Medicine* 24: 247–271; *Oxford DNB*.

Mark Jenner

CHANNING, WALTER (b. Newport, Rhode Island, USA, 15 April 1786; d. Brookline, Massachusetts, USA, 27 July 1876), *obstetrics.*

Channing was the son of William Channing, a lawyer and champion of American independence, and Lucy Ellery, whose father William Ellery was a signer of the Declaration of Independence. Walter's father died young and the family eventually moved to Boston where his brother, William Ellery Channing, was on the threshold of a career as a Unitarian minister and social reformer.

Channing was expelled from Harvard College in his junior year for participating in a student rebellion and refusing to apologize. Having decided on a medical career, he apprenticed to James Jackson and then attended medical school at the University of Pennsylvania, receiving the MD degree in 1809. He spent the following year studying obstetrics in London and Edinburgh.

Returning to Boston in 1811, he quickly established a general medical practice but gained a reputation for his obstetrical skills and compassion for parturient women who were often fearful of the pain of childbirth and the possibility of disability or death. Channing's practice preceded development of anesthesia and scientific understanding of infection, as well as medical technologies such as ultrasound and fetal monitors that make childbirth safer and easier today. He was frequently consulted by other physicians in difficult cases, especially when forceps and other instruments were needed.

He also established himself among the elite physicians who dominated medical practice in antebellum Boston. He was a founding editor of the *New England Journal of Medicine and Surgery* (1812), first lecturer in midwifery (1815) and first professor of midwifery and medical jurisprudence (1818) at Harvard Medical School, first Dean of the medical faculty (1819), and first assistant physician at Massachusetts General Hospital (MGH), where he served for eighteen years.

Channing was instrumental in the creation of the Boston Lying-in Hospital (1832) for poor or homeless women. Almost all babies were born at home and Boston's only other hospital, MGH, did not accept obstetrical patients. He served as attending or consulting physician for many years.

His primary contribution to obstetrics was his advocacy of anesthesia in childbirth. Although ether was first demonstrated as safe and effective in surgery at the Massachusetts General Hospital in 1846 and European obstetricians began to use it shortly thereafter, American physicians questioned its safety in childbirth, and clergy and laymen condemned it as a transgression of God's judgment upon Eve: 'In pain thou shalt bring forth children.' In the spring of 1847, proof of its safety was published by a Boston dentist who administered ether to Fanny Longfellow while a midwife delivered her baby. Soon after, Channing began to employ it, first in cases requiring the use of instruments, and eventually in normal childbirth when the patient requested relief from pain. He was impressed by the success of these events and felt compelled to disprove the critics. His *Treatise on Etherization in Childbirth*, published in 1848, included data from forty-five physicians who had used anesthesia in 581 cases without negative consequences. Channing concluded that women need not submit to suffering 'which is [as] unnecessary as it is . . . cruel'.

A physician who regularly witnessed disease and death in Boston's growing slums, Channing actively participated in the temperance movement and programs to relieve poverty. He was a committed Unitarian, an abolitionist, and an outspoken pacifist.

He retired from teaching in 1854 but continued to practice and write for medical journals for another ten years. In 1860, as Boston's most notable obstetrician, he was elected first president of the Boston Obstetrical Society.

Channing married twice. His first wife, Barbara Higginson, bore four children before her death in 1822. The second, Eliza Wainwright, died in childbirth, a devastating experience for Channing, who was the physician in the case.

Bibliography

Secondary: Kass, Amalie M., 2002. *Midwifery and Medicine in Boston, Walter Channing, M.D., 1786–1876* (Boston); *DAMB*.

Amalie M. Kass

CHAPIN, CHARLES VALUE   (b. Providence, Rhode Island, USA, 17 January 1856; d. Providence, 31 January 1941), *public health, epidemiology.*

Chapin was the only son of Joshua and Louise Value Chapin. His family was descended from Samuel Chapin, who emigrated from England to America in 1635. Although Chapin's more distant ancestors were Congregational ministers, Chapin, like his father, became a physician.

Chapin graduated from Brown University in 1876 and then enrolled in the College of Physicians and Surgeons in New York City. There he studied under William Henry Welch, who later became a founding teacher at the Johns Hopkins Medical School. From Welch, Chapin learned the techniques of laboratory research then being pioneered in Germany. Upon graduation in 1879, Chapin embarked on an internship at Bellevue Hospital, where he was affiliated with Edward S. Janeway, a pathologist and the Health Commissioner of New York City. Janeway was aware of the germ theory being developed by Louis Pasteur and Robert Koch, and Chapin saw these ideas implemented when he participated in the first antiseptic operation performed at Bellevue; antisepsis had been developed by Joseph Lister and was based on applying the germ theory of infection to surgery.

In October 1880 Chapin returned to Providence (where he would live for the remainder of his life) and began his medical career. In 1882 he was appointed to the staff of the Rhode Island Hospital and became a part-time instructor at Brown University. In 1884 Chapin became the Commissioner of Health of the City of Providence, whereupon he ceased private practice and resigned from the Rhode Island Hospital. This event signaled the beginning of his lifelong career in the field of public health; he would hold this position until his retirement in 1932. He taught at a number of institutions—including Brown University, Harvard Medical School, the Harvard School of Public Health, and the Massachusetts Institute of Technology School of Health Officers—and received numerous honors, such as president of the American Public Health Association in 1926 and the first president of the American Epidemiological Society in 1927.

Chapin illustrates the fundamentally new approach to public health that was ushered in by the discoveries of bacteriology. Unlike earlier generations of public health officials—who focused on general efforts at environmental sanitation—Chapin accepted the view that diseases were spread by specific germs. Consequently, Chapin believed that public health should be targeted at the specific populations most likely to be exposed to specific infecting agents. To this end, he established the first municipal bacteriological laboratory in 1888. In 1906 he delivered an address at the annual meeting of the American Medical Association entitled 'The Fetish of Disinfection', which criticized the view that generalized disinfection would prevent the spread of disease. Although initially met with skepticism, his views eventually prevailed; the city of Providence discontinued terminal disinfection for diphtheria in 1905 and for scarlet fever in 1908. Later, many other cities discontinued the practice until it eventually disappeared as a standard feature of public health practice. In 1910 Chapin published *The Sources and Modes of Infection*, which became a prominent early twentieth-century textbook in epidemiology.

Chapin embodied the ideal of a dedicated municipal health officer and epitomized the new scientifically trained public health professional who emerged in the early twentieth century.

Bibliography

Primary: 1934. *Papers of Charles V. Chapin, M.D., A Review of Public Health Realities* (New York); 1901. *Municipal Sanitation in the United States* (Providence); 1910. *The Sources and Modes of Infection* (New York).

Secondary: Terris, Milton, 1999. 'Charles V. Chapin (1856–1941), "Dean of City Health Officers."' *Journal of Public Health Policy* 20(2): 214–220; Goldowsky, Seebert J., 1979. 'Charles V. Chapin: His Influence on Concepts of Public Health.' *Rhode Island Medical Journal* 62(8): 313–323; Cassedy, James H., 1962. *Charles V. Chapin and the Public Health Movement* (Cambridge, MA); *DAMB*.

J. Rosser Matthews

CHARCOT, JEAN-MARTIN (b. Paris, France, 29 November 1825; d. Lac des Settons [Burgundy], France, 16 August 1893), *neuropathology, hysteria, medical psychology*.

Charcot was the eldest of four sons born to Simon-Pierre Charcot, a carriage and saddle maker of modest means, and Jeanne-Georgette Saussier. His mother, not quite seventeen at the time of the birth of her first child, died when Charcot was fourteen. After completing lycée,

Charcot began medical studies at the Paris Faculty in 1844. He was the only one of his brothers to pursue a liberal profession, choosing medicine over a career as an artist, although he would continue to make use of his artistic talent and had a proclivity to analyze works of art for their medical content.

During his internship (1849–52) in the Paris hospitals, Charcot spent his final year at the Salpêtrière, at the time a marginal medical institution, a *hospice des vieilles femmes* (a care institution for indigent elderly incapacitated women), rather than an active treatment hospital. Distant from the center of Paris, the Salpêtrière did not have a reputation for advancing a medical career. Charcot perceived, however, opportunities for the study of chronic ailments afforded by long-term presence of thousands of potential patients. From these, he selected the case histories for his MD thesis on gout and rheumatoid arthritis (1853).

While an intern, Charcot became a protégé of Pierre Rayer, a physician of Napoleon III's and future Dean of the Paris medical faculty. Rayer's patronage launched Charcot's career in academic medicine and medical practice: in the first instance by smoothing the way for membership in the newly founded Société de Biologie, where Charcot presented his early research, and in the second, by directing wealthy clientele to the young physician. (One such patient was Benoit Fould, a leading banker, whom Charcot accompanied on an Italian voyage and whose family he continued to serve throughout his career.)

In 1862 Charcot returned to the Salpêtrière as chief of medical service, a post he would hold for the remainder of his career that would be the institutional key to his remarkable success. He began clinical teaching at the hospice a few years later, leading to the publication of his first book, *Leçons cliniques sur les maladies des vieillards et les maladies chroniques* (1867). In 1872 Charcot finally secured a Faculty professorship, winning nomination on the day before his forty-seventh birthday to the chair of pathological anatomy, which had been vacated by Alfred Vulpian (1826–87), his long-time close friend and collaborator.

Professor of Pathological Anatomy

Charcot held the chair of pathological anatomy for nearly a decade, during which time he offered a biweekly course lasting four months. His lessons, subsequently published, focused on diseases of the lungs, kidneys, liver, and brain. Although the purpose of the course was essentially to review current knowledge and to carry on the Paris school's prestigious, if somewhat fading, reputation for anatomo-clinical medicine (the correlation of post-mortem findings with bedside observations), Charcot added some original contributions. He presented, for example, histological evidence in favor of Laennec's doctrine that tuberculosis was a unitary disease despite its various clinical manifestations. This countered the German school of thought, which argued for distinctive anatomical types.

In the years following France's humiliating military defeat by Prussia in 1870, Charcot (a patriot who remained at his post in Paris throughout the siege and refused thereafter to include Germany in his frequent travels abroad) took every opportunity to contrast the work of French investigators favorably against their German counterparts. This was evident when he used his Faculty podium to oppose the specialized 'institutes' of pathology found in the German universities that neglected what Charcot considered the physician's primary resource—the clinical investigation of disease.

Charcot was probably somewhat less than comfortable as professor of pathological anatomy. Although a useful career stepping stone toward a more prestigious clinical professorship, the chair of pathological anatomy lacked resources. Charcot was obliged to supplement the meager allotment of cadavers accorded to the Faculty with pathological specimens from the Salpêtrière. Often he had to limit his demonstrations to illustrations and models. Moreover, he had gained a considerable reputation for his work on diseases of the nervous system, a subject that accounted for an ever-growing majority of his publications. His course in 1875 dealing with brain diseases and cerebral localization proved the most original of his teachings in pathological anatomy. At the end of the decade he took a leave of absence from his professorship. All the while he had continued his 'unofficial' clinical conferences at the Salpêtrière on neurological topics. When he returned to Faculty teaching, it would be to a clinical professorship in that field.

Neuropathology

Charcot's contributions to identifying nervous system disorders began with his return to the Salpêtrière in the early 1860s. This work formed his most enduring legacy and, in large measure, led to the establishment of clinical neurology as a specialty. Charcot sought to establish criteria for defining archetypical expressions of various diseases. These 'types', as he referred to them, represented the most complete or full-blown manifestation of a given disease. General types emerged from the synthesis of partial versions ('formes frustes') observed in clinical and pathological studies of individual case histories. (Often these were relatively few, given the rarity of many neurological diseases.) In this manner, Charcot laid the basis for the classification of diseases of the central nervous system.

Locomotor ataxia, or tabes dorsalis, was the first of Charcot's investigations of diseases of the spinal cord. Building on Duchenne de Boulogne's classic clinical description (1859), Charcot, initially in collaboration with Vulpian in 1862 and later alone or with students, embarked on a series of publications resulting in a comprehensive account of this progressive and typically fatal malady. Their work determined the location of the spinal cord lesion (the posterior columns) responsible for the characteristic disorders in gait, coordination, and sensation. Charcot revealed the entire panoply of symptomatology that provided clues to the diagnosis and prognosis of locomotor ataxia, including the characteristic shooting pains and impairment of vision and gastrointestinal and bladder function. He reported cases in which destruction of the joints occurred, an original finding recognized by the eponym 'Charcot joints'.

In the late 1860s Charcot defined amyotrophic lateral sclerosis, a progressive paralytic disease previously unrecognized, also given his name. In another series of studies he differentiated multiple sclerosis and Parkinson's disease on the basis of close observation of differences in tremors and the scattered microscopic lesion in the spinal cord of MS patients. In contrast with ALS, which proved rapidly fatal, MS patients, Charcot noted, typically experienced periods of remission.

Charcot continued to study these and other diseases of the nervous system for the rest of his career. Unlike Vulpian, he remained at the Salpêtrière, where he concentrated his research on the new discipline. His clinical lessons featured meticulous examination of hospital patients and a comprehensive review of the literature. Manuscripts of the lectures, complete with Charcot's own drawings, were ready for publication nearly as given. These clinical lessons constituted the vast majority of his publications.

Charcot's Chair

In 1881 Charcot was named to a newly created Faculty chair in diseases of the nervous system. Shortly after coming to power, the republican national government, led by his friend, Léon Gambetta, established the clinical professorship at the Salpêtrière specifically for Charcot. (After his death, the post was known as 'Charcot's chair'.) Although some Faculty colleagues objected to the notion that a new chair should be created for a personality rather than a discipline (they believed that neurological disease did not merit a professorial chair of its own), the issue was never really in doubt. Charcot's manuscript notes contained an elaborate justification for a separate chair in nervous system disease based on the rapid progress in the discipline during recent decades. He consulted foreign colleagues in search of precedents elsewhere; except for combined positions in neurology and psychiatry, a union Charcot explicitly rejected, there were none. Charcot had to overcome his reservations about 'specialism'. While advocating specialization in research and teaching, he continued to see patients with a wide spectrum of medical problems in his enormous and lucrative private practice.

Charcot's new professorship represented official recognition and generous reward for his accomplishments in neurology. There were concrete advantages as well. He could now devote mornings exclusively to his hospital service; all his teaching would take place at the Salpêtrière. A clinical chair entitled the recipient to additional staff: a resident chef de clinique as well as interns. Additions to his facilities at the

Salpêtrière followed in rapid succession, including a new lecture amphitheatre, a ward for male patients (a first in the hospital's long history), an out-patient clinic, a pathology museum, and laboratories for histology, ophthalmology, otology, hydrotherapy, electrotherapy, and photography. The out-patient clinic became the site for Charcot's renowned Leçons du mardi (Tuesday lessons), two years of which were published in a unique format replicating examinations of selected patients who came to the clinic that day; the text consisted of Charcot's questions and his comments on the case histories and the patients' responses. On Fridays, Charcot presented his more formal public lectures, which attracted large audiences to the Salpêtrière. In 1882 in his inaugural lesson, Charcot gave particular attention to hysteria and he declared his intention to make the study of that ailment central to his ongoing investigation of nervous system disease.

The Great Neurosis

Charcot sometimes called hysteria the 'great neurosis', an allusion to the convulsive fits of the ailment and its apparent ability to mimic virtually every neurological deficit. Hysteria was a more prevalent diagnosis than the total of all forms of organic neuropathology. The ailment was classified as a neurosis because, unlike most of the diseases Charcot had previously studied, hysteria apparently involved no detectable material lesion of the nervous system. Moreover, hysterical deficits often did not conform to any known pattern of innervation. For example, the hysterical 'sleeve' displayed complete paralysis and anesthesia below a line around the wrist, a neuroanatomical impossibility. Faced with this anomalous situation, Charcot fell back on the paradoxical notion of a functional, or 'dynamic', lesion, most likely located, he supposed, in the cerebral cortex. For all practical purposes, however, he had to rely exclusively on clinical observation and hypotheses in investigating the 'great neurosis'.

Charcot's first lessons on hysteria (1870–72) coincided with an administrative transfer of patients within the Salpêtrière. In 1870 he received into his service a group of women suffering from epilepsy and hysteria who were judged not to be insane. (These patients had previously been housed with the severely mentally ill.) Charcot set about to construct the 'type' of hysteria according to his method of close observation of the variety of clinical signs displayed by the new arrivals. He observed muscular contractures and a spectrum of neurological as well as other somatic manifestations. Such chronic or long-lasting signs he termed 'stigmata'; they represented the formes frustes of hysteria. Some patients, indeed all of his recently admitted hysterics, also exhibited intermittent convulsive attacks, which, Charcot believed, completed the type-form of the 'great neurosis', also known as 'major hysteria' or 'hystero-epilepsy'.

In his initial series of four published lessons, Charcot demonstrated many features of hysteria in one particular patient, a forty-year-old woman. In addition to various stigmatic and periodic convulsive fits, Justine Etchevery suffered from ischuria, a chronic, nearly total urinary retention. By devoting an entire lesson to this extremely rare sign, Charcot evidently wished to show that hysteria could produce extraordinary somatic effects; he took elaborate precautions to make sure that the patient was not simulating her ailment, a frequent allegation in cases of hysteria.

Hysteria had a long history in the medical literature. Charcot acknowledged Pierre Briquet's *Traité de l'Hystérie* (1859) as his most noteworthy predecessor. Where Charcot claimed originality, however, was in showing hysteria to be a neurological ailment that conformed to regular recurring clinical patterns or laws. Hysteria was, he asserted, a disease to be investigated, not a marginal or even a suspect female problem, consigned by default to gynecologists or psychiatrists.

Charcot identified four phases of the full-blown attack of hysteria (*grande hystérie*) consisting in epileptoid seizures, contorsions with acrobatic postures (*grands mouvements*), emotional gestures and verbalizations (*attitudes passionelles*), and a final delirium. Although he sometimes spoke of hystero-epilepsy, a traditional label, Charcot noted numerous differences from true epilepsy.

Charcot's formulation of hysteria won wide recognition following the publication of the *Iconographie photographique de la Salpêtrière* (3 vols. 1876–78). Edited by D.-M. Bourneville, Charcot's chief assistant, the graphic case histories and dramatic photographs depicting the four phases of the hysterical attack testified to the objective reality of the phenomena. Paul Richer, Charcot's intern and a gifted artist, gave the most comprehensive account of Salpêtrière 'grande hystérie' in his MD thesis (1879, published in book form, 1881).

Richer's synthesis concluded a decade-long initial phase of investigation during which the Salpêtrière school established the nosography of hysteria. Toward the close of the 1870s, Charcot applied a similar methodology to the study of hypnotism. Identifying three progressively deeper hypnotic states: catalepsy, lethargy, and somnambulism, he proposed the experimental use of hypnotism to replicate hysterical stigmata. Other demonstrations involved the removal of hysterical signs and their transfer from one side of the body to the other, or even between hypnotized subjects. These clinical experiments indicated that hysteria derived from pathogenic ideas. Hypnotism, Charcot believed, was an artificially produced equivalent of hysteria. The mechanisms of each were analogous; in one process, the hypnotist/experimenter implanted ideas, whereas in hysteria, the patient's own mental processes acted. Indeed, Charcot held that only hysterics could be hypnotized.

Charcot made hypnotism a respectable scientific procedure in much the same way as he made hysteria a legitimate disease. Largely on the basis of this work, the Academy of Sciences elected him to membership in 1883. In so doing, the Academy reversed its long-held position that hypnotism was outside the realm of science. Confident that he now had a technique for investigating mental pathology, Charcot resumed his lessons on hysteria. During the 1880s, he developed the theory that psychological trauma was the most frequent precipitating cause (agent provocateur) of hysteria. Patients who had escaped railway or workplace accidents or other perceived trauma with slight injuries or no visible wounds at all sometimes developed hysterical paralysis or other stigmata days or weeks later. Many victims were working-class males, including robust artisans and construction workers, a type of individual who contrasted sharply with the women, effeminate men, and children commonly associated with hysteria in the popular and medical literature, including Charcot's earlier publications.

Charcot's work on cerebral localization and aphasia (language disorders) in the mid-1880s contributed to his psychological theory of hysteria. Affirming that psychology ultimately was reducible to cerebral physiology, he attributed hysterical mutism, for example, to dysfunction in the center for spoken language. Charcot's aspirations for an objective psychology, informed by pathology, led him to accept the honorary Presidency of the Société de psychologie physiologique founded in Paris in 1885. Influenced by the psychologist Théodule Ribot and by his own student, Pierre Janet, and others, he extended his concept of hysteria to more complex phenomena, including cases of doubling of the personality, amnesia, and fugue (unconscious wandering). Toward the end of his career, Charcot pointed to an important etiological role for purely emotional trauma, notably nightmares, in triggering hysteria.

Disease Theory and Therapy

Charcot strongly believed hereditary defects to be the underlying cause of neurological and rheumatologic disease. Taken collectively these chronic ailments formed two 'families' of interchangeable diseases, the predisposition to which was transmitted through families of patients. Thus a patient might inherit a predisposition toward a given disease from a parent or close relative with the same disease (similar heredity). More often, the predisposition might result in a different disease in the offspring (dissimilar heredity). Charcot viewed chronic diseases in universalistic terms, as existing throughout history, in all places, and among all peoples. Nonetheless he held that Jews displayed a particular predisposition to nervous and arthritic diseases.

Charcot's hereditary determinism gave scientific expression to a certain fatalism, doubtless related to the incurable and inexorable course of most organic neurological diseases. But he was not a therapeutic nihilist. He had recourse to hydrotherapy and electrotherapy as well as a wide range of drugs. He sent patients to spas, notably Lamalou-les-bains in the Languedoque, which specialized in the treatment of locomotor ataxia, and to which Charcot referred his friend, the writer Alphonse Daudet. He did not hesitate to experiment with novel, sometimes radical, therapies; for example, he adopted the Russian treatment of locomotor ataxia, suspending patients in a harness to exert traction on the spinal cord.

Charcot recommended isolation for cases of hysteria and neurasthenia; he noted several cures of anorexia in children whom he separated from their families. He also referred these kinds of patients to maisons de santé (private asylums). Charcot avoided hypnotic therapy, which he considered potentially dangerous. But he did practice moral (psychological) therapy in the form of asserting authoritarian persuasion. In his final year, Charcot wrote an essay for the general public in which he acknowledged the efficacy of religious healing. *La foi qui guérit* [The Faith Cure] (1892) attributed miracle cures primarily to the patients' own autosuggestion. Charcot did not explicitly refer to the popular sanctuary at Lourdes, but he was known to recommend a pilgrimage there for pious patients with intractable nervous disorders.

Fame

'People had come to realize that the activities of this man were a part of the assets of the nation's "gloire"' (Freud, 1893, p. 16).

During the 1880s, Charcot became a medical celebrity owing as much to the cultural milieu as to his medical achievements. Contemporaries invoked his name second only to Pasteur's among the reigning 'princes of science'. He enjoyed international recognition as the premier French clinician of the day; few if any rivals equaled during their lifetimes the prestige accorded Charcot by contemporaries. Consulted in private practice by patients around the world, Charcot's worldly success was reflected in his mansion on the Boulevard Saint Germain, where he and Madame Charcot hosted Tuesday soirées, the social pendant to his morning hospital lessons, attended, as were the lessons, by scientific and artistic elite as well as by colleagues and students.

Charcot's original contributions to neuropathology ensured his scientific stature. He personified a clinical and anatomical tradition, now in decline, which had during the first half of the century, made Paris the leading center for medical studies. In an era of nascent medical specialization, Charcot helped create a new hospital-based discipline, thus retaining, at least in the field of neurology, France's claim to leadership. His Salpêtrière school formed an outstanding cadre of French neurologists, and attracted foreigners from all over Europe, Russia, and the American continents. Many went on to distinguished careers, and trained, in their turn, the younger generation of neurologists well into the twentieth century.

His work on hysteria accounted for Charcot's wider cultural resonance beyond medicine. The hysteria diagnosis proved congenial to the secularizing agenda of the French Third Republic. Not content with a medical reading of contemporary cultural malaise, the Salpêtrière school retrospectively diagnosed demoniacal possession, witchcraft, religious convulsions and ecstasies, miracle cures, and the like as expressions of individual and epidemic hysteria. 'Stigmata', in the language of the physicians referred to signs of hysteria rather than miraculous replications of the wounds of the crucified Christ. Reducing phenomena, traditionally interpreted in supernatural terms, to positivist scientific explanation, Charcot's school provided discrete, but potent, support to Republican anticlericalism. Salpêtrière doctrine on hysteria found an echo in anticlerical novels like Emile Zola's *Lourdes* (1894), and Jules Claretie, another popular writer, simply appropriated the venue of the Salpêtrière (including Charcot's own name) and the theme of hysteria for his potboiler *Les Amours d'un Interne* (1881).

Awakening scientific interest in parapsychology and spiritualism, popular fascination with the supernatural, and simply fashionable curiosity drew journalists, literary and artistic figures, as well as medical onlookers to Charcot's public lessons on hypnotism and hysteria. This audience appreciated the theatrical aspects, the dramatic *mise en scène* presided over by Charcot, ably assisted by his senior staff. Sometimes, as in the famous group portrait presented at the Paris salon of 1887, the clinical lesson featured partially clad female hysterics. (The statuesque Blanche Wittman, depicted in the painting and in Salpêtrière photographs, was a frequent subject.) Here the sensational, the occult, and the erotic vied for attention. Ironically, these were the very aspects of hysteria that Charcot sought to demystify in the name of science. Admirers hailed him as a modern magus bravely exploring unknown mental terrain; detractors, including the Church, feminists, and authors of the caliber of Guy de Maupassant and Tolstoy, denounced the Salpêtrière lessons as dangerous, scandalous exhibitions. In either case, their notoriety was ensured.

Charcot's lessons on hysteria reached a peak in popularity with the general public at a time when his account of the ailment began to be challenged by his colleagues. Medical critics, beginning with Hippolyte Bernheim of Nancy, pointed out that the stages of hypnotism, in particular, and hysteria, as defined by the Salpêtrière school, did not appear elsewhere. They were cultural artifacts, likely the product of unintended suggestion acting upon susceptible patients who complied, unconsciously or not, with the expectations of Charcot and his assistants. Further, it was alleged that Charcot exaggerated the diagnosis of hysteria to the point where he perceived hysterical counterparts to almost all organic diseases. By the time of his death, most authorities, aside from his immediate entourage, had doubts about Charcot's conception of hysteria. Within a few years, Joseph Babinski, a former chief resident and active supporter, dismantled the elaborate taxonomy of hysterical symptomatolgy. Nonetheless Charcot's psychological formulation of hysteria would provide the point of departure for both Janet's and Freud's theories of psychopathology.

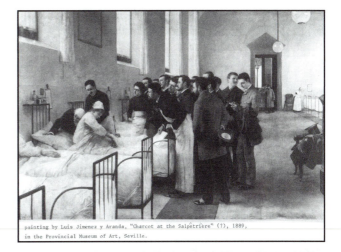

painting by Luis Jimenez y Aranda, "Charcot at the Salpêtrière" (?), 1889, in the Provincial Museum of Art, Seville.

Jean-Martin Charcot examines a patient at the Salpêtrière, Paris, 1889. From an oil painting by Luis Jimenez y Aranda, Wellcome Library, London.

Charcot died suddenly of congestive heart failure while on vacation with several colleagues in 1893. His marriage in 1864 to Augustine Victoire Durvis née Laurent, a wealthy widow, produced a daughter and son. The son, Jean-Baptiste, after completing medical studies—he served as his father's last intern—went on to a famous career as a polar explorer.

The dominant figure in late nineteenth-century French medicine, Charcot personified the ascendancy of the physician as cultural icon. Granted privileged access to the psyche, the image of the medical man replaced that of the priest in a secularizing society. As for Charcot's personal style, he was considered cold, authoritarian, even malevolent by professional rivals and enemies, while his many acolytes described him as a charismatic leader and teacher.

A statue of Charcot stood at the entrance to the Salpêtrière until, along with many others, it was melted down for scrap metal by the Vichy regime. Today, a large section of the vast hospital's grounds bears the name 'quartier Charcot'. His extensive personal library and papers are preserved for scholars. Remembered by neurologists as a founding figure, Charcot's work on hysteria remains a fertile source for historians of culture. Despite the eclipse of his theories and terminology, the phenomena Charcot observed are still seen and remain puzzling for neuroscientists and practicing neurologists.

Bibliography

Primary: 1877–90. *Oeuvres completes* 9 vols. (Paris) [English translations of vols. 1–4, 7]; 1887–89. *Leçons du mardi* 2 vols. (Paris) [English translation of selections. Edited by C. G. Goetz, 1987 (New York)]; 1892–93. *Clinique des maladies du système nerveux* 2 vols. (Paris); 1984. (with Richer, Paul) *Les démoniaques dans l'art* (1887) and *La foi qui guérit* (1892) [Reprint with introduction by Georges Didi-Huberman (Paris)].

Secondary: Goetz, Christopher G., Michel Bonduelle, and Toby Gel-fand, 1995. *Charcot. Constructing Neurology* (New York and Oxford); Harris, Ruth, 1991. 'Introduction' to *Clinical Lectures on Diseases of the Nervous System* by J.-M. Charcot, trans. Thomas Savill (London) pp. ix–lxviii; Micale, Mark, 1990. 'Charcot and the Idea of Hysteria in the Male: Gender, Mental Science and Medical Diagnosis in Late Nineteenth-Century France.' *Medical History* 34: 363–411; Goldstein, Jan, 1982. 'The Hysteria Diagnosis and the Politics of Anticlericalism in Late Nineteenth-Century France.' *Journal of Modern History* 54: 209–239; Freud, Sigmund, 1893. 'Charcot' in The *Standard Edition of the Complete Psychological Works*, 1966 (London). trans. and edited by James Strachey. vol. 3, pp. 7–23; *DSB*.

Toby Gelfand

CHARNLEY, JOHN (b. Bury, Lancashire, England, 29 August 1911; d. Manchester, England, 5 August 1982), *orthopedics.*

The son of a pharmacist father and a nurse mother, Charnley first chose dentistry as a career after finishing his grammar school education in Bury. Persuaded to read medicine instead, he graduated from Manchester University in 1932 with a BSc in anatomy and physiology. Three years later he gained his MB ChB, and in 1936 became FRCS. He became CBE in 1970 and, in 1975, became the first practicing orthopedic surgeon to be elected to a Fellow of the Royal Society. In 1977 he was knighted. Affable and outgoing, Charnley married late in life, to Jill Margaret Heaver, whom he met on a skiing holiday in Austria in 1957 and with whom he had two children.

Charnley had little thought of orthopedics until some years after qualifying. In April 1939 he became the resident casualty officer at the Manchester Royal Infirmary, where his responsibilities included the daily fracture clinic for outpatients. The post brought him into contact with one of the leading orthopedists and architects of the modern specialism, Sir Harry Platt (1886–1986). But it was only after August 1940 that he was more fully enrolled: Platt was then searching for medical officers for the military hospital at Davyhulme on the outskirts of Manchester, and Charnley (back in Manchester and depressed by his RAMC experience at Dunkirk) was available. Confirmation in the specialism occurred still later, when he was posted to No. 2 Orthopaedic Centre, Cairo, in 1941.

When he returned to Manchester after the war, Charnley obtained temporary attachments to the children's orthopedic hospitals at Oswestry and Biddulph Grange. For these appointments he was indebted to Platt, as for the 1946 appointment as lecturer in orthopedic surgery at the Manchester Medical School. In 1947 he was made visiting orthopedic surgeon to Park Hospital, Davyhulme, and to the Wrightington Hospital, Wigan, where his major biomechanical research was conducted in the 1960s. In 1947 he was also appointed assistant orthopedic surgeon to the Manchester Royal Infirmary, rising to full consultant in 1952.

From the early 1940s Charnley contributed to orthopedic literature, but it was his *The Closed Treatment of Common Fracture* (1950) that launched his reputation worldwide as an experience-based therapeutic innovator, experimentalist, and imaginative researcher who drew effectively on concepts from engineering. These were also the qualities that marked his work at the center for hip surgery that he established at Wrightington in 1961, where he came to concentrate all his (considerable) energies. It was here that he carried out careful studies of the biomechanics of hip-joint movement, the lubrication of joints, methods of fixing metal and plastic to bone, and not least, the prior causes of failure in hip-joint replacement operations. Ever single-minded in problem solving, Charnley perfected the materials necessary for, and the clean-air operating enclosure in which successfully to perform, total hip replacement. The former involved close cooperation with the surgical equipment company, Charles F. Thackray, whereas the latter involved Howorth Air Engineering. His first hip replacement was performed at the King Edward VII Hospital, Midhurst, Sussex, in 1969; by 1982 he had performed 1,400 such operations there.

Charnley succeeded Platt in the making of modern orthopedics, as Platt succeeded Sir Robert Jones, but he was never their political successor. Always more interested in perfecting technology than playing professional politics, his place in history lies above all with his perfecting the technology and techniques for hip replacement.

Bibliography

Primary: 1950. *The Closed Treatment of Common Fracture* (Edinburgh, 2nd edn., 1957, 3rd edn., 1961); 1961. 'Arthroplasty of the Hip: A New Operation.' *Lancet* i: 1129–1132; 1972. 'The Long-Term Results of Low-Friction Arthroplasty of the Hip Performed as a Primary Intervention.' reprinted (1995) in *Clinical Orthopaedics and Related Research* 319: 4–15.

Secondary: Waugh, William, 1990. *John Charnley: The Man and the Hip* (London); Platt, H. P., 1985. 'Sir John Charnley' in Elwood, W. J., and A. F. Tuxford, eds., *Some Manchester Doctors* (Manchester); Nisbet, N. W., and M. Woodruff, 1984. *Biographical Memoirs of Fellows of the Royal Society* 30: 117–137; *Oxford DNB*; *Plarr's Lives*.

Roger Cooter

CHAULIAC, GUY DE (aka GUIGO DE CHAULHACO, GUIDO DE CAULIACO, GUIGONIS DE CAULHIACO, DE CAULIACE) (b. Chauliac, France, *c.* 1300; d. Avignon, France, late July 1368), *medicine, surgery.*

Guy was born in Chauliac, a village in the Gévaudan, in south-central France, probably in the final years of the thirteenth century. According to legend, the son of peasants, Guy was assisted in his studies by the lords of Mercœur. In 1890 Nicaise, Guy's definitive biographer, admitted that there might be some basis for believing these lords assisted

Guy, particularly as Guy maintained a relationship with the family throughout his life. After studying at Toulouse, Guy went to Montpellier, where he studied under Raymond de Molières, probably in the 1320s. Guy received his title of *magister* in medicine at Montpellier, and it was with the teaching at Montpellier that he identified himself in his writings, particularly when comparing the procedures taught at Paris and Montpellier. From Montpellier Guy went to Bologna, where he studied anatomy with Niccolò Betruccio (a student of Mondino de' Liuzzi) and Alberto de Zancariis. He was briefly in Paris before settling in Lyon— as a physician, not a surgeon—sometime before 1344. In his *Inventarium*, Guy described himself as *cyrurgicus, magister in medicina*, surgeon and master in medicine; he was identified in charters from Saint-Just and in papal bulls as *physicus*. By 1348, Guy was in Avignon. He was the physician to three successive popes: Clement VI (1342–52), Innocent VI (1352–62), and Urban V (1362–70). A cleric from 1325, Guy was named the prévôt of the chapter of Saint-Just in Lyon in 1359; before then he had been a canon and held a prebend from the chapter at Reims. Guy was also a canon of the diocese of Mende. Several papal bulls refer to him as the papal capellanus (chaplain), implying that he might have been a fully ordained priest, though occasionally this title was honorific. His death date has been a matter of debate. At the end of April 1367, when Urban VI left for Rome, Guy was alive but unable to accompany him. When Urban returned to Avignon in September 1370, Guy was dead. A document from Lozère, identified by Nicaise, gives 23 July 1368 as the date of Guy's death. Nicaise presented several other records indicating Guy died later in July 1368. Records from 1369 describe Guy's nephew Étienne as donating toward anniversary commemorations of Guy's death. It seems safe to say that Guy died in 1368, probably in late July.

Four works are attributed to Guy: the *Inventory or Collection of Surgical Medicine* (given the title *The Great Surgery* by Renaissance editors and referred to here as the *Surgical Medicine*) and three smaller treatises, one each on astrology, cataracts, and hernias. Guy refers to the latter three within his *Surgical Medicine*. The treatises on cataracts and hernias have been lost; a manuscript of the astrology treatise was located in 1907. The work known as the *Little Surgery*, previously attributed to Guy, is actually a poor compilation of sections of his *Surgical Medicine*. Guy completed the *Surgical Medicine* in 1363 while living in Avignon; Nicaise claimed that he was no longer practicing medicine when he wrote the text. Guy himself wrote that it was done 'for the comfort of old age'. The *Surgical Medicine* was composed in Latin, but quickly translated into numerous vernacular languages, many before 1500. Nicaise identified twenty-two Latin manuscripts of the text as well as two in Provençal, four in French, three in English, and one each in Italian, Hebrew, and Dutch. Guy's most recent editor and biographer, Michael McVaugh identified another

English translation. Sixty printed editions were identified by Nicaise, the first a 1478 French translation by Nicolas Panis in Lyon. Laurent Joubert published the most influential of the Renaissance editions in 1579. This edition included a modernized Latin text, a French translation, and Joubert's identification of Guy's sources, notes, and indices. The text of *Surgical Medicine* had a long life; it was the authoritative surgical manual until the time of Amboise Paré (1510–90), went through at least seventeen editions in the seventeenth century, and was at its apex in the sixteenth century with at least thirty-eight editions.

Evidence for Guy's scholastic medical background is found throughout the *Surgical Medicine*. There are frequent references to other authors, particularly the Arabic authorities of Avicenna (Ibn Sīnā), Albucasis (Al-Zahrāwī), Rhazes (Al-Rāzī), and Haly Abbas (Al-Majūsī). McVaugh identified fifty authors to whom Guy referred, as well as procedures used by another dozen or so contemporaries. Guy would have been familiar with many of the authors from his studies at Montpellier and Paris, and his position at the papal court provided him with access to the latest translations. He referred to the works translated by Nicolas de Reggio in the first section of the *Surgical Medicine*. Margaret Ogden identified thirty-six Galenic works on anatomy, therapy, and pharmacology from which Guy drew; these included all of the major Galenic works translated into Latin before 1363. In the case of several works, Guy used multiple translations, from Arabic and Greek. Further evidence of his scholastic background is found in the style of the *Surgical Medicine*. Although Guy proclaimed the work to be a compilation, it was actually a scholastic analysis, which brought together various sources, with differing opinions, and attempted to reconcile them using methods drawn from the faculties of universities. Medical theory permeates the work, which fits into the learned surgical tradition in which Guy saw himself and also belongs to the more theory-based world of medicine at the universities. Guy was the last in a line of surgico-medical authors, such as William of Saliceto, Lanfranc of Milan, and Henry of Mondeville, who wrote trying to combine medicine and surgery.

The *Surgical Medicine* is divided into seven treatises, preceded by a prologue and a section containing a history of surgery in which Guy laid out his beliefs in a progressive development, culminating in his own work. Guy's formulation is still popular in current scholarship. Guy listed the four characteristics of a good surgeon, attributing them to Arnald of Vilanova: the surgeon must be educated, skilled, ingenious, and well behaved. As surgery is the third instrument of medicine, the surgeon must know the principles of medicine in order to practice surgery. The surgeon must know the naturals, the non-naturals, and the contra-naturals. Anatomy is the most important of the naturals. Guy also prescribed correct behavior for the patients and the doctor's assistants. The patient must obey the doctor, believe in the doctor, and be patient. The doctor's assistants must be peaceable, agreeable, faithful, and discreet.

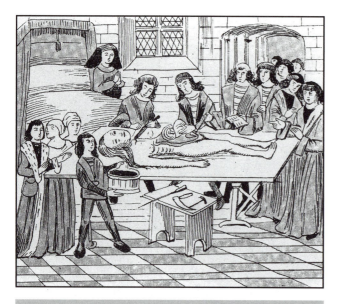

Autopsy of a woman in a bed chamber. Woodcut from *La grande chirurgie* . . . Tournon, 1611. Rare Books, Wellcome Library, London.

After the prologue and the section on the history of surgery, Guy included a list of the seven books and the various chapters of which they were composed. The first book or treatise of the *Surgical Medicine* deals with anatomy; there is no evidence that Guy participated in anatomical dissections. Guy based his discussion of anatomy on Galen's *On the usefulness of the parts of the human body*. The second book considers abscesses, ulcers, and pustules; it includes, in chapter five, his description of the 'great and unheard of mortality' which swept through Avignon in 1348 and 1360—the Black Death. Guy is most famous for this discussion of the plague.

He identified two forms of this plague, which 'affected the whole world'. The first version came at the beginning of the epidemics, involved bloody expectoration, and resulted in death within three days. The second version produced abscesses and buboes. The reaction of the people to the plague caused Guy to bemoan that 'Charity was dead, hope destroyed'. He argued that there were two causes of the plague: the universal cause was the heavenly conjunction of Saturn, Jupiter, and Mars in 1345; the particular cause was the disposition of the body of the patient. Guy himself suffered from and survived the plague in 1348. According to his own account, fear of infamy if he left his patients kept him in Avignon during the outbreaks. In 1360, he prepared a theriac based on recommendations taken from Arnald of Vilanova and the masters at Montpellier and Paris. Book III deals with wounds, including diets for those suffering from wounds. Book IV is on ulcers. Book V concerns fractures and dislocations. Book VI is on 'diseases which are not abscesses, nor ulcers, nor to do with bones' but which should be brought to a surgeon. Book VII is an antidotary including about 750

medical substances. Within each of the books, Guy included surgical and medical treatments, even describing the instruments that the practitioner should use.

Nicaise's French translation of the *Surgical Medicine* is based on Joubert's French translation of the Renaissance edition of the Latin text. The text was reworked to such an extent that Nicaise wrote, 'This is no longer Guy de Chauliac'. McVaugh's edition is based on a text found at the Vatican, which was completed in Montpellier in 1373, that is, within ten years of Guy's original composition. Björn Wallner has edited the first four books of the *Surgical Medicine* as well as the history of medicine section in five volumes based primarily on a Middle English manuscript located at the New York Academy of Medicine.

Bibliography

Primary: 1890. *La Grande Chirurgie* (introduction, translation, and commentary by E. Nicaise) (Paris); 1997. *Inventarium sive Chirurgia Magna. Vol. I: Text.* (McVaugh, Michael, ed.) *Vol. II: Commentary* (McVaugh, Michael, and Margaret Ogden, eds.) (Leiden).

Secondary: Wickersheimer, Ernest, and Danielle Jacquart 1979. *Dictionnaire Biographique des Médecins en France au Moyen Âge.* Nouv. édition, (Geneva) pp. 214–215; Ogden, Margaret, 1973. 'The Galenic Works Cited in Guy de Chauliac's *Chirurgia magna*.' *Journal of the History of Medicine and Allied Sciences* 28(1): 24–31; Gurlt, Ernst, 1964. *Geschichte der Chirurgie und Ihrer Ausübung: Volkschirurgie, Altertum, Mittelalter, Renaissance.* Vol. II. (Hildesheim) pp. 77–109; Mondor, Henri, 1949. 'Guy de Chauliac, 1300?–1370?' *Anatomistes et Chirurgiens.* (Paris) pp. 3–49; Nixon, J. A., 1907. 'Guy de Chauliac: A New MS. including the "*Practica Astrolabii*".' *Janus* 12(1): 1–6; *DSB*.

Michelle Garceau

CHÁVEZ SÁNCHEZ, IGNACIO (b. Zirándaro, Michoacán, Mexico, 31 January 1897; d. Mexico City, Mexico, 12 July 1979), *cardiology*.

Chávez said he had modeled his own biography. During the prime of his career he took advantage of his family and social circumstances during the era known as the 'Mexican miracle', a time of great economic and cultural development in Mexico. He was the fifth of ten children of a prosperous liberal merchant in a small Michoacán town who gave his offspring an excellent education by sending them to study in Morelia, the capital and an important late-nineteenth century cultural center.

Chávez studied at the Colegio de San Nicolás de Hidalgo, a unique institution in Mexico that inculcated in its students moral values, self-esteem, and group solidarity, providing solid training in science and the humanities. Chávez's friends from that period became intellectual and political leaders in Mexico. He graduated as a physician from the National University of Mexico and went to Paris, where he specialized in cardiology with Henry Vaquez and Charles Laubry (1926–27), also studying in Berlin, Prague, Vienna, Rome, and Brussels.

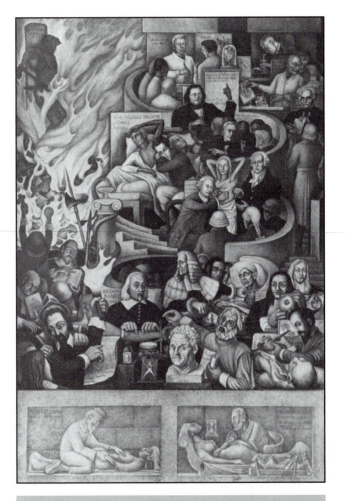

The history of cardiology. Mural painting by Diego Rivera in the Instituto Nacional de Cardiología, Mexico City, 1943. Wellcome Library, London.

He created the Mexican School of Cardiology, which was important nationally and internationally in the mid-twentieth century, and founded and directed the first cardiology service at the Hospital General, though his greatest merit was creating the National Institute of Cardiology in 1944, where he served as Director for many years. The Institute became an outstanding facility in cardiology and has maintained its prestige, due to its combination of medical care, basic research, and socio-medicine in cardiology. It also attracted as researchers first-class scientists, such as Arturo Rosenblueth, who worked for fourteen years with Walter B. Cannon at Harvard University. Chávez created and presided over several associations: the Mexican Cardiology Society, the Inter-American Cardiology Society, and the International Cardiology Society (1946), of which he became lifelong Honorary President in 1962. He founded and directed the Latin American Cardiology and Hematology Archives (1930) and the Archives of the Mexican Cardiology Institute (1944).

He was Director of the Hospital General, an important institution in Mexico because of its historical tradition and because medical specializations emerged there. Chávez modernized it and created a program for 'Hospital Physicians'. He wanted to make the hospital functional and pleasant for patients and doctors, to organize medical archives, and encourage clinical and basic research.

Chávez served as Rector of the University in his home state of Michoacán and as Director of the National Faculty (School) of Medicine. In the early 1960s, he was named Rector of the National University of Mexico. As in other areas of the world, this was an epoch of social conflict in Mexico, and Chávez had to confront serious problems with students that were a result of reforms he made in the programs of study and because he stiffened the rules for admission and continuation, all measures designed to improve the quality of instruction.

Chávez was President of the National Academy of Medicine. With distinguished Mexican intellectuals he founded the Colegio Nacional (1943). A member of the Consultative Committee of the WHO and the OAS, he imparted numerous courses and conferences in Mexico and abroad and was an honorary member of eighteen cardiologic and thirty-three scientific societies. He received twenty-one Doctorates Honoris Causa, was a corresponding or honorary member of fourteen academies of medicine, and received thirty-one decorations from foreign countries and eight in Mexico. A born leader, Chávez promoted the modernization of Mexican medicine. Universally respected as a teacher and creator of institutions, his success came from a fortunate conjunction of a historical moment with a man of great intelligence and ambition, a forceful personality, and an excellent education, who surrounded himself with capable, loyal collaborators.

Bibliography

Primary: 1931. *Lecciones de clínica cardiológica* (Mexico); 1945. *Enfermedades del corazón, cirugía y embarazo* (Mexico); 1947. *México en la cultura médica* (Mexico).

Secondary: Romo Medrano, Estela, 1997. *Un relato biográfico: Ignacio Chávez, rector de la UNAM* (Mexico).

Ana Cecilia Rodríguez de Romo

CHEN, SU LAN (b. Fuzhou, China, 13 February 1885; d. Singapore, 6 May 1972), *general practice, public health, politics.*

Chen Su Lan was born in the Chinese province of Fuzhou to a widowed mother, who was a devout Methodist. He spent his formative years in the Anglo-Chinese College in Fuzhou before pursing his medical education in Singapore, the key port city and administrative capital in British Malaya. He was among the first graduates of the King Edward VII College of Medicine, established in 1905. Considered the genesis of university education in Singapore, the college was the product of generous financial support of the Chinese merchant community in the British colony.

Aside from his private medical practice as a general practitioner, Chen also served on committees of several institutions in the colonial medical services: the Tan Tock Seng Hospital, the Central Midwives Board, and the Council of the King Edward VII College of Medicine. He was subsequently elected President of the Malayan Branch of the British Medical Association. His legacy as a health reformer became more visible in the late 1920s when he began to make public his views of the problems of diseases and poverty in the colony of Singapore. In his writings and lectures to both professional and public forums, Chen was instrumental in linking the surge in tuberculosis in Singapore with that of opium consumption and overcrowded and filthy living conditions in the city.

Complementing his words were also concrete actions on establishing the Anti-Opium Clinic in Singapore in 1933, a rehabilitation center to supplement its oversubscribed counterparts in government hospitals. A nonprofit body reliant on donations and token charges for patients, Chen declared that the spirit of the clinic would be 'charity to all and malice towards none'. Within a year, it catered to over 2,000 cases from all ethnic groups, cases that Chen claimed were regarded as hopeless by modern Western doctors and traditional healers. A more controversial stance taken by Chen was on the issue of public policy toward venereal diseases. Siding with the religious factions and temperance movements, Chen argued that the toleration of brothels and the compulsory medical examination of prostitutes were counterproductive and immoral.

The Japanese occupation in Malaya (1942–45) disrupted Chen's campaigns. After the war, Chen served briefly on the Advisory Council of the British Military Administration in Malaya. His crusades against opium and venereal diseases were superseded, however, by philanthropy when he founded the Chinese Young Men's Christian Association in 1945, a reformatory for juvenile delinquents. He subsequently established the Chen Su Lan Trust in 1947, which disbursed funds to Christian organizations. In 1968 the Wesley Methodist Church in Singapore established the Chen Su Lan Methodist Children's Home to provide for disadvantaged children. The purchase of land and the building of the Home were financed by the Chen Su Lan Trust. By this time Chen, in retirement, was turning toward theological issues. Even though he was away from the public limelight, Chen's contributions were continuously acknowledged. His alma mater conferred the Honorary Degree of Letters of Law (LLD) upon him in 1952.

Chen passed away on 6 May 1972, his funeral attended by about 500 people. As his obituary in the local newspaper two days later stated: 'His name will deservedly find a place in Singapore's history.' Chen was given a special mention as a member of the pioneering generation of medical personalities in the Centenary of the Medical Faculty of the National University of Singapore in October 2005.

Bibliography

Primary: 5 November 1931. 'Opium Smoking and Tuberculosis' *Straits Times* (Singapore); 1935. *The Opium Problem in British Malaya* (Singapore); 6 February 1941. 'No Brothels without Disease' *Straits Times* (Singapore); 1955. *Is Jonah a Myth?* (Singapore); 1958. *Is Lot's Wife a Myth?* (Singapore); 1969. *Remembering Pompong and Oxley Drive* (Singapore).

Secondary: Cheah, J. S., and B. Y. Ng, 2005. 'Centenary of the Faculty of Medicine, National University of Singapore and the National University of Singapore (1905-2005)' *Annals* 34(6): 1–3; Cheah, J. S., 2005. 'The First Graduates of 1910' *Annals* 34(6): 20–24C; Ho Tat Ming, 2000. *Doctors Extraordinaire* (Malaysia); Chen Su Lan Methodist Children's Home: http://www.cslmch.org.sg/our_history.htm

Kai Khiun Liew

CHESELDEN, WILLIAM (b. Somerby, Leicestershire, England, 19 October 1688; d. Bath, England, 10 April 1752), *anatomy, surgery.*

Cheslden was the third child and second son of George Cheselden, landowner and farmer, and his wife Deborah Hubbert. He probably attended the free grammar school in Leicester. At age fifteen he was apprenticed to James Ferne, surgeon for the stone at St Thomas's Hospital, London. He studied anatomy under William Cowper (1666/7–1710), with whom he lived. Cheselden passed the final examination of the Barber-Surgeon's Company on 29 January 1711. He remained extremely active in this company throughout his life and was at the forefront of the formation of the Company of Surgeons in 1745. In 1713 he married Deborah Knight (d. 1754), with whom he had a daughter Willhelmina.

Cheselden was the most successful exploiter of the space for a private anatomy and surgery course in early eighteenth-century London. Still young, and while there was no significant competition (the Barber-Surgeons' Company offered next to nothing in the way of teaching), he launched his distinguished career as surgeon, anatomical investigator, and teacher with a Latin abstract of his lectures in 1711. Clearly the way forward was in the vernacular, and in 1713 he published his immensely successful student manual, *The Anatomy of the Humane Body*, a work reissued and republished many times (including posthumously). Later, his lecture course was given for twenty years at St Thomas's Hospital, where he was appointed assistant surgeon in 1718 and, within a year, a principal surgeon. He resigned his hospital posts in 1737 to become resident surgeon at the Royal Hospital, Chelsea.

Becoming a model for later anatomists, notably William Hunter (1718–83), once he had achieved success in popular lecturing and publishing, he moved on to producing sumptuous volumes for subscribers. The *Osteographia, or the Anatomy of the Bones*, appeared in 1733. This magnificent folio containing fifty-six plates was intended as part of a comprehensive publication on human and comparative anatomy. Later anatomists presumably also learned from Cheselden's mistakes because, in fact, the *Osteographia* was a financial disaster. He broke up the sets and offered the plates separately.

If anatomy publishing proved unprofitable, he made operating surgery very lucrative. From about 1720 on, Cheselden developed his own operation for the stone, lithotomy. The most common procedure at this time was the high or suprapubic operation, developed by a surgeon at the Westminster Infirmary, John Douglas (d. 1743). Cheselden at first used this approach but, stimulated by French and Dutch work, investigated the lateral perineal procedure, which he gradually modified. John Douglas's brother James recorded the history of Cheselden's development of the operation. Eventually Cheselden could remove a stone in less than a minute and his method (if not speed) became the standard in Britain until the end of the nineteenth century. In the sixth edition of his *Anatomy* of 1741 he recorded performing 213 public lithotomies in which there had been twenty deaths. Of these latter, some he attributed to smallpox or whooping cough. Besides his reputation as lithotomist he was also widely sought out as an eye surgeon. As a child Cheselden broke his arm. It was splinted by a bonesetter in a hard case of rags dipped in egg white and flour. Cheselden modified this treatment and used it in fractures and clubfoot correction.

Cheselden was one of those surgeons whose public life promoted the acceptance of the manual operator in genteel society. He moved freely in the elite world of Enlightenment London, his activities facilitated by his sociable disposition. He was made FRS in 1711. He communicated an important paper in 1728 on a boy born blind that he couched (operated on) to restore his sight. He was a friend of Alexander Pope (1688–1744) and Sir Hans Sloane (1660–1753), and he attended Sir Isaac Newton near his death (1642–1727). In 1727 he was appointed surgeon to Queen Caroline (1683–1737). He had his portrait painted by Sir Godfrey Kneller (1722).

Bibliography

Primary: 1711. *Syllabus sive Index humani corporis partium anatomicus* (London); 1713. *The Anatomy of the Humane Body* (London); 1733. *Osteographia, or the Anatomy of the Bones* (London).

Secondary: Cope, Zachary, 1953. *William Cheselden, 1688–1752* (Edinburgh); Douglas, James, 1731. *An Appendix to the History of the Lateral Operation for the Stone* (London); *Oxford DNB*.

Christopher Lawrence

CHEYNE, GEORGE (b. Methlick, Scotland, 1671/2, baptized 24 February 1673; d. Bath, England, 13 April 1743), *medicine, nervous diseases.*

Cheyne was the son of James Cheyne, a tenant farmer; nothing is known of his mother. He attended Marischal College, Aberdeen, but left without a degree. In Edinburgh by 1699, he studied medicine with the Jacobite physician and iatromechanist Archibald Pitcairne (1652–1713). Cheyne's *New Theory of Fevers* (1701) defended Pitcairne's views; Cheyne declared that Newtonian natural philosophy would form the basis for a new system of medicine.

On 8 September 1701, with Pitcairne's sponsorship, Cheyne obtained his MD from King's College, Aberdeen, and moved to London, where he was elected FRS on 18 March 1702. He added a fuller account of Newtonian medical theory to the second edition of his *New Theory of Fevers* (1702) and appeared to establish himself as one of Newton's many acolytes at the Royal Society. But Cheyne did not succeed in establishing a medical practice.

Following the publication of his *Philosophical Principles of Natural Religion* (1705), Cheyne suffered a physical and emotional collapse and returned to Scotland. According to the autobiographical 'Case of the Author' appended to *The English Malady* (1733), he healed his body by a rigorous diet but healed his mind only by turning to religion.

He re-emerged to the public in 1715 with his *Philosophical Principles of Religion, Natural and Revealed*, emphasizing revelation over reason. Meanwhile he married Margaret Middleton of Aberdeen and established a medical practice in London and Bath. He moved to Bath with his wife and three children in 1718.

There he turned to writing popular medical works. His *Essay on Gout* (1720) established a pattern of practical advice coupled with moral exhortation. His audience, the upper classes frequenting Bath, suffered mainly from diseases of overindulgence. *An Essay of Health and Long Life* (1724) reached a seventh edition within a year. Organized around the Galenic 'six non-naturals', it emphasized diet and evacuations and their relationship to the passions. Failure to maintain one's own health was a sin; moderation in food and drink was the key to health. Diet and attention to spiritual needs could regulate the passions; uncontrolled, they would damage the nervous system.

He spoke as a fellow-sufferer, for in the 1720s his weight, always a problem, rose to thirty-two stone (448 pounds), and his health declined. *An Essay of Health and Long Life* made Cheyne famous. *The English Malady* (1733) offered advice on melancholy and those diseases known as hypochondria or hysteria. Although sympathetic to his fellow-sufferers, Cheyne relentlessly attacked their self-indulgence. He explained that melancholy centered in the fluids and fibers of the body, which a proper diet and moderate exercise could revive.

Letters from the 1730s to the novelist Samuel Richardson (1689–1761) and to the Countess of Huntingdon display Cheyne's methods. His final work, *The Natural Method* (1742), restated his therapeutic ideas, addressing women in particular. According to preformation theory, females contributed only nutrition to the fetus. Because women were weaker in body than men and more susceptible to luxury, they needed to be especially vigilant in regimen.

Cheyne's ideas about nervous function influenced David Hartley (1705–57) and Robert Whytt (1714–66), but did not long survive him. His works on regimen, however, were reprinted well into the nineteenth century and influenced many dietary reformers. John Wesley's (1703–91) popular *Primitive Physick* (1747) borrowed heavily from Cheyne and brought his ideas to another audience.

In the spring of 1743, he fell ill and died at Bath on 13 April. His wife and children survived him.

Bibliography

Primary: 1715. *Philosophical Principles of Religion, Natural and Revealed* (London); 1724. *An Essay of Health and Long Life* (London); 1733. *The English Malady* (London).

Secondary: Guerrini, Anita, 2000. *Obesity and Depression in the Enlightenment: The Life and Times of George Cheyne* (Norman, OK); Shuttleton, David E., 1992. 'My Own Crazy Carcase: The Life and Works of Dr George Cheyne, 1672–1743.' PhD thesis, University of Edinburgh; Rousseau, G. S., 1988. 'Mysticism and Millenarianism: "Immortal Dr Cheyne"' in Popkin, Richard, ed., *Millenarianism and Messianism in English Literature and Thought, 1650–1800* (Leiden) pp. 81–126; *DSB*; *Oxford DNB*.

Anita Guerrini

CHEYNE, WILLIAM WATSON (b. off Tasmania, Australia, 14 December 1852; d. Holloway Sanatorium, Surrey, England, 19 April 1932), *surgery*.

Cheyne was the son of Andrew Cheyne and Eliza Watson and, after his mother died when he was four years of age, relatives on the Shetland Island of Fetlar brought him up. He was educated at Aberdeen grammar school and Edinburgh University, graduating MB and CM (1875). He was a keen sailor and hoped to obtain a post as a ship's surgeon, but as a prize-winning student he pursued a more ambitious path. After graduating, he studied in Vienna with Theodor Billroth (1829–94) and Friedrich von Recklinghausen (1833–1910) before returning to Edinburgh to become Joseph Lister's (1827–1912) house surgeon at the Royal Infirmary. In 1877 he gained a Syme Surgical Fellowship and became lecturer in anatomy at the University.

In the same year Lister was offered the Chair of Surgery at King's College, London, and Cheyne was chosen as one of four assistants to accompany him. Cheyne's career then stalled as metropolitan hostility to Listerian antiseptic methods meant that the group had few opportunities for clinical work. However, this gave him time to study and undertake research, enabling him to become FRCS in 1879 and gain the Jackson Prize for his dissertation on antiseptic surgery, which was the basis for his influential book *Antiseptic Surgery: Its Principles, Practice, History and Results* (1882).

Around this time his career took off due to the growing acceptance and adoption of antiseptic methods, hence in 1880 he was appointed assistant surgeon at King's and went on to be surgeon in 1887, professor of the principles and practice of surgery in 1891, and professor of clinical surgery in 1902. He was active in the RCS, as Hunterian Professor in 1892, giving the Bradshaw lecture in 1908, giving the Hunterian Oration in 1915, and serving as President 1914–16.

Cheyne was and is best known as Lister's assistant and the most effective propagandist of Listerian antiseptic surgery. His *Antiseptic Surgery* was the first systematic treatise on new methods and was followed up in 1885 by his *Manual of the Antiseptic Treatment of Wounds for Students and Practitioners*. He maintained the role of 'Lister's Bull Dog' over many years, later defending antisepsis against the challenges of aseptic methods, which he regarded as desirable in principle but unachievable in most surgical settings.

Cheyne also reformed surgical teaching at King's College by introducing the systematic use of microscopy. His work and publications in the new science of bacteriology aided the acceptance of antiseptic surgery but were also crucial in their own right as Cheyne was acknowledged as one of the founders of the discipline in Britain. Cheyne's command of German enabled him to keep up with Continental work, and he translated Robert Koch's (1843–1910) important *Investigations into the Etiology of Traumatic Diseases* (1880, London). He then played a vital role in the communication of Koch's work on tuberculosis and the role of the tubercle bacillus to British audiences, repeating Koch's investigations and publishing his results in 1883.

He continued to make available the most important foreign language studies of microorganisms in English, editing two collections in 1886 and 1889 and translating C. Flügge's textbook *Micro-organisms: with special reference to the etiology of infective disease* (1890, London). Cheyne was elected FRS in 1894 for his work on suppuration and sepsis. Throughout this period he supported the development of bacteriological teaching, laboratories, and research and advocated a greater role for experimental science in medicine.

From the 1890s to the 1920s, Cheyne was one of the leaders of British surgery, playing a prominent role in profession organizations, in metropolitan societies, and in wider civil society. In the South African War he was a civil consulting surgeon and received the CB. He was made a Baronet in 1908 when he was appointed Surgeon in Ordinary to the King and created KCMG for his services to the Navy in World War I. After his retirement from surgery in 1917 he held a number of civic offices, such as MP for the Universities of Edinburgh and St Andrews and representing the combined Scottish Universities from 1918 to 1922. After leaving Parliament, he retired to Leagarth in Shetland, though he continued in public service as Lord Lieutenant of Orkney and Shetland from 1919 to 1930.

Bibliography

Primary: 1882. *Antiseptic Surgery: Its Principles, Practice, History and Results* (London); 1883. 'Report to the AAMR on the Relation of Micro-Organisms to Tuberculosis.' *Practitioner* 30: 240–320; 1884. *Public Health Laboratory Work* (London); 1885. *The Antiseptic Treatment of Wounds* (London); 1886. *Recent Essays by Various Authors on Bacteria in Relation to Disease* (London); 1889. *Suppuration and Septic Diseases* (Edinburgh); 1894. *The Treatment of Wounds, Ulcers and Abscesses* (Edinburgh).

Secondary: Worboys, M., 2000. *Spreading Germs: Disease Theories and Medical Practice in Britain, 1865–1900* (Cambridge); *Oxford DNB*; *Plarr's Lives.*

Michael Worboys

CHIARUGI, VINCENZIO (b. Empoli, Tuscany, Italy, 20 February 1759; d. Florence, Italy, 22 December 1820), *psychiatry.*

Chiarugi, the son of Anton Gregorio Chiarugi, a physician, and Margherita Conti, graduated in medicine from the University of Pisa summa cum laude (1779) after completing a humanities education in Empoli. He later moved to the medical school of Florence (1779), gaining there a license to practice medicine. During his training, he was able to benefit from the rich and lively scientific tradition in Tuscany, promoted by the Grand Duke Leopold who attracted many famous physicians to his court.

In 1782 Chiarugi started working at the hospital of S. Maria Nuova as a staff physician, and six months later, he was promoted to chief physician for the men's section. In 1785 he became senior physician and began to work as a psychiatrist in the old and overcrowded hospital of S. Dorotea, which hosted the mentally ill. It was their dreadful conditions that Chiarugi worked to change, as well as the practices used to treat the insane.

He first requested that a physician be permanently available to treat these patients. Second, he proposed that the Grand Duke Peter Leopold, who had previously decreed (in 1774) an enlightened reform for the hospitalization of the mentally ill, financially support the modernization of the old Bonifazio Hospital, in order to use it for the treatment of the mentally ill. The Grand Duke agreed to this second project in 1785, and in 1788 Chiarugi was named chief physician and director of the new Bonifazio Hospital, which now housed the insane, as well as invalids, people with incurable diseases, and patients suffering from skin diseases, many of whom—such as those with pellagra—had psychiatric symptoms. In 1789 Chiarugi was asked by the Grand Duke to draw up regulations for the S. Maria Nuova and Bonifazio hospital, emphasizing the physical and psychological respect of the ill.

Chiarugi's experience in the Bonifazio hospital led him to publish (1793–94) his three volumes devoted to classifying the mentally ill. This work can be considered as the first modern psychiatric treatise. In the first volume (later reprinted in German in 1808), he offered a general overview of the nature of insanity. In the second volume, he dealt with the symptoms, causes, and treatments of melancholia, mania, and amentia. In the third volume, he suggested a nosology of madness and described one hundred clinical cases. The treatise described the main advantages of the therapeutic method that Chiarugi had devised

In 1797 he was invited to draw up regulations for the lunatic asylum of San Servolo in Venice. In 1805 he lectured at the University of Pisa on physiology and medicine, which seems to represent the first academic course devoted to psychiatry. He became personal physician to Elisa Bonaparte, ennobled as Grand Duchess, after the French occupation of Tuscany. He participated in the medical commissions that studied the fever epidemics of 1804 and 1817, and observations arising from this work led him to publish an essay on Italian leprosy (1817).

In 1818 he was promoted as chief of the S. Maria Nuova Hospital while continuing to teach undergraduate students. He advocated a new regulation of medical courses and examinations (1819). In the same year, he described in a letter to G. Tommassini a case of pseudo male hermaphroditism.

Chiarugi contributed, like Pinel and the Tukes, to the modernization of the treatment of the insane and to so-called moral therapy.

Bibliography

Primary: 1789. *Regolamento dei Regi Spedali di S. Maria Nuova e Di Bonifazio*; 1793–94. *Della pazzia in genere ed in specie. Trattato medico-analitico con una centuria di osservazioni* (Florence).

Secondary: Cabras, Pier Luigi, 1993. *Uno psichiatra prima della psichiatria: V.C.* (Florence); Guarnieri, Patrizia, 1991. *La storia della psichiatria. Un secolo di studi in Italia* (Florence); Mora, George (trans.), 1987. 'Introduction' in Chiarugi, Vicenzo, *On Insanity and Its Classification* (Canton, MA) pp. i–lxxxiii.

Patrizia Guarnieri

CHOE, HAN'GI (b. Korea, 1803; d. Korea, 1870), *Korean medicine, medical philosophy.*

Biographical details for Choe Han'gi's life are scarce given the stature of his writings. Records tell us that he was born into the lower ranks of the ruling class. Despite passing the primary civil service examination in 1825, he decided not to go into the civil service, preferring neo-Confucian natural philosophy and technical subjects, such as astronomy, agriculture, mathematics, and medicine, which he studied from the 1830s onward. He was also very interested in Western science and technology. Throughout his life Choe Han'gi was a prolific writer, producing at least two treatises on astronomy, others on agriculture, geography, mathematics, and medicine, and two treatises each on mechanics and natural philosophy. Most of his work remains unpublished, but his early masterpiece *Ki'cheuk-che'ui* 氣測體義 [Principles for Measuring the Body using *Qi*] was printed in Beijing, which was rare at that time for a Korean work.

Sin'gicheonheo 身機踐驗 [Experimental Physiology], written in 1866, is a unique medical book demonstrating originality in the field of medical philosophy. Choe Han'gi brought modern Western medicine to Korea, and was also the first Korean who combined traditional East Asian with Western medicine.

Choe Han'gi learned Western medical knowledge from the books of Benjamin Hobson (1816–73), a missionary doctor. During the 1850s, Hobson published five important medical books on anatomy and physiology, medical treatments, pharmacology, gynecology and pediatrics, and internal medicine in Chinese. Choe Han'gi obtained the books through Korean envoys and translators. Hobson's books first introduced modern medical knowledge from the West, quite different from the Galenic medicine that had previously been available to Korean scholars.

Before this time Koreans could only read fragmented excerpts about Galenic physiology that Jesuit missionaries had chosen to translate into Chinese for the purpose of theological discussion. In contrast, the knowledge of Western medicine that Hobson presented seemed comprehensive, and was based systematically on scientific experiments. For the most part Choe Han'gi accepted Hobson's medicine and was impressed by his assumption that the human body could be measured just as other phenomena in the natural world.

Eulogizing the empirical basis of modern Western medicine, Choe Han'gi attacked both the assumptions and reasoning of traditional East Asian medical theories. He insisted that they could neither explain the true origin of diseases nor produce cures for the patients. He refuted both the five-agent theory, wherein the functions of the body were ruled by the movement of five phases of *qi* 氣, and the astro-medical notions about illness causation that suggested infectious disease was determined by the interaction between the *qi* of celestial bodies and the atmosphere.

Choe Han'gi proposed a compromise between traditional East Asian and Western medicine. According to him, Western medicine had an accurate knowledge of the human body but few useful drugs; on the other hand, Chinese and Korean traditional medicine had many useful drugs whose efficacy would eventually be verified, despite a misconceived physiology and pathology. Despite the fact that Choe Han'gi saw a need for a new medicine that balanced Western knowledge of physiology and East Asian knowledge of drugs, his views were far from simple.

On the one hand believing the body a material entity, Choe Han'gi attacked Hobson's Christian premise that God, as creator, was the origin of all spirituality of the body. Yet, on the other hand, he subordinated his own 'scientific' medicine to a grand philosophy that he styled *gi'hak* 氣學 [study of *qi*]. Since everything in the universe, including humanity, was united by the same *qi*, through their common condition, all peoples could come together in the creation of a better and more peaceful society. For Choe Han'gi, medicine was an important means for accomplishing this goal.

Bibliography

Primary: 1866. *Sin'gicheonheom* [Experimental Physiology] (Seoul).

Secondary: Dongwon, Shin, 2004. *Hoyeolja, Choson'eul Seup'kyok'hada: Momgoa Ui'hak'ui Hankuk'sa* [Cholera Invaded Korea: A Korean History of Body and Medicine] (Seoul); In-Sok Yeo and Jae-Hoon Rho, 1993. 'Choe Han-Kiui Uihak Sasang' [The Medical Philosophy of Choe Han-Ki] *Kor. J. Med. History* 2; Dujong, Kim, 1966. *Hankuk Ui'hak'sa* [History of Korean Medicine] (Seoul); Sakae, Miki, 1962. *Chosen Igakusi Kyu Sitsubeisi* [History of Korean Medicine and of Disease in Korea] (Osaka).

Dongwon Shin

CHOKSY, NASARWANJI HORMUSJI (b. ?, 7 October 1861; d. ?, 1 December 1939), *infectious diseases*.

Choksy was schooled at Elphinstone High School, Bombay, and entered Grant Medical College in 1879. After a brilliant academic career, during which he was awarded scholarships and prizes for proficiency, he topped his class in the final Licentiate of Medicine and Surgery examination. Principal Henry Van Dyke Carter appointed him assistant professor of anatomy, materia medica, and botany at Grant Medical College, which post he held for three years. He was then appointed secretary of the medical committee of the Indian Factory Commission (1884) set up to enquire into the physical condition of mill workers and the sanitary condition of the mills.

During the smallpox epidemic of 1888, Choksy was placed in charge of the smallpox hospital and was so competent at this job that he was made medical superintendent at the Arthur Road Hospital, which had been set up exclusively for infectious diseases (1892) and is still functioning today. He served there until 1922, his name becoming synonymous with this institution. His experience in treating cases of plague, smallpox, and cholera was considered unique. During the plague epidemic of 1896–97, Choksy worked single-handedly in the face of public apathy and suspicion. He also supervised the Maratha plague hospital (1902–21), which treated only plague patients. In fact, he fell victim to the disease (1897) but was saved by the timely use of Yersin's serum. He read a paper at the Bombay Medical Congress (1909) describing the treatment of 275 cases with the subcutaneous administration of this serum. In recognition of his work during the plague epidemics of the 1890s, the British gave him the title of Khan Bahadur. Choksy also diligently campaigned for smallpox vaccination, showing through carefully collated statistics that even one primary vaccination reduced case mortality in later life.

Associated with the establishment of the Acworth Municipal Leprosy Hospital, Bombay, Choksy was on the board of management (1897–1934) and a member of the Viceroy's Leprosy Relief Fund. He prepared special reports on plague, leprosy, fevers, and cholera.

In addition to his professional commitments, Choksy engaged in medical activism. He edited the *Indian Medico-Chirurgical Review* (1893–99) and contributed to *Lancet* and *Indian Medical Gazette*. The former was the voice of the Bombay medics and repeatedly expressed their demands for an improvement in their status and the opening of higher positions in government service to Indians. As president of the Bombay Medical Union, Choksy campaigned for recognition of the parity of Indian degrees with British degrees, so that holders of the former could qualify for government posts. He served as president, College of Physicians and Surgeons, Bombay, and was a member of the Bombay Medical Council (1912–32) and Council of State (1933–36).

With John A. Turner, Choksy was the initiator of a unique collaborative effort to promote public health in the early 1900s through semi-official organizations supported by the municipality, doctors, and philanthropists. This resulted in the establishment of the Bombay Sanitary Association (1903), which aimed at promoting sanitary consciousness through public lectures and the training of personnel. Choksy gave the first public lecture at the Bombay Sanitary Association entitled, 'Some common sense views on plague'. He was also connected with the Bombay Anti-Tuberculosis League (1912), which spread awareness of the disease and provided treatment.

Many distinctions were awarded to Choksy: Chevalier, Crown of Italy (1899); member of the Medical Society, Munich (1901), and the Medico-Physicians Academy, Florence (1903); MD honoris causa, Freiburg Germany (1903); Medalliste des Epidemies Republique Française (1906); and Commander of the Indian Empire (1922). He was knighted in 1929.

Bibliography

Primary: 1897. *Report on Bubonic Plague* (Bombay); 1909. 'The Serum Therapy of Plague in India' in Jennings, W. E., ed., *Transactions of the Bombay Medical Congress* (Bombay) pp. 120–125; 1915. 'The War and the Medical Profession in India.' *Report of the Bombay Medical Union* (Bombay) pp. 21–30.

Secondary: 1906. *Album of Men and Women of India* (Bombay).

Mridula Ramanna

CHOPRA, RAM NATH   (b. Gujranwala, Punjab, India, 17 August 1882; d. Srinagar, Kashmir, India, 13 June 1973), *pharmacology.*

Chopra, son of Raghunath Chopra, attended school in Jammu, Srinagar, and Lahore. Following his graduation from the Punjab University, Lahore, he was admitted to

Downing College, Cambridge, in 1903 from where he took the science tripos in 1905. In England he took the LRCP and MRCS in 1907; MB, BCh (Cantab) in 1908; and his MD in 1912 from St Bartholomew's Hospital Medical School. While in London, he took the Indian Medical Service examination and stood third. He served in the field service in East Africa and in Afghanistan, and in 1921 he returned to India as professor of pharmacology at the Calcutta Medical College, a position he held concurrently at the School of Tropical Medicine, Calcutta. Chopra was married to Parameshwari Devi, with whom he had three sons and two daughters.

While in Calcutta, Chopra single-handedly established a laboratory for modern experimental pharmacological work and pioneered the foundation of pharmacology as an independent scientific discipline in India. In 1922 he conceptualized a comprehensive study of the chemical composition and physiological action of indigenous drugs along with his colleague S. Ghosh, professor of chemistry at the School of Tropical Medicine, Calcutta.

Chopra was the first to publish papers on the cultivation of plants that yielded drugs, including aconitum, belladonna, and ephedra. His was the first pharmacological study of the now universally known *Rauwofia serpentina* (1933). The same year he also published a book-length study entitled *Indigenous Drugs of India: Their medicinal and economical value,* followed by *Medicinal and Poisonous Plants of India* (1949) and *A Glossary of Indian Medicinal Plants* (1956). His research interests stretched from topics in tropical medicine and therapeutics of poisons from snakes to problems of drug quality and pharmaceutical standardization.

In 1930 Chopra was appointed the chairman of the Drugs Enquiry Committee that examined the problem of drug adulteration and substandard drug manufacture in India. He was made a CIE in 1933, and soon afterward, he became the first Indian director of the School of Tropical Medicine, Calcutta (1935), where along with his colleagues he shaped and directed a medical research program that trained young students in understanding and addressing problems in tropical medicine, experimental pharmacology, drug standardization, toxicology, and drug addiction. The same year he was appointed Honorary Physician to the King of England and promoted to the rank of Brevet-Colonel.

Chopra was awarded a DSc by Cambridge University in 1937. The following year, he was elected FRCP (London) as well as Honorary Fellow of the American Society of Pharmacology and Experimental Therapeutics. He was knighted in 1941, which was also the year of his retirement from the School of Tropical Medicine, Calcutta. He spent the next twenty years as director of medical services and drug research in Jammu and Kashmir. During his tenure as director, he set up the Regional Research Laboratory at Jammu.

The recommendations made by the Chopra committee of 1930 were incorporated into the Drugs Act of 1940 and later, after Indian independence, into the Pharmacy Act of 1948. Chopra headed the Committee on Indigenous systems of Medicines (1948) that made two significant recommendations enabling the newly independent state to cope with health care. The committee suggested that modern medicine be integrated with indigenous medicines and furthermore, that graduates of the latter school be trained in modern medicine for a six-month period in order to work at the primary health care level.

Chopra witnessed interesting and immense political changes in his lifetime, but remained a steadfast and devoted educator and institution-builder dedicated to research in pharmacology and drug policy.

Bibliography

Primary: 1933. *Indigenous Drugs of India: Their Medical and Economic Aspects* (Calcutta) 1933. (with Gupta, J. C., and B. Mukherjee) 'The Pharmacological Action of an Alkoloid Obtained from *Rauwolfia serpentina*, Benth. A Preliminary Note.' *Indian Journal of Medical Research* 21: 261–271; 1936. *A Handbook of Tropical Therapeutics* (Calcutta).

Secondary: Mukerji, B., 1976. 'Sir Ram Nath Chopra.' *Indian National Science Academy: Biographical Memoirs* 4: 170–185; *Munk's Roll.*

Indira Chowdhury

CHRISTISON, ROBERT (b. Edinburgh, Scotland, 18 July 1797; d. Edinburgh, 27 January 1882), *toxicology, medicine.*

Christison, son of Alexander Christison, schoolmaster, and Margaret Johnstone, attended Edinburgh High School (1805–09/10), subsequently receiving his MA from Edinburgh University in 1815. He began taking medical courses in 1813 and graduated MD in 1819. From 1819–21 he studied chemistry, toxicology, and surgery in London and Paris under John Abernethy (1764–1831), William Lawrence (1783–1867), Guillaume Dupuytren (1777–1835), Pierre Jean Robiquet (1780–1840), and François Magendie (1783–1855).

In 1822 Christison's family connections aided him in obtaining the Regius Chair of Medical Jurisprudence at the University of Edinburgh. Once appointed, Christison studied medical jurisprudence in earnest and made toxicology his special study. In 1823 he published, with Charles W. Coindet, 'An experimental inquiry on poisoning by oxalic acid'. This was followed in 1824 by a series of publications describing chemical tests for arsenic poisoning. Christison's *Treatise on Poisons* (1829, German edition, 1831) was the standard English-language text for many years. The noted toxicologist Mathieu Orfila (1787–1853) was an admirer of his work. Though recognizing the limits of contemporary toxicology, Christison nonetheless maintained that 'the chemical evidence in charges of poisoning is generally, and with justice, considered the most decisive of all the branches of proof' (cited in Burney, 1999, p. 75.)

In 1827 Christison married Henrietta Sophia Brown of Stirling and the couple had three sons. Christison's first major court appearance came the same year, when he gave evidence in a trial involving Margaret Warden Smith, who was accused of poisoning her husband with arsenic. Two years later he testified at the trial of William Burke and Helen McDougal, who, with William Hare, committed sixteen murders and sold the bodies to the Edinburgh surgeon Robert Knox (1791–1862). He had a commanding presence as a witness and was frequently called for the prosecution. In 1839 Christison, with Thomas Traill (1781–1862) and James Syme (1799–1870), published *Suggestions on the Medico-Legal Examination of Dead Bodies.*

As a professor, Christison worked hard to successfully raise the status of medical jurisprudence as an academic subject. In 1825 the University of Edinburgh made it an optional course for medical degrees. He became a medical examiner for the Standard Assurance Company, and incorporated his experience into his teaching. He was wont to test his poisons on himself and incorporated that experience into his teaching as well. He also published a series of case studies on various aspects of medical evidence in the *Edinburgh Medical and Surgical Review.* In 1832, Christison was elected to the lucrative chair of Materia Medica and resigned that of medical jurisprudence. Though he lectured and published on the standard subject matter of material medica, his professional emphasis remained on toxicology. His *Dispensatory, or Commentary on the Pharmacopoieas of Great Britain* (1842, 1848) was especially valuable for its attention to the chemical analysis of the active principle in many common medicaments.

Christison was one of the leading lights of Edinburgh medicine, though by the end of his life his opposition to women physicians and to a national examination board for medical degrees rendered him anachronistic. He had an extensive practice, and his clinical writings are marked by their sympathetic understanding of the patients' point of view. He was elected president of both the RCPEd and the Royal Society (Edinburgh). He was physician-in-ordinary to the Queen in Scotland and was created a baronet in 1871. Though his work on toxicology was superseded by later achievements in pathology and chemistry, his reliance on scientific principles contributed to the increased importance of expert medical testimony.

Bibliography

Primary: 1842. *A Dispensatory, or Commentary on the Pharmacopoieas of Great Britain* (Edinburgh); 1845. *A Treatise on Poisons* (Birmingham, AL, rpt. edn., 1988); 1885–86. *The Life of Sir Robert Christison, Bart* 2 vols. (Edinburgh).

Secondary: Burney, Ian M., 1999. 'A Poisoning of No Substance: The Trials of Medico-Legal Proof in Mid-Victorian England.' *The Journal of British Studies* 38(1): 59–92; *Oxford DNB.*

Lisa Rosner

CHRISTOPHERS, SAMUEL RICKARD   (b. Liverpool, England, 27 November 1873; d. Broadstone, Dorset, England, 19 February 1978), *parasitology, tropical medicine.*

Samuel Christophers was the oldest of three children of Samuel Hunt Christophers and Mary Selina Christophers (née) Rickard; his father was head statistican of the Mersey Docks and Harbour Board. Samuel was educated at the Liverpool Institute and University College, Liverpool, where he studied medicine, graduating MB, ChB (1896).

After a spell as a medical officer on a steamer, which took him to the mouth of the Amazon, Christophers began to develop an interest in tropical medicine. From 1898 to 1902 he served on the joint malaria commission of the Royal Society and Colonial Office, where, together with his senior colleague John W. W. Stephens (1865–1946), he investigated malaria in West Africa and India. In 1902, after marrying Elise Emma Sherman, the daughter of a coffee planter in southern India, Christophers joined the IMS, where he was appointed director of the King Institute in Madras (1904) and of the Central Malaria Bureau (1910). His early work included some important observations on inherited and acquired immunity to malaria, as well as the classification of mosquitoes and tick-borne diseases.

Christophers was not merely a laboratory researcher but was also intensely interested in the practical side of antimalaria research. Together with some other IMS officers, he grew skeptical of Ronald Ross's (1857–1932) claim that malaria could be prevented by mosquito control and came to advocate mass prophylaxis with quinine. The role of quinine was then at the heart of a great controversy over the disease known as 'blackwater fever'. Some doctors, including the influential figure of Patrick Manson (1844–1922), believed it to be a disease in its own right, while others, including Christophers, maintained that it was a complication of malaria caused by the irregular administration of quinine. Together with Stephens, he was able to persuade the majority of the profession to accept his position.

During World War I, Christophers was given a commission as consultant on malaria with the army in Mesopotamia. A range of measures were taken to control malaria, but the apparent failure of quinine prophylaxis in some theaters began to tilt the balance of opinion back in favor of mosquito control. In 1920 Christophers was appointed director of the Central Research Institute (India) and remained in this post until 1932. There he concentrated on the taxonomy of malaria and other parasitic infections including the disease leishmaniasis, popularly known in India as kala-azar. His belief that the disease was transmitted to humans by the bite of infected sandflies was subsequently confirmed by his friend, H. E. Shortt (1887–1987).

In 1932 Christophers was appointed professor of malaria studies at the London School of Hygiene and Tropical Medicine. Here, in conjunction with J. D. Fulton, he conducted research on the respiratory biochemistry of malaria parasites and those causing sleeping sickness in humans. In 1938 he left London for Cambridge University, where he returned to entomological research.

Christophers did not retire from research until the advanced age of ninety and lived to be 104. He was extremely well liked, and the centenary of his birth was celebrated by the Royal Society of Tropical Medicine and Hygiene, of which he was president from 1939–43, and by the Royal Entomological Society of London. He was honored many times in Britain and overseas and was knighted in 1931; he was also honorary physician to king George V from 1927 to 1930 and was elected FRS in 1926.

Bibliography

Primary: 1904. (with Stephens, J. W. W.) *The Practical Study of Malaria* (London); 1904. 'Second report of the anti-malarial operations at Mian Mir, 1901–1903.' *Scientific Memoirs by Officers of the Medical and Sanitary Departments of the Government of India* 1–13; 1937. (with Stephens, J. W. W.), *Blackwater Fever: A Historical Survey of Observations Made over a Century* (London).

Secondary: Harrison, Mark, 1994. *Public Health in British India: Anglo-Indian Preventive Medicine 1859–1914* (Cambridge); Shortt, H. E., and P. C. Garnham, 1979. 'Samuel Rickard Christophers.' *Biographical Memoirs of Fellows of the Royal Society* 25: 199–207; *Oxford DNB.*

Mark Harrison

CHUNYU, YI 淳于意   (aka CANGGONG 倉公) (b. Qi Kingdom, Han Empire, Eastern China, 215 BCE; d. ?,?), *Chinese medicine.*

Chunyu Yi, or Master of the Granary as he is known to Chinese doctors to the present day, appears in the *Records of the Historian (Shiji* 史記) of c. 90 BCE, the first Chinese dynastic history composed by the Grand Historian and Astrologer Sima Qian 司馬遷 (c. ?145–86 BCE) of the Western Han (206–9 BCE). His biography, twenty-five medical case histories and eight answers to eight questions are recorded in the second part of the 105th chapter, after the biography of Bian Que 扁鵲 (also known as Qin Yueren 秦越人), which contains three medical cases and six principles of medical ethics.

Throughout medical history, Bian Que and Chunyu Yi were venerated for their knowledge in the study of *mai* 脈 (vessels and/or movements in the vessels, pulses). The concept of *qi* 氣, which related to airs, vapors, and breaths, was central to their medical theory, as was that of the five viscera (*wuzang* 五藏). Their Memoir is the earliest to record the pulse diagnostic method of *qie mai* 切脈 (pressing on the *mai*), and it testifies to medical knowledge and practice closely related to that in the manuscript literature of the second century BCE and the compilations of the received tradition, such as the *Suwen* 素問 [Basic Questions] and *Lingshu* 靈樞 [Divine Pivot], which together form the *Huangdi Neijing* 燒铂瘿籥 [Yellow Emperor's Inner Canon] that was composed for the first time between the

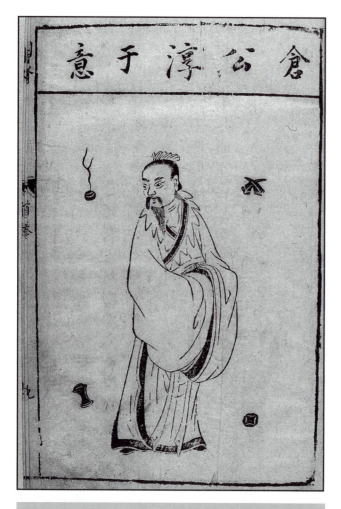

Chunyu Yi. Lettering on this woodcut reads 'Cang Gong Chunyu Yi' [Reverend Master of the Granary, Chunyu Yi]. From Chen Jiamo, *Bencao Mengquan* [Introduction to the Pharmacopoeia], 1573–1620. Library of Zhongguo zhongyi yanjiu yuan/Wellcome Library, London

third century BCE and 256/282, but its extant form dates to the Song dynasty (960–1279).

Chunyu Yi's Memoir can be divided into four sections, of which the first two are biographical. The first section may have been written by the Grand Historian himself or a member of his team. It recounts that in the fourth year of Emperor Wen (176 BCE) Yi was accused by a patient he refused to treat. He was brought to Chang'an, the capital of the Empire, where he was about to receive corporal punishment, when his fifth daughter (Yi had no sons), Tiying 緹縈, presented a document to the Emperor, who thereupon rescinded punishment. The second introductory section details some of the information previously provided, for example, the titles of the esoteric books Yi received. The third section is the longest and contains twenty-five medical case histories; the fourth section consists of eight questions and answers.

Yi was a Western Han official of the Qi kingdom who learned medicine late in life. His dates can be inferred from

two statements. The Memoir's first section states that he started studying with a new master, Yang Qing 陽慶, in the eighth year of Empress Gao 高 (180 BCE), and according to the second section, he was thirty-nine *sui* 矗, thirty-eight years old, after serving that master for three years. This gives a birth year of 215 BCE (although much scholarly ink has been spilled over this).

The Memoir

The introductory section of the Memoir ends with the following statement: 'An Imperial edict summoned him [Yi] and inquired about that which made him treat illnesses and [prognosticate] death and life. The cases proven true, how many were they? The main names among them were which ones?' (*Shiji* 1959: 2796) The second, third, and fourth sections are best read as a response to this edict, reporting on events that presumably happened before the Chang'an incident in 176 BCE. However, there is a controversy about the incident's exact date (which, according to some, was 167 BCE) and about whether the issuing of the edict actually related to this incident.

The third section of the Memoir is by far the longest, and for the medical historian it is a treasure of information on medical theory and practice in antiquity. Its historical significance parallels that of the *Epidemics* in the Hippocratic corpus for occidental traditions of medicine. The twenty-five medical case histories or, in Yi's terms, 'investigation reports' (*zhenji* 診籍), were formulaic in two respects. They recorded the patient's name, title of office (or relationship to a noble or king), and place of residence, much in the manner of the twenty-five legal case records of 217 BCE called 'Models for Sealing and Investigating' (Fengzhen shi 封診式). In recurrent phrases they provided systematic information about the name of the disorder, its cause, and the diagnostic pulse or color quality indicative of the disorder. In addition, they recorded in a less systematic fashion the disorder's signs and symptoms, details of its course and outcome, and medical management. Ten cases were prognosticated to end in death; the treatment of the other fifteen involved ingestion of hot liquids, application of poultices, fumigation, needling (acupuncture), cauterization, and other therapeutic measures. Among the hot liquids was a so-called *huoji tang* 炊布軸, which is best translated as a 'hot liquid made by the careful regulation of fire' (i.e., by simmering over a small fire). In all twenty-five cases, Yi's prognostications of death were accurate and his treatments led to a cure. He followed the instructions of the Imperial edict closely, if the above translation is correct. When, in section four, he disclaimed infallibility, he indicated that record taking in combination with the consultation of the so-called 'Model for the Study of *Mai*' (Maifa 脈法) had enhanced his esoteric knowledge. The case histories are formulaic in presentation and technical in language, yet they also have literary value, not least due to their narrative form.

The fourth section, which consists of eight questions and answers, concerned Yi's medical rationale, medical training, and teachings to his followers. In several respects it does not tally with the previous sections. There are differences in linguistic particles, details of medical theory, and statements about the transmission of knowledge regarding books and people. For instance, in his response to question six Yi named as his main teachers Gongsun Guang 公孫光 from Zichuan and Yang Zhongqing 楊中倩 from Linzi, who had an adult son called Yin 殷. Commentators identify the latter as Yang Qing 陽慶. However, according to the text in section one, Yang Qing had no sons, and sections one and four would therefore appear to blatantly contradict each other.

The Sociohistorical Cadre

Yi lived in the difficult times of the political division of the great Qi kingdom in Eastern China (present-day Shandong province), which was an integral part of the Han Empire. The Qi kingdom experienced a diminution in 193 BCE, 187 BCE, 181 BCE, and 178 BCE. In 164 BCE its original territory was split into seven kingdoms, and Liu Jianglü 劉將閭 (r. 164–53 BCE), who is mentioned in case twenty-three of Yi's Memoir, became king of a drastically reduced Qi. Yi said he relinquished his office and started studying medicine with Yang Qing in 180 BCE. Perhaps it was a coincidence that this was the year when Liu Xiang 劉襄, who then was King of Qi, attempted to usurp the Imperial throne after the Lü 呂 family had been eliminated. Perhaps Yi was a Lü loyalist.

Yi treated mainly nobility, mostly of the Qi kingdom. He also treated two slaves, three female attendants or concubines, a child, a wet nurse, a woman from his hometown, and at least one man en route from Qi to Chang'an. He also mentioned, in cases eleven to twenty-five, the King of Jibei, the former King of Jibei, the King of Zichuan, the King of Qi when he was the Noble of Yangxu (identifying him as Liu Jianglü), and, in section four, a certain King Wen and the Kings of Zhao, Jiaoxi, Jinan, and Wu, who all participated in a revolt of 154 BCE and who, perhaps not coincidentally, Yi refused to receive. If the Memoir were a single document written after 154 BCE, many years after the Chang'an incident, Yi would have been over sixty-six years old.

In spite of detailed calculations based on the names of his clientele, it is uncertain whether Yi could have had dealings with all the people mentioned in the Memoir. Case records in antiquity did not always mention names, and in Yi's Memoir, some surnames and given names were unusual; they sometimes rhymed or were nicknames. It is possible, if not probable, that a fairly coherent document on Yi's treatment of mostly Qi nobility was written in the year of the Chang'an incident, which was supplemented by further material of varied provenance. Cases one to ten form a unity in respect of formulaic structure and medical

rationale, which is partly at odds with that mentioned later. Naturally, it is possible that the case histories reflected a change in Yi's ideas over several decades. It is more likely, however, that material from related sources were assembled around one substantive document and selectively edited by Sima Qian and his team *c.* 90 BCE.

In this context, one wonders why detailed medical histories were recorded in a monumental work on the political history of the Han Empire. The Grand Historian gave hints as to how they should be read in his closing statement to the Memoir: he commented on Yi's fate of being a great physician, unfairly accused of a crime, by (mis)quoting Laozi 吩氛: 'Beauty and goodness are are instruments for [attracting] calamities' (*Shiji* 1959: 2817). His quote also applies to the famous Bian Que, who was ruthlessly killed by a despot and, as some have suggested, perhaps to Sima Qian himself, who was castrated as a punishment after taking sides in a political controversy during the reign of Emperor Wudi 武帝 (141–87 BCE). It may be for other than purely medical reasons that in Yi's Memoir about half of the cases were attributed to indulgence in 'wine' (probably a sort of beer; three cases), 'women' (five explicitly stated and three inferred cases), or 'wine and women' (two cases). Perhaps, in particular, the author of the initial ten cases, of which eight were attributed to 'wine' and 'women', was hinting at debauchery among the Qi nobility. The fact that Yi's medical case histories have survived in a dynastic history is not to be overlooked.

In contrast to Bian Que, whose extraordinary cognitive faculties, fabled ability of reviving the dead, and six precepts of medical ethics have become part of Chinese folklore, Yi was only known to later medical authors. Whereas he mostly was treated with great reverence and praised for his medical insight, there were authors, such as the legendary Hua Tuo of the Three Kingdoms (220–80), who deplored both Yi's ignorance and his abstruse reasoning.

It can be demonstrated beyond doubt that Yi's medical reasoning shows continuities with the early medical manuscript literature and canonical medical texts. Nevertheless, overall it has remained opaque to medical practitioners and historians alike, at least since Hua Tuo's times. It is primarily recent Western scholarship that has taken seriously Yi's Memoir as a valuable source for understanding early developments in the history of Chinese medicine. However, Yi's Memoir may well be a compilation of only loosely related primary source material and it forms part of a potentially heavily edited chapter of a dynastic history, therefore, its medical contents can be appreciated only with circumspection.

The Medical Contents

For the medical historian interested in medical rationale, Yi's Memoir represents the earliest extant document within which the medical theory of *qi* played a central role, both for diagnosis and treatment. Cases one to ten, in particular, show theoretical coherence in that they all referred to a fairly specified form of pulse diagnosis: Yi examined *mai* and felt *qi* coming from the viscera (*zang* 胴 and also other locations or aspects of the body); on the basis of this pulse quality, rather than of the cause of the illness, Yi named the disorders (*bing* 喃). His method of tactile examination was generally *qie* 暖, literally 'to cut', which probably meant 'to press down vertically'; in case nineteen, he mentioned *xun* 揩, which might have meant 'to stroke along the skin horizontally'. The word *mai* referred both to vessels and to movement in the vessels. In the early medical manuscripts from Mawangdui and Zhangjiashan, the courses of such vessels were described: they generally originated at the tip of an extremity and followed a distinct course on its surface to the trunk of the body. However, the eleven *mai* described in these manuscripts do not connect with the viscera, except to the heart/epigastrium and the liver/abdomen (or kidney/abdomen), and although there are fragments that suggest that the *mai* were investigated probably not at the wrist but at the ankle, *qi* is not mentioned in that context. Yi's method of *qie mai* provides the earliest evidence of *qi* being felt in the *mai* and the *mai* being connected to viscera.

The viscera, whose state of *qi* was detected through the examination of *mai*, were the liver, heart, spleen, lungs, kidneys, and bladder, the same five viscera common in the canonical writings and the bladder (which there was subordinate to the kidneys, as their outer aspect). There is little doubt that in case five the *pao*-bladder, which was originally situated in the center of the body and in some contexts designated the womb, was associated with water and the 'great *yin*' (as were the kidneys in the related tradition of 'inner alchemy'); in canonical writings, a different term for the bladder became predominant, namely *pangguang* 蠻腺, known as the outer aspect of the kidneys, which was associated with the 'great *yang*' (as were the kidneys in Yi's case seventeen). This indicates that the *mai* and viscera in Yi's Memoir were systemically related to those described in the medical canons, particularly if one avoids the temptation of presuming that Yi had an elaborate conception of body parts.

The *mai* were sometimes differentiated into *mai* of the foot or hand, and their names reflected three different degrees (or kinds) of either *yin* 憬 or *yang* 桄. They were called *yang* brilliance, minor *yang*, great *yin*, minor *yin*, and attenuated *yin*, as they are in early manuscripts and canonical writings. The great *yang* was also mentioned but only once (in case seventeen), and it is uncertain whether the text referred in that context to a *mai*, as it stated that 'the color [appearance] of the great *yang* is dry'. If the great *yang* did refer to a *mai*, the diagnostic methods by palpation of *mai* (*qie mai*) and inspection of color (*wang se* 初恢) were more intricately related than their occurrence in different cases of Yi's Memoir might suggest.

The concept of *qi* was not only central to diagnosis by palpation of *mai* or inspection of color but also to new

treatment methods: the needling/lancing (*ci* 刺) and cauterization (*jiu* 灸) of places (*suo* 所) or openings (*kou* 口) on the *mai* and the use of hot liquids (*tang* 湯). The former were akin to canonical acupuncture and moxibustion (i.e., cauterization with dried and crushed leaves of *Artemisia vulgaris*); also, insofar as they were applied within a framework of complex medical reasoning, the latter are best considered precursors of the water-based decoction.

Needling was mentioned four times in *Shiji* 105.2 (and once in *Shiji* 105.1). In cases eleven and sixteen, Yi needled a patient suffering from a 'heat *jue*' (*rejue* 擬鍼) and a '*jue* in the upper parts' (*jueshang* 鍼忙), respectively. In cases three and ten, other doctors, who clearly did not have as sophisticated a vocabulary and treatment rationale, and according to Yi were always mistaken, needled patients suffering from disorders that they diagnosed as 'the stone entering the interior' (*jue ru zhong* 鍼搨抵, translated here in line with the pre-modern European notion of urinary retention caused by kidney or bladder stones) and as 'wind entering the interior' (*feng ru zhong* 唓搨抵). It would be wrong to assume that in the *Shiji* needling was indicated only in the case of *jue* conditions (because case ten is not a *jue*). Nor were they by definition painful, and needling was not primarily used for treating pain (as is the prevalent belief about modern acupuncture). On the contrary, the *jue* condition that Bian Que treated was a state of numbness, like that of an inert stone ('stone' is the basic Chinese dictionary definition of *jue* 欅), or a coma in biomedical terminology. Needling brought the patient back to life.

Bian Que and the common doctors seem to have embraced an early understanding of *jue*, whereas the *jue* conditions Yi needled were conceived as inversions of *yin* and *yang* or hot and cold. Such inversions had much affinity with the idea expressed in later writings of *jue* arising from 'counterflowing *qi*' (*ni qi* 逆氣 was mentioned in case twenty-three, which other doctors diagnosed as *jue* but Yi considered *bi* 瘒, an obstruction). This would suggest that at first *jue* was used for describing conditions likened to the inertness of stone. These conditions of numbness were explained in terms of an inversion of *yin* and *yang*, or hot and cold, well before medical reasoning in terms of *qi* became explicit and predominant. Later, as *qi* physiology became fashionable, *jue* conditions were considered *qi* reversions and counterflows within the body.

Interestingly, all *jue* conditions Yi diagnosed had in common the symptom of fullness (*man* 燿). Yi's needling can thus be likened to the pricking of a balloon filled with *qi*. This may also explain why the other doctors needled the patient in case ten, whose replete (*shi* 沈) pulse indicated in Yi's terminology an amassment of *qi* (*shan qi* 醞烧). All *jue* conditions in *Shiji* 105 were curable, as were all *jue* in the early medical manuscripts.

In Yi's Memoir, cases nine and ten referred to cold conditions, whereas cases eleven and sixteen had symptoms of heat. The *jue* condition in case nine, marked by an excess of cold *yin*, was cured by making the patient drink an enormous amount of beer, with the result that he urinated the excess water and with it the cold. Yi cured the amassed *qi* in case ten, which was aggravated by exposure to the cold, by cauterization. So Yi needled only *jue* marked by heat. It is noteworthy that the rationale for Yi's needling and cauterizing reflected *yin yang* reasoning, as is characteristic of acupuncture and moxibustion in later medical writings.

Yi's case histories are also remarkable for their extensive use of hot liquids (*tang* 搾), which some consider precursors of the modern decoction (*tangye* 搾塼). Here we assume a broad definition of hot liquids, comprising water-based broths, alcoholic drinks, and gruel-like soups, which may have been simmered over a small fire and contained, particularly in later times, a variety of herbal, animal, or mineral ingredients. The term *huoji tang* may have originally referred to such a hot liquid produced over a carefully regulated fire, a meaning lost on later physicians (see case twenty-two). In eight cases Yi was explicit that he made his patient ingest a hot liquid (*tang*), gruel (*zhou* 姰), rice juice (*mizhi* 塼麤), or fermented alcoholic drink (*jiu* 屏). Four of the named drugs were also found in the early manuscript literature and later Chinese *materia medica*, namely, *banxia* 敫壞 (now identified as *Pinellia ternata*), *kushen* 嬞檽 (*Sophora flavescens*), *xiaoshi* 徠悍 (niter), and *yuanhua* 銑 壺 (*Daphne genkwa*); the fifth, *langdang* 莨礄 was perhaps *langdang* 莨菪 (*Hyoscyamus niger*).

Several names of the disorders are not found elsewhere in the medical literature. Yet constituents of those names are identical with those in early manuscripts and later texts, such as an abscess (*ju* 醋, conglomeration (*jia* 瘕), or state of overexertion (*dan* 癉). Excess of wind (*feng* 風) or heat (*re* 擬) figured in a third of the cases. With the information at hand, retrospective diagnoses can only be speculative, but they have been made, suggesting urinary retentions, terminal versus treatable diarrhea, dental caries, gout, sexual overexertion, sexual longing, lung injury, and a worm infection. Incidentally, particularly in the first ten cases, several patients had urinary tract problems. Since those are often aggravated by sexual intercourse, a medical rather than a moral rationale may be given for the many cases caused by sexual indulgence. If primarily urinary tract problems were treated by water-based decoctions, on the grounds of a *tong lei* 揮樱 (same kind) relationship of treating water with water, the case histories testify to an early stage in the history of the water-based decoction, which has been used as the main Chinese medical treatment method from the Eastern Han (23–220) to the present day.

Chunyu Yi's Impact on the History of Chinese Medicine

Bian Que was, and continues to be, celebrated as the initiator of the study of *mai*. However, it is Yi's Memoir that detailed medical rationale based on the palpation of *mai* for detecting the qualities of *qi* and the states of the internal viscera (*zang*). It is Yi whose therapy made use of both needling and cauterization, and of hot liquids, that is, the precursors of the modern decoction. Yi's Memoir thus referred to all the basic characteristics of China's elite scholarly medicine. However, Chinese medical history has not credited Yi for this, and in Chinese intellectual history Yi's daughter Tiying was more celebrated than her father.

Well-known commentators of the *Shiji*, for instance, Xu Guang 徐廣 and Wang Niansun 王念孫, commented on Yi's Memoir. Song dynasty works, such as the *Taiping yulan* 太平御覽 or the *Yishuo* 醫說, quoted it extensively. Most remarkable, however, is the output of eighteenth and nineteenth century Japanese commentators, including Ando Koretora 藤維寅 and his son, or Taki Motokata 愲娿沔窺 and his son, among others. In modern times, Takigawa Kametaro 戠愢伀爐 and Wang Shumin 壩迪洴 have made invaluable contributions to the elucidation of the text, and the renowned medical historian Fan Xingzhun 鑰峴弚 has an unpublished essay on it.

Because of the complications inherent to the recording of medical case histories in a dynastic history, modern Western scholarship has generally shied away from a medical exegesis; it would require finding either further early medical texts for comparison or useful methods of textual analysis. Although many aspects of Yi's medical rationale have parallels in the early medical literature and received tradition, several questions remain unresolved. Yi's Memoir is a text with many dimensions and refers with such freshness and detail to a form of medicine about which little is known that it will continue to attract the imagination of future historians of medicine.

Bibliography

Primary: *Shi ji* 组勉 [Records of the Historian] 1959. Han, *c.* 90 BCE. Sima Qian 巖攏憝 . (Beijing); Hübotter, F., 1927. 'Zwei berühmte chinesische Aerzte des Altertums Chouen Yu-I und Hua T'ouo.' *Mitteilungen der deutschen Gesellschaft für Natur- und Völkerkunde Ostasiens* 21A: 3–48; Hsu, E. and W. Nienhauser, (forthcoming). 'Chapter 105: The Memoir of Pien Ch'ueh and Ch'unyu Yi' in Nienhauser, W., ed., *The Grand Scribe's Records. By Ssu-ma Ch'ien*. Vol. 7 (Bloomington, IN).

Secondary: Hsu, E. (forthcoming). *The Telling Touch: Pulse Diagnostics in Early Chinese Medicine*. With an anthropological interpretation of the first ten medical case histories and an annotated translation of Chunyu Yi's Memoir in *Shiji* 105 (Cambridge); Yamada Keiji 1998. *The Origins of Acupuncture, Moxibustion, and Decoction* (Kyoto); Loewe, M. A. N., 1997. 'The Physician Chunyu Yi and his Historical Background' in Gernet, J., and M. Kalinowski, eds., *En suivant la voie royale. Etudes thématiques* 7. (Paris) pp. 297–313; Sivin, N., 1995. 'Text and Experience in Classical Chinese Medicine' in Bates, D., ed., *Knowledge and the Scholarly Medical Traditions* (Cambridge) pp. 177–204; Lu, G.-D., and J.

Needham, 1967. 'Records of Disease in Ancient China' in Brothwell, D., and A. T. Sandison, eds., *Disease in Antiquity* (Springfield, IL) pp. 222–237; Bridgman, R. F., 1955. 'La médicine dans la Chine antique.' *Mélanges Chinois et Bouddhique* 10: 1–213.

Elisabeth Hsu

CHURCHILL, EDWARD DELOS (b. Chenoa, Illinois, USA, 25 December 1895; d. Strafford, Vermont, USA, 28 August 1972), *surgery.*

Churchill was the son of Ebenezer Delos Churchill, grain merchant, and Maria Farnsworth Churchill, both college graduates and firm Presbyterians. He graduated from Northwestern University with a BS (1916) and an MA in biology (1917). Entering the second year class at Harvard Medical School, he received the MD, cum laude, in 1920.

He was surgical intern (1920–22) and surgical resident (1922–24) at Massachusetts General Hospital (MGH), and then rose through the ranks to assistant visiting surgeon (1927–28). The next two years were spent at Boston City Hospital, after which he returned to and remained at MGH until retirement (1961). In 1948 he became chief of the General Surgical Service. He was also surgical consultant and senior physician at the Rutland State Sanatorium (Massachusetts), where he introduced surgical treatment of tuberculosis.

Churchill joined the teaching staff at Harvard Medical School in 1922, becoming a member of the faculty in 1928. His students were encouraged to recognize the relationship of laboratory investigation to improved surgical methods. As a Moseley Fellow, he spent a year (1926–27) studying surgery in European medical centers. In 1931 Churchill was named John Homans Professor of Surgery.

During World War II, Churchill was a colonel in the Army Medical Corps and served in the North African–Mediterranean theater. For introducing improved procedures for management of wounded soldiers, he was awarded the Distinguished Service Medal. In 1953, as consultant to the Army Surgeon General, he visited military posts in the Far East. He also served on several advisory committees for the armed forces.

Early in his career Churchill became interested in diseases of the lung and was the first to use spirometry to measure lung ventilation following abdominal surgery. With Oliver Cope he described the reflex mechanism (rapid shallow breathing resulting from pulmonary congestion) now known as the Churchill-Cope reflex.

Churchill's major contributions lie in the development of surgical treatments for cancer of the lung and pulmonary tuberculosis, decortication of the heart for relief of constrictive pericarditis, and surgical treatment of hyperthyroidism. He demonstrated the safety of selectively removing diseased parts of the lung in chest diseases, beginning with successful resection for adenocarcinoma, and introduced segmental pneumonectomy for pulmonary

tuberculosis and bronchopulmonectomy in treatment of bronchiectasis. A daring pioneer, his work often caused widespread controversy until proven effective and safe.

As a Rockefeller grantee, Churchill went to India in 1958 to consult in several medical centers. He was also visiting professor of surgery at the American University of Beirut and acting director of the department of surgery at its hospital. He served on the advisory board of the American Hospital in Paris and was a consultant at the Shiraz Medical Center in Iran. He also served as consultant at the National Institutes of Health, chairman (1946–49) of the committee on surgery of the National Research Council, and twice (1948–49 and 1953–55) vice chairman of the task force on federal medical services of the Commission on Organization of the Executive Branch of the Government.

He was president of the American Surgical Association (1946–47), American Association for Thoracic Surgery (1948–49), and Society of Clinical Surgery (1949–50). An honorary member of more than a dozen foreign medical societies and an honorary fellow of the Royal College of Surgeons of England, he was also honored by the French, British, Italian, and Lebanese governments. Additionally, he received honorary degrees from universities in the United States and abroad.

Churchill and Mary Lowell Barton married on 7 July 1927 and had four children.

Bibliography

Primary: 1958. *To Work in the Vineyard of Surgery* (Cambridge, MA); 1971. *Surgeon to Soldiers: Diary and Records of the Surgical Consultant, Allied Force Headquarters, World War II* (Philadelphia); 1990. *Wanderjahr: The Education of a Surgeon* (Cambridge, MA).

Secondary: 2002. http://www.pbs.org/wnet/redgold/innovators; *ANB; DAMB.*

Amalie M. Kass

CILENTO, RAPHAEL WEST (b. Jamestown, South Australia, 2 December 1893; d. Brisbane, Queensland, Australia, 14 April 1985), *tropical public health, health administration.*

Cilento was born in the remote wheat-growing region of northeast South Australia, the son of Raphael Ambrose Cilento, a stationmaster, and Frances West. He studied medicine at the University of Adelaide, taking an early interest in the neo-Lamarckian physical anthropology taught by Frederick Wood Jones. He married Phyllis McGlew, a fellow medical student. Graduating in 1918, he joined the Australian Army Medical Services in Australian-occupied (formerly German) New Guinea. Recruited to the new Commonwealth Department of Health, Cilento was selected for a future in tropical medicine, completing a Diploma of Tropical Medicine at the London School of Tropical Medicine.

Cilento became a proponent of 'national hygiene', a view that Australia's population, cultural, and economic problems had a biological base: the problems of European acclimatization. As director of the Australian Institute of Tropical Medicine in Townsville (1922) he showed little interest in original research, but tirelessly promoted a rosy future for 'the White Man in the Tropics' if he would only embrace a sound diet, appropriate clothing and housing, and sound racial hygiene. Returning to New Guinea as director of health (1924), his programs mainly improved the health of white settlers. Appointed Director of the Commonwealth Department of Health's Division of Tropical Hygiene (1928–33), he developed an apocalyptic vision of a coming racial war with Asia. The prime duty of public health was to produce a white racial stock capable of winning this challenge.

In 1934 Cilento became Queensland's Director General of Health. He led the reform of the state's medical services, nationalizing hospitals, replacing the honorary system with salaried services under strong government control, and establishing the University of Queensland Medical School, where he was foundation professor of social medicine (1938). He pushed a radical scheme for centrally planned medical services built around group practice, raising the ire of the British Medical Association (BMA) but little interest from his political masters in the Queensland Labour Party, preoccupied with free admission to hospitals. Marginalized and frustrated at the state level, he prepared schemes to develop the Queensland model of nationalized health services Australia-wide—again based on central planning and group clinics. Members of the Federal Labour government showed no more interest than their Queensland colleagues and proposed a universal medical benefit scheme.

The war should have been a grand new opportunity for Australia's pre-eminent tropical health administrator. Instead, his enemies in the BMA ensured that doubts about his loyalty—based on prewar Italian fascist connections—denied him a commission. He finally left Australia at the invitation of Britain to become the United Nations Relief and Rehabilitation Administration's chief medical officer, working with refugees in occupied Germany. Success led him into the fledgling United Nations, directing the Division of Refugees and Displaced Persons (1945–46). He was sent to the UN Palestine Truce Commission (1948) as Director of Disaster Relief and Principal Medical Officer. Cilento's Middle East work was clouded by allegations of pro-Arab anti-Semitism. This, and disillusionment with the UN, led to his resignation in 1950.

Back in Brisbane, these rumors, hostile BMA memories of his reforming days, and his advancing years blocked further official appointments. His defenders have rejected charges of anti-Semitism as confusion over his pro-Arab sympathies. However, in his latter years he was active in extreme right wing politics, defending the embattled White Australia Policy and South African Apartheid while standing for Parliament with the support of the openly anti-Semitic far-right League of Rights.

He died an isolated and anachronistic figure.

Bibliography

Primary: Raphael Cilento Papers, UQFL44, University of Queensland; 1925. *The White Man in the Tropics* (Melbourne); 1944. *Blueprint for the Health of a Nation* (Sydney).

Secondary: Anderson, Warwick, 2002. *The Cultivation of Whiteness: Science, Health and Racial Destiny* (Melbourne); Fisher, Fedora, 1994. *Raphael Cilento* (Brisbane); Gillespie, James A., 1991. *The Price of Health: Australian Governments and Medical Politics* (Cambridge).

James Gillespie

CIUCĂ, MIHĂI   (b. Săveni, Dorohoi, Bukovina, 18 August 1883; d. Bucharest, Romania, 1969), *bacteriology.*

Ciucă studied at the 'Laurian' Lyceum in Botoșani. In 1901, after he obtained his baccalaureate, he enrolled at the Faculty of Medicine of the University of Bucharest, from where he received his doctorate in medicine (1907). Between 1907 and 1912, Ciucă was an assistant at the Laboratory of Experimental Medicine and worked as a doctor at the Military Hospital. During this period, he became interested in experimental medicine, immunology and infectious diseases, especially the streptococcal infections and tetanus. Between 1912 and 1913 he participated in the campaigns against cholera in Bulgaria under the leadership of Ioan Cantacuzino (1863–1934).

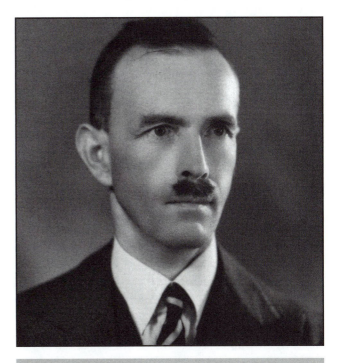

Mihăi Ciucă. Photograph, Iconographic Collection, Wellcome Library, London.

In 1914 he went to Paris and worked with Alphonse Laveran (1845–1922) at the Pasteur Institute. During World War I, he returned to Romania and was entrusted with the laboratory for serums and vaccines and the mobile hospitals for contagious diseases, which accompanied the Romanian army. In 1920 he went to the Pasteur Institute in Brussels and worked on the study of bacteriophage with Jules Bordet (1870–1961). In 1921 he was appointed to the Institute of Serums and Vaccines in Bucharest. In 1922 Ioan Cantacuzino recommended him for a professorship in hygiene at the Faculty of Medicine in Iași (eastern Romania). During this professorship, Ciucă researched the epidemiological aspects of diphtheria and created various vaccines with antitoxin, an antibody that is capable of neutralizing the specific toxin of diphtheria. Ciucă produced the antitoxin in animals and then used the resulting serum to counteract the toxin in other organisms. He also developed an antidiphtheria serum-therapy based on his observations of the epidemics of diphtheria, which plagued Europe in 1928 and 1930.

Malaria, and especially its immunogenesis, was Ciucă's main field of research. In 1924 he began his work for the League of Nations in Geneva as an expert for the Hygiene and Paludism Commission. In 1928 he became Secretary General of the International Commission on Malaria and was entrusted with epidemiological inquiries into diphtheria, malaria, and typhus as well as with organizing international anti-malaria campaigns, such as those in Spain, France, Italy, Greece and Soviet Russia (1924–25), and India, China, and Malaysia (1929–32). Ciucă also taught courses on malaria at various institutes in Europe, including the Institute of Hygiene in Paris (1929) and the Institute of Tropical Medicine in Hamburg (1930). In 1936 he became a corresponding member of the Romanian Academy and was elected an active member in 1938.

In 1934, after the death of Ioan Cantacuzino, Ciucă moved to Bucharest and became professor of bacteriology at the Faculty of Medicine. During this period, Ciucă researched widely on the bacteriophage (for instance, he discovered the phenomenon known as 'lysogeny') and refined the treatment of nervous syphilis (he applied various methods of treating venereal diseases using paludic (malarial) infection in the organism). In addition to Bordet's theories, which emphasized the relationship between the bacteriophage and its host cell, Ciucă adopted some of the theories about the role of microorganisms in nature introduced by Sergei Vinogradski (1856–1953).

Ciucă organized the first center of therapy for malaria in Romania and taught the first courses in microbiology at the Faculty of Medicine in Bucharest. In 1947 he became a member of the first Committee of experts of the Commission of Paludism of the World Health Organization and supervised the antipaludic campaigns in Romania between 1948 and 1949. Ciucă was a member of numerous institutions including the Romanian Academy of Medicine, the Société de Pathologie Exotique (Paris), and the Société de Médicine Tropicale (Brussels). His outstanding achievements in the study and prophylaxis of malaria were rewarded in 1966 with the 'Darling' Prize.

Bibliography

Primary: 1907. *Influence de l'hypothermie et de l'hyperthermie sur les infections expérimentales* (Bucharest); 1925. *Access pernicious mortal de malarie* (Iași); 1925. 'La malaria en Roumanie' C.H. Malaria/273, S.N.Org. d'Hyg; 1955. *Contribution expérimentale à l'étude de l'immunité dans la paludisme* (Bucharest).

Secondary: 1965. *Omagiu lui Mihăi Ciucă cu ocazia împlinirii a 80 de ani* (Bucharest).

Marius Turda

CIVIALE, JEAN (b. Salilhes, France, 5 July 1792; d. Garches, France, 18 June 1867), *surgery, urology.*

Civiale was born to peasant parents, Pierre Civiale and Jeanne Usse, in a village located in the elevated region of south-central France known as the Massif Central. Taking advantage of the educational opportunities created by the French Revolution and Napoleon, he went to Paris to study medicine in 1815. His teachers included the surgeon Guillaume Dupuytren, professor at the Paris Faculty of Medicine and surgeon-in-chief at the Hôtel Dieu hospital. After receiving his medical doctorate in 1820, Civiale went back to his native province to practice at Brioude. While there he married Marie-Dix-Août Faugère; his wife's given name recalled the uprising that overthrew the Bourbon monarchy on 10 August 1792. (Civiale himself evinced sufficient political flexibility to thrive throughout the successive regimes that followed the fall of Napoleon, though he remained a Free Mason, an affiliation associated with liberalism and anticlericalism.) Reportedly forced to leave Brioude because of a botched operation, Civiale returned to Paris, where he struggled financially in the early stages of his career.

Civiale owed his professional reputation almost entirely to the development of a surgical technique for removing bladder stones without the need for an incision. Lithotomy, or cutting for stone, was one of the oldest surgical operations. Even in the most skillful hands, it was a highly dangerous procedure, a last resort for patients wracked by unendurable pain. For centuries it was relegated to specialized operators, who lacked general medical or surgical training. The Hippocratic Oath required future physicians to foreswear lithotomy.

Civiale's technique, transurethral lithotrity, involved passing an instrument called a lithotrite through a cannula into the bladder, where it could crush the stones into pieces small enough to be evacuated via the urethra. He began experimenting on cadavers while still a medical student, first with solvents, which degraded the catheter used to inject them, and then with mechanical devices. In its perfected form, produced by the surgical instrument maker Joseph Charrière (1803–76), the lithotrite used pincers tightened remotely by a screw to locate, seize, and crush the stones; a large stone could be fragmented with a central drill rotated by a bow. In 1827 Civiale was appointed to the Necker Hospital and put in charge of a special service for bladder stone. He operated on more than 3,000 patients and claimed a mortality rate of less than 3 percent, as opposed to more than 20 percent for lithotomy. His study of the use of lithotomy and lithotrity in Europe was a prominent example of the statistical analysis of therapeutic outcomes, contemporaneous with Pierre Louis's more widely known research on the efficacy of bloodletting. In 1835 the Academy of Sciences appointed a special commission to assess and report on this work.

Despite continual priority disputes over the invention of the novel treatment for bladder stone, Civiale's contributions brought him fame, wealth, and honors, including a prize from the Academy of Sciences for developing lithotrity. The Academy of Medicine elected him to its section of operative medicine in 1834; he became a member of the Academy of Sciences in 1847. The government named him an officer of the Legion of Honor.

Civiale was a pioneer in the development of urology as a modern surgical specialty. His statistical work was an early contribution to what we would now call evidence-based medicine.

Bibliography

Primary: 1827. *De la lithotritie ou broiement de la pierre dans la vessie* (Paris); 1837–42. *Traité pratique sur les maladies des organes génito-urinaires* 3 vols. (Paris); 1847. *Traité pratique et historique de la lithotritie* (Paris).

Secondary: Bouchet, H., 1999. 'Chirurgie de la lithiase vésicale au XIXe siècle.' *Annales de chirurgie* 53: 908–914; Ramsey, Matthew, 1997. 'From *Expert* to *Spécialiste*: The Conception of Specialization in Eighteenth-and Nineteenth-Century French Surgery' in Kawakita, Yoshio, ed., *History of Ideas in Surgery* (Tokyo) pp. 69–117; Rames, J., 1899. *Étude sur le Dr Civiale* (Aurillac).

Matthew Ramsey

CLELAND, JOHN BURTON

CLELAND, JOHN BURTON   (b. Norwood, South Australia, 22 June 1878; d. Adelaide, Australia, 11 August 1971), *pathology, natural history, physical anthropology.*

Cleland, the son of William Lennox Cleland, a physician, and Matilda Lauder Burton, was educated at Prince Alfred College, Adelaide, and began medical training at the University of Adelaide, but conflict between the Adelaide Hospital honorary staff and the government compelled his transfer to the University of Sydney (MB 1900, MD 1902). He trained in pathology in Sydney and at the London School of Tropical Medicine and the London Hospital.

In 1905 Cleland became government bacteriologist and pathologist in Western Australia, where he investigated an outbreak of bubonic plague among humans and 'surra' among the camels that roamed the state's vast deserts. Nomadic by inclination, Cleland transferred in 1909 to the Bureau of Microbiology in Sydney. There he confirmed, using human volunteers, that *Aedes aegypti* transmitted dengue; and he identified the mysterious 'Australian X disease' as a transmissible encephalitis, distinguishing it from poliomyelitis. In 1920 Cleland returned to Adelaide as the first Marks professor of pathology, a post that encompassed microbiology. His days as an experimentalist were over, but his interest in observational and descriptive studies deepened with each passing year. At Adelaide he dissected more than 7,000 corpses in a series of meticulous autopsy examinations. The prospect of a body on the slab never ceased to stir and invigorate him; he regularly published his findings in the *Medical Journal of Australia* well into his eighties.

Cleland's interests and career reflected the distinctive culture of the Adelaide medical school, which was derived in part from its presence in a notably liberal and nonconformist city, its close connection to a natural history museum, and its proximity to the central deserts. Cleland eagerly embraced the natural history tradition of the medical school, shared with his colleagues an interest in the impact of the environment on human biology, and remained Lamarckian in his sympathies well into the twentieth century. Denying that the individual is merely a 'protective and nourishing envelope' for the germ plasm, he came to believe that humans possess hereditary potential that awaits a stimulating environment to call it forth and ensure its transmission as a phenotype to later generations. His liberal environmentalism led to an obsession with Aboriginal adaptation, and to speculation on the biologically correct means of absorbing 'half-castes' into the white community.

As chairman of the Board for Anthropological Research at Adelaide, Cleland traveled each year through the deserts around Alice Springs, bleeding 'full-bloods' and botanizing along the way. Repeatedly he demonstrated that Aborigines lacked blood group B, and therefore were related to Caucasians, a theory disputed since the 1890s. This biological affinity suggested that Aboriginal Australians might be absorbed into white Australia without 'throwbacks'. As a member of the South Australian Aborigines' Protection Board, Cleland frequently demanded the removal of 'half-caste' Aboriginal children from incompetent parents or communities and their adoption by white families, though he also urged the establishment of reservations for 'full-bloods' to delay their 'detribalisation' and demoralization. Mostly, he anticipated the day when 'nearly every inhabitant of Australia will have had an Aboriginal ancestor'—and it would not matter. In 1938–39, with E. A. Hooton of Harvard University, Cleland supported the optimistic 'half-caste' survey conducted by Norman 'Tinny' Tindale and

Joseph Birdsell. Thus the high-minded liberal environmentalism of Adelaide's medical circles helped to rationalize the 'stolen generations' of Aboriginal children.

Cleland also made major contributions to mycology and ornithology. He published extensively on the larger fungi and vascular plants of South Australia, and he presented a collection of nearly 30,000 plants to the South Australian Herbarium and hundreds of bird skins to the South Australian Museum. In his later years, he became committed to wildlife conservation and environmental protection.

Appointed CBE in 1949 and knighted in 1964, Cleland received numerous awards from a multitude of organizations. Cleland Conservation Park in the Mount Lofty Ranges is named for him.

Bibliography

Secondary: Anderson, Warwick, 2002. *The Cultivation of Whiteness: Science, Health and Racial Destiny* (Melbourne).

Warwick Anderson

CLOT BEY (aka ANTOINE BARTÉLÉMY CLOT)

(b. Grenoble, France, 7 November 1793; d. Marseille, France, 28 August 1868), *medicine.*

Son of a sergeant major in the Napoleonic army, Clot Bey's father and aunt provided his early education. In 1808 the Clot family moved to Brignoles, where he received his initial medical training from his father's comrade Sapey, a retired army surgeon. His first operation was the removal of a sebaceous cyst, which he preserved in alcohol and carried with him as a memento for the next twenty years.

In 1813 Clot Bey set off to Marseille, where a classmate, a medical student, helped him enter the Hôtel Dieu, the city hospital. He successfully passed the entrance exams and was admitted as a student *externe* and considered the best student. In 1817 he passed the examinations for the degree of Doctor of Medicine, but could still not earn enough money to support his widowed mother. In 1819, he attended the University of Aix-en-Provence and gained a Bachelor of Letters degree. He was accepted at the Montpellier medical school and in 1820 successfully defended his first thesis. Subsequently he was made assistant surgeon at the Hôtel Dieu in Marseille. In 1823, he returned to Montpellier, presenting his MD thesis on surgery. Probably because of his success, Clot Bey was dropped from the Academic Society of Medicine of Marseille and forbidden to give lessons in hospitals. In 1825, he joined the service of Muḥammad 'Alī the viceroy of Egypt, who was determined to keep his army in good health.

As Surgeon-in-Chief of the Armies, Clot Bey introduced French Army health regulations for the Egyptian army camps. To improve the health of the army, he convinced Muḥammad 'Alī to raise the health of the population and made smallpox vaccination mandatory for civilians. He also founded a medical school for 300 students at the 1,500-bed military hospital at Abou Zabel, outside Cairo.

He commissioned European doctors as teachers but faced two major obstacles: the language and religious opposition. He solved the first problem by introducing interpreters. The second was more difficult to tackle: religious fanatics even tried to kill Clot Bey while he performed an anatomy demonstration. However, he appealed to them, stating that by medical studies they could augment their influence and as a consequence several *Ulemā'* became medical students, and one even composed a medical dictionary. Clot Bey helped to assuage religious difficulties by making concessions to the Muslim religion, e.g., making the holy month of Ramadan the medical school's major holiday. The medical school soon developed four different curricula: medicine, veterinary medicine, pharmacy, and midwifery. In 1830 he arranged a very successful public examination for his students and brought an external examiner from Europe. This meant that in less than five years Clot Bey had founded a Western-style medical school and produced excellent Egyptian graduates. In 1831 Clot Bey successfully managed a cholera epidemic. He was made a general and the first Catholic to receive the title 'Bey'. A year later (1832), he departed for Paris with his best students. The trip was immensely successful. At the age of forty-seven he married Mlle. Gavoty and together they had a daughter. His mother came to stay with him in Egypt and died there. In 1849 Muḥammad 'Alī died. His successor, Abbas Pasha, discharged Clot Bey, who returned to Marseille.

Bibliography

Primary: Larousse, P., 1898. *Nouveau Larousse illustre dictionnaire universel encyclopedique* (Paris) contains a list of works by Clot Bey; 1949. *Mémoires de A.-B. Clot Bey* (publiés et annotés par Jacques Tagher) (Le Caire).

Secondary: Burrow, G. N., 1975. 'Clot Bey: Founder of Western Medical Practice in Egypt.' *The Yale Journal of Biology and Medicine* 48: 251–257.

Nikolaj Serikoff

CLOWES, WILLIAM (b. Kingsbury, Warwickshire, England, 1543/4; d. West Ham, Essex, England, 1604), *surgery, venereology.*

Clowes was the son of Thomas Clowes and Emma Beauchamp. His education and training remain obscure, but he fulsomely praised the instruction that he received from his 'Master', George Keble, who practiced both physic and surgery. In 1602 he wrote that he had been practicing surgery since 1563; that year he served as a surgeon on the military expedition to the French port of Le Havre and he then served as a naval surgeon for a number of years.

During the 1560s he engaged in civilian practice in Kent and in London; Clowes was admitted to the London Company of Barbers and Surgeons in November 1569. Around this time he began working in London hospitals; he was made one of the surgeons of St Bartholomew's Hospital in 1576 and apothecary-surgeon at Christ's Hospital. He received an episcopal license to practice in 1580 and was made middle warden of the Barber Surgeons four years later.

In 1585 he returned to military and naval service when he left his post at St Bartholomew's to serve as a surgeon with the Earl of Leicester's army in the Netherlands. He was also made one of the Queen's surgeons, and from 1586 he held a position as surgeon to the Navy, including being attached to Lord Howard of Effingham's flagship in the Armada campaign.

Thereafter, he developed a private practice across London, prospering sufficiently to purchase property in Fenchurch Street, to retire to the Essex village of West Ham, and to style himself a gentleman, displaying his family coat of arms.

In 1576 Clowes published a work on venereal disease, which was reissued in 1579 and 1585; he produced *A Prooved Practise for all Young Chirurgians*, with advice on the cure of wounds and burns in 1588 (it was reissued in 1591 and in an expanded form with his writing on the pox in 1596 and 1637) and a study of the treatment of the King's Evil in 1602. All were rooted in his personal experience and practice, giving vivid descriptions of particular cases he had attended. As a surgeon at St Bartholomew's he encountered many patients afflicted with venereal disease; he compared his military service with Hippocrates's advice that the surgeon should follow the wars; he included short notes so that a surgeon on board a ship without the advice of a physician would be able to purge his patients. All his books were, furthermore, published in English, and Clowes argued passionately against those who opposed vernacular medical works.

His emphasis upon his own service in the army and the navy and his condemnation of the poor quality of the surgeons attending English troops were clearly designed to present surgery as valuable to the state, and his publications more generally sought to elevate the surgeon's status. His books contain several bitter attacks upon unqualified healers, condemning those who 'foresake their trades' to practice physic and surgery and claiming that 'Roages, Ratcatchers [and] Runagetes' were abusing regular practitioners. Importantly his advice for surgeons advocated the use of ligatures before amputation, greatly reducing the loss of blood and increasing the likelihood of the patient surviving the operation. Moreover, he was one of the important advocates of chemical medicine in London during the 1570s and 1580s. Although he in no way rejected Galen or Hippocrates (and contributed to a partial translation of the medieval surgeon, Guy of Chauliac, c. 1300–68), he praised the works of Paracelsus (c. 1494–1541) and his treatise on the French Disease described and recommended mercurial treatment while recognizing its side-effects.

Bibliography

Primary: 1948. (Poynter, F. N. L., ed.) *Selected Writings of William Clowes* (London).

Secondary: Webster, C., 1979. 'Alchemical and Paracelsian Medicine' in Webster, C., ed., *Health, Medicine and Mortality in the Sixteenth Century* (Cambridge) pp. 301–334; Grell, O. P., 2004. 'War, Medicine and the Military Revolution' in Elmer, P., ed., *The Healing Arts: Health, Disease and Society in Europe 1500–1800* (Manchester) pp. 257–282; *Oxford DNB*.

Mark Jenner

COCHRANE, ARCHIBALD LEMAN (b. Galashiels, Scotland, 12 January 1909; d. Holt, Dorset, England, 18 June 1988), *epidemiology, clinical trials, health services research.*

Cochrane was born into a well-off Scottish tweed-making family, the first son of Walter Francis and Emma Mabel (née Purdom) Cochrane. His father was killed at the Battle of Gaza when Archie was only eight years old; one of Archie's brothers (Walter) died at age two from measles; and another (Robert) died at age twenty-one, after a motorcycle accident. Unsurprisingly, Archie's lifelong relationship with his older sister, Helen, was very close, and it was her son and daughter-in-law, Joe and Maggie Stalker, who cared for Archie at their home in Somerset in the years before his death.

That Archie's sister Helen outlived him was in part because he challenged a diagnosis of dementia made after she had been admitted to a psychiatric hospital. Further investigation led to the discovery that she—and Archie—had porphyria. Because he was concerned that other members of the family scattered around the world might unknowingly have the condition and put themselves at risk, he solicited urinary and fecal samples from 153 of them and succeeded in obtaining satisfactory specimens from 152 relatives.

In some ways this anecdote encapsulates the essence of Archie Cochrane. He was always ready to challenge medical (and non-medical) authorities to provide better evidence about the basis for their diagnoses and treatments. Although he had an epidemiologist's interest in the well-being of communities, he was also deeply concerned for the welfare of individuals. And, as reflected in the survey of his relatives, he was known particularly for achieving very high rates of participation and follow-up in his epidemiological and clinical studies.

Early Life

After attending a preparatory school at Rhos-on-Sea in Wales, Cochrane won a scholarship to Uppingham School (in Rutland, England) in 1922, where he became a school prefect and a member of the rugby football 1st XV. In 1927 he won a scholarship to King's College Cambridge, where he graduated in 1930 with first class honors in Parts I and II of the Natural Sciences Tripos, and also completed second MB studies. An inheritance enabled him to continue studying, and during 1931 he worked on tissue culture at the Strangeways Laboratory in Cambridge.

Richard Doll (1912–2005) (*Oxford DNB*) suggested that it was fortunate for medicine that Cochrane soon tired of what he concluded was trivial research and that he developed psychological symptoms leading him to abandon his research and seek medical help. In retrospect, it seems likely that his symptoms were due to porphyria. Be that as it may, Cochrane received little sympathy from the British doctors he consulted but found that doctors at the Kaiser Wilhelm Institute in Berlin were willing to take his problem seriously. Between 1931 and 1934 he underwent psychoanalysis with Theodor Reik (1888–1969), initially in Berlin, but then in Vienna and The Hague as Reik fled from Hitler. Cochrane did some medical studies in Vienna and Leiden during this time and published his first paper (*Elie Metchinikoff and his theory of an 'instinct de la mort'*). More significantly, these three years in Europe instilled in Cochrane a hatred of fascism and a skeptical attitude to all theories—including psychoanalysis—that had not been validated in experiments.

After returning to Britain in 1934, Cochrane enrolled as a clinical medical student at University College Hospital (UCH), London, but he abandoned his studies two years later in order to serve as a volunteer during the Spanish Civil War in a Field Ambulance Unit on the Aragon front and at the siege of Madrid. He resumed his clinical studies at UCH in 1937 and qualified MB, BCh (Cantab) in 1938. Until the outbreak of World War II he worked first as a house physician at the West London Hospital and then as a research assistant at the Medical Unit at UCH. As a captain in the Royal Army Medical Corps, he served first in Egypt as a hospital medical officer and then, after capture in Crete in 1941, as a prisoner of war medical officer in Salonica, Hildburghausen, Elsterhorst, and Wittenberg-am-Elbe (he was subsequently awarded MBE (military) in recognition of this service). Cochrane's experience as a prisoner of war medical officer reinforced his interest in testing unsubstantiated claims about the effects of medical treatments (he organized his first clinical trial during this time) as well as made clear to him the importance of care when there is no hope of cure.

Epidemiology

After leaving the army at the end of the war, Cochrane obtained a Rockefeller fellowship in preventive medicine. The first element of this involved attending the Diploma in Public Health course at the London School of Hygiene and Tropical Medicine, where he was greatly influenced by Austin Bradford Hill's (1897–1991) teaching on epidemiology and randomized clinical trials. In 1947, for the second element of the fellowship, Cochrane went to the Henry Phipps Clinic in Philadelphia, where he became interested in x-ray studies of pulmonary tuberculosis and developed what became a lifelong interest in inter-observer and intra-observer error.

Back in Britain in 1948, Cochrane joined the scientific staff of the Medical Research Council's Pneumoconiosis Research Unit in Penarth, near Cardiff (South Wales), and

two years later launched the Rhondda Fach ('two valleys') scheme to investigate the etiology of progressive massive fibrosis. Cochrane worked at the Pneumoconiosis Research Unit for over a decade, during which time his main interests were the x-ray classification of coal workers' pneumoconiosis and the relationship he demonstrated between x-ray categories, dust exposure, and disability. His interest in this field continued for the rest of his life, as reflected in the completion during 1974 to 1986 of twenty-year and thirty-year follow-up studies of the population of the Rhondda Fach.

Cochrane's research set very high standards for epidemiological studies because of his insistence on achieving very high response rates in surveys and follow-up studies and for his checks on the reproducibility of the measurements made. The meticulous quality of his work was reflected in the decision by the MRC to invite him to establish and direct a new epidemiology unit based in Cardiff. Cochrane took up this invitation in 1960 and was appointed the same year to the David Davies Chair of Tuberculosis and Diseases of the Chest at the Welsh National School of Medicine. He held the chair until 1969, when he was appointed CBE.

Under Cochrane's direction, the MRC Epidemiology Unit quickly established an international reputation for the quality of its surveys and studies of the natural history and etiology of a wide range of common diseases, including anemia, glaucoma, asthma, and gallbladder disease. These studies led naturally to Cochrane's interest in the validation of screening strategies within the National Health Service.

Clinical Trials

Although Cochrane himself was particularly proud that the quality of his epidemiological studies had set new standards for the specialty, he is probably most widely remembered for his advocacy of randomized controlled trials. He always acknowledged the important influence of Bradford Hill in introducing him to the principles of using these studies to obtain unbiased estimates of the effects of healthcare interventions, and the establishment of the MRC Epidemiology Unit under his direction provided him with the opportunity to put these principles into practice. The Unit coordinated a wide variety of randomized trials to evaluate pharmaceutical, surgical, and health service interventions. The trials with the most enduring and important implications for human health were those led by Cochrane's colleague Peter Elwood (who succeeded him as director in 1974), which first established that aspirin could reduce the incidence of cardiovascular diseases.

Randomized trials are of obvious relevance in guiding decisions about the use of resources in health services. An invitation from the Nuffield Provincial Hospitals Trusts to prepare the 1971 Rock Carling Lecture provided Cochrane with an opportunity to develop this theme, and he did so in a way that no one had done previously. His delivery of the lecture itself (on 20 March 1972, in Edinburgh) was apparently less than fluent; but the book that resulted from it, *Effectiveness and Efficiency: Random Reflections on Health Services*, promptly became an influential best seller.

Cochrane's little book was written in a very readable style, and covered important issues of general interest—the importance of using randomized trials to identify which health service interventions are more likely to do good than harm, the relevance of assessing the costs of the options available when deciding what to make available within the British National Health Service, and the importance of equitable access to effective treatments and to sensitive care when cure was not possible. The seminal importance of the book was recognized by the lay media as well as the medical press, and it was subsequently translated into many languages.

International Recognition

In the year the book was published, 1972, Cochrane became the first president of the new Faculty of Community Medicine (subsequently Faculty of Public Health). He received an honorary doctorate from the University of York the following year; was Dunham Lecturer at Harvard University in 1974; became an honorary fellow of the American Epidemiological Association in 1975; and, in 1977, received an honorary doctorate from the Rochester University, USA, and became an honorary fellow of the International Epidemiological Association.

In 1979, in a contribution to a book published by the Office of Health Economics, Cochrane wrote, 'It is surely a great criticism of our profession that we have not organised a critical summary, by speciality or subspeciality, adapted periodically, of all relevant randomised controlled trials.' A few years after his death, this proved to be the rallying point that led to the creation of the Cochrane Collaboration (www.cochrane.org). Over 10,000 people in many countries and specialties—most of them volunteers—are now preparing and maintaining systematic reviews of randomized trials, and reviews of other evidence when appropriate, within this international, non-profit organization and publishing the reviews electronically in *The Cochrane Database of Systematic Reviews*.

Cochrane was an accomplished gardener (his scree garden won an award from the Royal Horticultural Society) and a discerning collector of modern art and sculpture. He died of cancer in 1988 after a long illness. As he concluded in the obituary he wrote about himself for publication in the *British Medical Journal*, 'He was a man with severe porphyria who smoked too much and was without the consolation of a wife, a religious belief, or a merit award—but he didn't do so badly.'

Bibliography

Primary: 1951. 'Methods of Investigating the Connections between Dust and Disease' in *The Application of Scientific Meth-*

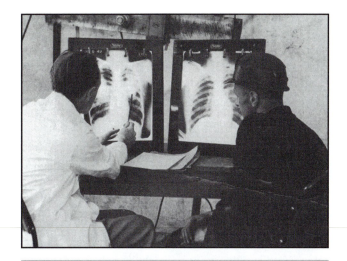

Archie Cochrane explaining progressive fibrosis of the lung to a miner at Ferndale colliery during the first Rhondda Fach survey. Halftone reproduction from *One Man's Medicine*, 1989. Reproduced with permission of Max Blythe.

ods to Industrial and Service Medicine (London) pp. 97–100; 1972. *Effectiveness and Efficiency: Random Reflections on Health Services* (London); 1979. '1931–1971: A Critical Review with Particular Reference to the Medical Profession' in *Medicines for the Year 2000* (London) pp. 1–11; 1989. (with Blythe, Max) *One Man's Medicine: An Autobiography of Professor Archie Cochrane* (London).

Secondary: Bosch, X., 2003. *Archie Cochrane: Back to the Front* (Barcelona); *Archie Cochrane Archive.* Centre for the History of Evaluation in Health Care, Cardiff University: http://www.cardiff.ac.uk/schoolsanddivisions/divisions/insrv/libraryservices/research/cochrane/index.html; Maynard, A., and Iain Chalmers, 1997. *Non-random Reflections on Health Services Research: On the 25th Anniversary of Archie Cochrane's 'Effectiveness and Efficiency'* (London); *Oxford DNB.*

Iain Chalmers

CODMAN, ERNEST AMORY   (b. Boston, Massachusetts, USA, 30 December 1869; d. Ponkapog, Massachusetts, USA, 23 November 1940), *surgery, orthopedic surgery.*

Codman was an early twentieth-century American surgeon who devoted himself to detailed and methodical record keeping as a means for improving medical practice. Early in his career, he compiled one of the first radiological atlases of human skeletal joints, furthering interest in the use of x-rays among his colleagues at Harvard Medical School. His most noted achievement was his controversial plan for compiling what he called End Results: a system for physicians to track the long-term outcomes from their treatments as a public record. Codman championed this idea against considerable resistance from his surgical colleagues and eventually found himself ostracized from the inner circles of Boston medicine. His End Result System is still widely praised and influential, though it is also still little used. Late in his career Codman made a final, lasting contribution to medicine by founding a national registry of cases of bone sarcomas to correlate clinical features, treatments, and outcomes for this rare disease.

Codman spent his life in Boston, Massachusetts, where he was, by his own account, 'a conventional enough Boston-Harvard boy, with relatives and acquaintances among the well-to-do' (Codman, 1934, p. vii). His parents, William Coombs and Elizabeth (Hurd) Codman, belonged to a cadre of elite families, nicknamed collectively the Boston Brahmins. His father began in business as an importer in the East India trade and later established a prosperous real estate and insurance firm. The couple sent Amory, as he was called, to St Mark's School, a boarding school founded and run by a physician and manufacturing chemist emphasizing the natural sciences. Amory Codman moved on to Harvard College and then to Harvard Medical School, graduating in 1895 after a year studying medicine abroad. Upon graduation he took a spot at Massachusetts General Hospital as a house officer and then went directly into practice, becoming an assistant surgeon under the tutelage of Francis Bishop Harrington at the hospital.

Codman won early recognition for his work on x-ray radiographs. In 1896, immediately following Roentgen's announcement of x-rays, Codman began to investigate their medical use. He made an extensive study of normal, human joints in different degrees of flexion, compiling a comprehensive atlas of x-ray photographs. In 1900 he followed with a detailed study of radial bone fractures using x-ray images, classifying what are known as Colles' fractures of the forearm into categories that remain part of the present-day classification. Codman also studied x-ray burns of the skin, which he experienced himself in his long exposures during research. In 1911 he contributed a chapter to a major textbook on the use of the x-ray in surgery.

By late 1914, Codman moved from assistant surgeon in the outpatient department at MGH to the regular staff and secured a post on the faculty of Harvard Medical School. At this point, however, Codman made a dramatic break with Boston's established medical community, sacrificing his reputation in a quixotic attempt to win acceptance for his End Result System.

The system was a simple method that he proposed for assessing and publicly ranking surgeons by tabulating their long-term therapeutic results from surgical operations. His major efforts to establish such a system were limited to surgery, but he aimed to apply the method to medical care as a whole. Codman asked simply that hospital administrators keep track of the long-term outcomes for patients treated by their surgeons and use that

information in promoting the surgeons on the hospital service.

An obvious source of resistance to Codman's system arose from its public nature. Codman was not suggesting that individual surgeons review their long-term outcomes privately as a road to self-improvement. He asked that hospitals track outcomes in order to rank surgeons. As Codman lobbied for the system, he contrasted it with the existing practice of rewarding surgeons according to seniority and reputation. The reigning system relied on criteria best evident to other surgeons, criteria that Codman mocked saying that he wanted 'to bury the old ideas of "nerve," "steady hand" and graceful'" operating (Codman, 1914, p. 136). Such terms were useful only in a hierarchy that judged and rewarded its members behind closed doors. The tabulation of actual long-term results would provide a valid, objective measure of skill. But getting surgeons to allow hospitals to collect and use such information proved difficult.

Codman realized early, partial support, instead, through alliance with surgeons working on the reverse project: to establish criteria for hospitals. He obtained some recognition for the End Result System in a national and influential movement within surgery to standardize hospitals. Codman's long-time friend, the gynecologic surgeon Edward Martin, used his presidency in 1912 in the Clinical Congress of Surgeons of North America to launch the new American College of Surgeons. Martin established Codman as the chairman of the Committee on the Standardization of Hospitals in the Congress of Surgeons and moved this group over as a permanent body in the new College. Codman was joined on the committee by several eminent surgical colleagues: William Mayo, Walter Chipman, Allen Kanavel, and John Clark. The first report from this group in November 1913 recommended requiring that all hospitals establish an End Result System for their surgeons. The Congress voted to mail out this report to 180 hospitals in the United States and Canada and to solicit word of progress toward this goal. Codman made sure to send out an early copy to the trustees at his own MGH. The response was weak, and no lasting reforms of the sort that Codman desired emerged from the effort.

Resistance to End Results began close to home. By the end of 1914, Codman had pushed his influence at the MGH to a breaking point. The hospital rebuffed his suggestion to appoint one of the hospital's lay trustees to oversee an End Result System. Codman recalled later that he handed in his letter of resignation to protest their obstinacy. He followed this letter with another to the trustees of the hospital, where he demanded, perhaps tongue-in-cheek, to be reinstated as the hospital's surgeon-in-chief, based on his own excellent record as judged by the End Results that he kept himself. In the end, he found his relationship with the hospital severed.

Codman's most extraordinary effort at propaganda for the End Result System came soon after in January 1915. He contrived to use his position in the Surgical Section of the Suffolk District Medical Society to make the group's January meeting a surprise showcase. Codman drew a crowd of substantial figures in Bostonian society and medicine, offering a panel of nationally known speakers to address the topic of hospital efficiency. At the conclusion of the speeches Codman appeared before the crowd and unveiled his surprise: a very large, three-paneled cartoon, broadly caricaturing the local resistance to his reforms. His prestigious audience found themselves the subject of Codman's ridicule. The cartoon depicted Boston's wealthy citizens as an ostrich with its head stuck in the sand. The ostrich could not look up to judge the ability of its doctors by End Results. On the left panel, these same doctors stood with their backs turned, ignoring 'medical science' embodied behind them in the buildings of Harvard Medical School. They occupied themselves instead catching the golden eggs of high medical fees that the ostrich kicked their way. The MGH appeared on the right panel, enshrining 'clinical truth'. The hospital's trustees sat ignoring this truth, while they pondered whether the wealthy ostrich would still lay golden eggs if Codman's End Result System revealed the truth about its physicians. Harvard University's President Lowell appeared in caricature presiding over the scene, worrying 'could my clinical professors make a living without humbug?' A caption explained that the End Result System threatened this cozy arrangement among the hospital, their elite physicians, and the medical school. The cartoon, of course, endeared Codman to none

of these groups. Codman was asked to resign from the section on surgery of the medical society, and he recalled later that he was also dropped as an instructor at Harvard Medical School.

Stripped of his affiliations with medical school, local surgical society, and hospital, Codman had one final avenue through which to promote his reforms. Although he could not persuade other hospital administrators to follow him, he might administer his own hospital according to his design. The Codman Hospital, which he had founded in August 1911, became a site for demonstrating the system in action. Efforts at the Codman Hospital peaked along with other reforms in 1914, when Codman published the first of three studies on hospital efficiency. These studies offered Codman Hospital as a model institution. The hospital was a modest endeavor, a townhouse that provided a site for Codman and a few other surgeons to perform roughly 300 operations during the six years that it remained open. For each operation, Codman recorded and published in the hospital reports an End Result card listing a preoperative diagnosis, the details of the operation, any complications, and the results after one year, with a frank account of any bad outcomes, including acknowledgement of personal errors. Codman hoped that his stringent honesty and the good economic performance of his hospital might demonstrate and promote the value of the End Result System. But after a few sound years, the hospital began to lose money. Codman absorbed the debts until the hospital shut down permanently in 1917, and Codman left Boston soon after to join the Medical Corps of the U.S. Army.

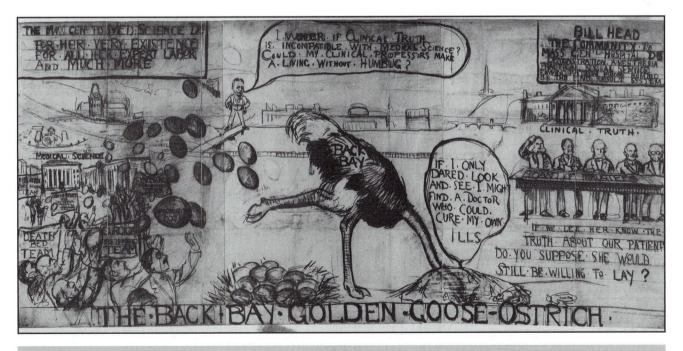

Back Bay Golden Goose Ostrich cartoon. (Courtesy of The Boston Medical Library in the Francis A. Countway Library of Medicine.)

Codman never abandoned his enthusiasm for the End Result System, but neither did he let other work lapse. After his return from the war effort in 1919, Codman received a gift from the family of a patient with their encouragement to study rare tumors of the bone called sarcomas. He set about the project with the same zeal that characterized his End Results. Using the gift and subsequent funding from the American College of Surgeons, Codman organized a national registry of cases of the disease, lobbying for surgeons to submit information on their cases to the registry. Codman quickly recognized that without such a mechanism, it was impossible to correlate among rare and widely dispersed individual cases. He found that nomenclature and treatment of the problem varied considerably. He promoted national efforts to standardize the classification of the tumors. Codman also tied his efforts back to his idea about End Results. He encouraged his colleagues to follow their patients who received treatment for bone sarcomas over the years to determine eventual outcomes and to report them to the registry. Perhaps insight about optimal treatment would emerge from this growing database.

Although isolated in his practice after the loss of his positions in Boston's prestigious medical institutions, Codman continued his surgical career. He gradually developed his interest and expertise in the surgical management of shoulder injuries and pathologies. In the final years of his career he summarized his extensive experience. Over the course of his practice, he compiled detailed information on 1,151 cases of shoulder disease, which formed the basis for a comprehensive book, *The Shoulder*, in 1934. The work was an extraordinarily complete survey of the anatomy, biomechanics, pathology, and treatment of the shoulder. This contribution to shoulder surgery has been widely acknowledged by present-day experts. A distinguished orthopedic surgeon specializing in the shoulder reported that the book was still being used in the 1990s as a reference (Mallon, 2000, p. 137).

Codman had a long, untroubled marriage with Katherine Bowditch Codman, who herself was involved with important medical movements. Katy Codman became a strong ally of the public health nursing program at Simmons College in Boston and rose to become Secretary and President of the Instructive District Nursing Association of Boston. She also became a close friend and political ally of Alice Hamilton, an influential professor at Harvard Medical School. Katy Codman worked closely with Hamilton in the cause of birth control and the abolition of capital punishment. The two may have met through the woman's suffrage movement. When Hamilton came to Boston to assume her position at Harvard Medical School, she moved in with Amory and Katy Codman on her arrival and later rented space from the Codmans in the building that had earlier housed the Codman Hospital.

Bibliography

Primary: 1898. 'Experiments on the application of Roentgen rays to the study of anatomy.' *J. Exper. Med.* 3: 383–391; 1914. *A study in hospital efficiency: The first two years of a private hospital* (Boston); 1922. 'Registry of cases of sarcoma of the long bones.' *Surgery Gynecology and Obstetrics* 34: 335–343; 1934. *The Shoulder* (Boston).

Secondary: Crenner, Christopher, 2001. 'Organizational Reform and Professional Dissent in the Careers of Richard Cabot and Ernest Amory Codman, 1900–1920.' *Journal of the History of Medicine and Allied Sciences* 56(3): 211–237; Mallon, William, 2000. *Ernest Amory Codman: The End Result of a Life in Medicine* (Philadelphia); Reverby, Susan, 1981. 'Stealing the Golden Eggs: Ernest Amory Codman and the Science and Management of Medicine.' *Bulletin of the History of Medicine* 55: 156–171; *DAMB*.

Christopher Crenner

COHNHEIM, JULIUS (b. Demmin, Pomerania, Germany, 20 July 1839; d. Leipzig, Germany, 15 August 1884), *pathology.*

Cohnheim was the son of a merchant. In 1856, he finished his school education, and between 1856 and 1860 he studied medicine in Berlin and Greifswald. In January 1861 he started to work under Rudolf Virchow (1821–1902) in the Pathological Institute of the Berlin Charité Hospital. In 1864 he was a military physician in Schleswig-Holstein during the German-Danish War. Thereafter he continued his collaboration with Virchow and became his 'first assistant'. In 1868, Cohnheim was appointed professor of pathological anatomy at the University of Kiel. The Franco-Prussian War interrupted his time in Kiel. During 1871–72, he worked again as a military physician, this time in Berlin. Between 1872 and 1878, Cohnheim had the chair of pathological anatomy in Breslau. After 1878 he worked in the same position at the University of Leipzig, where he died from a chronic disease in 1884.

Cohnheim cultivated and promoted experimental pathology in a morphological age, where scientific medicine learned from the static Virchowian investigation of organs, tissues, and cells in the dead room. The goal of experimental pathology, based on animal experimentation, was to uncover the processes of diseases and therewith complement the static view of pathological morphological changes. In principle, this was also Virchow's aim, but it was above all Cohnheim who put this idea into practice. Most important in this sense was his work on inflammation. This had long been a basic problem of medicine, and work on the subject was promoted in Virchow's institute. Many people, and above all the poor, died of infectious diseases, and elucidating the well-known phenomena of inflammation would improve medical diagnosis and treatment.

During his years with Virchow, Cohnheim developed a new theory. He worked on the role of the vessels in the course of the inflammatory process, performing experiments on the frog tongue, frog mesentery, and rabbit cornea. Cohnheim postulated that most of the inflammatory symptoms were caused by changes in blood circulation and that exudation occurred because of vessel damage. Moreover, he definitely showed that the so-called 'pus-corpuscles' (*Eiterkörperchen*) were not parenchymal products as Virchow claimed, but were leucocytes, which emigrated out of the blood stream through the vessel walls. This led to a conflict with Virchow, who never changed his views decisively.

Cohnheim supported the foundation of pathological physiology, the investigation of pathological *processes*, in his actual daily work. As it was also necessary to relate such laboratory results with knowledge achieved at the bedside, Cohnheim had close contacts with clinicians as early as his Berlin times, e.g., with Ludwig Traube (1818–76). Cohnheim's initiative to apply physiological thinking to practical medicine and to promote cooperation between pathologists and clinicians stemmed perhaps from his participation in the German-Danish War.

Cohnheim contributed to research on different areas of pathology, for example, the formation of tumors and the theory of infarct. Also, he had a decisive influence on other areas of medicine and on physicians outside of Germany. Paul Ehrlich (1854–1915) was among those who worked at his institute in Leipzig. Cohnheim (and also Ehrlich) were 'clinical pathologists' and they influenced the development of this new discipline especially in England after 1900. 'Clinical pathology' focused mainly on the examination of body fluids and tissue samples from the living patient. Morbid anatomy was only one method among others. The new strand of pathology came back to Germany only after 1945. With his work, which is underestimated by historians of medicine, Julius Cohnheim greatly influenced the character of twentieth-century medicine.

Bibliography

Primary: 1885. *Gesammelte Abhandlungen* (Berlin); 1867. 'Ueber Entzündung und Eiterung.' *Archiv für pathologische Anatomie und Physiologie und für klinische Medizin* 40: 1–79; 1873. *Neue Untersuchungen über die Entzündung* (Berlin).

Secondary: Prüll, Cay-Rüdiger, 2003. *Medizin am Toten oder am Lebenden?—Pathologie in Berlin und in London 1900 bis 1945* (Basel); Maulitz, Russell C., 1978. 'Rudolf Virchow, Julius Cohnheim and the Program of Pathology.' *Bulletin of the History of Medicine* 52: 162–182; Maulitz, Russell C., 1974. *A Treatise on Membranes: Concepts of Tissue Structure, Function and Dysfunction from Xavier Bichat to Julius Cohnheim* (Ann Arbor).

Cay-Ruediger Pruell

COINDET, JEAN-FRANÇOIS   (b. Republic of Geneva [now Switzerland], 12 July 1774; d. Nice, France, 11 February 1834), *therapeutics, endocrinology.*

Coindet was the son of Jean-Jacques Coindet and Catherine Gros. In 1796, while studying medicine at Edinburgh, he married Catherine Walker, who gave him two sons, the elder of whom (Jean-Charles, 1796–1876) also studied medicine in Scotland and later practiced medicine and psychiatry in Geneva.

Coindet received his doctorate in 1797 with a dissertation on smallpox. He spent the next two years in Paris, where he attended the meetings of the *Société philomatique* and published a French translation of Ms. Fulham's *Essay on Combustion* (1794). In 1799 he settled in his hometown, annexed in 1798 by France and whose fate was to be linked to Napoleon until 1813. In addition to his private practice, Coindet held the position of honorary physician at the Geneva Hospital from 1802 to 1831, was a member of several medico-social boards and commissions, and acted as physician for the prisons and contagious diseases for the *Département du Léman.* He also directed the local *Bureau de Bienfaisance.*

His publications are rather few. An article of 1800 dealt with methods of cowpox inoculation, not unexpectedly. In 1816, he won the prize awarded by the Royal Academy of Medicine at Bordeaux for the best entry on hydrocephaly, which appeared as a book in 1817, as well as in two lengthy excerpts in the *Bibliothèque universelle.* His three articles on iodine and goiter appeared in 1820 and 1821, to be followed in 1823 by a description of the properties and uses of quinine sulfate in intermittent fevers.

Around 1819 Coindet postulated that the active ingredient of sponge and of seaweed, successfully used in the treatment of goiter, was likely iodine, which had been discovered by Robert Courtois and Sir Humphry Davy in 1813. After chemical analysis had confirmed his conjecture, he prescribed iodine-containing solutions to patients and observed a softening and volume reduction of the goiter within a few weeks. In the summer of 1820, he was able to ascertain that with iodine modern chemistry had provided a powerful addition to therapeutics.

Iodine was actually so powerful that symptoms of iodine poisoning were reported and discussed first at the medico-surgical society and later at the faculty at the request of the government. The latter followed the advice that iodine could be obtained only by medical prescription from pharmacists, and the *Bibliothèque universelle*, where Coindet's first report had been published, issued a cautionary statement at the end of 1820. In February 1821 Coindet replied by stating that hundreds—if not a thousand patients—had been treated and that unwanted side effects were only seen exceptionally. These patients had shown accelerated heart rate, palpitation, insomnia, emaciation, and reduced vigor. For Coindet this syndrome, later characterized as iodine-induced hyperthyroidism or 'Jod Basedow' and often but not always associated with exophthalmia, was due to iodine saturation and could be alleviated by discontinuing the treatment and reinstalling it only after recovery at a lower dosage and under regular medical control. As an alternative way of administration, and to avoid stomach pain, Coindet reported favorable results in goitrous patients when rubbing the skin of the neck with an iodine-containing pomade.

Coindet was deeply disappointed by the criticism and opposed the conservative physicians by founding, with a few young colleagues, the still existing *Société médicale de Genève*. He must have been relieved when in 1831 he received a grand prize for his discoveries awarded by the French Academy of Sciences at Paris, which was accompanied by a sizable amount of money. He died in 1834, three quarters of a century before the discovery of the thyroid hormones, and their chemical structure, at last gave a rational explanation for the effects—beneficial or otherwise—of iodine on the function of the thyroid gland.

Bibliography

Primary: 1820. 'Découverte d'un nouveau remède contre le goitre.' *Annales de Chimie et de Physique* 15: 49–59 (also published in *Bibliothèque universelle, Sc. & Arts* 14: 190–198, 1820); 1821. 'Nouvelles études sur l'iode et sur les précautions à prendre dans le traitement du goitre par ce nouveau remède.' *Annales de Chimie et de Physique* 16: 320–327 (also published in *Bibliothèque universelle, Sc. & Arts* 16: 140–152, 1821); 1821. 'Note sur l'administration de l'iode par friction (etc.).' *Bibliothèque universelle, Sc. & Arts*, 16: 320–327.

Secondary: Greer, M. A., 1973. 'Jod-Basedow (or Jod-Coindet).' *New England Journal of Medicine* 288: 105–106; Oliver, Jean, 25 Juin 1948. 'Les origines de la Société médicale de Genève et le Dr J.-F. Coindet.' *Revue médicale de la Suisse romande* pp. 326–333.

Jean-Jacques Dreifuss

COLE, RUFUS (b. Rowsburg, Ohio, USA, 30 April 1872; d. Washington, D.C., USA, 20 April 1966), *medicine, clinical research.*

Cole, the son of Ivory Snethen Cole, a physician, and Ruth Smith, was encouraged from boyhood to study medicine, having two paternal uncles who were also doctors. He attended the University of Michigan, Ann Arbor (1892–96) and Johns Hopkins Medical School, Baltimore (MD, 1899), where he was taught by William Henry Welch, William Osler, and Lewellys Franklin Barker. At Johns Hopkins Hospital he served as Osler's resident house officer (1899–1900), assistant resident physician (1900–4), and instructor in medicine (1901–4). He spent a year in August Wassermann's laboratory at the Robert Koch Institut für Infektionskrankheiten, Berlin (1903–4), studying agglutination of various strains of typhoid bacilli, an infection he had suffered as a medical student. When Barker succeeded Osler as professor of medicine (1905), Cole was appointed resident physician. Barker restructured the teaching of clinical medicine on the German model by establishing laboratory research facilities adjacent to wards and promoted

Cole to head the Biological Division of the Clinical Research Laboratory (1906–9). Here he continued work on typhoid, pioneering the isolation of bacteria from the bloodstream and establishing the blood culture as a routine clinical procedure. Using the hospital laboratory to study disease rather than as a diagnostic facility was a radical concept in American medicine and paved the way for a new breed of full-time physician-scientist. Cole's appointment as first director of the proposed Hospital of the Rockefeller Institute for Medical Research, New York (1908), was inspired by a commitment of its Trustees to the future of biomedicine.

After his marriage to Annie Hegeler (1908), Cole traveled with her and their baby (they had three daughters) to Britain and Europe on a fact-finding mission (1909), taking ideas from university clinics to develop his state-of-the-art fifty-bed hospital, which opened October 1910. Under his directorship the working environment was comfortable, happy, productive, and internationalist. Cole was an excellent talent scout, 'discovering' among other distinguished scientists, Oswald Theodore Avery, Francis W. Peabody, Donald Dexter van Slyke, and George Draper. By his retirement (1937), nearly half the full-time chiefs of internal medicine in the United States had passed through the Rockefeller Hospital, including five recipients of the Kober Medal, the Association of American Physicians' highest award. The hospital's 'big science' ethos enormously influenced Western medicine, and it became the new mecca for young ambitious experimental physiologists and biochemists from around the world. Of the diseases selected for investigation in the hospital (pneumonia, poliomyelitis, syphilis, heart disease, and 'intestinal infantilism' (celiac disease)), Cole and his coworkers studied acute lobar pneumonia and one of its causative agents, the pneumococcus. They developed a serum therapy (1913) and investigated outbreaks of the infection among troops during World War I. This work, which classified the pneumococcus into three serotypes and related their pathogenic activity to substances later identified as complex polysaccharides, fed into basic and applied biological research on bacteria. It was always Cole's contention that the study of disease would impact the development of scientific biology, although he foresaw a time when laboratory science would dominate and determine clinical practice.

Cole was the recipient of many awards including the Médaille d'Honneur de l'Assistance Publique de la République Française (1926); the Kober Medal (1938); the Academy Medal, New York Academy of Medicine (1953); and the Kovalenko Award, National Academy of Sciences (1966). He was president of the Association of American Physicians (1909), the Society of Internal Medicine (1912–13), the American Society for Clinical Investigation (1915), the Harvey Society (1921–23), and the Practitioners Society (1940). He and his wife entertained colleagues in their upstate country house at Mount Kisco, a community to which Cole gave his expertise by chairing the Finance Committee; the District Nursing Association, Northern Westchester County (1930); and the Advisory Committee, Department of Welfare, Westchester County (1935). Cole's later years were spent researching and writing a two-volume English history, *Human History: The 17th Century and the Stuart Family* (1959)—a personal quest for a man whose ancestor, James Cole, had emigrated from England in 1633.

Bibliography

Primary: 1913. 'Treatment of Pneumonia by Means of Specific Serums.' *Journal of the American Medical Association* 61: 663; 1917. (with Avery, O. T., H. T. Chickering, and A. R. Dochez). *Acute Lobar Pneumonia: Prevention and Serum Treatment* (New York); 1926. 'The Modern Hospital and Medical Progress.' *Science* 64: 123–130; 1927. 'Hospital and Laboratory.' *Science* 66: 545–552; 1928. 'The Inter-relation of the Medical Sciences.' *Science* 67: 47–52; 1930. 'Progress of Medicine during the Past Twenty-five Years as Exemplified by the Harvey Society Lectures.' *Science* 71: 617–627; 1938. 'The Practice of Medicine.' *Science* 88: 309–316.

Secondary: Hirsch, Jules, 2004. 'Rufus Cole and the Clinical Approach' in Stapleton, Darwin H., ed., *Creating a Tradition of Biomedical Research: Contributions to the History of the Rockefeller University* (New York); Miller, C. Phillip, 1979. 'Rufus Cole.' *Biographical Memoirs, National Academy of Sciences* vol. 50 (Washington, DC); Corner, G. W., 1964. *A History of the Rockefeller Institute, 1901–1953* (New York); *DAMB*.

Carole Reeves

COLEY, WILLIAM BRADLEY (b. Saugatuck, Connecticut, USA, 12 January 1862; d. New York, New York, USA, 16 April 1936), *surgery, cancer immunotherapy.*

Coley's family traced its American roots back to relatives in the Massachusetts Bay Colony who arrived in 1631. At Yale, Coley was said to be a quiet student who did not participate in extracurricular activities. He entered Harvard Medical School in 1886 after reading the autobiography of J. Marion Sims, the celebrated woman's surgeon who helped found New York Cancer Hospital.

The work of Pasteur, Koch, and Lister had resulted in major advances in bacteriology and medicine. After graduating from Harvard, Coley became a surgical intern at New York Hospital and was promoted to house surgeon in 1890. He married Alice Lancaster in June of 1891. Coley became socially prominent and successful in his surgical practice at Memorial Hospital in New York City.

In 1891 Coley saw a seventeen-year-old girl with a sarcoma of the right arm associated with persistent inflammation. Despite surgery, recurrent tumor caused her death three months later. Coley searched for previous cases about this uncommon disease and discovered a patient with sarcoma who developed erysipelas, an infection due to the *Streptococcus*, postoperatively. After each attack of fever, the patient's tumor decreased in size and finally disappeared. Coley located

the patient some seven years after surgery and found he was well. Coley suspected that infection was responsible for the cancer regression and he began treating patients with streptococci, later adding *Bacillus prodigiosus* (*Serratia marcescens*). Patients treated with live organisms had erratic responses and so Coley switched to killed bacteria. These bacterial filtrates became known as 'Coley's toxins'. The dose was gradually increased depending on patient response, and the vaccine was injected directly into the primary tumor and metastases. Five-year survival of patients with inoperable sarcoma was reported to be between 30 and 50 percent and for patients with carcinoma, 15 percent. However, the potency and dosage were not standardized. Coley's toxins were criticized by many medical authorities, including James Ewing, a contemporary and the influential pathologist at the Memorial Hospital. Nevertheless, Coley is known as the 'father of immunotherapy' of cancer. The killed bacterial filtrates were manufactured by Parke-Davis pharmaceutical company from 1899 until the 1950s. Shortly after Coley died, the American Medical Association incorporated the vaccine into its list of new and nonofficial drugs. Coley's work was carried on by his devoted daughter, Helen Coley Nauts, who founded the Cancer Research Institute in New York City. She witnessed the rebirth of interest in immunotherapy of cancer during the latter part of the twentieth century. The active principle in Coley's toxins may have been lipopolysaccharide, which triggered release of tumor necrosis factor and other cytokines. Thus modern immunology provides a plausible explanation for the benefit Coley observed in some patients treated with his killed bacterial filtrates.

During Coley's professional career, vaccines were touted by others for treatment of various diseases. In 1906 Bernard Shaw's popular play *The Doctor's Dilemma* centered on immune therapy for infections. In the play, one of the physicians urges his colleagues to 'Stimulate the phagocytes', adding that 'drugs are a delusion'. A century later, advances in immunology unimagined by Coley and others of his time are finding promising application in cancer treatment.

Bibliography

Primary: 1893. 'The treatment of malignant tumors by repeated inoculations of erysipelas: with a report of ten original cases.' *American Journal of Medical Sciences* 105: 487–511; 1906. 'Late results of the treatment of inoperable sarcoma by the mixed toxins of erysipelas and Bacillus Prodigiosus.' *American Journal of the Medical Sciences* 131: 376–430.

Secondary: Hall, S. S., 1997. *A Commotion in the Blood* (New York); Starnes, C. O., 1992. 'Coley's Toxins in Perspective.' *Nature* 357: 11–12; Nauts, H. C., W. E. Swift, and B. L. Coley, 1946. 'The Treatment of Malignant Tumors by Bacterial Toxins as Developed by the Late William B. Coley, M.D., Reviewed in the Light of Modern Research.' *Cancer Research* 6: 205–216; *DAMB*.

Marvin J. Stone

COLOMBO, REALDO (b. Cremona, Italy, *c.* 1510; d. Rome, Italy, 1559), *anatomy, physiology, surgery.*

The son of Antonio Colombo, an apothecary, Realdo Colombo received his undergraduate education at Milan. He was apprenticed for seven years to Giovanni Antonio Lonigo, a leading Venetian surgeon, and consequently enrolled at the University of Padua, where his attendance as a student of surgery is documented in 1538. While still a student he occupied a chair of Sophistics at Padua in 1540. He probably received his degree in 1541, and then he returned to Venice to assist Lonigo. In 1543 he substituted for Andreas Vesalius, who had gone to Basel, and it was on this occasion that he pointed out some errors in Vesalius's teaching; in 1544 he took his place definitively. At the invitation of Cosimo I de' Medici (1519-74), Colombo left Padua in 1545 to teach anatomy at Pisa. In 1548 he moved to Rome, where he engaged in anatomical studies with Michelangelo and taught at the Sapienza. In 1556 he carried out the autopsy of Ignatius of Loyola. He remained in Rome for the rest of his life.

Colombo was the author (published posthumously) of an anatomical compendium entitled *De re anatomica* (1559), and although without illustrations, it became widely used as a textbook and was reprinted several times. Here he demonstrated his rich experience in dissection, vivisection, and the practice of surgery. Colombo's fame is above all due to his affirmation of the impermeability of the interventricular septum and to his description of the passage of the blood from the right heart to the left across the lungs (the so-called lesser or pulmonary circulation). Colombo also added the experimental demonstration, determined by vivisection, that the 'venous artery', i.e., the pulmonary vein, contains blood and not air, as had been sustained by Galenic doctrine. Colombo claimed that nobody before him had observed or described the passage of the blood across the lungs. However, the question of the discovery of the pulmonary circulation has been much disputed. In 1556 Juan Valverde de Amusco, Colombo's former student at Pisa, published in Rome a Spanish anatomy text entitled *Historia de la composición del cuerpo humano*, which was avowedly based on the Vesalius's *Fabrica* but which also incorporated many of Colombo's corrections and new discoveries, including the lesser circulation, which meant that Colombo had arrived at his own conclusions regarding the argument before 1553.

It is doubtful that Colombo was aware of the description of the pulmonary circulation of the blood contained in Michele Serveto's (or Severtus, *c.* 1509-53) *Christianismi Restitutio* (1553), considering the almost complete destruction of this unfortunate Spaniard's printed work. Nevertheless it would seem obvious that much importance would have been given to the manuscript copies of the work, one of which was found in Italy, thus giving weight to the hypothesis of a secret diffusion of Serveto's work, which was certainly more widespread than hitherto supposed. On the other hand, the Syrian physician Ibn al-Nafīs, in his commentary on Avicenna's (Ibn Sīnā's) *Canone* in 1268, had clearly outlined the lesser circulation, denying the possibility of a direct passage of the blood from the right heart to the left. In 1547 Andrea Alpago, a physician from Belluno, published in Venice a Latin translation of part of Ibn al-Nafīs's work. However, this did not include the sections discussing passage of the blood across the lungs, thus excluding the possibility that Colombo knew about Ibn al-Nafīs's opinion.

Bibliography

Primary: 1559. *De re anatomica libri XV* (Venice).

Secondary: Ongaro, Giuseppe, 1971. 'La scoperta della circolazione polmonare e la diffusione della "Christianismi Restitutio" di Michele Serveto nel XVI secolo in Italia e nel Veneto.' *Episteme* 5: 3–44; Wilson, Leonard G., 1962. 'The Problem of the Discovery of the Pulmonary Circulation.' *Journal of the History of Medicine and Allied Sciences* 17: 229–44; DSB.

Giuseppe Ongaro

CONCETTI, LUIGI (b. nr. Viterbo, Lazio, Italy, 6 March 1854; d. Rome, Italy, 6 December 1920), *pediatrics.*

Concetti, the son of Raffaele Concetti and Castori Teresa, was born into a family of humble origins and graduated from the medical school of the University of Rome (1879) after completing his humanities education in Viterbo. During his medical studies (1874–77) in Rome, he also benefited from training at the S. Giovanni pharmacy and at the medical clinic of Guido Bacelli, who was later appointed Minister of Italian State Education and who supported Concetti throughout his career.

After graduating, Concetti worked as assistant and later head physician in the children's ward of the Santo Spirito Hospital. There he studied pediatrics, and in 1883 he published his first volume: a collection of 562 pediatric clinical histories that would be followed by another eight volumes dealing with different aspects of clinical pediatrics.

Concetti became an assistant in the Vatican-owned Bambino Gesú Hospital in 1883, the first hospital for children in Italy founded in 1867. He was promoted to head physician in 1890. His clinical experience permitted him to identify various problems within the hospital, including the excessive length of the children's average duration of stay (three months), the risk of contracting chronic illness from contagion, the separation from the family, and finally, the inability to admit to the hospital children younger than two years old. To remedy these problems, Concetti worked with the hygienist Angelo Celli and a group of qualified female volunteers to set up a network of pediatric clinics and health care centers in poor areas in the Roman periphery, the first one of which was established in Trastevere district.

He also continued to work as a volunteer assistant at the Institute for Medicine and Experimental Pharmacology under the supervision of Guido Bacelli and in other institutions, such as the hygiene institute, the histology and general physiology institute, the clinical chemistry institute, and the institute of anatomy and histology of the nervous system, until 1895. In that year Concetti became the first full professor of clinical pediatrics in Italy, at the University of Rome, where he taught clinical pediatrics until 1920. Concetti, founder and organizer of the Italian Society of Pediatrics (1898), was a prolific author, with more than 120 publications devoted to various aspects of clinical pediatrics.

Throughout his long academic career, his work in the field allowed him to pioneer the field of childhood neuropathology. He was the first to introduce lumbar puncture to pediatric diagnosis. Concetti introduced important observations in the study of childhood splenic anemia, in the analysis of infective respiratory pathology, and in diphtheria, introducing antidiphtheritic serotherapy in Italy. He also studied meningitis in children and described postdiphtheric paralysis in children. As an expert on malaria, he contributed to the *Traité des maladies de l'enfance*, edited by J. Grancher, J. Comby, and A.-B. Marfan (Paris, 1904). Together with the pediatrician Giuseppe Mya, who worked in Florence, Concetti analyzed cerebral edema among newborns, which he divided into distinctive forms of infectious and toxic. Concetti's experience in the Roman children's hospital led him to publish the first manual devoted to the clinical care of children. This work can be considered as the first modern Italian pediatric treatise. In this volume he presented a general overview of the health of children.

He was the editor-in-chief of the *Rivista di clinica pediatrica*, with Giuseppe Mya, which was founded in 1903.

Bibliography

Primary: 1883. *Resoconto statistico-clinico di un biennio della nuova sala dei bambini infermi nell'Ospedale di S. Spirito in Sassia* (Rome); 1895. *Lo stato attuale della pediatria* (Rome); 1905. *L'igiene del bambino* (Rome and Milan).

Secondary: Guarnieri, Patrizia, 2001. 'Piccoli, poveri e malati. Gli ambulatori per l'infanzia a Roma nell'età liberale.' *Italia contemporanea* 223: 225–259; Latronico, Nicola, 1977. *Storia della pediatria* (Turin); Spolverini, Luigi, 1921. 'Commemorazione del socio prof. Luigi Concetti.' *Bullettino della Reale Accademia Medica di Roma* 47: 236–250.

Patrizia Guarnieri

CONI, EMILIO RAMÓN   (b. Corrientes, Argentina, 4 March 1855; d. Buenos Aires, Argentina, 4 July 1928), *public health.*

Coni, a physician, public health reformer, and one of his nation's top hygienists at the turn of the century, was the son of French-born parents who had immigrated to Argentina in the early nineteenth century. His father was a well-known publisher in Buenos Aires. After studies at the University of Buenos Aires medical school, where he was among the first generation to graduate, in 1878 with a specialization in hygiene and public health, he embarked on a career of social and medical reform and public service. Coni was best known for his institutionalizing efforts in public health and for leading government campaigns against tuberculosis and venereal disease. He also played a large role in professional medical organizations of the time; among his many offices were President of the Argentine Medical Association from 1891 to 1893 and founder of the Argentine Anti-Tuberculosis League.

Early in his career, Coni excelled in the collection and publication of medical and epidemiological statistics, helping to establish Argentina's reputation in that field. He was director of the *Bulletin mensuel de demographie* and his many health surveys of Argentine provinces and cities included tabulations of prison populations, hospital services, legitimate and illegitimate births, prostitution, and venereal disease. Coni published widely in Argentine medical journals, such as *Semana médica* and the *Revista medica-cirurgica*, and served for many years as an editor of the former and a director of the latter.

In 1883 Coni helped to found the *Asistencia Publica*, or Welfare Department, which was based on the French model, its purpose to organize and regulate the city's hospitals and asylums. In 1901 Coni helped to organize the Argentine Anti-Tuberculosis League, funded by the Interior Minister and private donors and modeled after similar institutions in Europe and the United States. As a public health crusader and advocate for social welfare programs, Coni focused on poverty and the living conditions of the poor. Together with his wife, Gabriela Laperrière de Coni, a feminist and social reformer, he warned that the substandard environment of Argentina's factories would destroy the reproductive health of women and the health of their future children. Some industries, such as match-making, used noxious chemicals with detrimental health effects. The Conis took a special interest in the health of women because they believed that through women one could control the health of children and the future population.

Control of venereal disease and prostitution was another of Coni's top public health concerns. Coni argued persuasively that limiting the movement of prostitutes would lower rates of venereal disease, and he helped to implement a series of syphilis clinics for prostitutes throughout Buenos Aires. He supported municipal legislation regulating the space and free movement of prostitutes that gave physicians broad authority over prostitutes and the urban poor. In 1907 Emilio Coni formed the Argentine Society for Moral and Sanitary Prophylaxis, the first concerted effort to combat both tuberculosis and venereal diseases. Although his plan did not get support from the state, it served as a model for the Argentine Social Prophylaxis League, which was founded in 1920.

Despite his tireless efforts to establish and fund a comprehensive public health system, many of his plans, including an extensive 1917 proposal to create a national system of primary care institutions, were not adopted by the Argentine government. He died in 1928, openly bitter about Argentina's, in his view, lack of progress in public health, especially for communicable diseases such as tuberculosis.

Bibliography

Primary: 1880. *Higiene pública: El servicio sanitario de la ciudad de Buenos Aires* (Buenos Aires); 1887. *Progres de l'hygiene dans la Republique Argentine* (Paris); 1918. *Memorias de un médico higienista* (Buenos Aires).

Secondary: Guy, Donna, 1989. 'Emilio and Gabriela Coni: Reformers, Public Health, and Working Women' in Ewell, Judith, and William Beezley, eds., *The Human Tradition in Latin America* (Wilmington, DE) pp. 233–248.

Julia Rodriguez

CONOLLY, JOHN   (b. Market Rasen, Lincolnshire, England, 27 May 1794; d. Hanwell, Middlesex, England, 4 March 1866), *medicine, psychiatry.*

Conolly was the second son of Jonathan Conolly, an impoverished Anglo-Irish gentleman, and his wife Dorothy Tennyson, a distant relative of the poet Alfred Tennyson. His father's death during Conolly's childhood deprived him of the chance to receive a formal and extended education. His early military career terminated with the end of the Napoleonic War. Conolly's marriage to Elizabeth Collins (1817) at the tender age of twenty-three necessitated the search for a stable source of income. In 1819 he matriculated at Edinburgh University to study medicine and graduated MD in 1821. In the following seven years, Conolly tried to establish a medical practice at Lewes, Chichester, and Stratford-upon-Avon, successively, achieving at best moderate success in each abode. His struggle to scrape an income and a semblance of social status in the provinces was temporarily rewarded in 1828, when he was appointed as professor of medicine at a newly created University College London, mainly due to the patronage of George Birkbeck (1776–1841) and Henry Brougham (1778–1868), the future Lord Chancellor. However, Conolly's professional life in the metropolis was short-lived, and in 1830 he resigned from the professorship. Conolly once again retreated to the obscurity of provincial practice, this time in Warwick. In 1838 he applied for the post of superintendent at the Hanwell County Asylum in Middlesex, which became vacant after the asylum's governors fired the incumbent, William Ellis. He could not get even this little-coveted position, defeated by an army surgeon, J. R. Millingen. Up to this point, Conolly's professional career had been one of struggle and failure.

The turning point came in 1839. The governors of the Hanwell Asylum fired Millingen, unsatisfied at his slovenly performance of the duties, and appointed Conolly instead. The second choice turned out to be a spectacular and celebrated success. Conolly followed the example of Robert Gardiner Hill (1811–78) at the Lincoln Asylum in abolishing all mechanical restraints, such as chains, manacles, and straitjackets, making Hanwell the second asylum conducted under the principle of nonrestraint. In so doing, Conolly was greatly assisted and encouraged by reform-minded governors of the Hanwell Asylum. He was also helped by the favorable attention of influential medical and general organs of the mass media, such as *Lancet* or *The Times*. Success in nonrestraint almost overnight brought the middle-aged and minimally experienced alienist to the center of the nation's excited attention. Conolly served as testimony to the progress of civilization and the fight against barbaric practices of the past.

Conolly stayed in the office for about five years. In 1844 he was forced to resign from the post, due to the new arrangement of the organization conceived by the governors, and assumed a new position of a visiting physician to the asylum. He kept this honorary position until 1852. He supplemented his income by running a private asylum, The Lawn at Hanwell, as well as involving himself in the running of another private asylum, Moorcroft House. The latter institution became the focus of notorious scandal for wrongful confinement in the case of *Nottidge v. Ripley and another* (1849). Although this incident had the potential to irrevocably damage his reputation, Conolly's status among the psychiatric profession survived. For the psychiatric profession, which badly needed a public figure to improve its lowly status, Conolly's celebrated achievement at the Hanwell was too impressive and important to discard. He remained a highly revered figure among psychiatric practitioners. For those outside the profession, however, Conolly's standing was not so certain. Charles Reade's *Hard Cash* (1864), a sensational novel with barely concealed lampooning of Conolly, might have lowered his standing in the eyes of the general public. The irreverent and iconoclastic obituary of Conolly by Henry Maudsley (1835–1918), his son-in-law, published in the year of his death (1866), caused a visible unrest among the psychiatric profession.

Bibliography

Primary: 1830. *An Enquiry concerning the Indications of Insanity* (London) [reprint, 1964]; 1847. *The Construction and Government of Lunatic Asylums and Hospitals for the Insane* (London) [reprint, 1968]; 1856. *The Treatment of the Insane without Mechanical Restraint* (London) [reprint, 1973].

Secondary: Scull, Andrew, Charlotte Mackenzie, and Nicholas Hervey, 1996. *Masters of Bedlam: Transformation of the Mad-Doctoring Trade* (Princeton); Suzuki, Akihito, 1995. 'Politics and Ideology of Non-Restraint: The Case of the Hanwell Asylum.' *Medical History* 39: 1–17; *Oxford DNB.*

Akihito Suzuki

CONSTANTINE THE AFRICAN (b. Carthage, North Africa, ?; d. the Abbey of Monte Cassino, Italy, before 1098/9), *translation.*

Constantine was the first figure in the West to render a large body of Arabic medical literature into Latin, thereby stimulating the recovery of Greek traditions preserved in Arabic and unavailable to the West since the close of antiquity. Moreover, he initiated European scholarly interest in Greco-Arabic medicine, a trend furthered by medieval scholasticism, which endured well into the Renaissance and beyond.

Three versions of his biography survive: one attributed to 'Matthaeus F[errarius?]', a twelfth-century Salernitan physician; one anonymously preserved in a manuscript now redated to the twelfth century; and one by Peter the Deacon, chronicler and librarian of Monte Cassino (*c.* 1110–50). Matthaeus's version is generally accepted as the most reliable; it tells that Constantine, working as a spice or pharmaceutical merchant, arrived in Lombard in southern Italy, where he learned of the poverty of the Latin medical tradition. After returning to Africa for a period of study, Constantine carried a corpus of Arabic medical texts back to Salerno for translation. Regrettably, some of the books were damaged in a storm off Cape Palinuro.

At Salerno, Constantine was befriended by Archbishop Alfanus I, who was himself a scholar of medical traditions and a former monk of Monte Cassino. Around 1077 Constantine met Robert Guiscard at Salerno, and Prince Richard of Capua granted him the Church of St Agatha at Aversa. Constantine transferred this property to the Abbey of Monte Cassino upon joining the community. While at the Abbey, and perhaps beginning at Salerno, Constantine rendered his texts into Latin with the aid of at least two assistants: Johannes Afflacius, a converted Saracen physician, and Atto, former chaplain to the Empress Agnes. The date of Constantine's death has been debated, with the *terminus ante quem* established by the mention of Constantine 'monk and physician' in the calendar of Leo Marsicanus *c.* 1098/99; according to the calendar, Constantine was to be memorialized by his brethren in prayers for the dead offered every 22 December. Peter's version states that, following Constantine's death, his assistant Johannes Afflacius continued his teacher's work, eventually taking all of Constantine's books with him to Naples, where he died some years later. This seems to explain the near-absence today of Constantine's corpus in the surviving collection at Monte Cassino; survivors include a draft of the *Isagoge*, a section of *Pantegni*'s surgery, and a brief collection of anatomical/physiological concepts very recently discovered.

No complete list of his textual corpus has yet been established, but a number of his works have received concentrated attention. Most notable among his translations or adaptations were the mammoth *Pantegni* or 'total art of medicine', inspired by the encyclopedic *Kitāb al-mālikī* of 'Alī ibn al-'Abbās al-Majūsī (d. *c.* 994); the *Viaticum* or 'traveler's handbook', derived from the *Zād al-musāfir* of Ibn al-Ǧazzār (d. 1009); the *Isagoge* of Johannitius (809–73); the books *On Diets, On Fevers,* and *On Urines* of Isaac Isreali (Isaac Judaeus); the *Megategni,* a synopsis of Galen's *De methodo medendi;* and the Hippocratic *Aphorisms* and *Prognostics* with Galen's commentaries. Several shorter texts include the *De genecia, De gradibus, De elephancia, De stomacho, De coitu, De melancholia, De humana natura,* the *Antidotarium, Liber de oculorum,* and *Liber de oblivione.* Constantine was probably involved also in the translation of *De spermate.* Several works contain prefatory dedications to Abbot Desiderius of Monte Cassino (the *Pantegni*), Archbishop Alfanus I of Salerno (*De stomacho*), Atto (the *Aphorisms*), and Johannes Afflacius (*Megategni, De urinis, De febribus* and *Liber de oculorum*). The order of Constantine's production has not yet been determined, but it appears that the *Isagoge* was the earliest; it survives in two working drafts written in the Beneventan script. The *Isagoge's* early circulation is demonstrated by the library catalogue of St Angelo in Formis, a house closely associated with both Monte Cassino and St Agatha at Aversa.

Constantine's significance for later ages was profound. The five-text curriculum at Salerno established early in the twelfth century, which later became known as the *Articella,* opened with his *Isagoge* and included both the Hippocratic *Aphorisms* and *Prognostics* with their accompanying commentaries by Galen. The *Articella* was expanded to include more texts after *c.* 1150 and remained a central component of medical education across Europe through the Renaissance. In particular, the introduction of Hippocratic-Galenic medical theory in these texts, and their rational formatting, made the philosophical aspects of medicine a priority for later ages. The hundreds of surviving and largely unstudied manuscripts of Constantine's many *oeuvres* testify to the enthusiasm of later ages for his textual productions.

Bibliography

Primary: 1515. *Omnia opera Ysaac* (Lyons); 1536, 1539. *Constantini opera* (Basel).

Secondary: O'Boyle, Cornelius, 1998. *The Art of Medicine: Medical Teaching at the University of Paris, 1250–1400* (Leiden); Bloch, Herbert, 1986. *Monte Cassino in the Middle Ages* (Cambridge, MA); Burnett, Charles, and Danielle Jacquart, eds., 1994. *Constantine the African and 'Alī ibn al-'Abbās al-Maǧūsī: The 'Pantegni' and Related Texts* (Leiden); Wack, Mary, 1990. *Lovesickness in the Middle Ages: The 'Viaticum' and Its Commentaries* (Philadelphia); Von Falkenhausen, Vera, 1984. 'Costantino Africano.' *Dizionario Biografico degli Italiani* XXX: 320–324.

Florence Eliza Glaze

CONTI, LEONARDO AMBROSIO GIORGIO GIOVANNI

(b. Lugano, Switzerland, 24 August 1900; d. Nuremberg, Germany, 6 October 1945), *Nazi medicine, Reich's health administration.*

Conti belonged to the generation of those in German-speaking countries who were extremely vulnerable to seduction by the Nazi party. Born around 1900, without any positive identification with Imperial Germany and without experience of the trenches of World War I, many of them were in search of a sense of life and new duties in the 1920s—a time of unemployment and economic as well as political upheaval.

Conti was the son of a post director in Lugano. After his parents divorced, his German mother took him back to Germany, where he finished his schooling in 1918. In the same year, he served in the German Army. After the German defeat and the end of World War I, he was involved in the revolutionary street fights against left-wing parties and groups. From his student days, Conti had an anti-Semitic attitude and was engaged in the German nationalistic right wing movement. Although he studied medicine in Berlin and Munich (1919–23), the city of Berlin denied his employment as doctor in the city administration in 1925 because of his nationalistic views (*völkische Gesinnung*). In 1920, as a student, Conti had participated in protests of nationalistic students against the pacifist Jewish Berlin professor of physiology, Friedrich Nicolai (1874–1964). These student protests lead to the expulsion of Nicolai from Berlin University and then Germany altogether.

After he got his medical degree in 1923, Conti worked as a general practitioner and started his career in the National Socialist Party (NSDAP). In that year, he became a member of the SA, where he built up a medical service in the following years. In 1927 he became a party member, and in 1929 he founded with other colleagues the Nazi Physicians' League (NSDÄB, *Nationalsozialistischer Deutscher Ärztebund*). In 1930 he shifted from the SA to the SS. In 1932 Conti became a member of the Prussian Parliament.

In 1933 Hermann Göring (1893–1946), then Prussian Minister of Internal Affairs, gave Conti the post of commissioner for special duties (*Kommissar zur besonderen Verwendung*) for 'cleansing the health system' ('*Säuberung des Gesundheitswesens*'). In this function, Conti became predominantly responsible for the discrimination and expulsion of Jewish physicians. In 1936 he organized the medical service of the Olympic Games in Berlin.

Conti took his most important step on the career ladder in the Nazi movement in 1939. After the death of the Reich's physicians' leader Gerhard Wagner (1888–1939), Hitler gave Conti Wagner's post, now entitled 'Reich's health leader' (*Reichsgesundheitsführer*), with expanded responsibilities. Furthermore, he became head of the NSDÄB, and Hitler made him State Secretary for Public Health in the Reich's Ministry of Internal Affairs. With this amalgamation of power, Conti was responsible for health measures in the Nazi party and for those of the state regarding the whole Reich. In this function he supported ideas of racial hygiene and was involved in several Nazi crimes. For example, he advocated human experiments in concentration camps, and in 1940 he pleaded for mass sterilization of Sinti and Roma.

Conti remained in this post for four years. In 1943 Hitler gave his personal physician, Karl Brandt (1904–48), leadership of the medical and health system in the Reich. This was a setback for Conti, whose power was curtailed. Conti then furthered his career in the SS and educated physicians in the State Academy of Public Health in Berlin-Charlottenburg. In 1945 he was imprisoned by the Allied Forces and—in a state of agony—committed suicide in the Military Prison in Nuremberg.

Bibliography

Primary: 1943. 'Gesundheitsführung und Leistungssteigerung.' *Die Gesundheitsführung. Ziel und Weg* 5: 57–61; 1944. 'Zehn Jahre Hauptamt für Volksgesundheit der NSDAP.' *Die Gesundheitsführung. Ziel und Weg* 6: 109–112.

Secondary: Maggi, Flavio, 1999. *Un medico ticinese alla corte di Hitler: Leonardo Conti (1900–1945)* (Locarno); Kater, Michael H., 1989. *Doctors under Hitler* (London); Kater, Michael H., 1985. 'Doctor Leonardo Conti and His Nemesis: The Failure of Centralized Medicine in the Third Reich.' *Central European History* 18: 299–325; Labisch, Alfons, Florian Tennstedt, 1985. *Der Weg zum Gesetz über die Vereinheitlichung des Gesundheitswesens vom 3. Juli 1934*, Part 2 (Düsseldorf).

Cay-Ruediger Pruell

COOK, ALBERT RUSKIN

(b. Hampstead, London, 2 March 1870; d. Kampala, Uganda Protectorate, 23 April 1951), *missionary medicine, medical education.*

Cook was born to a large, well-connected family. His father, William Henry Cook, was a family physician, initially in Tunbridge Wells and later in London, and his mother, Harriet Bickersteth, was the daughter of Edward Bickersteth, Rector of Watton in Hertfordshire, and sister of Edward Henry Bickersteth, Bishop of Exeter. Significantly, Cook's grandfather and uncle both had strong connections with the Church Missionary Society (CMS), which was to become the focal organization of Cook's own professional life.

Cook was educated at St Paul's School, London (1881–89), after which he went up to Trinity College, Cambridge, to take a double first (BA 1893). Although initially favoring an Arts education, he decided that he wanted to focus his career on medicine and continued his training as a Shuter scholarship student at St Bartholomew's Hospital, London, graduating MB in 1895. It was during these university days that his interest in Africa began to take shape. He was said at this time to have read several important colonial works, including *Through the Dark Continent*, which influenced him to the extent that he attended a talk by its author, the explorer Henry Morton Stanley, in 1890 (who had been

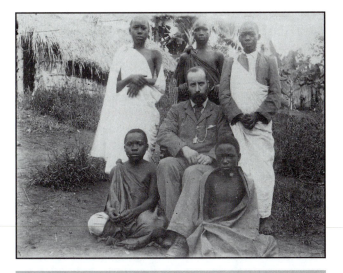

Sir Albert Ruskin Cook with (standing L–R) Behindi, Simoni, Mayanya; (sitting L–R) Yosen and Albert, Mengo Hospital, Uganda, 1897. Photograph, Archives and Manuscripts, Wellcome Library, London.

invited up to Cambridge to receive an honorary degree). He was also said to have been deeply affected by the life of Bishop James Hannington, who had been a prominent CMS missionary murdered while pursuing his vocation in East Africa. Cook's interest in doing work in Africa was further stimulated during his membership in the Cambridge Inter-Collegiate Christian Union. In this forum, Cook came into contact with a variety of medical missionaries, so it seemed like a natural step when, in 1895, he and his younger brother (John Howard Cook) signed up for the next CMS mission to East Africa, which departed in 1896.

Bound for Uganda Protectorate, Cook and his brother comprised part of a small party of CMS missionaries, one of whom, Katherine Timpson, a nurse, was to become Cook's wife (they married in 1900) as well as a key player in his health care initiatives. Not only was she to become Matron of their hospital (1897–1911) but also the Principal of the first Ugandan training college for midwives and nurses that they both helped establish in 1921: the Lady Coryndon Maternity Training School. As the Ugandan railway was still being constructed at this time, the newly arrived team had to make the arduous journey on foot from their port of arrival, Mombassa, to Mengo, near Kampala, finally arriving at their destination in February 1897. It was said that Cook and his party attended to 2,230 patients on this long overland route (Foster, 1968, p. 325).

It did not take very long before Cook started shaping organized medical care in the region. By May of the same year, he opened the first hospital in the Uganda Protectorate, Mengo Hospital, which grew so rapidly that by the 1930s it was one of the most important medical facilities in sub-Saharan Africa. In addition to its in-patient beds, Mengo Hospital was organized from very early on with appropriate (if rudimentary) facilities so that doctors could perform basic laboratory analysis of blood and urine as well as record disease incidences throughout the region. Cook was fastidious in taking case notes and, whenever he could, he conducted autopsies on his patients. Although the hospital buildings were initially only of mud and wattle construction, after lightning destroyed the original in 1902, they were rebuilt in brick. By 1908 the hospital had grown to such an extent that it was dealing with 1,500 in-patients and over 80,000 outpatients a year—a far cry from the first ward of six beds that opened in 1897.

Mengo also maintained a training school for African medical assistants and a radiological department that contained the country's only complete x-ray apparatus. In 1917, Mengo Medical School opened with seventeen African students in the first class training to be African dressers and dispensers. Significantly, the courses that were first offered at Mengo to train African medical assistants were the forerunners of those that later were established at Mulago (where it moved in 1924) and finally at Makerere College, eventually the University College of East Africa, the undisputed center of medical education in sub-Saharan Africa.

Cook's passionate interest in medical education was revealed not only through his training initiatives established at Mengo but also by his schemes within the realms of maternal and child health. He published several pamphlets in local African languages in order to help medical education in the region. He published *Amagezi Agokuzal-isa*, a Lugandan language textbook for midwifery students (1923) and some time later a *Handbook of Midwifery for Teaching Native Midwives* (1931). Also during the early 1920s he embarked on a project to set up local healthcare centers staffed by midwives throughout Uganda, a project that was immensely successful and allowed for the establishment of dozens of new regional stations. Dedicated to his faith throughout his life Cook also was instrumental in the establishment of several other medical missions—most notably the mission centers at Bor, Acholi, and Fort Portal.

In addition to his hospital and teaching duties, Cook was actively involved in scientific research. Most famously in 1901 he and his brother were involved in diagnosing the first cases of sleeping sickness (trypanosomiasis), which went on to take nearly a quarter of a million lives in the Lake Victoria region of Uganda. It was this early identification that led to a direct appeal by Cook to the Royal Society in London, resulting in the setting up of the famous 1903 investigative commission to look into the disease, recruiting both Major David Bruce and Aldo Castellani to the cause. After the investigations, organisms discovered in the cerebrospinal fluid of patients helped to prove the link between the external agents (tsetse flies) and infection. This discovery led Cook to become intimately involved with several population-evacuation and bush-clearance campaigns over the next decade.

Cook had other medical scientific interests, however; he was also, for example, one of the first to identify the treponema of relapsing fever, publishing his findings on this and other numerous cases widely in both regional and international medical journals. With his wife, he also participated in a vigorous campaign against venereal disease, working tirelessly for the government-sponsored Social Purity Campaign during the 1920s that promoted sexual education as a means of eradicating venereal disease.

It was chiefly for his establishment and development of Mengo Hospital, however, that Cook became, within his own lifetime, something of a figurehead for western medical endeavors in East Africa. A prominent local presence from quite early on, he became the first President of the Uganda Branch of the British Medical Association (1914–18) and he was awarded the Silver Medal of the Royal African Society and the Order of Leopold by Belgium, both in 1928.

Already awarded the OBE in 1918 and the CMG in 1922, in 1932 Cook was knighted in recognition of his immense contribution to the development of Western medicine in Uganda. He officially retired from his duties in March 1934 but continued to work as a consultant to Mengo Hospital for many years. During his supposed retirement, he also became, for the second time, the president of the Uganda Branch of the British Medical Association (1936–37); he was also President and later honorary Vice-President of the Uganda Literary and Scientific Society. An avid diarist throughout his life, he spent his latter years corresponding and writing reminiscences as well as continuing his scientific interests. His wife died of malaria-related illness in 1938, after which point he was alleged to have become addicted to morphine in order to help him sleep and to help fill the gap that her death had created.

As a tribute to his achievements, in 1945 the Uganda Society published his autobiography, *Uganda Memories*. He died in his home at age eighty-one. He was survived by his only daughter, Margaret Ellen Cook, although he also had an adopted son, David, who was killed on active service during World War II.

Bibliography

Primary: 1934. 'The Journey to Uganda in 1896.' *Uganda Journal* 1: 83–95; 1934. 'Further Memories of Uganda.' *Uganda Journal* 2: 97–115; 1945. *Uganda Memories, 1897–1940* (Kampala).

Secondary: Iliffe, John, 1998. *East African Doctors; the History of the Modern Profession* (Cambridge); Ofcansky, Thomas P., 1982. 'The Life and Times of Sir Albert Ruskin Cook.' *Journal of the History of Medicine and Allied Sciences* 37: 225–228; Foster, Derek W, 1978. *The Church Missionary Society and Modern Medicine in Uganda: The Life of Sir Albert Cook, K.C.M.G., 1870–1951* (Prestbury); Foster, Derek W., 1968. 'Doctor Albert Cook and the Early Days of the Church Missionary Society's Medical Mission to Uganda' *Medical History* 12: 325–343.

Anna Crozier

COOPER, ASTLEY PASTON (b. Brooke, Norfolk, England, 23 August 1768; d. London, England, 12 February 1841), *anatomy, surgery.*

Cooper was the fourth son of a clergyman-poet and author father and a novelist mother. His grandfather had been a surgeon in Norwich, and his uncle was a surgeon to Guy's Hospital, London. He was first apprenticed to the latter in 1784 but soon transferred to study under Henry Cline (1750–1827), surgeon to St Thomas's Hospital, London, who had attended John Hunter's (1728–93) first lectures in surgery.

Cooper studied anatomy and surgery at the Borough Schools (the combined Guy's and St Thomas's Hospitals) and later for seven months at Edinburgh. Appointed a demonstrator in anatomy at St Thomas's in 1789, he joined Cline as chief lecturer in anatomy and surgery in 1791. The following year he spent some time in Paris, helping the wounded in the French Revolution and becoming friends with several of the principal surgeons of the day, including Dominique J. Larrey (1766–1842) and Guillaume Dupuytren (1777–1835). On his return to London he started separate courses in anatomy and surgery and served as a lecturer in the latter at the Surgeons' Hall (later the RCS) from 1793 to 1796. A cofounder of the new medical school at Guy's Hospital, which was formed when the two hospitals separated, he was appointed surgeon there in 1800.

Cooper was obsessed with dissection: 'a day without dissection is a day lost' is a quotation frequently associated with his name. Nor did he content himself with examining and lecturing on the bodies of executed criminals (and there were suggestions that he was associated with the resurrectionists). He helped John Hunter dissect a whale and was always ready to examine animals that had died in the menagerie at the Tower of London—activities that led to his subsequent appointment as professor of comparative anatomy at the RCS (1813). But his research was equally devoted to treating human disease. His name is associated with ligature of the arteries for aneurysm, including the common carotid and the abdominal aorta, the repair of hernia, and the suggestion that breast cancer be treated by radical mastectomy, which was included in his *Lectures on the Principles and Practice of Surgery* (1824-7), one of several of his successful books.

All this led to a large private practice, claimed by some to have been the largest any surgeon has ever had. Cooper's largest fee (1,000 guineas, £1,050) came from a successful operation for stone in a West Indian planter, and in 1813 his annual income was no less than £21,000. The seal on his fame came when he removed a cyst from the head of King George IV and was created a Baronet. A public figure, he took an active part in the formation of the Medico-Chirurgical Society, becoming its first Treasurer, and he was elected President of the RCS on two occasions (1827, 1836).

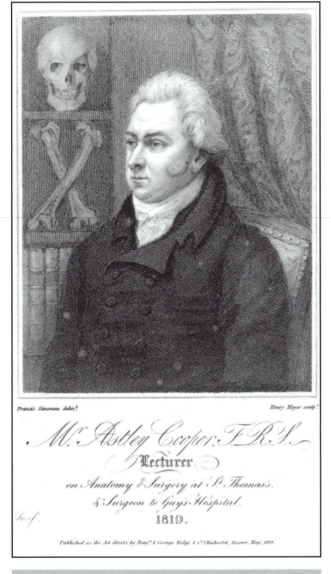

Francis Simonau delin.   Henry Meyer sculp.

M.ʳ Astley Cooper, F.R.S.

Lecturer

on Anatomy & Surgery at S.ᵗ Thomas's
& Surgeon to Guy's Hospital.

1819.

Published as the Act directs, by Benj.ⁿ & George Ridge & C.ᵒ Chichester, Sussex, May, 1819.

Sir Astley Paston Cooper with skull and cross bones. Stipple engraving by H. Meyer after Francis Simoneau, 1819. Iconographic Collection, Wellcome Library, London.

With several others, Cooper had a major role in raising the status of surgeons from handymen sawbones to gentlemen professionals. His high standing was based on dexterity and a firm theoretical underpinning, leading him to achieve results that many had doubted were feasible. He was also an inspiring teacher but combined this with a smiling public presence. A debonair man of the world, who had married a wealthy heiress (their only child died in infancy, but they subsequently adopted a son and daughter), he was as much at home in the great mansions as in the fetid public wards of the London teaching hospitals. Once anesthesia was introduced, surgeons could carry his painstaking methods forward, and Joseph Lister's (1827–1912) subsequent work on antisepsis removed much of the danger and terror of surgical treatment prevalent when

Cooper was born. At his request he was buried in the crypt of Guy's Hospital Chapel, adjacent to the tomb of Thomas Guy (*c.* 1645–1724).

Bibliography

Primary: 1822. *A Treatise of Dislocations, and on Fractures of the Joints* (London); 1830. *Observations on the Structure and Diseases of the Testis* (London); 1832. *The Anatomy of the Thymus Gland* (London); 1840. *The Anatomy of the Breast* (London).

Secondary: Brock, R. C., 1952. *The Life and Work of Astley Cooper* (Edinburgh); Cooper, B. B., 1843. *The Life of Sir Astley Cooper* 2 vols. (London); *Oxford DNB*.

Stephen Lock

COPPLESON, VICTOR MARCUS (b. Sydney, Australia, 27 February 1893; d. Sydney, 12 May 1965), *surgery, medical education, military medicine, surf lifesaving.*

Coppleson, an Anglican in later life, was the son of Russian Jewish émigrés Sarah Middlemass née Sloman and her second husband Albert Abram Coppleson, an itinerant hawker then a general merchant. Victor received his primary schooling at Wee Waa, a wheat and sheep town on the Namoi River in northwest New South Wales. He boarded at Sydney Grammar School and then studied medicine at the University of Sydney, graduating MB ChM (1915). He enlisted in the Australian Naval and Military Expeditionary Force immediately after graduation and served in New Guinea, Belgium, and France, where he was wounded at the Battle of Bullecourt (1917). In World War II, he served in Greece (April 1941) with the rank of Lieutenant Colonel and as senior surgeon at the Concord Repatriation Hospital in Sydney.

Coppleson trained as a surgeon at three London hospitals—St George's, the Westminster, and the North Middlesex—gaining his FRCS (England) in 1921. He was made a foundation Fellow of the Royal Australasian College of Surgeons when that body was formed in 1928. He practiced as a surgeon based in Sydney, especially at St Vincent's Hospital in Darlinghurst and at his Macquarie Street surgery, from 1922 until his death. An assertive and authoritarian workaholic, he was respected and 'held with curious affection', not only in the clinical and collegiate worlds of medicine but also in the military, sporting, and lifesaving arenas as well.

In addition to his professional *centrum* of surgery, Coppleson's two great contributions were in the fields of postgraduate medical education and in surf lifesaving. His role as a medical teacher, particularly in anatomy and surgery, dated from his University of Sydney appointments as Honorary Curator of the Wilson Museum of Anatomy (1923–56), Lecturer in Surgical Anatomy (1925–34) and Lecturer in Clinical Surgery (1926–65). He was an influential personality in surgery and medical education at St Vincent's Hospital, the Royal North Shore Hospital, and Prince

Henry Hospital, where he was named as a member of the Board of Directors. He wrote the *Clinical Handbook for Residents, Nurses and Students* (1928), producing new editions of this major work in 1936 and 1946.

Victor Coppleson was a leading advocate and promoter of the Australian surf lifesaving movement for forty years. In 1926 he was appointed honorary medical adviser to the Surf Lifesaving Association of Australia. With his colleague, Justice Sir Adrian Curlewis (President of the Association from 1933–74), Coppleson promoted the concepts of service, professional competence, altruism, and gallantry that characterized SLSAA and that in twentieth-century Australia was one of the nation's proudest images.

Following Peter Safar's 1956 demonstration in Pittsburgh that expired air resuscitation ('mouth-to-mouth') was the most effective emergency way of sustaining life by lay bystanders treating the unconscious nonbreathing victim, Coppleson became the leading Australian advocate for the universal teaching and introduction of expired air resuscitation. He was co-convenor of the first International Convention on Lifesaving Techniques, a major international symposium held in Sydney in 1960. Coppleson was also a keen naturalist. He was an international authority on shark attacks, and in his submission for his entry in the *Medical Directory of Australia*, he listed his book, *Shark Attacks in Australian Waters* (1958), as the most significant of his many published works. He was the Australian correspondent from 1930 for *Lancet*. His other publications included a surgical booklet entitled *Treatment of Varicose Veins by Injection* (1928, with a second edition in 1929).

Coppleson was the leading figure in the formation of the Australian Postgraduate Federation in Medicine (1948) and his many memorials include the Victor Coppleson Institute of Postgraduate Medical Studies (opened in 1977) at the University of Sydney.

Bibliography

Secondary: 1965. 'Sir Victor Coppleson.' *Australian Zoologist*, 13(2): 216.

John Pearn

CORNARO, LUIGI (aka CORNARO, ALVISE) (b. Venice, Italy, *c.* 1484; d. Padua, Italy, 8 May 1566), *hygiene.*

The son of Antonio di Giacomo and Angeliera Angelieri, it is now thought that Cornaro was born in 1484. This date is drawn from an official declaration he made to the Republic of Venice in 1540, where he stated he was fifty-six years old, and it is confirmed by his documented presence at the University of Padua as a student of law in 1504 and 1505, when he was aged about twenty. Cornaro, convinced that nature had assigned man a lifespan of *c.* ninety to one hundred years, modified his age several times apparently providing personal support for his views. He lived in Padua with his maternal uncle, but he left university without taking a degree.

Cornaro lived in a splendid palace in Padua, surrounded by artists and men of culture from the worlds of architecture, literature, and the theatre, such as Giovan Maria Falconetto and Angelo Beolco, called Ruzante. He wrote a *Trattato dell'architettura*, published posthumously (1952), in which he claimed, among other things, that living in a well-designed and comfortable building contributed significantly to prolonging one's life. His treatise on agriculture is lost. He had promoted the reclamation of some of the valleys near the Venetian lagoon, stressing also the advantages to the salubrity of the air, but Venice did not give him permission to carry out his project. He repeated the importance and validity of this plan in his *Trattato di acque* (1560).

In 1558 Cornaro published his *Trattato de la vita sobria* [A treatise on sober life], the first of a series of writings printed in Padua on longevity and the methods of achieving it. He followed this with the *Compendio breve della vita sobria* (1561), a *Lettera* to Daniele Barbaro (1563), and the *Amorevole esortatione . . . a seguire la vita sobria* (1565). The four writings were later published together under the general title *Discorsi intorno alla vita sobria* and quickly enjoyed great success. According to Cornaro, only a regular and sober life could guarantee good health and the possibility of the maximum lifespan assigned to man by nature. He discovered the benefits of sobriety in his late thirties when he was in very poor physical condition: as soon as he reduced the amount of food and drink consumed, his health improved. Cornaro recommended moderation in everything, but especially in eating and drinking. His diet consisted of bread, broth with an egg, meat—namely, veal, kid, or chicken—and wine. When life had reached its natural end, death came not from disease, but by the dissolution of the humors of which the body consisted. Galen's physiology underlay Cornaro's views on nutrition.

Certainly he lived a long time, even though it was not as long as he would have had others believe. He lived according to the principles he taught: the common sense and gentleness with which he counseled the sobriety and ethical values of his arguments explained his book's persuasiveness and extraordinary success. It went through many editions and is reprinted and read today. Leonard Leys, or Lessius, made the first translation into Latin. He wrote his own book on the same subject (1613), and it was often issued with Cornaro's. Cornaro's treatise was also translated into French, Dutch, English, and German.

Bibliography

Primary: 1965. *Discorsi intorno alla vita sobria* in Fiocco, Giuseppe, *Alvise Cornaro, il suo tempo e le sue opere* (Vicenza) pp. 169–190. (English trans., 1634).

Secondary: Rippa Bonati, Maurizio, 2004. 'L'"ars vivendi" di Alvise Cornaro', in Scortegagna, Renzo, ed., *Vivere a lungo e bene* (Venice) pp. 217–234; Menegazzo, Emilio, 1980. 'Alvise Cornaro: un veneziano del Cinquecento nella terraferma padovana' in *Storia della cultura veneta*, III/II (Vicenza) pp. 513–538; Puppi, Lion-ello, ed., 1980. *Alvise Cornaro e il suo tempo* (Padua); Lüth, Paul, 1965. *Geschichte der Geriatrie* (Stuttgart) pp. 133–136; Sigerist, Henry E., 1956. *Landmarks in the History of Hygiene* (London) pp. 36–46; Walker, William B., 1954. 'Luigi Cornaro, a Renais-sance writer on personal hygiene.' *Bulletin of the History of Med-icine* 28: 525–534.

Giuseppe Ongaro

CORRIGAN, DOMINIC JOHN   (b. Dublin, Ireland, 1 December 1802; d. Dublin, 1 February 1880), *medicine.*

With Robert Graves (1796–1853) and William Stokes (1804–78), Corrigan formed a triumvirate of physicians who made Dublin an international center of clinical excel-lence and medical pedagogy between the 1820s and 1880s. Graves and Stokes came from leading families of the Anglo-Irish protestant ascendancy closely linked with Trinity Col-lege Dublin, but Corrigan's background was native Irish and Catholic. Raised in one of the poorest areas of Dublin, he was the son of a successful merchant. He was schooled at the lay college attached to the seminary at Maynooth. Introduced to medicine by the local practitioner who attended the college, Corrigan attended the School of Physic at Trinity, where he was taught anatomy and pathol-ogy by James Macartney (1770–1843), for whom he also snatched corpses for dissection.

In the 1820s it was necessary for the Catholic Corrigan to complete his MD at Edinburgh University, where he was a contemporary of the postgraduate William Stokes. His first Dublin appointment was as physician to the Meath Street Sick Poor Institution, then the city's largest dispen-sary. Corrigan's series of papers on heart conditions in *Lan-cet* helped secure his first hospital position as physician to the Charitable Infirmary, Jervis Street, which was followed by appointments at the Cork Street Fever Hospital and House of Industry Richmond Hospital. His own practice prospered and facilitated a move (1834) to fashionable Merrion Square. He flourished as private physician to the aristocratic and professional elite, becoming the wealthiest practitioner of Victorian Dublin and the most successful Irish Catholic medical man since Thomas Arthur (1593–1675) in the seventeenth century. At his peak he earned over £9,000 per annum and built a Dalkey coastal villa with a private harbor and aquarium.

Although Corrigan did not publish as extensively as Graves or Stokes, he produced several classic descriptions of cardio-logical symptoms and pathology. His 1832 paper on visible pulsation in the neck resulted in that symptom of aortic dys-function becoming known as Corrigan's Pulse or Sign, despite the earlier description of its significance by Raymond Vieus-sens (1635–1715). Armand Trousseau (1801–67) in *La Lancet Française* (1838) established the use of the term 'Corrigan's Disease' to characterize the pathology of aortic deficiency as described by Corrigan. His work on what he called cirrhosis of the lungs became paradigmatic for subsequent under-standing of pulmonary fibrosis. The circular metal plate he designed for treating sciatica—Corrigan's Button—joined the ranks of Irish medical eponyms.

As a practitioner and Irish nationalist Corrigan became involved in public health issues, warning in 1829 that famine and disease would likely follow any failure of the potato crop. As the Great Famine worsened in 1846, he lamented the export of Irish corn while so many of the peasantry starved or died from famine fever. But while he and Robert Graves agreed on the crucial role of nutrition in the treatment of the latter, Corrigan differed from Graves about the need for enforcing isolation to combat contagion. This disagreement hardened into personal enmity when Graves blamed Corrigan for the desultory scheme of payment allowed by the Board of Health to remunerate famine doctors.

Graves prevented Corrigan's election as honorary fellow of the College of Physicians in 1847, although Dublin Castle made him the first Catholic physician-in-ordinary to the Queen in Ireland the same year. Eventually (1859) he became the College's first Catholic president, acquired its present pre-mises from the Kildare Street Club, opened the fellowship to graduates of any university, and opened the license examina-tion to women, who were thereby eligible for entry on the medical register. He was first president of the Irish Pharma-ceutical Society, president of the Royal Zoological Society, and Commissioner for Lunacy. Always a keen traveler, his *Ten days in Athens* (1862) arose from one of his journeys. He was knighted in 1866. As Liberal MP (Dublin City, 1870–73) Cor-rigan had a public platform for support of nondenomina-tional education, opposition to Isaac Butt's campaign for Irish home-government, and the opportunity to dine fre-quently and extensively at the Reform Club. Having long been involved with the Queen's University as a senator, he became its vice-chancellor in 1871. He largely retired to his Dalkey retreat after 1873 but continued to practice until par-alyzed by a stroke in late 1879. Corrigan's funeral was one of the greatest in a great age of Dublin funerals.

Bibliography

Primary: 1832. 'On permanent patency of the mouth of the aorta or inadequacy of the aortic valves.' *Edinburgh Medical and Surgical Journal* 37: 225–245; 1838. 'On cirrhosis of the lung.' *Dublin Jour-nal of Medical Science* 13: 266–286; 1846. *On famine and fever as cause and effect in Ireland; with observations on hospital location and the dispensation in outdoor relief of food and medicine* (Dublin).

Secondary: Coakley, Davis, 1992. 'Dominic Corrigan 1802–1880: Fundamental Observations in Cardiology' in *Irish Masters of Medicine* (Dublin) pp. 106–115; O'Brien, Eoin, 1983. *A Con-science in Conflict: A Biography of Sir Dominic Corrigan, 1802–1880* (Dublin);Lyons, J. B., Eoin O'Brien, et al., 1980. 'Sir Dominic Corrigan (1802–1880).' *Journal of the Irish Colleges of Physicians and Surgeons* 9: 9–57; *Oxford DNB*.

James McGeachie

CORVISART DES MARETS, JEAN-NICOLAS (b. Dricourt, France, 15 February 1755; d. Paris, France, 18 September 1821), *medicine, clinical diagnosis, pathological anatomy, heart disease.*

Corvisart was born on a small family property in the Ardennes region of Champagne, east of Paris. He was the second son of Pierre Corvisart, an attorney of the *Parlement* (high court) of Paris who had returned to his birthplace when that body was exiled from the capital by Louis XV. Pierre's wife, Madeleine-Louise Scribot, was also a native of the Ardennes, having been born in a nearby village.

When the *Parlement* was later recalled by the king, Pierre returned to Paris with his family. Jean-Nicolas, however, was not taken with them but instead, possibly for reasons of economy, was sent to Vimille near Boulogne on the Straits of Dover to live with one of his maternal uncles, the village priest. This uncle, the abbé Pain-Dubuisson, was responsible for the young Corvisart's education until he reached the age of twelve.

In 1767 Pierre Corvisart brought his son to Paris and enrolled him in the college of Sainte-Barbe. Jean-Nicolas found the constraints of this institution uncongenial after the freedom he had enjoyed in Vimille, and he acquired the reputation of being a restless and often rebellious student. His time at Sainte-Barbe was also clouded by the death of his mother in 1771. When he completed his secondary education the following year, at the age of eighteen, his father insisted that he study law and again his rebelliousness appeared, leading to a temporary break with his family.

Although Corvisart enrolled in the faculty of law as his father demanded, he neglected his studies and spent much of his time in other activities. On one occasion he attended a lecture in the Faculty of Medicine given by the anatomist Antoine Petit (1718–94), and this experience seems to have determined him to pursue a career in medicine. He began attending other medical lectures, and when his father discovered what was happening, he was faced with the choice of returning to his legal studies or being disowned. Refusing to abandon his interest in medicine, he left home and persuaded the director of the Hôtel-Dieu, the largest hospital in Paris, to take him on as an orderly.

Faced with this display of independence, Pierre Corvisart eventually became reconciled to the prospect of a medical career for his son, and Jean-Nicolas was welcomed back into the family. The young man was not following in his father's profession, but both his grandfather Jacques Corvisart (1688–1738) and his great-grandfather Jean-René Corvisart (1647–1724) had been surgeons, so his interests were consistent with some aspects of family tradition.

Although one of Corvisart's military ancestors had been ennobled by Louis XIV in 1669, it was more by affectation than by right that Jean-Nicolas enrolled in the Faculty of Medicine as 'Corvisart des Marets'. He began his formal

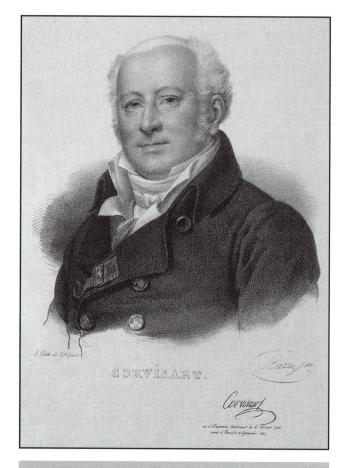

Jean-Nicolas, Baron Corvisart. Lithograph by Bazin le jeune after F. P. S. Gérard, 1832. Iconographic Collection, Wellcome Library, London.

medical studies in November 1777 and received his license in July 1782, finishing first in his cohort although he was the youngest among them. After passing further examinations and defending two additional theses, he was awarded the title of Doctor-Regent in November 1782, the Faculty's highest recognition and one conferring the right to teach. The good impression made by Corvisart's academic performance was undermined, however, at the customary banquet that he subsequently hosted for his professors, because his speech at this event was considered highly disrespectful toward the Faculty.

With a similar disdain for tradition, Corvisart lost the opportunity of being appointed to a hospital recently founded by Madame Necker, wife of the eminent financier, by refusing to wear a wig. Instead, he took the less remunerative post of parish physician in 1783, with responsibility for treating the poor in their homes.

To develop his clinical skills after completing the largely theoretical curriculum of the Faculty, Corvisart began following the surgical rounds of Pierre-Joseph Desault (1738–95) at the Charité hospital. Desault, who became chief surgeon at the Charité in 1782, systematized the clinical teaching of surgery and provided a model that Corvisart would later develop for his own clinical teaching of medicine. In particular, the combination of instruction at the bedside, student involvement in patient care, and systematic autopsy of all patients who died served as the hallmark of both Desault's and Corvisart's teaching.

When Desault moved from the Charité to the Hôtel Dieu in 1785, Corvisart stayed at the Charité and began following the medical rounds of Louis Desbois de Rochefort (1750–86). It was Rochefort's example that persuaded Corvisart that Desault's clinical teaching could be applied to medicine as well as surgery. With the premature death of Rochefort at the beginning of 1786, Corvisart was appointed as 'expectant' physician at the Charité, the position vacated by Rochefort's successor.

Corvisart delivered the eulogy of Rochefort at a meeting of the Faculty of Medicine in November 1786, and early in the following year published Rochefort's text on materia medica, which had been left incomplete at the time of the author's death. Corvisart's work on both these projects was interrupted by a serious wound infection that he contracted in August 1786 while conducting an autopsy. For several days his life was in danger, but he was successfully treated by Desault and rapidly recovered.

In 1788 Corvisart attained the position previously held by Rochefort. Although this promotion made Corvisart second physician, as Rochefort had been, the elderly chief physician gave Corvisart the same freedom that Rochefort had previously enjoyed. Corvisart therefore undertook a comprehensive reorganization of the medical service at the Charité. He divided patients into separate groups according to their symptoms, he applied the teaching methods of Desault as described previously, and he introduced the technique of thoracic percussion as a regular feature of clinical examination.

The outbreak of the French Revolution toward the end of 1789, and the radical political climate in the years immediately following, induced Corvisart in 1790 to change the aristocratic tag 'des Marets' at the end of his name to 'Desmarest', and then a year or so later to abandon it altogether. He maintained good relations with the municipal authorities in his district of Paris by providing advice on public health as a demonstration of his patriotism. Because his teaching was based in the Charité rather than in the Faculty of Medicine, his activities were not disrupted in 1793, when the government closed the Faculty along with other teaching and scientific institutions of the old regime. Only the name of the hospital was changed, from Charité to Unité, to indicate that responsibility for its administration had passed from the church to the state.

In 1794, when the most radical phase of the revolution had passed, the legislature established a new medical school to replace the suppressed Faculty. Corvisart was named professor of clinical medicine at the Unité from the beginning of 1795. Early in 1796 he was also appointed to the Chair of Medicine at the College of France. As professor of clinical medicine he continued to teach at the bedside and in the autopsy room, as he had done prior to the revolution, excelling in diagnostics and educating virtually an entire generation of French physicians. At the College of France, however, where traditional lectures were expected, he soon wearied of lecturing on medical theory and instead gave presentations on individual cases from his hospital wards—thus introducing a clinical perspective.

Although Corvisart advocated that patients, rather than printed volumes, were the 'books' from which medical students should learn, he came under pressure from colleagues to publish some learned works to secure his reputation. Suspicious of theoretical systems, he turned to collections of aphorisms, which he valued as summaries of the clinical experience of eminent medical predecessors. Thus in 1797 he published a French translation of the aphorisms on fevers that the Austrian clinician Maximillian Stoll (1742–87) had originally published in Latin a decade earlier. Stoll's work incorporated some aphorisms of the eminent Dutch medical teacher, Herman Boerhaave (1668–1738), and in 1802 Corvisart published a French translation of Boerhaave's aphorisms as well.

Both Boerhaave's clinic at Leiden and the Viennese clinic where Stoll taught were recognized as forerunners of the much larger-scale teaching clinics of the Paris medical school. Although Corvisart's translations were relatively minor contributions to the profession, they were helpful for students because knowledge of Latin was no longer required for medical study. Of more direct utility to the profession was Corvisart's revival in 1801 of the *Journal of Medicine, Surgery and Pharmacy*, which had ceased publication seven years earlier; but here again he was facilitating the dissemination of other writers' contributions to medical knowledge rather than making contributions of his own.

Corvisart's career took an unexpected turn in 1801, when he was called to treat Napoleon Bonaparte (1769–1821), then First Consul of the Republic. Corvisart's therapeutic success on this occasion and his generally skeptical disposition appealed to Napoleon, who distrusted medicine, and Corvisart was soon appointed 'government physician' (a republican euphemism for 'personal physician to the First Consul'). When the Empire was proclaimed in 1804, Corvisart became First Physician of the Imperial Court. In this capacity he oversaw the medical service of the Imperial household and personally attended Napoleon and his immediate family. Corvisart's court appointment also brought him a large influx of private patients from the upper echelons of Parisian society. When titles of nobility were reintroduced by Napoleon, Corvisart was made a Baron of the Empire.

Despite the pressure of his official duties, it was during the early years of the Empire that Corvisart brought out his two most valuable publications. In 1806 his *Essay on the*

Diseases and the Organic Lesions of the Heart and Large Vessels appeared, compiled from his lectures by one of his students. This work set a new standard for the diagnosis, treatment, and pathological anatomy of heart conditions, many of which had previously been confused with diseases of the lungs. It also introduced the diagnostic tool of percussion to the medical profession at large.

The technique of thoracic percussion was developed by the Austrian physician Leopold Auenbrugger (1722–1809) in the previous century and was described by him in his *Inventum Novum*, published in 1761. This Latin text attracted little attention outside Vienna, however. Corvisart, for example, first learned of Auenbrugger's discovery through reading Stoll. The success of Corvisart's *Essay* stimulated widespread medical interest in percussion, thus prompting Corvisart to publish a French translation of Auenbrugger's work in 1808. Unlike his previous translations, this one carried an extensive commentary by Corvisart himself, which for many readers was more valuable than the original text.

With the fall of Napoleon in 1815, Corvisart retired to private life. His failing health and feelings of political disillusionment caused him to withdraw from medical practice, and he refused a number of overtures from the restored Bourbon regime. At the end of 1820, however, he agreed to accept appointment to the newly established Royal Academy of Medicine, most of whose members were his former students. A series of strokes prevented him from taking an active role in this organization, and he died in September of the following year.

Bibliography

Primary: 1806. *Essai sur les maladies et les lésions organiques du cœur et des gros vaisseaux* (Paris) [Translated by Jacob Gates, 1812, *An essay on the organic diseases of the heart and great vessels* (Philadelphia)]; 1808. 'Commentaire' in Auenbrugger, Leopold. *Nouvelle méthode pour reconnaître les maladies internes de la poitrine par la percussion de cette cavité . . .; ouvrage traduit du Latin et commenté par J. N. Corvisart* (Paris); 1929. *Aphorismes de médecine clinique, recueillis par F.-V. Merat* (Paris).

Secondary: Albury, W. R., 1998. 'Corvisart and Broussais: Human Individuality and Medical Dominance' in Hannaway, Caroline, and Ann Le Berge, eds., *Constructing Paris Medicine* (Amsterdam) pp. 221–250; Ganière, Paul, 1985. *Corvisart, médecin de l'Empereur* (Paris [new edition, augmented; originally published as *Corvisart, médecin de Napoleon* in 1951]); Albury, W. R., 1982. 'Heart of Darkness: J. N. Corvisart and the Medicalization of Life' in Goubert, Jean-Pierre, ed., *La médicalisation de la société française, 1770–1830* (Waterloo, Ont.) pp. 17–31; DSB.

W. R. Albury

COTTON, HENRY ANDREWS

COTTON, HENRY ANDREWS (b, Norfolk, Virginia, USA, 18 May 1876; d, Trenton, New Jersey, USA, 8 May 1933), *psychiatry*.

Cotton, the son of George Adolphus Cotton, occupation unknown, and Mary Delha Biggs (daughter of U.S. Senator Asa Biggs), studied medicine at Johns Hopkins and the University of Maryland, from which he received his MD (1899). Six months of service in the Army Medical Corps and at the Baltimore Lunatic Asylum was followed by an appointment as an assistant physician to the Worcester, Massachusetts, State Hospital, where he worked under Adolf Meyer (1866-1950). Three years later, after Meyer had left to head the New York Psychiatric Institute, Cotton moved to a post at the Danvers (Mass.) State Hospital. During 1905–6, with Meyer's sponsorship, he spent a year in Munich, working under Alois Alzheimer (1864–1915) and Emil Kraepelin (1856–1926) and, following his return to the United States, quickly obtained a position as superintendent of the New Jersey State Hospital at Trenton. He remained at this post until 1930, when he was appointed as the hospital's honorary director of research.

Cotton was appointed to Trenton in the aftermath of a scandal involving mistreatment of patients and a cover-up of an epidemic of typhoid fever. Within two months, he had eliminated all mechanical restraint at the hospital, and thereafter he made sustained efforts to bring psychiatry into closer relation with general medicine. Convinced that insanity was a somatic disorder, he employed a series of physical treatments—hydrotherapy, salvarsan for syphilitics, and glandular extracts, all without much success.

In 1916, however, he became aware of the notion of focal sepsis, a doctrine then enjoying a vogue in some respectable medical circles, which attributed a variety of mysterious systemic diseases, such as arthritis, to the effects of chronic low-grade infections. Cotton adapted this theory to psychiatry, suggesting that the symptoms of mental disorder were the epiphenomenal manifestation of the impact of the toxins produced by focal sepsis on the brain. In a preantibiotic era, the therapeutic conclusion he drew was that these sites of infection must be located and surgically eliminated.

Cotton began by removing teeth and tonsils, and when this failed to produce the desired improvements, he summoned outside specialists, such as bacteriologists and abdominal surgeons, and began the task of searching for sepsis elsewhere in the body; stomachs, spleens, uteri, gall bladders, but especially colons were soon targeted for elimination. Aggressively trying to obtain both lay and professional attention for his work, he claimed that he had shown both the biological origins of major mental disorders and the way to treat them. His claimed cure rates approached 85 percent.

Within the profession, there was mixed reaction to Cotton's claims, though few of his American colleagues attacked his 'findings' in print or questioned his program of abdominal surgery, which he acknowledged produced a mortality rate of 30 percent (the true figure was closer to 45 percent). He visited Britain on two occasions, in 1923 and again in 1927, and was hailed by many of the great and good in British medicine as a 'new Lister', the man who had brought psychiatry into the medical mainstream.

Despite his personal ties to Cotton, Adolf Meyer agreed to provide oversight for a systemic assessment of the work at Trenton. This was carried out over a twelve-month period by one of his chief assistants, Phyllis Greenacre. Greenacre's findings were a devastating indictment of Cotton's claims, showing that his interventions were not only useless but also actively harmful, even fatal, in their effects. Meyer, however, suppressed Greenacre's findings, allowing Cotton to continue his experiments unchecked for several more years. Though Cotton lost his superintendency when local physicians complained that he had developed a lucrative private practice to supplement his income from the state hospital, he continued to perform colectomies on wealthy mental patients until his unexpected death from heart disease. Even then, Meyer protected his protégé, eulogizing him in the pages of the *American Journal of Psychiatry* as a brave psychiatric pioneer.

Bibliography

Primary: 1921. *The Defective Delinquent and Insane* (Princeton); 1922. 'The Etiology and Treatment of the So-Called Functional Psychoses.' *American Journal of Psychiatry* 79: 157–194.

Secondary: Andrew Scull, 2005. *Madhouse; A Tragic Tale of Megalomania and Modern Medicine* (London and New Haven); Meyer, Adolf, 1934. 'In Memoriam: Henry A. Cotton.' *American Journal of Psychiatry* 90: 921–923.

Andrew Scull

COTUGNO, DOMENICO FELICE ANTONIO   (b. Ruvo, Italy, 29 January 1736; d. Naples, Italy, 6 October 1822), *anatomy, physiology.*

Cotugno, son of Chiara Assalemme and Michele, humble peasants in Apulia, grew up with his aunt Anna Antonia. Because of his intelligence he was sent to study Latin at the Episcopal seminary of Molfetta. Back at Ruvo he learned about metaphysics, physics, and natural sciences and made his first dissections. In 1753 he enrolled at the University of Naples and engaged with Newtonian science and the recent medical literature. At the age of eighteen he was appointed assistant (and later director) of the Ospedale degl'Incurabili, one of the biggest hospitals in Italy. In 1756 he obtained his degree at the Medical School of Salerno and, not succeeding in entering upon an academic career, he dedicated his free time to research.

Cotugno united some of the most important medical and physiological trends of the second half of the eighteenth century: Marcello Malpighi's tradition of studying the fine anatomy of the hidden mechanisms of living organisms, Giovanni Battista Morgani's doctrine of the anatomical localization of the seat of disease, and Albrecht von Haller's concept of physiology as *anatomia animata*. In 1761 Cotugno discovered the nasopalatine nerve, responsible for sneezing. In the same year he published *De aquaeductibus auris humanae internae*, describing the anatomy of one of the finest organs: the inner ear. He identified the (Cotunnius') aqueduct and the columns in the osseous spiral lamina of the cochlea. Since Aristotle, scientists had been convinced that sound propagated only through the air, whereas Cotugno, studying fresh instead of old specimens, showed that the labyrinth was filled with liquid. This revolution of the concept of hearing was discussed and verified by the main European anatomists and established Cotugno's celebrity, consolidated by a trip to the main centers of Italian medicine (1765).

In *De ischiade nervosa commentarius* (1764) he distinguished arthritic from nervous sciatica. He showed that the second is an inflammation caused by an excess of 'Liquor Cotunni', describing for the first time in detail the cerebrospinal fluid. He also noted the relationship between edema and proteinuria. Cotugno's third great work was *De sedibus variolarum* (1769). Dissecting thirteen persons of different sex, age, and class who had died of smallpox, he described the anatomy of the pustules and localized the seat of the disease in the Malpighian layer of the skin. He demonstrated the uselessness of hot baths and proposed grafts and, later, Jennerian vaccination, thus pioneering epidemiology.

In 1766 Cotugno became professor of anatomy (1766–1818). Besides his engagement in the University and the hospital, he made his fortune as physician of the Neapolitan nobility. In 1794 he married Ippolita Ruffo, widow of the duke of Bagnara. They had no children. Cotugno then concentrated on institutional and didactical reforms. In the tradition of Giovanni Maria Lancisi he aimed at a strong alliance between scientific investigation and clinics, practice, and constant update of the medical literature, and between medicine, politics, and social progress. He was one of the founders of the Academy of Science and Letters, cultivated a huge correspondence with the provincial doctors, and possessed one of the biggest personal collections of medical books and manuscripts, art, and antiquities.

During the Jacobin revolt Cotugno maintained a moderate position. This saved him from the persecutions of the Restoration of 1799 that saw many Neapolitan intellectuals executed or exiled. During the French decade (1806–15) he was appointed president of the Reale Istituto d'Incoraggiamento (1806–08), rector of the University (1811–13), and president of the Scientific Academy (1810–17), and he held other important institutional offices. In 1818 he suffered a cerebral embolism and died four years later at the age of eighty-eight.

Bibliography

Primary: 1761. *De aquaeductibus auris humanae internae* (Naples); 1764. *De ischiade nervosa commentarius* (Naples) [English trans. 1775. *A Treatise on the Nervous Sciatica* (London)]; 1769. *De sedibus variolarum* (Naples and Vienna, 1771); 1774. *Dello spirito della medicina* (Florence).

Secondary: Borrelli, Antonio, 2000. *Istituzioni scientifiche, medicina e società: biografia di Domenico Cotugno (1736–1822)* (Florence); Ongaro, Giuseppe, 1975, 'Cotugno, Domenico' in *Scienziati e tecnologi dalle origini al 1875* vol. 1 (Milan) pp. 341–343; *DSB*.

Ariane Dröscher

COUNCILMAN, WILLIAM THOMAS (b. Pikesville, Maryland, USA, 1 January 1854; d. York Village, Maine, USA, 26 May 1933), *pathology*.

Councilman was born on a farm outside Baltimore, Maryland, to John T., a farmer and country doctor, and Christiana Drummond Mitchell, a judge's daughter. When he was thirteen, he attended St John's College in Annapolis, Maryland. He left at the end of his sophomore year (1870), spending the next six years living an 'independent existence' in which he 'raised side whiskers . . . and did pretty much as he chose' (Cushing, 1933, p. 614). Eventually, however, he returned to his father's example, entering medical school at the University of Maryland. During the standard two-year, lecture-intensive program, he was particularly drawn to dissections, supplementing his training with self-directed comparative animal anatomies at his father's farm. Councilman graduated MD in 1878.

America's new model medical institution deflected him from his intended career path in country practice. The Johns Hopkins University had opened, and his father, present at T. H. Huxley's opening address (1876), was impressed by the promise of autonomous research it offered. Shortly before graduation, son William met Hopkins's physiologist Henry Newell Martin, who offered him space in his laboratory for a brief period of study. Councilman learned microscopy and found himself drawn to histology. He used the wages he earned as Baltimore's assistant quarantine officer to buy a microscope and the wages he earned subsequently, both in that job and in his position at Bay View Asylum, to save money for study at Europe's top pathological laboratories. The trip abroad, which commenced in late 1880, included study in Vienna, Leipzig, and Strasbourg. Returning to Baltimore, Councilman continued to work at Bay View; he also taught at local medical schools, acted (briefly) as the city's coroner, and helped John Shaw Billings prepare the *National Medical Dictionary*. All the while, he continued his research, publishing his first widely recognized study—on malaria—in 1885. The next year, he joined William Welch's laboratory at Johns Hopkins as an associate in pathology.

At Hopkins, Councilman delighted in his excellent collaborators, completing an acclaimed study of amoebic dysentery with H. A. Lafleur (1891). He was an associate professor of pathology when he left Baltimore to take up the Shattuck professorship of pathological anatomy at Harvard (1892). In Boston, he continued his collaborative studies, publishing important work on epidemic cerebrospinal meningitis (1898), diphtheria (1901), and small-pox (1904). He also married Isabella Coolidge (1894). When Peter Bent Brigham Hospital opened (1913), he was named its pathologist. Councilman was an influential teacher; indeed, Wolbach argued that teaching was 'his most important work at Harvard' (Wolbach, 1933, p. 117). Many of his students and collaborators eventually became noted pathologists. He played a founding role in the American Association of Pathologists and Bacteriologists and served as its first president (1901). Despite his love of the laboratory, Councilman never abandoned his enthusiasm for nature, accompanying A. Hamilton Rice's Expedition to the Amazon (1916) and attending personally to the horticultural improvement of Brigham Hospital. After retiring from Brigham (1917), he held a two-year appointment (from 1919) as temporary professor of pathology at Peking Union Medical College. Councilman resigned his Harvard professorship in 1923. One of the three daughters who survived him (Elizabeth) became a medical doctor.

Bibliography

Primary: 1891. (with Lafleur, Henri Amadée) 'Amoebic Dysentery.' *Johns Hopkins Hospital Reports* 2: 395–548; 1898. (with Mallory, Frank Burr, and John Homer Wright) *Epidemic Cerebrospinal Meningitis and Its Relations to Other Forms of Meningitis* (Boston); 1904. (with Magrath, G. B., W. R. Brickerhoff, Ernest Edward Tyzzer, Elmer Ernest Southard, Ralph Leroy Thompson, I. R. Bancroft, and Gary Nathan Calkins) 'Studies on the Pathology and on the Aetiology of Variola and Vaccinia.' *Journal of Medical Research* 11: 1–361.

Secondary: Cushing, Harvey, 1933. 'William Thomas Councilman, 1854–1933.' *Science* 77: 613–618; Wolbach, S. B., 1933. 'William Thomas Councilman, 1854–1933.' *Archives of Pathology* 16: 114–119; *DSB*; *DAMB*.

Kim Pelis

CRILE, GEORGE WASHINGTON (b. Chili, Ohio, USA, 11 November 1864; d. Cleveland, Ohio, USA, 7 January 1943), *surgery*.

The fifth of eight children of a prosperous farmer, Crile followed the tradition that one family member should bear the first names of George Washington. He left school at the age of 14 to teach in a district school, subsequently combining this with study at the Northern University, Ohio, and later with medical training. Crile first studied with a preceptor before entering Wooster Medical School in Cleveland, Ohio, where qualification with the highest honors guaranteed him a house officer's post at the University Hospital.

After experience in private surgical practice Crile intended to join the U.S. Navy. But he contracted typhoid, thus remaining in the practice and undertaking training tours to surgical units in Europe in 1892 and 1895. Well before this, however, he had started a lifelong series of research projects, in both animals and humans. His early studies focused on problems in head and neck surgery: tracheostomy for the highly prevalent diphtheria and total laryngectomy, then a hazardous procedure, as well as developing a carotid clamp. Two specific lifelong interests also started then; the first was goiter surgery, then the only effective treatment for severe thyrotoxicosis. The second was the physiology and management of shock—which culminated much later in developing a pneumatic suit to prevent peripheral pooling of fluid (subsequently used in World War II to prevent the effects of high G forces in fighter pilots).

This evaluation of shock continued in 1898 (the year after he was appointed professor of surgery at Cleveland), when Crile served as a brigade surgeon in the Spanish-American War. It continued in civilian practice in experiments on blood transfusion in dogs and an attempt in 1905 in a patient using a sutured anastomosis between the blood vessels of donor and recipient. His first successful transfusion occurred the following year, with Crile subsequently developing a cannula for linking the vessels, and he published a monograph on transfusion in 1909 (one of twenty-seven books he authored). He further contributed to surgical safety by starting the training of specialist nurse-anesthetists.

Crile's expertise and worldwide contacts came to the fore in World War I. He established an American Military Hospital in late 1914, introducing blood transfusion into the British Army and advising on resuscitation and base hospital organization. Serving in the first U.S. contingent to enter the war in 1917, he operated tirelessly on casualties, characteristically also finding the time to research the effect of war gas. Promoted to Colonel, he became research director for the American Expeditionary Force.

The postwar years were largely centered on the Cleveland Clinic, developed by Crile and his colleagues and opened in 1921. With an emphasis on research (especially into chronic conditions, such as diabetes and hypertension), this clinic subsequently added a hospital and acquired a worldwide reputation. Crile continued his hyperactive life, becoming increasingly prominent in surgical politics yet persisting with research, which extended into dissecting large animals shot on safari. By the end of his life, with his colleagues he had performed no fewer than 27,000 thyroid operations, and only the onset of blindness prevented his continuing at the same pace. He died of bacterial endocarditis, which failed to respond to sulfonamides and the small doses of penicillin then available. His achievements show how rapidly an individual can contribute to a discipline's evolution given the right seed (an exceptionally inquiring mind) and soil (similarly talented colleagues without the subsequent constraints of, say, randomized trials and research ethics committees).

Bibliography

Primary: 1921. (Rowland, Amy, ed.) *A Physical Interpretation of Shock, Exhaustion and Restoration* (London); 1934. (Rowland, Amy, ed.) *Diseases Peculiar to Civilized Man: Clinical Management and Surgical Treatment* (New York); 1947. *An Autobiography.* (Philadelphia).

Secondary: English, Peter C., 1980. *Shock, Physiological Surgery and George Washington Crile: Medical Innovation in the Progressive Era* (Westport, CT); *DAMB*.

Stephen Lock

CRUVEILHIER, JEAN   (b. Limoges, France, 9 February 1791; d. Sussac, France, 10 March 1874), *pathological anatomy.*

Cruveilhier was the son of Léonard Cruveilhier, a military surgeon who served in the armies of the Rhine and Moselle and who was chief surgeon in the military hospital of Choisy-le-Roi. His early education was at the Collège de Limoges. Cruveilhier was a pious young man and he initially thought of becoming a priest. But his father wanted him to be a physician, and he began his medical studies in Paris at age nineteen. Cruveilhier had an introduction to the surgeon Guillaume Dupuytren, another Limousin native, and became his protégé. The future leader in pathological anatomy was initially repelled by dissection of the cadaver. He considered reverting to a career in the Church, but his father persuaded him to resume medical studies. His doctoral thesis (1816) was on general pathological anatomy. Cruveilhier then returned to take over his father's practice in Limoges for seven years.

In 1823, as part of a reorganization of medical education by Catholic royalists, positions of *professeurs agrégés,* or junior professors, were initiated. Encouraged by his father to enter the public competition, Cruveilhier obtained a post. Dupuytren recommended Cruveilhier for a professorship in surgery at the University of Montpellier, but it was not to his liking. The death of Pierre-August Béclard opened up the professorship of anatomy at the Paris Faculty of Medicine. With the patronage of the Abbé Frayssinous, the grand master of the university, Cruveilhier was appointed to this chair in November 1825. In 1836, after the death of Dupuytren, he became the first holder of the new chair in pathological anatomy founded by Dupuytren's bequest. Cruveilhier held this chair for thirty years.

Cruveilhier was very methodical in his anatomical and physiological research. He spent entire days dissecting and set great store on making his own observations of healthy and diseased organs. His reputation largely rests on his two great illustrated treatises of pathological anatomy published over a period of thirty-five years (1829–64). Although Cruveilhier believed that phlebitis dominated pathology, he followed Bichat's doctrines and sought the causes of disease in the tissues of the body. In his discussion of puerperal fever, Cruveilhier expressed his often-quoted belief that these murderous epidemics would be prevented if large maternity hospitals were broken up into small ones of only fifteen or twenty women housed in private rooms.

He held hospital positions at La Maternité, the Salpêtrière, and later at La Charité. The large numbers of autopsies at the Salpêtrière provided him with material for his extensive investigations in pathological anatomy.

Cruveilhier reconstituted the Société Anatomique, the creation of Laennec and Dupuytren, in January 1826 with himself as president, and he kept this position for forty years. The society was a forum for presentation of anatomical ideas, especially for young physicians. Cruveilhier became a member of the Academy of Medicine in 1836 and its president in 1839. He is noted today for his studies of multiple sclerosis, progressive muscular dystrophy, gastric ulcers, and colon diverticulosis, as well as brain tumors.

Cruveilhier had a large practice and was known for his charity to poor patients. His most famous client was the statesman Talleyrand, whose physician he became in 1835. He died in his native region, near Limoges, at the age of eighty-three.

Bibliography

Primary: 1816. *Essai sur l'anatomie pathologique en générale, et sur les transformations et productions organiques en particuliers* (Paris); 1828–1842. *Anatomie pathologique du corps humain, ou descriptions avec figures lithographiées des altérations morbides dont le corps humain est susceptible* 6 vols. (Paris); 1849–1864. *Traité d'anatomie pathologique générale* 5 vols. (Paris).

Secondary: Béclard, Jules, 1878. 'M. Cruveilhier' in *Notices et portraits, éloges lus à l'Académie de Médecine* (Paris) pp. 259–287; *DSB*.

Caroline Hannaway

CRUZ, OSWALDO GONÇALVES

(b. São Luiz do Paraitinga, Brazil, 5 August 1872; d. Petrópolis, Brazil, 11 February 1917), *public health, microbiology, tropical medicine.*

Cruz was born in a small town in the State of São Paulo, where he spent his first years and where his father practiced medicine. In 1877 his family moved to Rio de Janeiro, then capital of Brazil, where his father assumed the post of hygiene inspector. In 1887, at the young age of fifteen, Oswaldo entered the School of Medicine of Rio de Janeiro. During his medical training Cruz was interested in the renewal of medical knowledge by microbiology, which coexisted with a strong hygienist tradition in Brazil. He worked as an assistant at the laboratory of the hygiene university chair (1888–90) and at the National Institute of Hygiene (1890–92). His MD thesis, presented in 1892, was about water as a vehicle of microbe transmission.

In 1893 he married the daughter of a rich Portuguese tradesman with whom he had six children. He kept his interest for research by installing a small microbiology laboratory at his residence. He started his medical practice at the consultation office that had belonged to his father; he also worked as a doctor at a textile industry. Between 1894 and 1897 he was the head of the laboratory of clinical analyses of

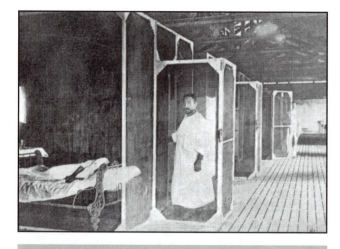

Wire-walled isolation cubicles for nursing patients with yellow fever at the Hospital St Sebastiao, Rio de Janeiro. Halftone reproduction from *Os Serviços de Saúde Publica no Brasil...*, Rio de Janeiro, 1909. Wellcome Library, London.

the General Policlinic of Rio, an important medical assistance institution, where he made contact with a group of doctors strongly influenced by bacteriology and German medicine.

In 1897 Cruz traveled to France with his family to specialize at the Pasteur Institute in microbiology and its applications to public health, at a time of many discoveries related to pathogenic microorganisms, the development of sera therapy, and the consolidation of tropical medicine. He was dedicated to the study of bacteriology and the techniques of microscopy, learned to produce the glassware needed for setting up laboratories, and deepened his knowledge of the production of sera. Being aware that he would need a medical specialization upon his return to Brazil, Cruz also studied urology and trained at the Toxicology Laboratory of Paris.

Cruz returned to Brazil in August 1899; two months later he took part in a federal commission sent to the port of Santos, in the state of São Paulo, to investigate a possible bubonic plague epidemic identified by Adolfo Lutz and Vital Brazil but nevertheless denied by local doctors and tradesmen. Once the suspicions that the plague had arrived in Brazil were confirmed, Cruz remained in Santos to combat the disease that threatened other ports, particularly the port of Rio de Janeiro. This episode, besides raising his prestige, brought him closer to Emílio Ribas, a pioneer in the adoption and diffusion of the theory of the mosquito as a yellow fever transmitter. In that same year, Cruz was elected to the prestigious National Academy of Medicine.

The episode alerted the federal government to the need for its own sera production institute. Cruz was invited to be the technical director of the Federal Serum Therapy Institute (ISF) that was under construction at the Manguinhos farm on the outskirts of Rio. The ISF was initially under the general direction of the Baron of Pedro Afonso, owner of the Municipal Vaccine Institute, which produced the vaccine against smallpox. The ISF was inaugurated in May 1900; by October it already supplied the federal health services with vaccine and antiplague serum. In 1902, Oswaldo Cruz assumed the general direction of the Manguinhos Institute that he progressively transformed into a center of studies in tropical diseases and experimental medicine, which, similar to the Pasteur Institute, associated scientific research, biological product output, and teaching.

The Sanitation of Rio de Janeiro (1903–09)

In 1903 Rodriguez Alves assumed the presidency of the Republic; the main focus of his government program was urban renewal and the sanitation of the federal capital. In that year Cruz was appointed Director General of Public Health, with the task of fighting yellow fever, smallpox, and bubonic plague that paralyzed the federal capital and the other ports of the country, cost thousands of lives, and threatened the reputation and the economy of the country. From that time on, Cruz's life, public health, and the Manguinhos Institute would become inseparable.

Amidst a radical urban renewal program executed with the intention of 'civilizing and Europeanizing' the city of Rio de Janeiro, in April 1903 the Service for the Prophylaxis of Yellow Fever was created. With resources and ample power, Cruz executed an enormous campaign against the disease, based on the strategy of exclusively combating the yellow fever transmitter mosquito (*Stegomya fasciata*, today *Aedes aegypti*) in its larval and adult forms, at the same time that he sought for the adhesion to that perspective of the medical community and of the population by means of the distribution of sanitary education pamphlets. The federal capital turned into a test field for the mosquito theory under authoritarian conditions, though not under military occupation as had been the experience of the North Americans in Cuba. The absence of previous sanitation of the city was another important element to verification of the results of Cruz's strategy. The campaign against bubonic plague included obligatory notification of cases, isolation of sick people, treatment with the serum produced at Manguinhos Institute, and the extermination of rats.

In June 1904 Cruz presented at the National Congress a law aimed at again making obligatory anti-smallpox vaccination and revaccination all over the country, with draconian clauses that would guarantee its execution. The coercive aspects of this law and the sanitary services' actions unified the different groups that opposed the government and those unsatisfied with the deep changes in life and housing conditions of the lower-income classes in Rio de Janeiro. In the beginning of November 1904, there was a huge popular rebellion, known as the Vaccine Revolt, which paralyzed the city and was controlled by the government over a week later.

The sanitary campaigns directed by Cruz established a long-term model in Brazilian public health, characterized by the centralization of actions, strong regulations, and the election of one disease and its transmission forms as specific and exclusive targets. The success of Cruz's actions, many times strongly criticized, may be evaluated by the drastic decline of cases and mortality caused by those diseases, particularly yellow fever (from 584 deaths in 1903 to 4 in 1908) as well as the recuperation of the country's and its capital's image. The international recognition of Cruz for the extinction of yellow fever in its epidemic form in Rio de Janeiro happened when he was granted the golden medal at the Fourteenth Congress of Hygiene and Demography in Berlin in 1907. He returned to Brazil as a national hero. In March 1908 the ISF was named the Oswaldo Cruz Institute (IOC).

At the end of 1905, Cruz visited twenty-four ports from north to south on the Brazilian shoreline in order to get to know the sanitary conditions in order to propose measures for the country's defense against cholera and bubonic plague, in accordance with the international sanitary conventions of which Brazil was a signatory. From 1906 he was dedicated to the execution of a plan to combat tuberculosis, which affected above all the poor segments of the population. In 1909, due to a law that forbade the accumulation of civil service positions, Cruz opted to remain director of IOC and left the sanitary services.

The Direction of Oswaldo Cruz Institute (1902–17)

Since his adhesion to the theory of the transmission of yellow fever by the mosquito, Cruz became interested in tropical medicine and stimulated at Manguinhos Institute the studies on malaria, filariasis, beriberi, hookworm disease, schistosomiasis, and leishmaniasis. For this undertaking Cruz gathered a group of young doctors and researchers who were enthusiastic about the renewal of biomedical sciences and which he referred to as the 'kindergarten of science'.

His interests were reaffirmed after the cycle of the great sanitary campaigns in the country's capital—which gave him the epithet of public health hero—when he had the opportunity to study pathologies that were until then little known. Private and public enterprises requested help to combat diseases, especially malaria, at the construction sites of hydroelectric plants and railways in the most remote regions of the country. An example is his participation, in 1910, in malaria control among the workers of the railway Madeira-Mamoré, built by a North American company in the Amazonian jungle near the Bolivian border.

The development of tropical medicine was stimulated by study trips of IOC researchers to Europe and the United States. Besides this, between 1908 and 1909, European researchers were hired, such as Stanislas von Prowazek and Gustav Giemsa, from the School of Tropical Medicine in Hamburg, and Max Hartmann, from the Institute of Infectious

Diseases in Berlin. It became a permanent and main field of investigation from 1909, when Carlos Chagas—who succeeded Oswaldo Cruz as the director of IOC—discovered a new tropical disease, Chagas' disease. Tropical medicine was further developed by a large amount of information and material related to Brazilian pathologies and the population's health and life conditions proceeding from the observations made by several researchers from Manguinhos during their trips through the Brazilian mainland in 1912–13.

From its creation, IOC had teaching activities, initially on an informal basis, in bacteriology, parasitology, anatomy, and pathologic histology. Those courses were basically of practical and experimental character and nonexistent at the School of Medicine. They were attended by medical students, who from 1901 used the Institute's laboratories to prepare their theses, and also by graduate professionals. Many of those students took part in the Institute's research projects initially on a voluntary basis; some of them became members of its cadre. Others later on occupied positions in the public health services of the Federal Capital and of other states. In 1907 a course in veterinary medicine was created, comprising pathology, hygiene, and therapeutics; the following year, the Institute started courses on bacteriology and parasitology as applied to veterinarian pathology, hygiene, and therapeutics.

Shortly before Cruz's death, the institution he had created was huge: a scientific complex composed of a series of buildings and modern laboratory infrastructure on the same level as similar institutions in more developed countries. It had also diversified the production of therapeutic and prophylactic products, both human and veterinarian. The income of the commercialization of those products allowed Cruz to implement his plans. Manguinhos Institute had accumulated significant knowledge related to the prophylaxis of malaria, the evolution of parasites in their hosts, and the systematics and biology of insect transmitters of human and animal diseases. The confluence of tropical medicine and microbiology—that expressed Cruz's intellectual path—led to an original scientific organization that articulated the interests of knowledge production with public health issues. This model distinguished the institution created by Cruz from other public research institutions. Recognized by his contemporaries for his achievements, Cruz was awarded with several distinctions, such as the French Legion of Honor and membership in the prestigious Brazilian Academy of Literature, which he entered in 1913.

Oswaldo Cruz died at forty-five years of age, in Petrópolis, Rio de Janeiro, where he had been appointed mayor in mid-1916, after leaving IOC because of the worsening of a chronic renal insufficiency. The myth of Oswaldo Cruz has been worshiped by successive generations of doctors and sanitarians and by Brazilian society. He is regarded as a national hero, public health reformer, founder of Brazilian experimental medicine, and responsible for the Brazilian renewal of science.

Bibliography

Primary: 1917. *Opera Omnia* (Rio de Janeiro).

Secondary: Britto, Nara, 1995. *Oswaldo Cruz: A Construção de um Mito na Ciência Brasileira* (Rio de Janeiro); Benchimol, Jaime Larry, ed., 1990. *Manguinhos do sonho à vida. A ciência na belle époque* (Rio de Janeiro); *DSB.*

Gilberto Hochman and
Nara Azevedo

CRUZ-COKE LASSABE, EDUARDO (b. Valparaíso, Chile, 22 April 1899: d. Santiago, Chile, 18 March 1974), *social medicine, endocrinology.*

Cruz-Coke was a prominent medical researcher on metabolism, a promoter of scientific research as the basis of medical education, a pioneer of Chilean national health policies based on nutrition studies, and a supporter of social medicine. Born to a French mother, Cruz-Coke was a member of a family with solid European culture. He studied at the University of Chile Medical School (1915–21) and shortly after became professor of physiological chemistry at the same university. He also practiced medicine privately, an activity that soon put him in contact with the elite of Santiago, the capital of the country.

He traveled to Europe in 1926 to study and work in German, French, and English laboratories under reputed medical scientists such as the French Luis Lapicque. Upon his return to Chile (1927) he became a professor at the Medical School during a period of social and political turmoil and participated actively in an effort to renew the scientific activities at the University of Chile. During the period 1930–40 he played a key role in the formation of a generation of physicians and researchers that made a lasting contribution to the development of biomedical sciences in the second half of the twentieth century.

Cruz-Coke made his own original research mark in this context by examining metabolism, nutrition, and endocrinological processes. His physical-chemical approach to these processes was meant to transcend the limited clinical knowledge that prevailed among Chilean medical doctors in the first decades of the twentieth century. However, without doubt, his most important contribution to medicine was his studies on nutrition, which became the basis for social policies in his home country oriented to the protection of mothers and children. Cruz-Coke designed and applied national surveys on nutrition to examine the chemical quality of food intake. He concluded that the excess of products rich in wheat and the lack of milk constituted the principal factors in people's malnutrition. Cruz-Coke also created a journal on medicine and nutrition (*Revista Chilena de Medicina y Alimentación*) and a national council on nutrition and health. These activities were carried out during the 1930s, especially when Cruz-Coke was Secretary of Health and Social Assistance (1937–38). This was a ministerial position in charge of the national public health activities as well as medical establishments in the country. From this position he designed crucial legislation on nutrition and preventive medicine.

Cruz-Coke is also widely recognized in his country for his promotion of a type of medicine that emphasized the prevention of diseases: social medicine. He adapted the meaning of a term originated in Europe to emphasize prevention, social security legislation for the working classes, defense of Chilean family health, and state intervention and implied that clinical medicine was of limited use in solving the health problems of his country. He supported social medicine and public health also as a Senator and member of the Conservative Party (1941–57).

Bibliography

Primary: 1942. *La corteza suprarenal; química, fisiopatología, clínica.* (Santiago); 1946. *Medicina Preventiva y Medicina Dirigida* (Santiago).

Secondary: Huneeus, Carlos, and María Paz Lanas, 2002. 'Ciencia política e historia. Eduardo Cruz Coke y el Estado e Bienestar en Chile, 1937–1938.' *Historia* 35: 151–186; Cruz-Coke M., Ricardo, 2001. 'Historia de la obra científica de Eduardo Cruz-Coke Lassabe.' *Revista Médica de Chile* 129: 447–455.

Soledad Zárate

CULLEN, WILLIAM (b. Hamilton, Lanarkshire, Scotland, 15 April 1710; d. Edinburgh, Scotland, 5 February 1790), *medicine, medical education.*

Cullen was the second son of William Cullen, an attorney and agent for the duke of Hamilton, and his wife Elizabeth. The elder Cullen's legal expertise and a small estate in nearby Bothwell ensured that the family would be ranked among the professional classes. But with seven sons and daughters, the Cullens, like many other Scottish professional families, looked toward education as the path for advancement for their male offspring. William's education was entirely typical for a Scots 'lad of parts'. He began his studies at a local grammar school, and at the age of sixteen he went to the University of Glasgow for the Arts course, which included mathematics. He was briefly apprenticed to John Paisley, a surgeon in Glasgow, and then followed the path of many an ambitious Scotsman going to London in 1729. He obtained a post as ship's surgeon, probably through the patronage of the captain, a relative, and spent a year on the West Indies circuit, including six months in Portobello (now in Costa Rica). In the 1720s the position of ship's surgeon was barely respectable: it was poorly paid, and the surgeon, though nominally an officer, had little authority. But for many eighteenth-century medical men,

the position was a necessary rite of passage. Cullen never undertook another voyage, but his lifelong interests in medical geography and in teaching practical forms of diagnosis and treatment may well have arisen out of his experience.

After returning to Britain, Cullen spent a few months working in an apothecary's shop in London. The death of his father and elder brother made him the head of the family, and he moved back to Shotts, near Hamilton, Scotland, to set up general practice and provide for his younger siblings. A small legacy allowed him to pursue his own education. He first went to Northumberland, in northern England, to study literature and philosophy, and then spent the winter sessions 1734–35 and 1735–36 studying medicine at Edinburgh.

In 1734 the Edinburgh medical school was still very new, having only been formally instituted in 1726, though medical teaching had existed in the city before then. Still, Cullen turned the opportunity to his advantage, demonstrating abilities and aspirations that would set him apart from the typical country practitioner. Together with like-minded students, such as Francis Home (1719–1813), later professor of materia medica, he founded what became the Royal Medical Society, a medical self-improvement club promoting essay writing and public debate. It became a magnet for ambitious students and a model for many subsequent student societies. Membership was considered a badge of honor for the elite of the medical school.

Cullen returned to practice in Hamilton in 1736. He acquired the Duke of Hamilton as both a patient and patron; the patronage of other prominent families soon followed. In 1740 Cullen acquired his MD from the University of Glasgow in order to practice as a physician. In 1740 he married Anna Johnstone, the daughter of a minister, and the couple had seven sons and four daughters. Mrs Cullen was widely admired for her charm and intelligence, and throughout her life she was hostess to her husband's wide circle of colleagues, friends, and students.

But Cullen was not content to remain a county physician. Moreover he, like his father, had to support a large family and at a higher social rank. He had hoped that the Duke would build him a laboratory and botanical garden, but the latter died unexpectedly. Deprived of his best patron, Cullen moved to Glasgow in 1744 in order to try medical teaching. The University of Glasgow was much older than the University of Edinburgh and had the legal privilege of granting medical degrees. However, it had very few medical lectures. For several years, Cullen was almost a one-man medical curriculum. He began with lectures on the theory and practice of medicine (1746), added materia medica and botany (1747), and by 1748 offered courses on chemistry.

By mid-century, chemistry was established across Europe as both a branch of experimental philosophy, revealing basic truths about the structure and function of

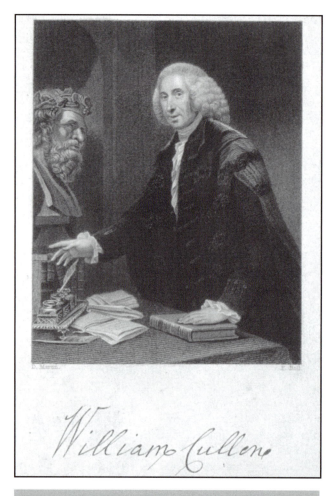

William Cullen. Stipple engraving by F. Holl after D. Martin. Iconographic Collection, Wellcome Library, London.

the natural world, and a subject from which private individuals as well as public institutions could derive economic benefits. Chemistry chairs were founded in all the major universities, and it became incorporated into the many academies of science in cities throughout Europe and the new world. Cullen was the contemporary of Frenchman Pierre Joseph Macquer (1718–84) and Prussia's Andras Sigismund Marggraf (1709–82), and like them he sought to strip chemistry of any vestiges of alchemical language and concepts. The accepted method of teaching was lecture and demonstration because professors were required to provide their own supplies and it would not have been practicable for Cullen to equip an entire laboratory out of his own pocket. But Cullen, throughout his teaching career, was on the lookout for particularly promising students and invited one of these, Joseph Black (1728–99), to be his assistant. He 'treated me with the same confidence and friendship and direction in my studies, as if I had been one of his children', Black later recalled (cited in Doig et al., p. 17). The two became close friends and frequent collaborators. Cullen's lectures became the basis of Black's subsequent work on

carbon dioxide and latent heat, and they influenced research by Torbern Bergman (1735–84) and Antoine Lavoisier (1743–94) on pneumatic chemistry and elective attraction.

In 1751 Cullen was appointed to the professorship of medicine at Glasgow. His chemical interests, particularly as they related to improving agriculture, gained him influential friends, among them the prolific author and indefatigable improver, Henry Home (Lord Kames, 1696–1782), and also the most influential man in Scotland, Archibald Campbell, the third Duke of Argyll (1682–1761). As a result of their patronage, in 1755 the Edinburgh Town Council offered Cullen the position of joint professor of chemistry when the incumbent, Christopher Plummer, was incapacitated—over the objections of Plummer and other members of the medical faculty. His former student, Black, took over his position as professor of chemistry at Glasgow. When Plummer died the following year, Cullen became the professor of chemistry and medicine at Edinburgh.

Welcomed or not, Cullen quickly became one of the leading lights of Edinburgh medicine. He had many distinguished colleagues, such as Alexander Monro secundus (1733–1817), John Gregory (1724–73) and his son James Gregory (1753–1821), Joseph Black, Andrew Duncan senior (1744–1828), and Daniel Rutherford (1749–1819). Yet Cullen's name stands out among the many student letters and diaries from the second half of the eighteenth century. 'The inimitable Dr Cullen', his students called him, 'the Scotch Hippocrates', 'that shining oracle of physic', and 'the great the unrivalled Dr. Cullen' (cited in Rosner, 1991, p. 51). The reason is that Cullen, even more than the other members of the faculty, devoted his energy to the organization and smooth functioning of the medical school. We can trace his reforming, modernizing spirit in administrative details of matriculation and graduation records, in his yearly revisions of his courses adapted for students at a variety of levels, in his benevolent, if strict oversight of graduation theses, and in his voluminous correspondence with former students as they left to set up practice or teaching on their own. The result was that the catchment area for Edinburgh University medical school expanded to include Scotland and northern England, the American colonies, and students from Continental medical schools. British Dissenters, barred from Oxford and Cambridge, gravitated naturally toward Edinburgh, whereas Church of England medical students matriculated at one of the prestigious English universities but attended medical courses at Edinburgh.

As the most junior member of the Edinburgh medical faculty for his first few years, Cullen would have been responsible for keeping track of student fees, and it may have been at his suggestion that the medical faculty began keeping matriculation records from 1762. It is likely that he played an important role in the 1767 statute, the first in Britain requiring 'a course of study in all the branches of

Medical teaching in this or some other University' for graduation (cited in Rosner, 1991, p. 63). In 1777 the University amended the statute to specify three years of study, attendance at a wide range of courses, a thesis, and an examination. Versions of the Edinburgh regulations were adopted by Glasgow University and Trinity College, Dublin, as well as the new medical schools in Philadelphia and New York. No national or regional regulations specified graduation as a prerequisite for medical practice until the 1850s, but an MD based on extensive course attendance and examination became the hallmark of an elite practitioner from the 1760s. Cullen's own views on the value of strict standards for medical examination were expressed in a graduation address: 'It is essential that the title of Doctor of medicine ensures that its owner is both learned and skilful. . . . In Edinburgh University the best regulations are faithfully observed to that end' (cited in Doig et al., p. 94).

Cullen brought his discerning eye and experience in materia medica to the revision of the *Edinburgh Pharmacopoeia*, which he worked on for thirty years with other Edinburgh colleagues. He applied the same modernizing views he had applied to chemistry teaching, removing obvious anachronisms such as vipers, toads, and powdered skulls, and recommending simpler, more palatable remedies: 'He used existing remedies—tartar emetic, James's powders, hyoscyamus (black henbane), cicuta (hemlock)—with care, noting their physiological effects' (*Oxford DNB*). The *Pharmocopoeia* of 1783 was a model of Enlightenment materia medica, and like other aspects of Edinburgh medicine, was readily copied throughout Britain and America.

One of the most important aspects of the Edinburgh medical school was its clinical lectures. John Rutherford, professor of the practice of medicine, carried out clinical teaching at the Royal Infirmary of Edinburgh from 1729. Rutherford based his lectures on those of his own teacher, Herman Boerhaave (1668–1738) at Leiden, retaining much of Boerhaave's Hippocratic language. By 1757 Cullen began giving clinical lectures as well, but though he retained the classic form of the case history he once again stripped it of what he thought of as unnecessary reliance on traditional language as well as theory. 'I allow we derive much knowledge from the Ancients', he told his students, 'but they have many deficiencies from their Ignorance of Anatomy, Chemistry, and natural knowledge. They therefore cannot give us much instruction. The confusion also that prevails in their writings is such that I cannot set them up as Models in our studies' (cited in Rosner, 1991, p. 37). Rutherford as well as other professors complained, and Cullen agreed to moderate his views, always speaking respectfully of Boerhaave as 'a philosopher, a physician, and the author of a system more perfect than any thing that had gone before, and as perfect as the state of science in this time would permit of' (cited in Doig et al, p. 31). But students approved of Cullen's modern approach and straightforward style, and as more and more enrolled in clinical lectures, additional

faculty members agreed to teach the course. By the 1760s clinical lectures were taught in rotation by two professors per year, each taking a three-month course. These clinical lectures, like other aspects of the Edinburgh curriculum, became a model for new medical school foundations in Britain and abroad.

Cullen hoped to be appointed to the chair of practice of medicine when Rutherford resigned in 1766, but Rutherford made it clear that John Gregory was his preferred successor. Cullen was appointed professor of the theory of medicine on the death of the incumbent later that year, and his old friend Joseph Black took over his appointment as chemistry professor. Though from an academic family, Gregory was an outsider in Edinburgh, and Cullen's students petitioned the Town Council for his appointment. The two men compromised by alternating the teaching of theory and practice of medicine until Gregory's death in 1773, when Cullen was appointed sole professor of the practice of medicine.

A number of students took Cullen's practice of medicine course more than once, and to these Cullen offered private, less formal discussion classes. 'What I greatly admire is the manner in which Cullen gives these lectures', noted Samuel Bard (1742–1821), who later founded the Medical College in New York: 'we convene at his own house once or twice a week, where after lecturing for one hour, we spend another in an easy conversation upon the subject of the last evenings lecture, & every one is encouraged to make his remarks or objections with the greatest freedom and ease' (cited in Rosner, 1991, p. 58).

Cullen arranged his lectures on medical practice according to the principles of his nosology, the organization of diseases into classes, orders, genera, and species according to their symptoms, which he published as *Synopsis nosologiae methodicae* (1769). It went through four Latin editions during his lifetime, and editions were published in English, French, and German. Learned opinion varied as to whether the classification reflected real differences in the cause of disease or was simply a convenient way of organizing and teaching pathology. In this as in other areas of teaching, Cullen took a pragmatic approach. He considered his nosology to be a 'history of diseases', which he compared with divisions in natural history. The four classes were *pyrexia* (fevers), *neuroses* (diseases of the nervous system), *cachexia* (wasting diseases), and *locales* (local diseases). Diseases in each class had a set of features in common; they were further grouped into nineteen orders and 132 genera. Each disease was considered a distinct species, with characteristics that set it apart from all other diseases. The distinctive feature of the pyrexia was the inflammation of the whole body, and this group included smallpox, pneumonia, and scarlet fever. The distinctive feature of neurosis was injury of the sense and motion, without fever or local inflammation. In Cullen's usage, it included not only what we would now call psychiatric disorders, such as insanity or depression, but also coma, apoplexy, and diabetes. The distinctive feature of the third class, the cachexia, was the wasting-away of either the whole body, or of individual limbs. And the distinctive feature of the fourth, locales, was that it was 'an affection of some part, but not of the whole body' (*Synopsis*, 1792, p. 95).

What distinguished Cullen's nosology from those of his contemporaries Carl Linnaeus (1707–78) and Boissier de Sauvages (1710–95) was not its theoretical framework but its impact on generations of students. In studying pathology, whether in lecture courses or during Cullen's clinical rounds at the Royal Infirmary, students learned to associate each disease entity with a class, order, genus, and species, much as botanists and zoologists do with their subjects. Associating a set of symptoms as they appeared in the patient with a species of disease required observation, judgment, and attention to differential diagnosis.

Like his contemporaries Friedrich Hoffmann (1660–1742) and Albrecht von Haller (1707–77), Cullen believed the nervous system played a fundamental role in health and disease, stating that 'in a certain view, almost the whole of the diseases of the human body might be called NERVOUS' (cited in *Oxford DNB*). So closely associated was Cullen with this view that many of his students, such as Benjamin Rush (1745–1813), felt he had given the definitive explanation of nervous disorders. Scholars have noted connections between Cullen's ideas on medical theory and those of his close friends and leading lights of the Scottish Enlightenment, Adam Smith (1723–90) and William Robertson (1723–93), on political economy. Smith's 'invisible hand' regulating political economy has resonances with Cullen's view that the nervous system was the great integrative system of the body. Though Cullen did not believe the animal economy, as he termed it, to be entirely self-regulating, he did make cautious use of the concept of the 'healing power of nature', or *vix mediatrix naturae*, which 'has continued in the schools of medicine from the most ancient times to the present' (*First Lines*, 1793, p. xxi). And Robertson gave to his essentially economic theory of the development of European civilization a physiological twist, suggesting that the more advanced the economic system, the more impressions assaulted the nervous system of its constituents, leading to a population both more sensitive and more cultured but also less hardy, more vulnerable to nervous disorders. Lay authors as well as physicians picked up the latter concept. It became the basis for the late eighteenth-century ideas of sensibility, the starting point for nineteenth-century physicians, such as George M. Beard (1839–83), interested in the physical basis of nervous disorders.

Cullen did not recommend that students take detailed notes on his lectures: as he told them, 'With respect to taking notes there can be nothing more useful and proper', 'but as the attention is abstracted by them, therefore make them short, otherwise you will lose more than you gain'. In other words, notes were aids to active engagement with the

material, not substitutes for a textbook. 'Those taken in shorthand', Cullen added, 'are often grossly erroneous and are always imperfect' (cited in Rosner, 1994, p. 75). He had other reasons for objecting to this practice, for in Edinburgh students made a practice of buying professors' lectures. Cullen's lectures on material medica were pirated and published, without his permission, in 1772. Only when he was unsuccessful in preventing their sale did he agree to their correction and reissue. It may have been this experience that led him to issue *Institutes of Medicine* (1772) and, over the next twelve years, *First Lines of the Practice of Physic* (1777–84). Characteristically, he made a virtue of student's insistence on a text in his advice on how to study: 'I suppose you are divided into two classes', Cullen noted in the introductory lecture to his course, 'those who come here for the first time, and those who have learned some system. The business of those in the first class, is to form a system and learn one system only, the attending to a variety of opinions must be perplexing'. For that reason Cullen did not recommend a whole series of books. Instead, he told his beginning students, 'in your situation you are at the mercy of the professor, and must take the system which he explains. The [textbooks] which I have published are far from being perfect, but they are the best I can offer, and they are now received over the whole of Europe'. That was straightforward enough, but Cullen went on to explain 'the most proper method of using this book'. 'I would advise you', he said, 'to read over carefully as much as you expect that I will consider at my next lecture. If you do not understand every part, those that are difficult will engage your attention during the Lecture. . . . [then] As the particulars of an hour's lecture are with difficulty remembered, read over the text after, and endeavour to recollect what hath been heard' (cited in Rosner, 1994, p. 75). The student would thus have been actively engaged with the material three times in succession.

First Lines became a classic as soon as it was issued, with many translations into Latin, French, German, and Italian, and Spanish European and American editions. Like his nosology, it accompanied medical men around the globe, and many a shipboard surgeon, country practitioner, or newly minted MD, when confronted with an unfamiliar disease, reached first for his copy of Cullen's text. *First Lines* 'display Cullen at his clinical best, alert to the complexities of disease, concerned to do his best for his patients, and aware of the strengths and weaknesses of what he had to offer' (*Oxford DNB*).

These qualities enabled him to establish an extensive private practice as the most prominent physician in Scotland. He also carried on a voluminous consulting practice via post, extending throughout Great Britain and beyond, to Europe and America. His letters indicate how seriously he took the task of eliciting information from his patients and adapting his suggestions for treatment to each individual case. Though of necessity he had to be more restricted in his prescriptions for the charity patients in the Royal Infirmary, he still made it a point to study their cases and adapt, where practicable, their points of view: 'Do not imagine that we may use more freedom in this house [the Royal Infirmary] than in private practice', he told his students, 'for physicians who prescribe medications that run counter to their patients' convictions 'do so at their peril'. In such a case, he noted, 'I would rather let a Disease kill a patient than kill him by my medicine' (1772–73, 'Clinical Lectures').

Cullen watched over the required medical theses at Edinburgh with a more-than-paternal eye, giving advice on topics, reading through drafts, and occasionally admonishing the more tardy students. He also continued his involvement with the Royal Medical Society. His nosology formed the starting point for the many medical theses and Royal Medical Society essays, which dealt with clinical subjects, and no thesis on apoplexy, acute rheumatism (rheumatic fever), or diabetes was complete without a definition taken from either Cullen's *First Lines* or his *Nosologia*.

By the 1770s Cullen's ideas on medicine came under attack from his former protégé, John Brown (1735–88). Brown had been a tutor to Cullen's family, and Cullen seems to have treated him as he did other promising students. But Brown felt that Cullen should have supported him for a professorial chair; when this support was not forthcoming, he developed his own medical system in explicit opposition to Cullen's. He acquired a student following, and the ensuing conflict dominated the Royal Medical Society in the 1780s. Students followed Brown's lead in attacking nosological systems, calling them the 'pride of classification', as well as Cullen's observations on fevers, referring to these as 'useless theories . . . chargeable with falsehood and absurdity' (cited in Rosner, 1991, pp. 133, 131). Cullen's supporters among the medical students rose to his defense. There is no sign that Cullen himself was greatly perturbed by this. He was, by this point, an established professor, whose Europe-wide reputation was assured.

Cullen, like some of his improving friends, lost more money than he gained by adopting scientific principles to management of his own estate. He kept teaching until November 1789, when he resigned his chair in medical practice in favor of James Gregory.

Cullen exemplified Enlightenment medical principles, and he contributed to the rise and prominence of one of the premier medical centers. The combination ensured his fame during his lifetime. Many of the ideas he taught, on the nervous system as an integrating structure, on the body as a self-regulating mechanism, and on the systematic classification of disease, survived into modern medical practice only in altered form. But his attention to how to teach medicine—on the creative interplay between lectures, notes, and text, on importance of differential diagnosis, on the therapeutic consequences of treating even charity patients as individuals, and on the need to imbue students with medicine as both science and art—remain an integral part of medical education.

Bibliography

Primary: 1827. (Thomson, J., ed.) *The Works of William Cullen* 2 vols. (Edinburgh); Thomson, John, W. Thomson, and D. Cragie, 1859. *An account of the life, lectures, and writings of William Cullen* (Edinburgh) [1997. Reprinted with an introduction by Michael Barfoot (Bristol)]; 1772–73. 'Clinical Lectures' in *Royal College of Physicians Library* (Edinburgh); 1773. *Lectures on the Materia Medica* (New York) [reprint 1993]; 1792. *First Lines of the Practice of Physic* (Philadelphia).

Secondary: Rosner, Lisa, 1994. 'Student Culture at the Turn of the Nineteenth Century: Edinburgh and Philadelphia.' *Caduceus* 10(2): 65–86; Doig, A., J. P. S. Ferguson, I. A. Milne, and R. Passmore, 1993. *William Cullen and the Eighteenth Century Medical World* (Edinburgh); Rosner, Lisa, 1991. *Medical Education in the Age of Improvement* (Edinburgh); Donovan, Arthur, 1975. *Philosophical Chemistry in the Scottish Enlightenment: The Doctrines and Discoveries of William Cullen and Joseph Black* (Edinburgh); Rush, Benjamin 1790. *An eulogium in honor of the late Dr. William Cullen, Professor of the practice of physic in the University of Edinburgh* (Philadelphia); *DSB*; *Oxford DNB*.

Lisa Rosner

CULPEPER, NICHOLAS (b. probably at Ockley, Surrey, England, 18 October 1616; d. Spitalfields, London, England, 10 January 1654), *medical astrology, popular medicine, herbalism.*

Culpeper was the son of Nicholas Culpeper, rector of Ockley, and his wife, Mary Attershole. The family was an eminent one, owning country estates. His father was buried nineteen days before the young Nicholas was born. After the birth Culpeper returned with his mother to her father's home. William Attershole, Culpeper's grandfather, was rector of St Margaret's at Isfield, Sussex.

Culpeper went up to Cambridge in 1632 intended for the ministry. In 1634 the woman with whom he planned to elope was struck dead by lightening. Culpeper, apparently on this account, left Cambridge. He began work with a Mr White, apothecary, near Temple Bar, London. After a year, the business having failed, Culpeper became an apprentice apothecary to Francis Drake of Threadneedle Street. When Drake died in 1639, Culpeper went into business with Drake's former partner, Samuel Leadbetter. In 1640 he married Alice Field (b.1625). On Alice's modest fortune (Culpeper having been effectively disinherited for not entering the ministry) they had a house built in Red Lion Street, Spitalfields. They had seven children, but only the fourth, Mary, survived her father. Culpeper lived there until his death.

Culpeper had a keen interest in physic, astrology, and hermetic philosophy. As well as making up prescriptions, he was diagnosing and prescribing, practicing medicine from his house. Culpepper, however, had no license from the RCP. The details of his life during the first years of the Civil War (1639–44) are unclear, but on 17 December 1642 he was apparently tried for witchcraft and acquitted. In 1643 Leadbetter was warned twice by the Society of Apothecaries about employing an unlicensed assistant. In this year Culpeper, a fervent republican, fought on the side of parliament and was seriously wounded in the chest by a musket ball. He saw the death of Charles I as presaging the millennium and denounced organized religion and Oliver Cromwell. He committed himself to serving the sick poor.

Culpeper dedicated himself to writing and translating books for the poor so that medicine might be in their hands rather than that of monopolies—apothecaries and physicians. Culpeper first translated the *Pharmacopoeia* of the College of Physicians as *A Physicall Directory* in 1649. Besides the translation, he added instructions for use and directions for preparation of medicines. Not surprisingly, Culpeper was attacked by College and Royalist interests. In later editions he explicitly criticized the College and added astrological material. Culpeper also produced a text for midwives and translations of learned works of anatomy and physic, including Francis Glisson's (1597–1677) *Treatise of the Rickets* (1651). As well as his medical texts, Culpeper also published overtly political works. His major work, *The English Physician* (1652) was a comprehensive guide to common illnesses and their treatment. Its philosophy was hermetic and astrological rather than the Galenic one favored by orthodoxy. Over one hundred editions appeared. A reprint of it was the first medical book published in the American colonies (1708). Works under Culpepper's name continued to pour from the presses after his death. *Mr Culpeper's Treatise of Aurum Potabile* (1656) was the source of much controversy. The aurum potabile was a universal secret remedy prepared by Culpeper. In 1655 Alice Culpeper (who remarried to an astrologer), was selling it from the Culpeper home. Culpeper, as in his own day, still remains beyond the pale of orthodoxy. He is remembered today by the later editions of his herbal.

Bibliography

Primary: 1649. *A Physicall Directory, or, A Translation of the London Dispensatory Made by the Colledge of Physicians in London* (London); 1651. *A Directory for Midwives or, a Guide for Women, in Their Conception, Bearing, and Suckling their Children* (London); 1652. *The English Physician or an Astrologo-Physical Discourse of the Vulgar Herbs of this Nation Being a Compleat Method of Physick, whereby a Man May Preserve his Body in Health* (London).

Secondary: Tobyn, G., 1997. *Culpeper's Medicine: A Practice of Western Holistic Medicine* (Shaftsbury); Thulesius, O., 1992. *Nicholas Culpeper: English Physician and Astrologer* (New York); Poynter, F. N. L., 1962. 'Nicholas Culpeper and His Books.' *Journal of the History of Medicine and Allied Sciences* 17: 152–167; *Oxford DNB*.

Christopher Lawrence

CUMPSTON, JOHN HOWARD LIDGETT

CUMPSTON, JOHN HOWARD LIDGETT (b. Melbourne, Victoria, Australia, 19 June 1880; d. Canberra, Australian Capital Territory, Australia, 9 October 1954), *public health.*

Family Background and Education

Born into a strongly Methodist family, with a mother who conducted one of the first kindergartens in Australia and a father who was a lay preacher as well as a successful commercial traveler, Cumpston was educated at New College and Wesley College, Melbourne. At the age of twenty-two, he graduated from the University of Melbourne in medicine.

As a resident at Melbourne Hospital, he saw wards full of typhoid cases and, impressed by the triumphs of the new bacteriology, he became committed to preventive medicine, a commitment reinforced by seeing, soon after, the reduction in smallpox and cholera in the Philippines achieved by American public health doctors such as Victor Heiser, later Director for the Far East of the Rockefeller Foundation's International Health Board.

As was common at this time for Australians bent on a career in public health, Cumpston traveled to England for postgraduate training and was awarded the London diploma of public health in 1906. In 1907 he received the MD of Melbourne University for work on diphtheria and scarlet fever carried out at the Lister Institute, London. While in Europe, he attended international conferences on infant health and on hygiene, talked to Albert Calmette about tuberculosis, and on the way home to Australia, spent time in India studying plague, leprosy, and smallpox. He wrote to his future wife, Gladys Maeva Walpole, daughter of a Tasmanian general practitioner, that having decided against a career in the Indian Medical Service or general practice, he would pursue one in Australia in preventive medicine, 'the medicine of the future'.

He married Gladys in Fremantle in 1908 and they had seven children, all of whom went on to successful careers in science, medicine, diplomacy, health, or academia. Howard Cumpston has been described as a 'strict disciplinarian . . . [who expected] those around him . . . to aspire, labour and achieve'. A former subordinate, public health doctor-bureaucrat Sir Raphael Cilento observed that 'Cumpston was a remarkable organizer who fell short of personal greatness by a streak of . . . meanspiritedness amounting to ruthlessness whenever he met resistance'.

Career and Achievements

Cumpston began his long career in public health as medical officer to the Western Australia Central Board of Health in 1907, transferring to the Federal Quarantine Service in 1910. He went back to Melbourne in 1913 as Acting Director of the Service and was soon made Director. For the first two decades of nationhood, control of quarantine was an area of conflict between the State and Federal governments. Cumpston's assertion of Commonwealth control during an outbreak of mild smallpox in Sydney in 1913

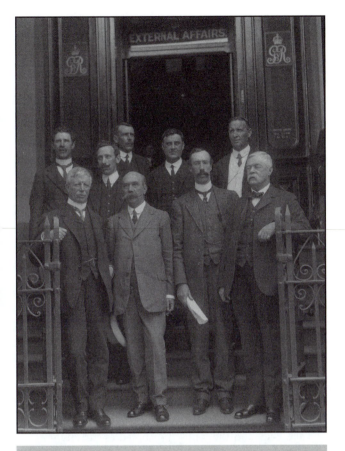

Cumpston (back row, second left) at the conference of Federal and State Medical Officers to consider the lifting of quarantine restrictions at Sydney. Photographed outside Parliament House, Melbourne, c. 1913. Medical History Museum, University of Melbourne.

much provoked the NSW Premier, W. A. Holman, but Cumpston weathered the political storm with the firm backing of his Minister, E. L. Groom.

Cumpston's *The History of Smallpox in Australia, 1788–1908* (1914) was the first of a series of histories of infectious diseases he published over the next decade and a half. This corpus of scholarly work on historical epidemiology culminated in the production in 1927–28 of his magnum opus, *Health and Disease in Australia: A History*. It was not published at the time probably because of the financial stringencies resulting from the Depression of the early 1930s; so serious were these cutbacks that Cumpston had to fight hard to stop abolition of the Federal Health Department itself. There was a practical as well as an intellectual purpose behind his historical investigations. He held that historical knowledge of infectious diseases was central to better understanding of epidemics and thus more efficient management of future crises.

Public health development in Australia in 1850–1950 may be divided into four phases. The first saw the colonial governments building public health administrations of the classic English type and encouraging often reluctant local

authorities to carry out their sanitary duties. The second covers the era from Federation in 1901 to World War I, when public health began to concern itself with the health of individuals in particular groups identified as especially significant for national development: mothers, children, and industrial workers.

The third spans the interwar years, when Cumpston, having persuaded the Commonwealth government on the narrow platform of its constitutional power over quarantine to establish a Federal Health Department, used his considerable political and intellectual skills to promote public health nationally through cooperation with the States, ever jealous of their constitutional prerogatives.

The fourth covers the 1940s, when the concept of a national health service was extensively discussed in the context of widespread acceptance that greater collective responsibility for health care was necessary. Cumpston and colleagues produced in 1941 an innovative plan for a service that was publicly financed, offered universal access, and organizationally integrated the traditionally separate areas of preventive and curative medicine. Cumpston retired as founding Commonwealth Director General of Health in 1945 before the political conflict over the shape of the national health service was resolved. Later he distanced his 1941 plan from the 'socialist' aims of the Federal Labor governments of the day, but there is no doubt centralized state control was a large part of the plan.

In 1919 Cumpston had pressed the Commonwealth to assume sole control of public health. The States would not transfer powers. A Federal Health Department was finally secured in 1921 after the Rockefeller Foundation offered to fund training of Australians to fill the leading posts. The Department would persuade and educate the States but not directly execute policy except in the Federal Territories.

As in other countries where Europeans worked in the tropics, since the late nineteenth century there had been concern about disease barriers to white settlement of the tropical north. This issue (and concern about possible importation of infections from Asia and the Pacific Islands) had preoccupied the Department until the late 1920s, when research had shown whites could safely work in the north. Thereafter the focus shifted to health in the temperate south where the bulk of the population lived.

Lobbying by Cumpston and his allies saw the establishment of the first national inquiry into health status and services, the Commonwealth Royal Commission on Health in 1925. It endorsed two Cumpston proposals: a Federal Health Council and a national public health scheme. The Commonwealth-run, public health scheme failed to materialize, but the idea did reappear as part of the 1941 plan for a national health service. The Health Council, operative from 1927, was hobbled by State fears of loss of power. However, the proposal for a national school of public health to train medical officers of health was taken up, and the school opened at Sydney University in 1930.

The 1925 inquiry called for a health research council. The National Health and Medical Research Council (NHMRC), established in 1936, was an organizational compromise between the medical profession's wish to see medical research funded through an independent body and that of Cumpston to relate research closely to the improvement of public health practice.

From 1943 the Federal labor government turned to postwar planning. The Treasury began to influence health planning, and the objective shifted from 'socialization' to payment of cash benefits to be used to purchase medical services from private practitioners. This also meant the end of the ambitions of Cumpston and allies to integrate preventive and curative services in a centrally run system, as expressed in the 1941 plan.

When the High Court held pharmaceutical benefits provision was unconstitutional, the Commonwealth obtained by referendum power to provide medical and dental services (and social benefits), but not so as to authorize civil conscription of doctors. This proviso remains an insuperable barrier to nationalization of medicine in the British mode. Under Labor's national health service legislation, 1948-9, the great bulk of the population was to continue to purchase fee-for-service medicine and be part-reimbursed through government benefits. After the Liberal-Country Party Coalition came to power in 1949, it introduced its own form of national health service. This involved subsidization of those citizens willing (and able) to take out private insurance.

Conclusion

Two great themes run through the career of J. H. L. Cumpston, the doyen of Australian public health professionals in the twentieth century: the struggle for power between Commonwealth and States, and the balance of power between private and public medicine. At the outset of his career, public health began to offer services to individuals, notably infants and children. But then and subsequently, the organized medical profession ensured curative services were not provided through public facilities. At the end of his career, he was centrally involved in the battle over the nature of the national health service. Here the two themes interacted dramatically. The constitutional limits on Commonwealth power frustrated efforts to shift the balance toward public medicine. Then, as time passed, the wartime push for 'nationalization' lost momentum, and the Coalition government, highly valuing individual responsibility, delivered a national health service acceptable to a profession wedded to fee-for-service, private practice. To realize his life-long vision of a robustly healthy Australia, Cumpston was always ready to do what he could to advance Commonwealth influence and he also sought to shift the emphasis from privately organized, curative medicine to public health and preventive medicine.

Bibliography

Primary: 1914. *The History of Smallpox in Australia, 1788–1908* (Melbourne); 1926. (with F. McCallum) *The History of Plague in Australia, 1900–1925* (Melbourne); 1927. (with F. McCallum) *The History of Intestinal Infections (and Typhus Fever) in Australia, 1788–1923* (Melbourne); 1927. *The History of Diphtheria, Scarlet Fever, Measles and Whooping Cough in Australia, 1788–1925* (Melbourne).

Secondary: Lewis, M. J., 2003. *The People's Health. Public Health in Australia, 1788–1950* (Westport CT and London); Cumpston, J. H. L., 1989. (ed. Lewis, M. J.) *Health and Disease in Australia: A History* (Canberra); Spencer, M., 1987. *John Howard Lidgett Cumpston 1880–1954. A Biography* (Tenterfield, NSW).

Milton James Lewis

CUSHING, HARVEY WILLIAMS (b. Cleveland, Ohio, USA, 8 April 1869; d. New Haven, Connecticut, USA, 7 October 1939), *surgery, neurosurgery, endocrinology.*

Cushing was the tenth child born to Henry Kirke Cushing, MD, and Betsey Maria Williams Cushing. Both parents were descended from Puritan families that had migrated westward from New England in search of opportunity. In 1835 his grandfather Erastus Cushing established a medical practice in the village of Cleveland, situated on the shores of Lake Erie, and the family prospered as the city grew to become an American metropolis.

Harvey enjoyed an unremarkable, happy boyhood. In 1887 he graduated near the top of his class from Cleveland's Central High School and was admitted to Yale College in New Haven, Connecticut, which had historic ties to Cleveland. He received a good liberal education at Yale and was a regular on Yale's very good baseball team. Influenced by family tradition and an older brother, Edward Cushing, Harvey never seriously considered anything but a medical vocation. After graduating from Yale in 1891 he followed his brother's path through the Harvard Medical School in Boston and in 1895–96 took a surgical internship at the Massachusetts General Hospital.

Noted for his manual dexterity—he had considerable artistic ability—Cushing naturally gravitated into surgery, whose possibilities had recently been revolutionized by the effective anesthesia and asepsis. After his internship he applied to train in the new residency system that was being developed at Johns Hopkins Hospital in Baltimore and began working there under William S. Halsted in 1896. He soon became Halsted's chief resident, and by 1900 had emerged as one of America's most promising surgeons, already doing pioneering work on disorders of the nervous system.

Cushing was deeply influenced by Halsted's doctrine of surgical respect for tissue, which involved rigid asepsis, elaborate hemostasis, exceptionally careful wound closing, and, to achieve these goals, disregard for surgeons'

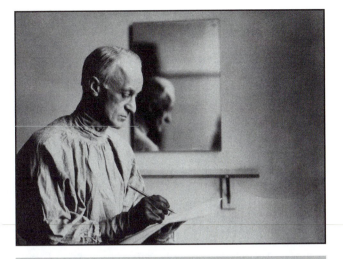

Harvey Williams Cushing in the operating room. Photograph, Iconographic Collection, Wellcome Library, London.

traditional obsession with haste. Unhappy experiences with ether anesthetic led Cushing to experiment with cocaine as a local anesthetic, and he developed an expertise in nerve-blocking that led him through general surgery into attempts to relieve facial nerve pain, culminating in his 1900 publication of a new surgical procedure for reaching and severing the gasserion ganglion in cases of trigeminal neuralgia or 'tic doloreux'. An intensely hard and dedicated worker from medical school days, Cushing drew inspiration and professional companionship from Johns Hopkins' chief physician, William Osler, who recognized the young man's potential and advanced his career at a time when Halsted was distracted and deeply troubled by morphine dependency.

In 1900–01 Cushing went to Europe for a traditional graduate *Wanderjahr*. His diary indicates that he was disappointed with the quality of surgery in Great Britain and on the continent, finding little to learn from Old World surgeons and being particularly appalled by operators' callous treatment of their patients. On July 4, 1900—the symbolism is striking—the young American watched Victor Horsley of London, a noted pioneer in intracranial surgery, crush bone with crude forceps to enter patients' skulls. Unimpressed, Cushing abandoned plans to do further work with Horsley.

Instead he did productive research in Bern, Switzerland, under the surgical guidance of Theodor Kocher and with physiological help from Hugo Kronecker. Assigned to study the effects of intracranial pressure, Cushing built windows in the craniums of experimental animals, became fascinated by the central nervous system, and, with apparently coincidental encouragement from Halsted, decided to make neurological surgery a specialty. He spent a few weeks working on cerebral localization with C. S. Sherrington in Liverpool and also brought back to America an early blood-pressure cuff, developed by Scipi-

one Riva-Rocci, that he had observed in clinical use in Italy.

Cushing returned to Baltimore in 1901, where he entered private practice and was appointed a surgical 'Associate' at Johns Hopkins, with responsibility for surgery of the nervous system. In 1902 he married Kate Crowell, a high-school sweetheart from Cleveland; living next door to the hospitable Oslers, they began raising a family. Private practice was not important to Cushing. His family's properties in Cleveland made him independently wealthy, freeing him to develop the techniques that were to make him the founder of effective neurosurgery.

By 1908 Cushing had become the first surgeon in history who could open what he referred to as the 'closed box' of the skull of living patients with reasonable certainty that his operations would do more good than harm. He brought to the previously crude and bloody field of craniotomies and craniectomies Halsted's obsession with hemostasis and caution, his own dexterity and obsessive attention to detail in every aspect of the surgical experience, and a particularly sophisticated understanding of problems of intracranial and vascular tension. By 1905 he had developed a procedure for subtemporal decompression that largely vitiated the problems of herniation and fungus cerebri in brain surgery, gave palliative relief to victims of tumor, and facilitated further exploratory procedures aimed at locating tumors. Operating before antibiotics, Cushing almost never lost patients to secondary infection.

Lacking effective imaging devices, brain tumor localization was extremely difficult, leading Cushing into extensive study of signs and symptoms, particularly optical disorders. By 1908 he was beginning to be able to locate and remove benign subdural tumors in human patients, including a spectacular excision carried out while talking to a fully conscious subject. With student help at Hopkins's Hunterian Laboratory of Experimental Medicine, whose creation he had fostered, he was developing techniques to approach the hitherto-mysterious pituitary gland, situated deep in the brain. In 1910 Cushing removed a 200-gram meningeal tumor from the head of Leonard Wood, ranking general of the United States Army and a noted military/political leader. He was also beginning surgical and clinical treatment of pituitary conditions and making pioneering contributions to the understanding of the gland's physiology, as outlined in his 1912 monograph, *The Pituitary Body and Its Disorders*. Cushing was the first to glimpse the pituitary's role in secreting hormones that influenced growth.

It can be said that by 1910 Harvey Cushing had, virtually single-handedly, created neurosurgery as a special field, with a population of one. His operative results so far exceeded all others, including Horsley's, so as to be noncomparable. Europeans were now coming to America to observe Cushing and such other surgical stars such as William and Charles Mayo in Minnesota, George Crile in Cleveland, and Alexis Carrel at the Rockefeller Institute in

New York. With the surgical world at his feet, Cushing decided that year to accept the senior chair in surgery at Harvard and the surgical headship at Boston's new Peter Bent Brigham Hospital. He relocated to Boston in 1912.

Cushing continued his pituitary and ophthalmological studies in Boston. His transphenoidal route to the pituitary was for many years the standard surgical approach. In 1917 he published the first detailed study of acoustical tumors, *Tumors of the Nervus Acusticus*. But World War I seriously disrupted his career. In 1915 he interrupted his work to lead a Harvard surgical unit that spent several months treating wounded soldiers at an American-sponsored hospital in a Paris suburb. When the United States formally entered the war, in May 1917, Cushing's previous experience in France had led to a degree of preparedness that resulted in his expanded Brigham/Harvard unit, U.S. Army Medical Corps Base Hospital No. 5, being one of the first American contingents to cross the Atlantic and begin serving in France.

Seconded to work with British medical units, Cushing experienced several months of intense battlefield surgery at a casualty clearing station during the terrible battle of Passchendaele, August–October 1917. Specializing in head cases, and under pressure to speed up, he developed techniques of wound debridement that were recognized as state-of-the-art by both the British and American medical corps. Coincidentally, Cushing was one of a team of American surgeons that was unable to save the life of Sir William Osler's son, Revere, killed that August by enemy shrapnel while serving in a British artillery unit.

Cushing served in France until war's end as military surgeon, consultant, administrator, and gadfly to both the British and American medical corps. In 1936 excerpts from his very detailed war diaries were published to favorable reviews under the title *From a Surgeon's Journal, 1915–1918*. After a bout of influenza in the summer of 1918, Cushing began suffering from a form of polyneuritis, probably Guillain-Barré syndrome; it may have been superimposed on a form of Buerger's disease in his legs, accentuated by many years of cigarette smoking. At war's end Cushing was not sure that he would be able to recover his health or his career.

When he could not find support for an ambitious plan to create a U.S. national neurological institute in Washington or New York, Cushing returned to Boston and gradually rebuilt his team at the Brigham. During the 1920s Cushing operated on several hundred patients a year, almost exclusively tumor cases, with continually impressive results—except for General Leonard Wood, who died following a second operation in 1927. By 1930 Cushing had driven his case mortality rate below 10 percent in an era when most other neurosurgeons still reported mortality in the range of 30–45 percent—although all statistics were crude and unreliable. Some of his former students also began attempting more sophisticated, pioneering studies of the quality of life of his patients. On 15 April 1931, Cushing

operated on his 2,000th case of verified brain tumor. Seriously troubled by recurrent vascular problems in his legs, he retired from active surgery, in accordance with hospital rules, aged sixty-three in 1932.

During the 1920s Cushing collaborated with numerous assistants and visitors on several ongoing research projects. Histological work on tumors with Percival Bailey led to a series of articles and monographs that established the basic classification of brain tumors in use today. Cushing's interest in an electric scalpel developed by W. T. Bovie resulted in the first applications of electricity to neurosurgery in 1926. Cushing's team continued their study of pituitary conditions, attempted vainly to isolate growth and other pituitary hormones, and often operated on dwarfs, acromegalics, and others suffering from pituitary tumors.

In a spectacular last triumph before retirement, Cushing in 1932 brilliantly synthesized clinical observation and theorizing in his paper 'The Basophil Adrenomas of the Pituitary Body and Their Clinical Manifestations (Pituitary Basophilism)', in which he outlined what would quickly become known as Cushing's syndrome (the consequences of hypersecretion from the adrenal cortex) and Cushing's disease (when the syndrome is caused by a basophilic pituitary adenoma). He daringly based his hypothesis on only three clear cases of pituitary basophilism and then led a successful search for vindication with other examples.

Although Cushing became a legend during his surgical lifetime—men came from around the world in the 1920s to work with or observe the brilliant American—some younger neurosurgeons began to see him as an establishment figure, cautious and conservative to a fault. One of his former students, Walter Dandy, who succeeded him as Johns Hopkins's most prominent neurosurgeon (Cushing had declined to return to Hopkins as Halsted's successor), developed ventriculography as the first imaging technique useful in locating brain tumors and was much more aggressive than Cushing in attacking acoustic and other deep-seated tumors. The Cushing-Dandy relationship was often tense, complicated, and personal, as a surgical father figure tried to temper the enthusiasms of a brilliant but rough-hewn surgical offspring.

Virtually everyone who studied or worked with Cushing found him a hard-driving, sometimes mean-spirited, credit-seeking, and ultra-competitive taskmaster. Dandy excepted, Cushing's students and associates, such as Kenneth McKenzie, Hugh Cairns, Norman Dott, and Geoffrey Jefferson, eventually came to respect and cherish the man who taught them how to work and survive on the treacherous alpine slopes of neurosurgery. Companionable and charming when he chose to be, and very interested in the development of the specialty, in 1920 Cushing was a moving spirit in the creation of the exclusive Society of Neurological Surgeons. In 1932 a group of his former students founded the slightly more accessible Harvey Cushing Society, which in 1965 changed its name to the

American Association of Neurological Surgeons. At the end of the twentieth century it was still a mark of distinction among neurosurgeons to have worked with anyone who had worked with Harvey Cushing.

Cushing was often torn between the urge to devote himself single-mindedly to neurosurgery and his catholic interests in general surgery, medicine, and medical literature. When he came back from Europe in 1901 he became an ardent advocate of blood pressure monitoring in all forms of surgery. In 1903 he was one of the founders of the Society of Clinical Surgery. He served terms as president of the Society for the Study of Internal Secretions (now The Endocrine Society) in 1920–21, the American College of Surgeons in 1922–23, the American Surgical Association in 1926–27, and other medical and surgical societies. In 1934–35 he sat on a medical advisory committee charged with reporting on health insurance to President Franklin D. Roosevelt's Committee on Economic Security. Cushing, a proud champion of traditional medical values and practitioner independence, resisted any insurance scheme not acceptable to American physicians. The committee fizzled. Cushing's involvement in the issue also reflected his easy access to the White House because of the marriage of his daughter Betsey to James Roosevelt.

In 1920 Sir William Osler's widow asked Cushing to write the official biography of her husband. Writing early in the morning before going into the operating room, and then late in the night after surgery, Cushing in 1925 published with Oxford University Press the two-volume, 1,400-page *Life of Sir William Osler*. It was immediately hailed as a classic of medical biography and in the United States won the 1926 Pulitzer Prize for biography. Many of Cushing's other biographical, inspirational, and reflective essays were anthologized in *Consecratio Medici and Other Papers* (1929) and *The Medical Career and Other Papers* (1940). He championed old-fashioned medical values, idolized the humble country practitioner, and endorsed Stephen Paget's confession of medical faith: 'If a doctor's life may not be a divine vocation, then no life is a vocation, and nothing is divine'.

Cushing never felt totally comfortable in Boston, clashing fairly often with colleagues and administrators at Harvard and its various teaching hospitals. He was too prickly to be a medical school team player, and he was not entirely in sympathy with new-fangled emphases on science, research, and preventive medicine in the training of physicians. In 1933 he passed up repeated offers of a chair in medical history at Johns Hopkins and instead became Sterling Professor of Neurology at Yale, the edenic college of his youth.

Continuing circulatory problems precluded a hoped-for return to active surgery at Yale. In 1937 Cushing retired again to become Yale's titular Director of Studies in Medical History. From early in his career he was showered with numerous honorary degrees and other recognitions, culminating in Fellowship in the Royal Society. In 1938 Cushing published with his assistant, Louise Eisenhardt, a 741-page study, *Meningiomas: Their Classification, Regional Behaviour, Life History, and Surgical End Results*. The highly technical monograph could also be read as a professional autobiography. Cushing died in his seventy-first year following a severe heart attack in October 1939.

Cushing's surgical perfectionism included the keeping of elaborate patient records, with photographs, as well as the preservation of tumor specimens. He hoped that his collection, the Cushing Tumor Registry, which he had moved to Yale from Boston, would become a center for the pathological and histological study of tumors. Louise Eisenhardt became custodian of the registry at Yale after his death. It fell into disuse in the 1950s, but at the end of the century was rediscovered and reappreciated as a rare treasure-trove of medical Americana.

Cushing was also a lifelong bibliophile and sophisticated collector of medical and surgical books, specializing in the works of Vesalius and other anatomists. Impressed by Osler's donation of his library to McGill University, Cushing willed his books and papers to Yale, where, along with the libraries of Arnold C. Klebs and John F. Fulton, they formed the basis of what has become the Historical Library of the Harvey Cushing/John Hay Whitney Medical Library.

Harvey Cushing was a conservative man, very conscious of family tradition and his family's and his own role in American medical history. His hopes that one of his sons would follow in the family's medical footsteps were dashed when his eldest child, William, a junior at Yale, was killed in an automobile accident in 1926, and his second son, Henry, dropped out of Yale for a career in business. As a neo-Puritanical, Victorian father, Cushing did not encourage his talented daughters to attend university. The 'fabulous Cushing sisters'—Betsey, Mary, and Barbara—collectively garnered much publicity as tasteful members of New York high society in the 1940s and 1950s. Kate Crowell Cushing, who had found it difficult to live with a compulsive workaholic who was really married to medicine and surgery, had been by the standards of the time a model medical wife and mother. Her stewardship of the Cushing household was part of the foundation of her husband's success.

Cushing's personal conservatism, very much in the tradition of his physician father and grandfather, and perhaps of their Puritan forebears, was, ironically, in large part responsible for the radical breakthroughs he achieved as a surgeon. To do intracranial surgery in Cushing's day required a temperament attuned to care, attention to detail, deliberation, small achievements, and great patience, all combined with a willingness to break from convention and journey into unknown surgical territory. Cushing identified with explorers and the pioneers of America's westward migration, once calling work on the brain the equivalent of surgery's Northwest Passage. Remarkably talented and utterly dedicated—like Osler he looked on doctors as a secular priesthood—he was the first to negotiate that hazardous passage.

Cushing's personal achievement was also neatly representative of the rise of North American medicine and medical research. Its social bases rested on the American prosperity that made the Cushing family independently wealthy and that underlay the merchant Johns Hopkins's magnificent endowment of a hospital and university mandated to achieve international excellence. Its educational roots lay in the residency system that Halsted and Osler established at Hopkins, in their explicit relocation of Old World training standards to the New. The high standards of medical care and service that American patients expected from their physicians and the modern world's determination to create medical progress through advanced research also contributed to American progress. Thus Theodor Kocher of Bern, Switzerland, sent his son to observe Harvey Cushing in Baltimore, Maryland, in 1907, writing 'the United States are the place where we have to go and learn more than we are able to show to the many men coming over to see us. Our turn now to admire others.'

Bibliography

Primary: 1912. *The Pituitary Body and Its Disorders* (Philadelphia and London); 1925. *The Life of Sir William Osler* (Oxford and New York); 1926. *Studies in Intracranial Physiology and Surgery* (Oxford); 1928. *Consecratio Medici and Other Papers* (Boston); 1935. *From a Surgeon's Journal, 1915–1918* (Boston); 1938. (with Eisenhardt, Louise) *Meningiomas: Their Classification, Regional Behaviour, Life History, and Surgical End Results* (Springfield, IL); 1940. *The Medical Career and Other Papers* (Boston).

Secondary: Bliss, Michael, 2005. *Harvey Cushing: A Life in Surgery* (Toronto and New York); Greenblatt, Samuel H., ed., 1997. *A History of Neurosurgery, in Its Scientific and Professional Contexts* (Washington, DC); Matson, Donald D., et al., eds., 1969. *Harvey Cushing: Selected Papers on Neurosurgery* (London and New Haven); Thomson, Elizabeth H., 1950. *Harvey Cushing: Surgeon, Author, Artist* (New York); Fulton, John, 1946. *Harvey Cushing: A Biography* (Springfield, IL); *DSB; DAMB.*

Michael Bliss

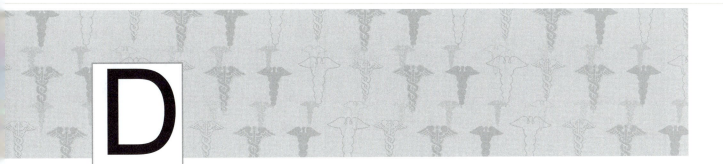

D

DA COSTA, JACOB MENDEZ (b. St Thomas, West Indies, 7 February 1833; d. Villanova, Pennsylvania, USA, 11 September 1900), *cardiology, medical education.*

Da Costa's parents were Jonathan Mendes Da Costa (described in contemporary accounts as a 'gentleman of leisure' descended from planters and bankers) and Rama Levy. The family left the Caribbean when Da Costa was four; he attended gymnasium in Dresden. In 1849 he moved to Philadelphia and enrolled at Jefferson Medical College. There he served as demonstrator for professor of surgery Thomas Dent Mütter, displaying Mütter's pathological specimens to other students twice weekly. After completing his MD in 1852, he returned to Europe for eighteen months, visiting the great clinics of Paris, Prague, and Vienna.

Back in Philadelphia in 1853, Da Costa began practice at a poorhouse dispensary. He was soon engaged to teach physical diagnosis at an independent auxiliary summer medical school that enrolled students from the South and West as well as Philadelphia. Within a year he was established as a general internist with particular interest in diseases of the heart and the lungs. At this point he began publishing on yellow fever and typhoid, and translating and editing works from other languages. He published the first of several editions of *Medical Diagnosis* (regarded by some as the best treatise in the field until the end of the century) in 1864.

Da Costa married Sarah Frederica Brinton in 1860. They had two children, one of whom died in infancy; the other became a notable lawyer in Philadelphia. As an 'Acting Assistant Surgeon' during the Civil War, Da Costa worked part-time at a military hospital in Philadelphia. His observational skills in this position led him to the clinical work for which he remains best known, on the 'irritable heart'.

Da Costa's career followed a common nineteenth-century Philadelphia pattern. After establishing himself as a private teacher, he was appointed lecturer in clinical medicine at his alma mater and, in 1872, professor of the theory and practice of medicine—a position he retained until he retired from Jefferson in 1891. His first hospital appointment was at Episcopal Hospital; later he joined the staffs of the more prestigious Pennsylvania Hospital and Philadelphia General Hospital. He was also a consulting physician at the Children's Hospital of Philadelphia.

Da Costa was regarded as one of Philadelphia's leading medical teachers and consultants and was known to have had particularly great influence on residents who served under him at the Pennsylvania Hospital. A Fellow of the College of Physicians of Philadelphia beginning in 1858 (and twice its president), he wanted the College to exert more influence over health matters in Philadelphia. He chaired the College's committee on the threatened cholera epidemic in 1892, and he advocated filtration of the city's water supply. He was an early participant in the tuberculosis movement.

Da Costa was a gentleman consulting physician known for his diagnostic skill and powers of observation. His work in clinical cardiology and his ability as a clinical teacher were major contributions to the medicine of his day.

Bibliography

Primary: 1864. *Medical Diagnosis, with Special Reference to Practical Medicine: A Guide to the Knowledge and Discrimination of Diseases* (Philadelphia); 1867. 'Observations on Diseases of the Heart Noticed Among Soldiers, Particularly the Organic Diseases' in *Sanitary Memoirs of the War of the Rebellion* vol. 1 (New York) pp. 360–382; 1871. *On Irritable Heart: A Clinical Study of a Form of Cardiac Disorder and Its Consequences* (Philadelphia).

Secondary: Woolsey, Charles F., 2003. 'William Osler and Jacob Mendez Da Costa: Philadelphia Medicine, 1884–1889.' *Journal of Medical Biography* 11: 65–73; Woolsey, Charles F., 2002. *The Irritable Heart of Soldiers and the Origins of Anglo-American Cardiology: The U.S. Civil War (1861) to World War I (1918)* (Aldershot); Wilson, J. C., 1902. 'Memoir of J. M. Da Costa.' *Transactions of the College of Physicians of Philadelphia* 24: lxxxi–xcii; *DAMB*.

Edward T. Morman

DA MONTE, GIOVANNI BATTISTA   (aka MONTANUS or MONTANO) (b. Verona, Italy, 1489; d. Terrazzo, near Verona, 6 May 1551), *medicine, medical education.*

Da Monte was the eldest son of Conte, a professional soldier and nobleman whose family originated from Monte San Savino (Arezzo), hence the family name. A man of lively intelligence, Da Monte was drawn not only to medicine, but also to philosophy, literature, botany, chemistry, and archeology. In Padua he was the pupil of Marco Musuro, who tutored him in Latin and Greek, and Pietro Pomponazzi, who taught him philosophy. From Padua he went to Ferrara, where he became friendly with Giovanni Manardi and where he graduated in philosophy and medicine under the guidance of Nicolò Leoniceno (1428–1524). After practicing as a physician at Brescia for several years, he set out on his travels, which took him to Rome and Naples—where he met Pontano and Sannazzaro—and then to Palermo. Subsequently he stayed at Venice, at Verona, and finally at Padua, where on 7 December 1539 he was offered the first chair of ordinary practical medicine *in paritate loci* with Francesco Frigimelica. On 9 October 1543 he was given the first chair of ordinary theoretical medicine, a post which he held with great success until his death.

Very few of the works that bear his name were actually written by him and published in his lifetime: only the Latin translation of ten of the sixteen books of medicine by Aëtius of Amida, that is, the first seven and last three (1543); *Tabulae in tres libros artis parvae Galeni* (1538); and *Metaphrasis summaria* (1550). The other works are collections of his lectures and consultations put together by his pupils, who sometimes altered the texts and therefore rendered them somewhat unreliable. Da Monte himself, when he promised to publish his commentaries on Avicenna (Ibn Sīnā), complained about the boldness and impudence of some of his pupils.

In 1808 the Italian physician and patriot Giovanni Rasori credited Da Monte with the introduction in *c.* 1543 of clinical teaching at the bedside as an indispensable part of his students' medical studies at the Hospital of San Francesco Grande in Padua, notwithstanding that this was completely unknown to all the historians of the University of Padua. Rasori's claim was accepted by most medical historians without any critical verification. The truth is that the Hospital of San Francesco and the University were two completely independent institutions, and Rasori's assertion was based on his erroneous interpretation of some clinical consultations published by Da Monte's pupils. The first mention of a connection of the Hospital of San Francesco with the activity of the Studio, in an unofficial form, was during the period 1577–78, thanks to Marco degli Oddi, head physician in the San Francesco Hospital, and Albertino Bottoni, who held the first chair of extraordinary practical medicine.

Da Monte, however, must still be considered as one of the leading personalities in medical education at Padua in the sixteenth century. He placed great importance on the method in medicine, as can be seen from his posthumous works *Opuscula varia* (1558) and *Medicina universa* (1587), in which he dealt with the interpretative problems of the three Galenic doctrines (resolutive, compositive, and definitive), with a view more didactic and clinical than theoretical, following the interpretations of Leoniceno (1508).

Bibliography

Primary: 1538. *Tabulae in tres libros artis parvae Galeni* (Padua); 1550. *Metaphrasis summaria eorum quae ad medicamentorum doctrinam* (Padua); 1558. *Opuscula varia et praeclara, in quibus tota fere Medicina methodice explicatur* 2 vols. (Basel); 1587. *Medicina universa* (Frankfurt).

Secondary: Ongaro, Giuseppe, 1994. 'L'insegnamento clinico di Giovan Battista Da Monte (1489–1551): una revisione critica.' *Physis* 31: 357–369; Muccillo, Maria, 1986. 'Da Monte, Giovanni Battista' in *Dizionario biografico degli Italiani*, XXXII (Rome) pp. 365–367; Cervetto, Giuseppe, 1839. *Di Giambatista Da Monte e della medicina italiana nel secolo XVI* (Verona); *DSB*.

Giuseppe Ongaro

DALE, HENRY HALLETT   (b. London, England, 9 June 1875; d. Cambridge, England, 23 July 1968), *physiology, pharmacology.*

Born to a father who was the manager of a manufacturing firm, Dale was one of seven children. He won a scholarship to Trinity College, Cambridge, graduating with first class honors in 1898 and remaining there for another two years to work in John N. Langley's (1852–1925) department of physiology. A further scholarship took him to St Bartholomew's Hospital, where he qualified in 1903. Thereafter he resumed his physiology studies at University College, London, also spending a few months at Paul Ehrlich's laboratory in Frankfurt-am-Main, Germany. At the end of the following year, he accepted a post as pharmacologist at the Wellcome Research Laboratories, becoming its director eighteen months later.

At Sir Henry Wellcome's suggestion Dale started his rewarding studies on ergot. First, in 1906, he showed that ergotoxine reversed the hypertensive effect of adrenaline. Second, in 1910, together with George Barger (1878–1939) he isolated histamine from ergot, proceeding to compare its actions with the features of anaphylactic shock and later showing that during the latter the antibodies become fixed to the cell surface. Third, in 1914, he isolated acetylcholine, finding that it had a muscarinic effect on smooth muscle, gland cells, and the heart, and a nicotinic effect on autonomic ganglion cells and the adrenal medulla. These were not his only research interests; in 1908, for example, he had found that an extract of the posterior pituitary caused the uterus to contract (resulting in the isolation of oxytocin in 1928, which was then developed for therapeutic use). Nevertheless, his findings on ergot were to be part of a continuum. Thus Dale's discovery of acetylcholine continued his interest in the autonomic nervous system fostered in Langley's department, while it also persisted into further research showing that acetylcholine was released at certain nerve endings (including those in the muscles—thereby delineating the first neurotransmitter to be identified). In 1936, together with Otto Loewi (1873–1961), Dale received the Nobel Prize for this work, and he was to coin the terms *cholinergic* and *adrenergic*. He had also continued his work on histamine, showing that it, as well as acetylcholine, was normally present in animal tissues.

The last developments had been carried out within the Medical Research Council (initially Committee), where Dale had moved in 1914, first as pharmacologist and, from 1928, as the director of the National Institute of Medical Research, where he remained until 1942. In 1938 he became chairman of the Wellcome Trust, and in 1940 president of the Royal Society. He was knighted in 1932 and received the Order of Merit in 1944. Well before this, however, he had become an important figure both internationally and nationally. Soon after the end of World War I, he had lobbied for standards to be established for hormones, vitamins, and drugs—pressing the League of Nations to undertake this task and providing the first standard for insulin himself.

After World War II, in which he had served as chairman of an advisory scientific committee to the cabinet, Dale was prominent in arguing for the nonpolitical application of science, and in particular the peaceful use of atomic energy.

And the Wellcome Trust, where he had played such an important part, was to evolve into a continuing prominent source of funding for medical research. His career illustrates how, given a broad approach, a distinguished researcher can have an equally critical role in setting the direction of and implementing research policy.

Bibliography

Primary: 1953. *Adventures in Physiology* (London).

Secondary: Tansey, E. M., 1995. 'What's in a Name?: Henry Dale and Adrenaline. 1906.' *Medical History* 39: 459–476; Feldberg, W. S., 1970. 'Henry Hallett Dale, 1875–1968.' *Biographical Memoirs of Fellows of the Royal Society* 16: 77–174; DSB; Oxford DNB.

Stephen Lock

DAMESHEK, WILLIAM   (b. Semliansk near Voronezh, Russia, 22 May 1900; d. New York, New York, USA, 6 October 1969), *hematology*.

Dameshek was the son of Isadore Dameshek, a hatmaker, and Bessie Muskin. To escape anti-Semitism, the family emigrated to the United States in 1903, settling in Medford, Massachusetts. Dameshek attended public schools, spent two years at Harvard College, served a year in the Army, and graduated from Harvard Medical School in 1923. That same year he married Rose Thurman of Worcester, Massachusetts.

During a two-year internship at Boston City Hospital (1923–25), he began an association with Ralph C. Larrabee, who had established a blood laboratory in a corner of the hospital basement. Hematology was an emerging science and the blood laboratory an innovation. Dameshek became fascinated by blood diseases, studied acquired hemolytic anemia, and published his first hematologic paper, 'The Reticulated Red Blood Cells—Their Clinical Significance' (*Boston Medical and Surgical Journal*, 1926).

Following his internship, Dameshek began work at the Boston Dispensary, started a highly successful private practice, and initiated his teaching career by assisting with Larrabee's course on laboratory medicine at Tufts Medical School. In 1928 he was appointed hematologist at the recently founded Beth Israel Hospital, where he established the Hematology Laboratory and did some of his most important experimental work.

In 1939 he moved to the Pratt Diagnostic Hospital (later New England Medical Center), where he was chief of hematology and organized the Blood Research Laboratory. He also re-affiliated with Tufts, first as clinical professor, then as full professor of medicine. Upon retirement in 1966 he joined Mount Sinai Medical School in New York as attending hematologist and professor of medicine emeritus, and remained there until his death.

A major contributor to the transformation of hematology from its early emphasis on morphology to a biomedical discipline incorporating physiology, biochemistry, and nuclear physics, Dameshek is often called the 'father of modern hematology'. He developed bone marrow aspiration for clinical diagnosis of hematological disorders, which led eventually to bone marrow transplantation. His studies revealed the relationship of autoimmune diseases to development of hematological diseases and the pathogenesis of radiation-induced leukemia. Other research interests included hypersplenism, pancytosis, leukosarcoma, and myeloproliferative and immunoproliferative disorders.

Dameshek was a prolific writer, publishing more than 450 journal articles and six books; *Leukemia* (1958) was coauthored with Frederick Gunz and became a standard reference. Recognizing the need for a specialized journal in a field of increasing importance, he was the founder of *Blood* (1946) and served as its editor until his death.

As a clinician he excelled in the management of patients with blood diseases and attracted a large practice that included many foreign patients. As a teacher his lectures were always carefully prepared and clear. However, his most significant teaching occurred on the wards, where he stimulated lively discussion among the students, house staff, and visiting physicians who followed him from bed to bed. Never one to avoid controversy, he advanced theories of disease that often annoyed his colleagues but served as catalysts for thought even among those who disagreed.

Dameshek's energy and creativity were also expressed in professional organizations, including founding roles in the International Society of Hematology (1946) and the American Society of Hematology (1956). A strong advocate of the importance of international scientific understanding, he successfully enabled hematologists from the Communist countries to attend meetings despite the Cold War mentality of the era. Dameshek trained more than 300 hematologists, many of whom became outstanding in the field. His influence through his writing, lectures, and travels contributed to the advancement of hematology throughout the world, especially in Russia, South America, and Israel.

Dameshek died unexpectedly during open-heart surgery to repair a dissecting aneurysm, and was survived by his wife and daughter.

Bibliography

Primary: 1955. *The Hemorrhagic Disorders* (New York); 1958. (with Gunz, Frederick W.) *Leukemia* [3rd edn. 1970] (New York).

Secondary: Gunz, F. W., 1970. 'William Dameshek, 1900–1969.' *Blood* 35: 577–582; Crosby, William H., 1960. 'Dr. William Dameshek: A Biographical Comment.' *Blood* 15: 580–584; 1960. 'Publications of Dr William Dameshek, 1922–47.' *Blood* 15: 585–589; 1960. 'Publications of Dr William Dameshek, 1948–1959.' *Blood* 15: 589–595; ANB; DAMB.

Amalie M. Kass

DANARAJ, THAMBOO JOHN (b. Ipoh, Perak, Malaya [now Malaysia], 1 February 1914; d. Kuala Lumpur, Malaysia,

20 March 1996), *tropical eosinophilia, Danaraj's disease, medical education.*

Education and Training

Born of South Indian heritage in 1914 in Ipoh, Perak, in what was then British Malaya, Danaraj received his early education in English-medium schools before going to the King Edward VII College of Medicine in Singapore in 1905. He graduated in 1938 with a diploma Licentiate in Medicine and Surgery (LMS) and joined the Straits Settlements Medical Service, serving in government general hospitals in Melaka, Singapore, and rural Dungun in Terengganu. He returned to Singapore in mid-1940 and married Winifred Lewis, who had been a fellow student at the College. They both served at the General Hospital at Outram Road.

When the war in the Pacific (1941–45) broke out, Danaraj, then a doctor in Penang, was forced to evacuate with the retreating British forces to Singapore. During this experience, he witnessed the discriminatory practices of the British colonial government toward its Asian subjects. Before the war, only Europeans were appointed as Medical Officers, the title of doctors in the Colonial Medical Service. Asians, no matter how illustrious their academic qualifications and training, could only be Assistant Medical Officers. Frustrated with such overt racial prejudice, Danaraj devoted his life after the war to medical education to ensure that Asians did not suffer discrimination.

After the war, Danaraj returned to serve in the General Hospital in Singapore and later became a member of the teaching staff of the College.

Research Work

Danaraj established his research expertise in the field of tropical eosinophilia, achieving a breakthrough discovery of its etiology—primarily a parasitic that results in the observed symptoms of wheezing and breathlessness. In recognition of this work, he was awarded a Master of Medicine by the University of Malaya at its inaugural convocation in 1950. For his contribution to research on eosinophilic lung disease, he was elected FRCP (Edinburgh) in 1960, the first Malaysian to be so honored.

Danaraj also had interests in the fields of neurology and cardiology. He embarked on investigations relating to primary arteritis of the aorta, commonly referred to as Takayasu's arteritis, which most frequently afflicts young (under forty) females in Asia, although there are recorded incidences of male sufferers and sufferers in other parts of the world. His work on this vascular disease was undertaken together with his second wife, Dr Wong Hee-Ong. Because of his contributions, he became associated with this ailment, which is now called 'Danaraj's disease'.

Medical Education

In 1960 Danaraj was elected Dean of the Faculty of Medicine at the University of Malaya in Singapore. Then, in February 1963, he became Foundation Dean of the Faculty of Medicine, University of Malaya at Kuala Lumpur.

Danaraj's determination to ensure the establishment of a medical school with its own teaching hospital led him to approach the then prime minister of Malaya, Tunku Abdul Rahman Putra Al-Haj (1957–1970), who was also the Chancellor of the University of Malaya. Subsequently funds were made available for the school. The first batch of students that commenced in mid-1963 graduated in June 1969. He remained Dean and professor of medicine until his retirement in 1975. He was also instrumental in establishing a teaching hospital at the King Abdulaziz University, Jeddah, Saudi Arabia. Upon his return home in 1980, he became Emeritus Professor of Medicine at the University of Malaya.

As a teacher, Danaraj emphasized the importance of having a disciplined and systematic approach to recording patient histories, undertaking clinical and physical examinations, attending to laboratory investigations, offering treatment, and handling case presentations. He felt that it was imperative that a doctor gain the confidence, respect, and trust of his patients, and hence that proper grooming, including attire, was as important for a physician as one's deportment.

For his contribution to medicine and medical education, the king of Malaysia bestowed on Danaraj the title Tan Sri, the Malaysian equivalent of a British knighthood. He was elected a Distinguished Honorary Member of the Academy of Medicine of Malaysia in 1987, and was the inaugural recipient of Royal College of Physicians of London–Academy of Medicine of Malaysia Medal in 1989 in recognition of his research and his encouragement of research activities among his students and peers.

At the time of his demise, Danaraj, then aged eighty-two, was Honorary Consultant at the University of Malaya, Kuala Lumpur.

Bibliography

Primary: 1959. (with D'Silva, L. S., and J. F. Schacher) 'The Serological Diagnosis of Eosinophilic Lung and Its Etiological Implications.' *American Journal of Tropical Medicine and Hygiene* 8: 151–159; 1960. (with Khoo, F. Y.) 'The Roentogenographic Appearance of Eosinophilic Lung (Tropical Eosinophilia).' *American Journal of Roentogenology* 83: 251–260; 1963. (with Wong, H. O., and M. A. Thomas) 'Primary Arteritis of Aorta Causing Renal Artery Stenosis and Hypertension.' *British Heart Journal* 25: 153–165; 1988. *Medical Education in Malaysia: Development and Problems* (Petaling Jaya); 1990. *Japanese Invasion of Malaya and Singapore: Memoirs of a Doctor* (Kuala Lumpur).

Ooi Keat Gin

DANDY, WALTER EDWARD (b. Sedalia, Missouri, USA, 6 April 1886; d. Baltimore, Maryland, USA, 19 April 1946), *neurosurgery.*

Dandy was the only child of John Dandy and Rachel Kilpatrick Dandy, who had immigrated to the United States from England in the 1880s and settled in the railway town of Sedalia, Missouri. The hard-working, blue-collar parents encouraged their son to strive to excel in everything he did. He graduated as class valedictorian from Sedalia High School, began medical studies at the University of Missouri, then was admitted into the second-year medical class at Johns Hopkins Medical School in 1907.

While still an undergraduate, Dandy began doing research for Harvey Cushing, who was in process of becoming the father of effective neurosurgery. Upon graduation in 1910 he was first invited to be Cushing's research assistant in Hopkins's Hunterian Laboratory, then in 1911 to be his neurosurgical resident. Dandy both absorbed his master's pioneering techniques and aspired to replace Cushing as America's greatest brain surgeon. Dandy was bitterly disappointed when Cushing decided he was not socially and professionally mature enough to be included in the group. Cushing relocated to Harvard and the Peter Bent Brigham Hospital in 1912. Dandy stayed at Johns Hopkins, finishing his surgical training under W. S. Halsted, and from 1919 onward held various appointments at Johns Hopkins Hospital and Medical School that made him the effective head of neurosurgery.

As a young man Dandy made two major contributions to his field. Research assigned to him by Cushing on the circulation of cerebrospinal fluid led Dandy to develop by 1913 the distinction between 'obstructive' and 'communicating' forms of hydrocephalus, along with a practical diagnostic test. He also discovered, learning partly from abdominal and thoracic surgery, that by replacing cerebrospinal fluid with an equal volume of air in the ventricles of the brain he could create contrasts that made possible effective x-ray studies of ventricular conditions. 'Ventriculography', announced by Dandy in 1918, was a giant first step forward in the development of intracranial imaging. In 1919 Dandy began refining the technique with the development of encephalography, which involved more extensive injection of air into subarachnoid spaces.

Dandy was an ambitious, aggressive operator, who believed that Cushing was too conservative, and in the early 1920s developed techniques for the total removal of encapsulated acoustic tumors, a procedure Cushing had thought too risky. Dandy's tendency to claim huge diagnostic and surgical breakthroughs with his innovations, based on very few cases, plus his obvious disdain for most other neurosurgeons, considerably irked Cushing and other senior figures. Cushing rebuked Dandy publicly and privately for exaggeration and other professional discourtesies, further exacerbating a rivalry that continued until the former's retirement in 1932. Dandy saw himself as a maligned outsider in American neurosurgical circles, despised Cushing, and tended to isolate himself from the evolving profession. Nevertheless he was the leading figure among younger, radical neurosurgeons, who tended to be less cautious than Cushing's generation in their willingness to sacrifice healthy brain tissue, when necessary, in the hope of progressing beyond palliation in difficult cases.

Although he could be irascible in the operating room to the point of instrument-throwing, Dandy was happily married to Sadie Martin and was the devoted father of four children. Like Cushing, he tended towards workaholism and conservative political views. His publications included 159 articles and five books, and his contributions were wide-ranging, including innovations in spinal cord surgery and the surgical handling of Ménière's disease. At the time of his death in 1946 from myocardial infarction, Dandy had succeeded Cushing as America's most prominent neurosurgeon. Debates about the famous rivalry of teacher and student continue to the present, but Dandy's niche in neurosurgical history as the father of ventriculography is undisputed.

Bibliography

Primary: 1914. (with Blackfan, K. D.) 'Internal hydrocephalus, an experimental, clinical and pathological study.' *American Journal of Diseases of Children* 8: 406–482; 1918. 'Ventriculography following the injection of air into the cerebral ventricles.' *Annals of Surgery,* 68: 5–11; 1957. (comp. by Troland, Charles E., and Frank J. Otenasek) *Selected Writings of Walter E. Dandy* (Springfield, IL).

Secondary: Bliss, Michael, 2005. *Harvey Cushing: A Life in Surgery* (Toronto and New York); Fox, William Lloyd, 1984. *Dandy of Johns Hopkins* (Baltimore and London); Fairman, David, 1946. 'Evolution of Neurosurgery through Walter E. Dandy's Work.' *Surgery* 19: 581–604; *DAMB*.

Michael Bliss

D'ARCY, CONSTANCE ELIZABETH   (b. Rylstone, NSW, Australia, 1 June 1879; d. Sydney, Australia, 25 April 1950), *obstetrics, gynecology.*

D'Arcy, daughter of police constable Murty D'Arcy and his wife Bridget (née Synnott), was one of eight siblings, and she shared a house with two of her sisters for most of her adult life. She graduated from the University of Sydney in 1904 (the twelfth woman to do so); she was ranked fourth in her class in her final year after having achieved consistently high marks throughout the five-year course.

Although D'Arcy's university results qualified her for a residency at Sydney's most prestigious general hospitals, neither the Sydney nor the Royal Prince Alfred had yet developed a definite policy on accepting women doctors. Instead, D'Arcy traveled to Adelaide for her first residency. In 1905 she was appointed the first RMO at the Sydney Benevolent Society's Royal Women's Hospital, with which she maintained a professional connection throughout her career. She became an honorary member of staff in 1908, the first woman to gain such a post in Sydney, and established a successful private practice in Macquarie Street.

Catholicism was an important influence in D'Arcy's life and work, and she was a long-standing supporter of the Guild of St Luke's, the Catholic medical association. In 1923 she became the first medical woman appointed to St Vincent's Hospital, where she used radium for the treatment of gynecological cancers. She became a member of the University of Sydney's Cancer Research Committee in 1929.

D'Arcy had joined the local branch of the British Medical Association in 1906 and was active in a range of separatist women's professional bodies: the NSW Medical Women's Association (foundation vice-president 1928–33, president 1933–34), the Australian Federation of Medical Women (whose founding meeting she chaired in 1929), and the Medical Women's International Association. This commitment led her to participate in the movement to found the Rachel Forster Hospital, the women doctors' hospital for women. Opened in 1922, 'The Rachel' later became a crucial path for women's professional advancement. D'Arcy provided the fledgling body with credibility, and with links to the world of private patronage on which most hospitals then depended.

Another organization of great importance for D'Arcy was the University of Sydney. She was a stalwart supporter of the Catholic women's college, Sancta Sophia; a member of the University Senate, 1919–49 (the first woman elected to this body); and a lecturer in clinical obstetrics, 1925–39. In 1943 she became the university's Deputy Chancellor, the first woman to occupy this post.

D'Arcy was one of the earliest women to develop a successful career in Sydney's world of consultant surgery. Many recalled her 'feminine' style, particularly her jewelry and hats, with a mixture of fondness and awe. She was described as 'a large-hearted woman with an opinion of her own which she was always prepared to defend . . . It was sometimes thought that her judgments were harsh, but those who knew her felt that she tried to temper mercy with justice' (*Medical Journal of Australia* 1950, p. 275).

Constance D'Arcy received numerous honors. In 1935 she was admitted MRCOG and became a DBE; in 1940 she was honored by the Pope; in 1941 the 'Rachel' named its new surgical ward in her honor; and on her death the Royal Women's memorialized her in the same way. She was a Foundation Fellow of the RACS. Constance died in the hospice run by the Sisters of Charity across from the hospital where she had helped to establish the legitimacy of women in the profession.

Bibliography

Primary: 1935. 'The Anne McKenzie Oration: The Problem of Maternal Welfare.' *Medical Journal of Australia* 1: 385–399.

Secondary: McCarthy, Louella, 2001. 'An Uncommon Practice: Medical Women in New South Wales, 1885–1939.' PhD thesis, University of New South Wales; Radi, Heather, 1991. 'Constance

D'Arcy' in Radi, H., ed., *200 Australian Women. A Redress Anthology* (Sydney) p. 121; (Anon.), 1950. 'Constance Elizabeth D'Arcy—Obituary.' *Medical Journal of Australia* ii: 274–275.

Louella R. McCarthy

DARWIN, ERASMUS (b. Elston, Nottinghamshire, England, 12 December 1731; d. Breadsall, Derbyshire, England, 18 April 1802), *medicine, natural history, poetry.*

Darwin, the youngest of the seven children of Robert Darwin, a wealthy lawyer, and Elizabeth Hill, was educated at Chesterfield School and Cambridge University (1750–53), reading mathematics and classics but also attending lectures at William Hunter's (1718–83) anatomy school in London. He studied medicine at Edinburgh University (1753–56), took his MB at Cambridge (1755), and practiced briefly in Nottingham before moving to Lichfield (November 1756). Of his three sons by his marriage to Mary Howard (1757), the youngest, Robert Waring, went on to become a physician and father of Charles Darwin.

Erasmus's patients were largely drawn from the rising entrepreneurs of the industrializing midlands (he refused requests to become George III's physician). Busy, successful, and innovative, he had an interest in mind/body medicine, a gift for history-taking, and a penchant for 'heroic' remedies, using steel, opium, and later the pneumatic medicine of Thomas Beddoes (1760–1808). A polymath of prodigious energy, often seen as embodying the spirit of the English Enlightenment, his interests included geology, meteorology, gas chemistry, scientific agriculture, and all mechanical contrivances. His inventions included a carriage steering mechanism (1759), a mechanical voicebox (1771), a 'bi-grapher' copying machine, canal lifts, and a horizontal windmill used by Josiah Wedgwood (1730–95), whose leg he amputated in 1769, to grind pottery pigments. He was elected FRS (1761). As one of the founding members of the Birmingham-based Lunar Society (*c.* 1765), which brought together important industrialists, inventors, and thinkers, including James Watt (1736–1819), Matthew Boulton (1728–1809), Joseph Priestley (1733–1804), and Benjamin Franklin (1706–90), Darwin became involved in iron mills, steam power, and the building of transportation canals.

After his wife's death (1770), he took a mistress, Mary Parker. They had two daughters, Susan and Mary, whom Darwin helped establish a girls' boarding school (1794). His ideas on the education of (middle-class) women included exercise (which he disliked himself) and knowledge of sciences, languages, and arts and manufactures (1797), a curriculum designed to produce fit wives and mothers to men of industry. With Brooke Boothby (1743–1824), he founded the Botanical Society at Lichfield and established a botanical garden (1778); Darwin was largely responsible for translating the works of Carl Linnaeus (1707–78), which were published as *A System of Vegetables* (1783) and *The Families of Plants* (1787). In his anthropomorphic poem *The Loves of*

the Plants (1789), concerned with plant sexuality and reproduction, Darwin proposed that nature worked progressively toward 'greater perfection'. A later epic poem, *The Economy of Vegetation* (1791), celebrated the new industrial achievers. In essence, it claimed that man raised himself by his own energies and the material world contained everything necessary for him to do so. His verse, in heroic couplets, briefly influenced Romantic poets such as S. T. Coleridge (1771–1834) and William Wordsworth (1770–1850). Darwin married Elizabeth Pole (1781), a widow and daughter of the Earl of Portmore, and the family moved to Derby. Their eldest daughter (of six surviving children) became the mother of Francis Galton (1822–1911).

Darwin's largest work, *Zoonomia* (1794, 1796), was an ambitious attempt to unite Albrecht von Haller's (1707–77) physiology of nervous stimulus and response with the utilitarian associationism of John Locke (1632–1704) and David Hartley (1705–57), and to explore the interplay of mind and body in the generation of diseases. He recognized four physiological powers or faculties as being fundamental to life: irritation, sensation, volition, and association. These, working on the organism from conception to death, had the power to produce changes that could, he argued, be transmitted to offspring. The idea that the natural world developed and progressed over time was further explored in his poem *The Temple of Nature* (1803). In common with many of his friends, Darwin was sympathetic to the causes of the French and American Revolutions, decried slavery, and argued for freedom of the press and religious toleration. Contemporaries described him as a large man with strong views, witty and ebullient despite a stammer, and a lover of food but a teetotaler. Darwin fell ill with pneumonia in the spring of 1801, after which he retired from medical practice, and died the following year. His life and work were animated by a faith in reason and progress.

Bibliography

Primary: 1791. *The Botanic Garden: A Poem in Two Parts, Part I Containing the Economy of Vegetation; Part II the Loves of the Plants, with Philosophical Notes* (London); 1794–96. *Zoonomia; or, the Laws of Organic Life* (London); 1797. *A Plan for the Conduct of Female Education in Boarding Schools* (Derby); 1803. *The Temple of Nature or, The Origin of Society: A Poem with Philosophical Notes* (London).

Secondary: Uglow, Jenny, 2003. *The Lunar Men: The Friends Who Made the Future* (London); King-Hele, Desmond, 1999. *Erasmus Darwin: A Life of Unequalled Achievement* (London); Browne, Janet, 1989. 'Botany for Gentlemen: Erasmus Darwin and 'The Loves of the Plants.' *Isis* 80: 593–621; Porter, Roy, 1989. 'Erasmus Darwin: Doctor of Evolution?' in Moore, James R., ed., *History, Humanity and Evolution: Essays for John C. Greene* (Cambridge); McNeil, Maureen, 1987. *Under the Banner of Science: Erasmus Darwin and His Age* (Manchester and Wolfeboro); *DSB*; *Oxford DNB*.

Carole Reeves

DAVAINE, CASIMIR JOSEPH (b. Saint-Amand-les-Eaux, France, 19 March 1812; d. Garches, France, 14 October 1882), *medicine, bacteriology.*

Davaine's mother died when he was nine. He was educated by his father, a wealthy brewer, and later studied medicine in Paris. His family was Catholic, but as an adult he became a freethinker. He had a son with an English woman, Maria Georgina Forbes.

Davaine made a living out of private practice in Paris, with famous patients, among whom were Emperor Napoleon III, Claude Bernard, and the consumptive courtesan Marie Duplessis, who was the model of Verdi's *La Traviata.* He organized his research on his own, with the help of colleagues who showed him their pathological findings. He made numerous observations on parasites of plants and animals and became a founding member of the Société de Biologie in 1848. He had a strong interest in teratology, although he felt that the absence of unambiguous criteria for normality deprived the science of firm foundations. But the work for which he is best known is his contribution, through his studies on anthrax, to the development of the germ theory of disease and the emergence of bacteriology.

The story started when, with his mentor Rayer, Davaine observed tiny motionless rods in the blood of two sheep. One sheep had died of a disease called *sang de rate* because of the purplish color of the blood, and the second had been inoculated with the former's blood. In 1863, influenced by Pasteur's work on the link between living ferments and fermentations, Davaine extended his first, casual observations by means of a whole series of experimental studies. He regularly found the bacteria to be present in anthrax cases, including in the human malignant pustule, and called it *bacteridia.* In 1869 he dismissed the notion of any concomitant virus or poison in the genesis of the disease.

Davaine's work is fairly typical of the French style of research in early bacteriology. While German researchers tried hard to isolate and cultivate the germs on appropriate media, Davaine focused on elucidating the transmission by sequentially inoculating the pathological fluids into various animals. He showed that most experimenters failed to transmit the disease because they confused anthrax with septicemia caused by putrefied blood.

Davaine also experimented, *in vivo* and *in vitro,* on the effects on the bacteridia of various drugs derived from a range of sources, from plant material such as walnut leaves to old chemicals such as mercury and iodine and to new compounds such as carbolic acid.

Davaine wrote an epoch-making article entitled 'Bactérie' for Dechambre's *Dictionary.* In these early days, when the very existence of germs and their role in the production of disease were still highly controversial, he broke fresh ground. He listed thirty bacteria and suggested supplementing morphological characters in classifications with physiological criteria, such as the reproductive mode and relationship with the medium.

Although Davaine never explicitly referred to the methodology, subsequently known as Koch's postulates, he sought to prove that the microbes observed under the microscope were the cause, both necessary and sufficient, of anthrax. His work alerted Louis Pasteur to the importance of using bodily fluids from living animals and of careful sterilization of instruments. Pasteur acknowledged his debt by helping Davaine to receive several awards during his lifetime.

Davaine hoped that the mysteries of anthrax would be unraveled by science, which would lead to eradication of the disease. He died in 1882, one year after the successful trial of anthrax vaccination, at Pouilly-Le-Fort, at the outset of a decade that would see the identification of numerous microbial diseases. His work on anthrax prepared the way for the first vaccine and the beginning of modern methods of immunization.

Bibliography

Primary: 1863. 'Recherches sur les infusoires de sang et de la maladie connue sous le nom de sang de rate.' *Comptes rendus de l'Académie des Sciences* 57: 101–115, 220–223, 351–353; 1868. 'Bactérie, bactéridie' in Dechambre, A., ed., *Dictionnaire encyclopédique des sciences médicales* (Paris) 8: 8–39; 1870. *Études sur la genèse et la propagation du charbon* (Paris).

Secondary: Wrotnowska, Denise, 1975. 'Pasteur et Davaine d'après des documents inédits.' *Histoire des sciences médicales* 9: 213–230; Theodorides, Jean, 1968. *Un grand médecin et biologiste, Casimir-Joseph Davaine (1812–1882)* (Oxford).

Anne Marie Moulin

DE GIOVANNI, ACHILLE (b. Sabbioneta, Italy, 28 September 1838; d. Padua, Italy, 9 December 1916), *medicine, anthropometry.*

De Giovanni never knew his father Mario, a district doctor, but he inherited his passion for religion, which was very strong in De Giovanni's youth. His mother, Rosina Traversi, attended to his education. She discouraged her son's youthful sacerdotal ambitions and persuaded him to study pharmacy at Pavia University. Early on, however, he decided to change his initial choice of study and graduated in medicine in 1862. During and after his studies, he took part in the Independence movement; in 1859 he joined the Cacciatori delle Alpi as a volunteer and in 1866 he followed Garibaldi's expedition to Trentino as an army medical officer. He remained active in Italian politics throughout his lifetime and became a senator in 1902.

After his degree, he moved first to Bologna, then to Milan. However, his scientific and clinical activity was hampered by his poor health. He suffered from tuberculosis, and later his only child died from the same disease while completing his medical education. Tuberculosis thus became a personal challenge for him, and this played a decisive part in the foundation of the first *Lega Nazionale contro la Tubercolosi* (1899).

In 1867 he received his first position at the University of Pavia, and in 1879 he was called to the prestigious chair of clinical medicine at the University of Padua, where he remained until his death. For a few months in 1881 he was in Paris at the Salpêtrière Clinic, led by Jean-Martin Charcot (1825–93), where he became familiar with the anatomic-clinical method. His most important work, *La morfologia del corpo umano* (1891; English edition, 1909), was dedicated to Charcot.

De Giovanni has been portrayed as the father of constitutionalism in Italy. The fundamental ideas in his medicine were the concepts of constitution and predisposition. The main instruments of his clinical activities were anatomical observation and anthropometry. Against the analytic tendency dominating medicine in the second half of the nineteenth century, he focused his attention on the problem of individuality. The empirical evidence that the same disease could develop differently in different individuals led him to consider that individuality was predominant in human pathology. As a clinician, he insisted on the fundamental principle that medicine must treat individuals, not diseases.

In conflict with the newly emerging medical paradigm of microbiology, which insisted upon identifying the external agents considered responsible for infectious diseases, De Giovanni, referring explicitly to the ancient Hippocratic and Galenic doctrine of temperaments and constitutions, upheld the importance of constitutional factors in the causal process of many diseases. He considered that tuberculosis, for example, was due not to Koch's bacillus but to a specific morphological makeup that predisposed an individual to it.

He was convinced of the existence of certain specific morphological 'predispositions' to certain specific diseases. Thus, he distinguished and described three fundamental 'morphological combinations' predisposing an individual to three different groups of diseases. Believing in a strong relationship between form and function, he put forward the hypothesis that morphological imbalances corresponded to physiological dysfunctions. Therefore, he drew on anthropometry as an auxiliary science of fundamental importance for his clinical and scientific activity. His therapeutic approach was based upon the idea that it was possible to change the individual constitution in order to rid the body, when and where possible, of its predisposition to disease. His conception of medicine was hence mostly preventive.

He played a fundamental role in the systematic introduction of anthropometry in the clinical field. Using a series of anthropometric instruments and measurement methods that he himself had invented specifically toward that aim, he elaborated a method to determine individual morphologic value. His ambition was to transform clinical medicine, with the help of numbers and measurements, from an empirical into an exact science.

Bibliography

Primary: 1891. *Morfologia del corpo umano* (Milan); 1909. *Clinical Commentaries Deduced from The Morphology of Human Body* (London).

Secondary: Albrizio, Angelo, 2005. 'La "clinica col metro". L'antropometria di Achille De Giovanni.' *Medicina e Storia* 10: 5–27; Pogliano, Claudio, 1983. 'Filosofia dei medici e medicina filosofica: due 'casi' tra Ottocento e Novecento.' *Giornale critico della filosofia italiana* LXII: 349–359; Viola, Giacinto, 1904. 'L'indirizzo individualistico in medicina e il metodo morfologico del De Giovanni.' *A. De Giovanni. Lavori dell'Istituto. Studi di morfologia clinica* 2: 3–44 (Padua).

Angelo Albrizio

DE GRAFT-JOHNSON, SUSAN (b. British Gold Coast [now Ghana], 1917; d. London, England, 1985), *maternal health, nutrition.*

Ghana's first female medical doctor, de Graft-Johnson (née Ofori-Atta) was instrumental in extending medical services to urban families there. As a member of the emerging medical profession in Ghana at its independence, she participated in the creation of the Ghana Medical Association, Ghana Medical School, and Ghana Planned Parenthood Association. She worked to eliminate childhood malnutrition and optimize perinatal care, thereby strengthening confidence in Western medicine among Ghanaian women and children.

De Graft-Johnson was the daughter of Agnes Akosua Doudu and the renowned indigenous king and statesman, Nana Sir Ofori-Atta I (1881–1943), Omanhene of the Akan state of Akyem Abuakwa in the British Gold Coast. Knighted by Great Britain in 1928, her father excelled in early mission schools and served on the Executive Council of the Gold Coast. De Graft-Johnson was a beneficiary of her family's strong emphasis on education, despite the fact that she was a female child among at least one hundred of her father's offspring. Her early education was at Catholic schools in Elmina attached to the St Mary's Convent. Later she was among the first female students at the Prince of Wales College in the Gold Coast (now Achimota). Excelling in her studies, de Graft-Johnson discovered a love of biology and chemistry. Her mentors at Achimota included Agnes Savage, the British medical officer in charge at Achimota hospital, who encouraged her to train first as a nurse midwife at the nearby Korle Bu Midwifery Training School, and then to extend her studies in medicine in Edinburgh in 1937. After two years, she completed a premedical course and decided to join other Gold Coast students, including R. A. Quarshie, M. A. Barnor, H. S. Bannerman, and E. Evans-Anfom at the University of Edinburgh Medical School. In 1949 she qualified as a physician, becoming one of sub-Saharan Africa's first black female doctors.

After her return to the Gold Coast that year, de Graft-Johnson played a leadership role in the institutionalization of medical services, emerging as what Ghanaian writer Kojo Vieta has termed one of 'The Flagbearers of Ghana' (Vieta, 1999, pp. 279–282). In 1950 she was accepted into the Gold Coast Medical Service, becoming one of eighteen African physicians in a service of eighty-five. She headed Kumasi Hospital in 1951, and subsequently the Princess Marie Louise Children's Hospital. As a founding member of the Ghana Medical Association, de Graft-Johnson was active in the establishment of the country's first medical school and headed the pediatrics department. A strong Catholic, de Graft-Johnson nonetheless decided to participate in Ghana's family planning movement, attending early meetings of the fledgling Ghana Planned Parenthood Association pioneered by her Edinburgh classmate Mathew Barnor during the 1960s. Recognition for her contribution to medicine in Ghana included *The Royal Cross* from the office of Pope John Paul II in 1980, membership in the Ghana Academy of Arts and Sciences, and an honorary Doctor of Science degree from the University of Ghana in 1974.

De Graft-Johnson was active in improving the status of Ghanaian women, in both the political and medical spheres. Her private Accra clinic, established during the 1960s, was known to welcome female patients from all walks of life, and it provided services at very low costs. De Graft-Johnson worked particularly among urban market women wary of institutionalized medicine. At the political level, she was active in the Women's Society for Public Affairs and lobbied for legislation to improve inheritance rights of women and children under pre-existing customary Akan laws. Her siblings included William Ofori-Atta, a member of the 'Big Six' who led Ghana to independence. De Graft-Johnson took a similar interest in politics, working on the committee to draft a new Constitution in 1969.

De Graft-Johnson spent her later years in the United Kingdom. Her marriage to the Ghanaian academic and politician E. V. C. de Graft-Johnson was in part responsible for the family's exile by the 1980s. De Graft-Johnson sustained injuries in a car accident in 1971, which led to debilitating health conditions before her death in 1985.

Bibliography

Primary: 1972. 'Problems of Social Status and Education for Ghanaian Women.' *Proceedings of Ghana Academy of Arts and Sciences*, 9/10: 95–101.

Secondary: Barnor, Mathew Anum, 2001. *A Socio-Medical Adventure in Ghana: Autobiography of Dr. M.A. Barnor* (Accra, Ghana); Vieta, Kojo, 1999. *The Flagbearers of Ghana* (Accra, Ghana); Addae, Steven, 1996. *The Evolution of Modern Medicine in a Developing Country: Ghana 1880–1960* (Durham, NC).

Abena Dove Osseo-Asare

DE LA RIVE, CHARLES-GASPARD (b. Republic of Geneva [now Switzerland], 14 March 1770; d. Republic of Geneva, 18 March 1834), *medicine, psychiatry, natural philosophy.*

De La Rive was born to one of Geneva's leading families, the son of a lawyer, Jean-Ami De La Rive, and Jeanne-Elisabeth Sellon. He first studied at Geneva's College (Collège) and Academy, where he gained a doctorate in law on 25 May 1789. In 1794 he was arrested and then banished by Geneva's Revolutionary Tribunal because of his conservative background. He consequently emigrated first to England and then to Scotland, where he studied medicine. He graduated at Edinburgh as a doctor in medicine three years later, on 24 June 1797, having defended a thesis on animal heat: *Tentamen physiologicum de calore animali.*

De La Rive then visited British asylums and worked as an assistant physician for the London dispensary of Cary-Street for over a year (1798–99). In 1799 he returned to Geneva, where he set up a practice and developed a long-lasting passion for chemistry and physics. Three years later, he was appointed honorary professor of pharmaceutical chemistry (1802–19) to Geneva's Academy. In 1819, when Geneva was free from French rule, De La Rive was appointed honorary professor of chemistry to the restored Academy (1819–34). He refused an ordinary chair in chemistry in 1831.

An important aspect of De La Rive's activities was his role as physician to Geneva's mental asylum, then established in the Discipline, a section of the town's hospital. He took care of the mentally impaired on a voluntary basis from 1802 until his death in 1834. As a physician, he was in favor of removing the patient from his or her environment, although he believed in sending inmates home as soon as possible. De La Rive used gentle methods and suppressed a series of coercive practices, including chairs of restraint, turnstiles (tourniquets), and surprise baths. The presence of noisy inmates in the vicinity of one of Geneva's popular squares was considered inappropriate at a time when medical theorists voiced the importance of isolation, quiet, good air, and farm work for the healing of diseased minds. Where should one house the insane? De La Rive played an important role in commissions of inquiry into the possibility of building a new asylum in the countryside. He believed Geneva too small for an institution devoted to the insane, and he spoke out against the government's project to finance a new building and in favor of moving most incurable inmates to a farm in the countryside, while retaining a handful of those deemed curable in the hospital. His patients finally left the center of town for a farm in the countryside during the 1832 cholera epidemic and remained there until 1838.

Alongside his duties as a physician, De La Rive set up a laboratory where he built a Volta battery, copied from the one belonging to Humphry Davy in England, which he had seen in London in 1818. In 1820 he demonstrated in public the influence of electricity on a magnetic needle by using Hans Christian Oersted's experiment (1819). He was both an admirer and a friend of André-Marie Ampère and reproduced the latter's experiments in his own laboratory. De La Rive contributed a number of articles to the *Bibliothèque britannique* and, later, to the *Bibliothèque universelle*. His research areas included animal heat, nitric acid, batteries, and electricity. He was a member and later president of the Royal Society of Edinburgh, and a founding member of Geneva's Reading Society (Société de lecture), Natural History Museum, and Botanical Gardens.

In 1813 De La Rive was called to be a member of the Conseil Provisoire, which monitored the restoration of the old Republic. He was an active member of the Conseil Représentatif (1814–32) and of the Conseil d'État (1814–18), and was the first syndic of the Republic in 1817 and 1818.

Bibliography

Primary: 1797. *Tentamen physiologicum inaugurale, de calore animali.* Doctoral thesis, University of Edinburgh; 1830. 'Sur la statistique des affections mentales' in *Bibliothèque universelle*.

Secondary: Fussinger, Catherine, and Deodaat Tevaerai, 1998. *Lieux de folie, monuments de raison: architecture et psychiatrie en Suisse romande, 1830–1930* (Lausanne); Benguigui, Isaac, 1990. *Trois physiciens genevois et l'Europe savante, les De la Rive 1800–1920* (Geneva); Reverdin, Frédéric, 1915. 'Notes biographiques.' *Actes de la société helvétique des sciences naturelles* 97: 290–291.

Philip Rieder

DE LANGE, CORNELIA CATHARINA   (b. Alkmaar, the Netherlands, 24 June 1871; d. Amsterdam, the Netherlands, 28 January 1950), *pediatrics, clinical genetics, nutrition.*

De Lange, daughter of a distinguished family in Alkmaar, was the first girl who entered the local high school (HBS) in 1886, taking her exam in 1889. As her father, who was a lawyer and a member of the Dutch parliament, objected to her going to university, she was sent to Switzerland in order to finish her education. However, after returning to Alkmaar she took the university entrance exam in 1891 and enrolled to study chemistry at the University of Amsterdam. From 1892 onward she studied medicine. In 1897 she passed her medical qualifying examination, becoming the fourth woman in the Netherlands to write a medical thesis.

After specializing in pediatrics in the Kinderspital in Zurich (with Oskar Wyss), she started a private practice for children in Amsterdam. From 1907 onward she worked in the Amsterdam children's hospital 'Emma Kinderziekenhuis', where she supervised the new ward for infants, which also served for the nurses' training. Her work in the hospital offered better opportunities for scientific work. The majority of her patients suffered either from poor nutrition and hygiene or from infectious disease. Fevers and dehydration were among the main causes of infant mortality. No remedies existed for patients with congenital anomalies such as heart diseases, metabolic disorders, or anomalies of the central nervous system. During these years her interests

gradually shifted to pathological anatomy, and in cooperation with Bernard Brouwer (1881–1949), a professor in neurology, she specialized in the anatomy of the brain.

After the death of Jacob de Bruin (1861–1927), she was appointed to the chair of pediatrics at the University of Amsterdam, becoming the first female medical professor in the Netherlands. In her inaugural address she mentioned the treatment of encephalitis, hydrocephalus, convulsions and tuberculosis, the problems of nervous children, pathological anatomy, and genetics as the topics for the future. In 1933 and again in 1938, she published on a new syndrome, the 'typus Amstelodamensis', later named the Brachmann–De Lange syndrome, in remembrance of her description of the characteristic features of the patients, such as low birth weight, microcephaly, hirsutism, confluent eyebrows, long eyelashes, and small head and feet.

From 1929 to 1935, she was president of the Dutch Association of Pediatricians, again the first female in this position. She was valued for her experience, knowledge of the literature, and synthetic approach. She was member of the editorial boards of the *Nederlandsch tijdschrift voor geneeskunde*, the *Acta paediatrica scandinavica* and the *Annales paediatrici*. For the lay public, she published popular books on child care.

She resigned as professor in 1938 but continued to work as a pediatrician and during World War II was superintendent of the 'Emma Kinderziekenhuis'. The governing body of the hospital awarded her an honorary membership. In 1947 she received a knighthood from the Dutch government.

De Lange's work as a pediatrician covered half a century, during which pediatrics emerged as a specialism. Her influence on this development was substantial. Because of her position at the university and in the Pediatric Association, she was able to consolidate pediatrics as an academic discipline and to educate a new generation of physicians.

Bibliography

Primary: 1904. (with de Bruin, J.) *De voeding van het kind in het eerste levensjaar* 2 vols. (Amsterdam); 1933. 'Sur un type nouveau de dégénération (typus Amstelodamensis).' *Archives de médecine des enfants* 36: 713–719; 1941. *Ziekteleer van den pasgeborene* (Amsterdam); 1943–1946. *Zieke kinderen. (Twintig) clinische voordrachten voor artsen en studenten* 3 vols. (Amsterdam).

Secondary: De Knecht-van Eekelen, A., and R. C. M. Hennekam, 1994. 'Historical Study: Cornelia C. De Lange (1871–1950)—A Pioneer in Clinical Genetics.' *American Journal of Medical Genetics* 52: 257–266; De Knecht-van Eekelen, A., 1990. *Cornelia Catharina de Lange (1871–1950)* (Nijmegen).

Annemarie de Knecht-van Eekelen

DE SANCTIS, SANTE   (b. Parrano, Terni, Italy, 7 February 1862; d. Rome, Italy, 20 February 1935), *psychiatry, child neuropsychiatry.*

De Sanctis graduated in medicine at the University of Rome (1886) with a dissertation on aphasias in neuropathology.

Afterward he worked as a physician in the Orvieto countryside. Moving to Rome in 1891, he worked at the laboratory of pathological anatomy in the S. Maria della Pietà mental hospital, and was promoted to assistant physician in the psychiatric clinic (1892), where he was involved in research on psychopathology. In the same period, he also collaborated with the institute of physiology, which was directed by Luigi Luciani, in work on the nervous system, and with the institute of anthropology, which was under the guidance of Giuseppe Sergi. De Sanctis followed with interest Wilhelm Wundt's experiments on physiological psychology, applying Wundt's experimental technique in Rome.

De Sanctis taught general psychopathology and practical semiotics from 1893 to 1895. He traveled to Zurich (1893) to study the phenomenon of hypnosis with Auguste Forel, and thence to Paris to improve his psychiatric training at the Salpêtrière. His initial research on dreams and sleep, in which he supported the hypothesis of the clinical and etiological connection between dreams and psychosis, would later be cited by Théodule Ribot and Carl Gustav Jung. In his *Die Traumdeutung* (Vienna, 1900), Sigmund Freud criticized De Sanctis's book *I sogni* [Dreams] (Turin, 1899). Nevertheless, after 1900, Freud and De Sanctis corresponded and they met in 1906.

De Sanctis was also founder of the Roman Association for the Medical-Pedagogical Treatment of Mentally Ill Children (1898). He opened the first Italian nursery school for poor and mentally disturbed children in Rome, where he collaborated with Maria Montessori. Although the Superior Council of the Italian State Education Ministry rejected his application to teach experimental psychology in 1901, only a year later (1902) he was given permission to teach psychology in the Faculty of Philosophy at the University of Rome, and Luciani asked him to teach physiological psychology in his institute. After having worked in the mental hospital asylum of Nocera Inferiore, De Sanctis started practicing as a psychiatrist on the committee overseeing the private and public asylums in the Siena area. In 1904–05 he took over the direction of the psychiatric clinic from Ezio Sciamanna.

De Sanctis organized the fifth international congress of psychology in Rome (1905) and won the first national competition in Italy for the chair in psychology at the University of Rome. He was named head of the psychological institute, and he worked there for the following twenty-three years. He became head of the Italian Society of Psychology as soon as it was founded in 1910, and he held the position until his death.

De Sanctis identified a new pathological condition that he called dementia praecocissima ('prematurely precocious dementia'), which was confirmed by Emil Kraepelin and became known later as infantile autism. He also described a kind of senile aphasic syndrome in 1916. De Sanctis was the only Italian to participate in the *Handbuch der vergle-*ichenden Psychologie (Munich, 1922), edited by G. Kafka. In 1925 De Sanctis published a book devoted to child neuropsychiatry. He opened the first neuropsychiatry ward for children in Rome, and is in fact considered the father of this specialty in Italy. Moreover, he held the first chair in criminal and judicial psychology and, on the basis of his long experience as a forensic psychiatrist, he was appointed co-director of the Italian Society for Criminal Anthropology in 1933.

Other central themes in his research agenda were infantilism, mongolism, epilepsy, and neurosis.

Bibliography

Primary: 1925. *La neuropsichiatria infantile* (Rome); 1929–30. *Trattato di psicologia sperimentale* 2 vols. (Rome); 1936. 'Autobiography' in Murchison, Carl, ed., *History of Psychology in Autobiographies*, vol. 3 (Worcester, MA) pp. 83–120.

Secondary: Cimino, Guido, and Giovanni Pietro Lombardo, 2004. *Sante De Sanctis tra psicologia generale e psicologia applicata* (Milan); Guarnieri, Patrizia, 1998. 'I rapporti tra psichiatria e psicologia in Italia' in Cimino, Guido, and Nino Dazzi, eds., *La psicologia in Italia*, vol. 2 (Milan) pp. 581–608.

Patrizia Guarnieri

DEBRÉ, ROBERT (b. Sedan, France, 7 December 1882; d. Kremlin-Bicêtre, France, 29 April 1978), *pediatrics, medical education.*

An exceptional person in many ways, Debré was one of the rare doctors to have been both a key organizer of public health as well as a remarkable clinician. In this respect, he deserves recognition as one of the principal modernizers of French medicine in the twentieth century.

Debré was born to a family of Alsatian rabbis who resettled in France after the Franco-Prussian War in 1870. He studied medicine in Paris, passing the 'internat' in 1906. His medical thesis was on the treatment of cerebrospinal meningitis with antimeningococcal serum as discovered by Simon Flexner, director of the Rockefeller Institute for Medical Research. Debré was drafted in 1914 as a lieutenant and served as doctor for an artillery regiment, and after the armistice in 1918, he was hired by the Director of the Institute of Hygiene in Strasbourg. In the early 1920s he succeeded Antonin Marfan at the Hôpital des Enfants Malades, where he established the modern French school of pediatrics. Working with Gaston Ramon of the Pasteur Institute, Debré developed a new smallpox vaccine, and demonstrated the value of antidiphtheria vaccination using anatoxin. Debré's principal focus of attention, however, was tuberculosis in children. Working with Marcel Lelong, he began by demonstrating the fallacy of hereditary transmission, then quickly became a strong supporter of BCG vaccine. Based on immune reactions, he favored repeated use of the tuberculin tests discovered by the pediatrician Clemens von Pirquet. In order to avoid maternal-child transmission, he established a facility in the countryside to raise newborns away from the risk of contagion in the family residence. This public health measure brought him into contact with the work of Ludwik Rajchman of the League of Nations Health Organization, which became UNICEF after World War II. With French government support, Debré founded the Centre International de l'Enfance (CIE) in 1948, where he continued his work with BCG in collaboration with René Dubos of the Rockefeller Institute. At this same time, Debré was one of the first clinicians to do therapeutic trials with tubercular children using the newly developed streptomycin.

Debré is equally famous for his proposals to incorporate biology into French medicine by encouraging hospital research. In the mid-1930s, with the support of the French government along with that of American foundations (Macy and Rockefeller), he incorporated laboratories into the new pediatric clinic at the Hôpital des Enfants Malades. As he recalled later in his memoirs, '[at the time] we protested this use of complementary laboratory examinations, as if they were a supplement to pediatric clinical study rather than a fundamental part of modern medicine.' These activities expanded dramatically after World War II. For example, he adopted modern perinatal techniques learned by one of his interns, Alexandre Minkowski, whom he had sent to the United States. Likewise, he established a laboratory for another of his interns, Georges Schapira, which became one of the centers of biochemistry and medical genetics in France.

During World War II Debré began plans for a major reorganization of the French medical system, which was finally achieved in 1958 when De Gaulle returned to power. Avoiding major reprisals or restrictions from the Vichy regime, Debré presided over the Comité National de la Résistance, which discussed an ambitious program of postwar modernization of the health system, one of whose recommendations was adopted after Liberation with the creation of a Ministry of Population and Health. In 1954, at the instigation of Jean Dausset, the government of Mendès France formed an Interministerial Committee for the Reform of Medical Studies, which led to the laws of 30 December 1958 that implemented the rest of Debré's recommendations despite the opposition of some of his colleagues, who blamed him for 'the disappearance of the elite'. Actually, by attacking the privileges of 'la Médecine Libérale', the French private practitioners, the Debré reforms resulted in integrating the medical schools with the hospital system by creating Centres hospitalo universitaires (CHU). This established in France the famous system of 'bedside teaching by full-time practitioners', which was recommended a half century earlier in the United States by Abraham Flexner.

Bibliography

Primary: 1938. *Quelques vérités premières sur les maladies des enfants* (Paris); 1946. (with Sauvy, A.) *Des Français pour la France, le problème de la population* (Paris); 1974. *L'honneur de vivre, Témoignage* (Paris).

Secondary: 1982. *Commémoration du centenaire de la naissance de R. Debré* (Catalogue de l'exposition) (Paris); 1982. 'Centenaire de naissance de Robert Debré.' *Bulletins de l'Académie Nationale de Médecine* 166: 1257–1303; Dausset, Jean, 1978. 'Notice nécrologique sur Robert Debré . . .' *Comptes rendus de l'Académie des sciences.*

Jean-François Picard

DÉJERINE, JULES   (b. Geneva, Switzerland, 3 August 1849; d. Paris, France, 6 March 1917), *neurology.*

Déjerine studied biology and comparative anatomy in his native Switzerland before moving to Paris in 1871 to advance his entry into academic clinical medicine. His mentor, Prévost, provided him with a letter of introduction to E. Vulpian, the distinguished professor at the Paris Medical School, who engaged the young researcher, resulting in collaborations that were extensive and highly fruitful for the young provincial. His most extensive collaborations, however, were with the American-born Augusta Klumpke, whom he married in 1888, the pair forming a life-long team that developed their own French school of neurological study and research.

Déjerine is distinctive among nineteenth-century neurologists in France because he never studied or worked with Jean-Martin Charcot. In contrast to the Charcot-led Salpêtrière school of neurology, Déjerine developed his interest in neuroanatomy under the guidance of Vulpian, whose primary post was not neurological, and his ascent in international circles pitted him inevitably against Charcot's own protégé, Pierre Marie. After Charcot's death, this rivalry accelerated in a series of debates between the two men on the importance of the left third frontal convolution to language production. The bitterness that was engendered reached far beyond a single neurological issue and led to a fragmentation within French neurology in the early twentieth-century, with two distinct and antagonistic schools.

Déjerine made several seminal discoveries in both clinical neurology and neuropathology. Like Silas Weir Mitchell, who studied victims of the American Civil War, Déjerine studied a variety of nerve lesions consequent to the battle injuries of World War I. He studied hereditary neuropathies and trauma-related plexopathies that are today linked to his name. His studies of aphasia were detailed and authoritative, leading to his international reputation as an expert on cortical control of language. His research on pure word blindness became an archetypal example of highly localized cortical language deficits. Déjerine's name is linked to the early descriptions of olivo-ponto-cerebellar atrophy and to hemianesthetic syndromes associated with thalamic lesions.

Déjerine conducted most of these studies in the Salpêtrière hospital. From the mid-1890s onward he directed a neurological service that gradually came to eclipse the larger service that had formerly belonged to Charcot. Déjerine's interests also included psychotherapy. He established an isolation ward in his service for the treatment of working-class patients suffering from neurasthemia and hysteria, using a technique that combined reasoning and emotional persuasion.

With the death in 1910 of F. Raymond, who had held the professorial chair of Charcot, Déjerine was named to the chair of diseases of the nervous system. This move simultaneously honored Déjerine's leading role in French neurology and blocked a resurgence of the Charcot school. He and his wife moved across the Salpêtrière courtyards to establish their own unique unit with increased funding. For seven years, the program thrived under the leadership of neurologists who were trained by Déjerine and Déjerine-Klumpke and who trained future leaders in neurology, including Roussy, Lhermitte, Ajuriaguerra, André-Thomas, and Alajouanine, among several others. After his death, as a reflection of the unresolved hostility between the Charcot legacy and the Déjerine School, Madame Déjerine and her colleagues were forced to vacate their clinical and laboratory units at the Salpêtrière with the ascent of Pierre Marie to the professorial chair of clinical neurology.

Bibliography

Primary: 1883. 'Sur le nervo-tabes périphérique (ataxie locomotrice par névrites périphériques avec intégrité absolue des racine postérieures, des ganglions spinaux et de la moelle épinière).' *Comptes rendus de l'Académie Sciences Paris* 97: 914–916; 1895. (with Déjerine-Klumpke, A.) *Anatomie des centres nerveux* (Paris); 1900. (with Thomas, A. A.) 'L'atrophie olivo-ponto-cérébelleuse.' *Nouvelle Iconographie de la Salpêtrière* 13: 330–370; 1913. (with Gauckler, E.) *The psychoneuroses and their treatment by psychotherapy,* trans. Smith Ely Jeliffee (Philadelphia).

Secondary: Goetz, Christopher, Michel Bonduelle, and Toby Gelfand, 1995. *Charcot. Constructing Neurology* (Oxford); Gauckler, E., 1922. *Le Professeur Déjerine* (Paris).

Christopher Goetz

DEL GARBO, DINO (aka ALDOBRANDINO, DINUS DE GARBO, DE FLORENTIA, FLORENTINUS) (b. Florence, Italy, c. 1280; d. Florence, 30 September 1327), *surgery.*

The son of a Florentine surgeon, Bono del Garbo, Dino studied arts, philosophy, and medicine at Bologna, at least in part under Taddeo Alderotti. About a year into his study of medicine, probably in the 1290s, Dino's education was interrupted by warfare in Bologna. He returned to Florence, where he was practicing medicine by 1297. By 1305 Dino had completed his studies at Bologna and began lecturing there. In 1306 a papal interdict drove Dino from Bologna, and he accepted a salaried chair of medicine at Siena. The rest of his career was spent teaching medicine intermittently at Bologna, Siena, and Padua, and practicing medicine in Florence.

Dino was a prolific medical writer. As noted by Siraisi, he was among the first to undertake commentaries on large parts of the *Canon* of Avicenna (Ibn Sīnā), and is credited for his impact on the full assimilation of Avicenna's ideas by the medical faculties. His first major work was his *Surgery,* a commentary on selected sections of Book IV of the *Canon.* The text, which treats wounds and injuries, was begun in Florence probably c. 1296 and completed c. 1308. Between 1311 and 1319 he commented on *Fen* 4 of Book I in his *Clarification of the Entire Practice of Medical Science,* dealing with disease and therapy, and in 1325 he completed *On the Virtues of Medicines,* a commentary on Book II, regarding medicinal simples. He also produced commentaries on Hippocrates and Galen.

Dino's work reflects the gradual introduction of surgical education into the medical faculties of northern Italy. In his *Surgery,* Dino expanded the definition of surgery to include the body of principles necessary for the correct performance of manual operations, placing knowledge of theory alongside practical experience. For Dino, surgery was a learned discipline, a *scientia,* rather than a mere series of manual treatments. Through a series of scholastic *quaestiones* [questions], Dino evaluated Avicenna's ideas against authorities such as Galen and Abulcasis (Al-Zahrāwī), as well as against contemporary surgical practice. As noted by Siraisi, Dino adopted this academic format in order to place surgery alongside the tradition of learned medicine.

In addition to his achievements in medicine, Dino shared Taddeo Alderotti's interest in the liberal arts and vernacular literature. He was the author of a commentary on Guido Cavalcanti's *Donna mi prega* [A lady asks me], a *canzone* dealing with the nature of love. Dino was praised by fourteenth-century biographer Filippo Villani for excellence in philosophy as well as in medicine.

That Dino was renowned in his day for his medical achievements is attested by the adulation of the chroniclers Filippo and Giovanni Villani, the generous salary of 350 florins he earned during his second professorship at Siena, and the patronage of Robert of Anjou, king of Sicily. His career was not, however, unmarred by controversy: Giovanni Villani relates that Dino was accused of plagiarizing the work of contemporary physician Pietro Torrigiano de Torrigiani, and that he was involved in the condemnation of astrologer and poet Cecco d'Ascoli, burned for heresy in 1327. These claims have been challenged by modern scholarship.

Bibliography

Primary: 1489. *Expositio super tertia, quarta, et parte quintae fen IV. libri Avicennae* (Ferrara); 1502. *Scriptum Dini super libro de natura fetus Hypocratis* (Venice); 1514. *Dyni florentini super quarta fen primi Avicenne preclarissima commentaria . . .* (printed with *Expositio Dini super canones generales de virtutibus medicinarum simplicium secundi canonis Avicenne*) (Venice).

Secondary: McVaugh, Michael, 2000. 'Surgical Education in the Middle Ages.' *Dynamis* 20: 283–304; Siraisi, Nancy, 1994. 'How to Write a Latin Book on Surgery: Organizing Principles and Authorial Devices in Guglielmo da Saliceto and Dino del Garbo' in García-Ballester, Luis et al., eds., *Practical Medicine from Salerno to the Black Death* (Cambridge) pp. 88–109; Siraisi, Nancy, 1981. *Taddeo Alderotti and His Pupils: Two Generations of Italian Medical Learning* (Princeton).

Caroline Hillard

DELAY, JEAN (b. Bayonne, Basses-Pyrénées, France, 14 November 1907; d. Paris, France, 29 May 1987), *neuropsychiatry.*

Delay's career rise was meteoric. He passed his baccalaureate at the precocious age of fifteen, and he won his internship at twenty. By thirty, he was a *médecin des hôpitaux*, and he arrived at the highest rank, clinical professor, at thirty-nine. Delay also obtained a philosophy degree and a doctorate in letters in 1942, eventually writing three novels based on his experience in caring for the sick.

In 1945 Delay was called to the Nuremburg Trials to examine Rudolph Hess, former right-hand man of Hitler who fled the Third Reich in the middle of the war to attempt a peace initiative with the English. He also examined Jules Streicher, the Nazi anti-Semitic ideologue. In 1947 Delay was named to the clinical chair of mental illness and encephalitis and as director of the Psychological Institute at Sainte Anne Hospital. In 1950 he organized the First World Congress of Psychiatry, which drew more than 2,500 participants to Paris.

Two years later Delay achieved notable milestones in both his literary and medical careers. He began a biography of the novelist André Gide, and with his collaborator Pierre Deniker he used a treatment based on a new molecule developed by Henri Laborit at Val de Grâce Hospital to induce artificial hibernation in patients with certain mental illnesses. The efficacy of chlorpromazine, the first of the major tranquilizers, marked the debut of psychotropic medications. As a result, brutal restraints, such as straitjackets, and more intrusive therapeutic interventions, such as electroshock (ECT), were largely replaced. This also initiated a movement toward deinstitutionalization of psychiatric asylums. His contributions to neuropharmacology brought Delay admission to the Academy of Medicine in 1955 and the Académie Française in 1960. At Delay's reception, the grandson of Pasteur, Vallery-Radot, thanked him as follows: 'one can compare the revolution in psychiatry brought by synthetic chemicals to that which occurred in infectious medicine because of antibiotics, and thanks to you, sir, we owe a large part of this revolution.' Among his extensive scientific publications were *Les astéréognosies, étude de la pathologie du toucher* (1935); *Les ondes cérébrales et la psychologie* (1941); *Les dissolutions de la mémoire* (1942); *Les dérèglements de l'humeur* (1946); *Méthodes biologiques en clinique psychiatrique* (1950); *Études de psychologie médicale* (1953); and *Aspects de la psychiatrie moderne* (1956).

Though only a moderate subscriber to the psychoanalytic theories of Freud and Jung, Delay found himself considered 'a doctor by psychologists, a psychologist by psychiatrists, and a psychiatrist by neurologists'. In May 1968 the antipsychiatry student movement pushed for the separation of psychiatry and neurology and occupied his office at the hospital. Although bitter, he resigned his duties discreetly to devote himself full-time to writing. He wrote a sociobiography of France, focusing on the family and mother. As a specialist in historical consciousness, Delay wanted to break through what Charles Péguy called 'the wall of four grandparents'. *Avant mémoire*, published by Gallimard in four volumes from 1979 through 1986, symbolized a new literary genre: psychosocial biography.

Bibliography

Primary: 1942. *Les dissolutions de la mémoire* (Paris); 1950. *Méthodes biologiques en clinique psychiatrique* (Paris); 1979–1986. *Avant mémoire* 4 vols. (Paris).

Jean-François Picard

DEMOCEDES OF CROTON (b. Croton, Italy; fl. 500 BCE), *natural philosophy, medicine.*

Son of Calliphon and born in Croton in South Italy, Democedes was known around 500 BCE as the best doctor and had an adventurous life, which is recorded by Herodotus (*Histories*, 3.125 ff.). He started by practicing in Croton, and then was employed as a community physician in Aegina and later at Athens; this is the first example of a community physician in the Greek world. From Athens, he moved to Samos, always in search of higher payment, and there he acted as doctor to the tyrant Polycrates. After his master's assassination, he was taken prisoner by the Persian king Darius. Nevertheless, he distinguished himself again through a successful, though more gentle, surgical treatment of the king's injured ankle, thus achieving new status at the Persian court in Susa, at the expense of the highly reputed Egyptian doctors. Eventually he escaped to Italy and returned to his native Croton, where he married the daughter of Milon the wrestler and settled.

Nothing is known about Democedes' doctrines and conception of medicine. Yet he is an important figure in two ways. He is a spectacular case of professional success in the rough world of archaic tyranny and the nascent Greek city and, as such, bears witness to the spread of the reputation of Greek surgeons as far as Persia. Even more importantly, he provides the earliest extant evidence for the salaried employment of doctors on behalf of the community in the Greek world.

Bibliography

Primary: Diels, H., and W. Kranz, eds., 1952. *Die Fragmente der Vorsokratiker* (Berlin) I: 110–113; Longrigg, J., 1998. *Greek Medicine. From the Heroic to the Hellenistic Age. A Source Book* (London) pp. 61, 180.

Secondary: Nutton, V., 2004. *Ancient Medicine* (London) pp. 48–49; Longrigg, J., 1998. *Greek Medicine. From the Heroic to the Hellenistic Age. A Source Book* (London) pp. 79, 188; Griffiths, A., 1987. 'Democedes of Croton: a Greek Doctor at the Court of Darius in Sancisi–Weerdenburg' in Kuhrt, H., and A. Kuhrt, eds., *Achemenid History, II: The Greek Sources* (Leiden) pp. 37–51.

Manuela Tecusan

DEMOCRITUS OF ABDERA   (b. Abdera, Thrace (now Greece); fl. 420 BCE), *natural philosophy, biology, medicine, cosmology.*

Democritus, the long-lived 'laughing philosopher', was one of the key Pre-Socratics. Together with his teacher Leucippus he formulated ancient atomism in response to the attack of the Eleatics on the possibility of motion and change; his disciple Nausiphanes taught Epicurus, who developed atomism further. Leucippus probably introduced the notion of void, but his and Democritus's doctrines can hardly be separated.

Ancient authorities ranked Democritus, with Pythagoras and Empedocles, among the famous first philosopher-doctors, who proved that medicine was founded in the study of nature. Democritus had already in antiquity acquired a legendary reputation, as the supposed teacher of Hippocrates and Pythagoras. Even more legends proliferated throughout the Middle Ages and Renaissance, when he was considered the equal of Hippocrates and spurious Latin works circulated under his name (e.g., the *Prognostic of Democritus* foretelling death, or a *Medical Book* excerpted from Oribasius). The iconic role he played in the history of medicine until the seventeenth century reflects his eminence in both philosophy and medicine and the impact of atomism on medical thought. Although it remains a big question whether Democritus himself explained biological phenomena in atomistic terms, his construction of the physical world was a powerful counterweight to the dominating Aristotelian model. He wrote on cosmology, astronomy, and meteorology, as well as on medical, biological, and psychophysiological topics (*Medical Opinions, Causes Concerning Animals, On Those in Hades*).

In Democritus's physics, the ultimate constituents were *atoma* ('atoms', the smallest 'indivisible' units of matter), separated by void. Indestructible, invisible, and homogenous, they were infinite in number and movement. Destruction of a compound only released the constituent atoms to their motion in void, from which they associated into new compounds. They had spatial extension and the primary qualities of size, shape, and arrangement (within compounds), all other qualities being derivative. This distinction between primary and secondary qualities was a momentous contribution to philosophy. Further, his philosophy led to the demarcation of the classical positions of skepticism and relativism, as evidenced by the dispute since antiquity over whether Democritus conceived of secondary qualities as depending on a subjective perceiver or as existing in their own right as a result of atomic contacts within the compound.

Democritus accorded the brain a leading role in cognition and sensation (e.g., the production of hearing). However, he regarded the soul not as seated there but as distributed throughout the body in the form of spherical atoms. Like Diogenes of Apollonia and others, he attached importance to air (*pneuma*), considering it to be the vehicle of life and perception, the source of motion and warmth, and the essence of soul. The shape he gave these views, linking the notions of soul, air, and fire, and the theory of perception he constructed out of them, had a profound influence on Stoicism.

Democritus provided the main alternative to Aristotle's physiology, in which respiration cooled the innate heat: he claimed that soul was constantly fed through breath, having its round atoms replaced by *pneuma* from outside. He explained sleep and death as depletions-without-renewal of the soul-atoms, carried to different degrees; functions like the growth of hair continued after death because depletion was gradual—thus even resurrection was possible. But there was no final survival of soul, which dispersed into its pneumatic-fiery constituents. The air was thus pervaded by soul-atoms, which accounted for strange phenomena like visions and prophecies.

Perceptions and sensations were alterations determined by the predominant configuration of atoms in the stimulus and produced by images that either affected the percipient through contact (touch and taste) or imprinted the air and traveled through it to the sense-organ (sight, hearing, and smell). This influential notion of an imprinted *pneuma* was to be especially developed in the analysis of sight. Thought was an alteration consequent upon sensation and unable to exist without it, yet it led to genuine knowledge of invisibles—which Democritus contrasted to the 'bastard' knowledge of sensory items.

In explaining reproduction, Democritus adopted, like Empedocles, a pangenetic theory of the seed, represented as drawn from all the parts of the bodies of both parents. He also claimed that the seed transmitted the *pneuma* of the soul, a view that had great influence on Aristotle. His interests extended to the anatomy of the womb and sex organs, which may be the origin of medieval representations of Democritus as a champion of animal dissection.

In medicine, he placed emphasis on preventive measures rather than therapy, arguing for a healthy lifestyle. His name is associated to a type of pulse, which he called 'worming'.

Bibliography

Primary: Diels, H., and W. Kranz, eds., 1964. *Die Fragmente der Vorsokratiker* (Zurich, Berlin) II: 81–230; Luria, S., 1970. *Demokrit* (Leningrad); Kirk, G. S., J. E. Raven, and M. Schofield, eds., 1983. *The Presocratic Philosophers* (Cambridge).

Secondary: Kahn, C., 1985. ˙ ˙Democritus and the Origins of Moral Philosophy.' *American Journal of Philosophy* 106: 1–35; Barnes, J., 1979. *The Presocratic Philosophers* (London, Henley, Boston) I: 19ff.; Cole, T., 1967. *Democritus and the Sources of Greek Anthropology* (Chapel Hill, NC); Vlastos, G., 1945, 1946. 'Ethics and Physics in Diogenes.' *Philosophical Review* 54: 578–592, 55: 53–63.

Manuela Tecusan

DEPAGE, ANTOINE

DEPAGE, ANTOINE (b. Bosvoorde, Belgium, 28 November 1862; d. the Hague, the Netherlands, 10 June 1925), *surgery, hospital reform.*

Depage was the son of a Flemish farmer and burgomaster, Frederic Depage. After obtaining his medical degree in Brussels, he went to Leipzig, Prague, and Vienna to specialize in surgery. After returning to Brussels, he engaged in research with Edmond Destrée, creating the first Belgian hospital laboratory in 1889. In 1895 Depage was appointed surgeon in the Hospice de l'Infirmerie in Brussels; in 1899 he became surgeon-in-chief of St John Hospital, and, in 1901, *Chargé de cours* ('lecturer') for special surgical pathology at Brussels University. In 1904 he was appointed surgeon-in-chief at St Peter Hospital, and, in 1909, professor at Brussels Free University. Two years before (1907), he had become a member of the Academy of Medicine.

Depage used his great organizational talents to professionalize both surgery and nursing. In 1890 he founded the first private surgical hospital in Brussels, together with Verhoogen, Slosse, and his tutor Jules Thiriar. In 1892 he participated in the founding of the Belgian Society for Surgery. Ten years later, he was cofounder of the Société Internationale de Chirurgie. Together with his wife, Marie Picard, a nurse whom he married in 1893, Depage founded the first Belgian nursing school in 1907, which was directed by the English nurse Edith Cavell. Together with Jules Bordet, Depage was the first to establish a Belgian cancer institute. Initially founded in 1921 as a Radium Institute, it later came under the auspices of the 'Ligue nationale Belge contre le cancer'.

Depage published widely on surgical pathology and new operative techniques, including an annual anthology of surgical publications called *L'année chirurgicale*. He improved hospital conditions for surgical patients by not only constructing a new private clinic, which opened in 1907, but also, as a member of the Brussels town council, by changing the infrastructure of civil hospitals. In 1912, during the Balkan War, Depage set up the first 'ambulance' for wounded soldiers in Istanbul, including medical and nursing personnel, surgical instruments, bandages, and drugs. This experience proved to be of great importance during World War I. When Germany invaded Belgium in August 1914, Depage was asked to command the medical services of the Belgian Red Cross and to organize a great 'ambulance' for the wounded at the Royal Palace. However,

he left Brussels in order to deploy surgical activities closer to the front. With the support of Queen Elisabeth of Belgium, Depage succeeded in setting up a field hospital in a former hotel in a town called De Panne. 'Hôpital l'Océan' was to become a model for war surgery. Originally equipped with 1,200 beds, by the end of the war his hospital could hold 3,000 patients. Depage's speed and insight in initiating medical action were unanimously praised. Treatment of patients, scientific organization, and especially war-oriented surgery attracted doctors from all Allied countries. Depage organized several scientific meetings in De Panne. The well-known French surgeon Alexis Carrel became one of Depage's best friends. Early in May 1915 Depage suffered a great loss: while returning from a fundraising mission in the United States, his wife perished in the waves when the Germans torpedoed the *Lusitania.*

After World War I, Depage was widely honored by the Belgian Society for Surgery (in the presence of H.M. Queen Elisabeth), by the American Society of Medicine (in 1919), and by the fifth congress of the Société Internationale de Chirurgie in Paris. Depage received the five-yearly prize of the Belgian Royal Academy of Medicine, and King Albert awarded him the rank of General. Two universities—Budapest and Sheffield—made him *doctor honoris causa.*

During a trip to Morocco in April 1923, Depage contracted bacterial pneumonia, complicated by bilateral thrombophlebitis. He was operated upon several times, but to no avail: he succumbed in a hospital in the Hague on 10 June 1925.

Bibliography

Primary: 1898/1899. *L'année chirurgicale. Revue encyclopédique de chirurgie générale et spéciale* (Brussels); 1913. 'Ambulance Belge à Constantinople pendant la guerre des Balkans.' *Bulletin de l'Académie Royale de médecine de Belgique* 4th series, 27: 35–53; 1917–18. *Ambulance de 'l'Océan': La Panne* (Paris).

Secondary: Colard, A., 1970. 'Antoine Depage' in *Biographie nationale* vol. 35 (Brussels) pp. 171–180; Custers, J., M. Leroy, L. Cooremans, et al., 1962. 'Commémoration du centenaire de la naissance d'Antoine Depage.' *Bulletin de l'Académie Royale de médecine de Belgique* 7th series, 2: 683–723; Depage, H., 1956. *La vie d'Antoine Depage* (Brussels).

R. van Hee

DESAULT, PIERRE-JOSEPH

DESAULT, PIERRE-JOSEPH (b. Vouhenans [Haute-Saône], France, 6 February 1738; d. Paris, France, 1 June 1795), *surgery.*

Desault was born in a hamlet in the Franche-Comté, the youngest of five children in a peasant family of modest means. (Contemporary eulogies misstated his year of birth as 1744). After studying in a Jesuit school, he apprenticed under a barber-surgeon and then worked for three years at the military hospital in nearby Belfort. In the mid-1760s Desault came to Paris where he attended courses at the College of

Surgery and, at the same time, offered his own private lessons in anatomical dissection, as enterprising young surgeons often did. The considerable success of Desault's teaching attracted influential patronage from Germain Pichault de la Martinière, first surgeon to King Louis XV and President of the Academy of Surgery, and Antoine Louis, the Academy's permanent secretary.

In 1776 la Martinière selected Desault to be the first candidate to sustain a thesis (in Latin) for the mastership in surgery, in a lavish ceremony at the magnificent new surgical buildings (now the Paris Medical Faculty) that had been designed by the king's architect, Jacques Gondoin. The promising young surgeon occupied various positions in new institutions created by the Crown for the Paris surgical profession. In collaboration with François Chopart, Desault taught for six years at the *école pratique*, the College of Surgery's school for anatomical dissection, and at the College's *hospice*, a small hospital for innovative surgical operations. As consulting surgeon to the *hospice*, Desault acquired practical experience with challenging procedures. Until then his contributions to surgery had derived primarily from anatomical studies.

In 1782 Desault was named chief surgeon at the Charité, the second most prestigious hospital in Paris after the Hôtel Dieu. He had climbed the ranks of the Paris surgical profession, availing himself of collegial connections and opportunities afforded by academic institutions. For the remainder of his career Desault would work largely independently, eschewing these earlier affiliations and devoting himself exclusively to creating his own school at the Charité and then at the Hôtel Dieu, where he became chief surgeon in 1786. (He had in effect assumed these duties in 1785 as assistant to the aged incumbent.)

Reforming Surgical Instruction at the Hôtel Dieu

During the 1780s, numerous projects for a modern central hospital or hospitals for Paris were presented in the aftermath of a destructive fire at the Hôtel Dieu. Given the deteriorating financial context of the pre-Revolutionary years, none came to fruition. The construction of a new Hôtel Dieu would be put off for almost another one hundred years. But the deplorable conditions of the largest institution in France for treating all forms of disease became a focus for Enlightenment reform. Already singled out as a deadly institution by the philosopher Denis Diderot, the Hôtel Dieu became the object of critical reports by the Academy of Sciences (1785) and especially by Jacques Tenon in his *Mémoires sur les hôpitaux de Paris* (1788). Tenon drew attention to the horrors of surgery in the ancient hospital. Operations took place amid other patients, who thus witnessed the sight and heard the screams of the 'torture' while waiting their turn or recuperating.

Desault too was appalled at this state of affairs. Overcoming the inertia of the hospital administrators and determined opposition from the Augustine nuns responsible for patient care, the chief surgeon succeeded in removing major operations from the wards to a newly constructed, spacious amphitheater. Desault was not indifferent to improvements in the nutrition and hygienic conditions for his surgical patients, but his primary objective was pedagogical. In the amphitheater, students could observe him at work and be instructed in the performance of surgical operations. Together with teaching at the bedside, the amphitheater instruction introduced clinical surgical teaching on a scale unprecedented in France and probably in the rest of Europe as well. As an integral part of instruction, the chief surgeon delegated to students considerable responsibility for presentation of patients, record-keeping, and treatment.

In 1791 Desault himself provided the most vivid description of his innovation. With the Revolution well under way, a deputation of 'citizen-students' accused the chief surgeon of excluding them from his clinical lessons. Desault pointed to the irony that, just a few years earlier, the hospital's nursing sisters had attacked him for admitting too many outsiders to his lessons in the amphitheater. According to the nuns, the chief surgeon's public lessons on female patients were indecent. Desault countered that the patients undergoing surgery not only consented but appreciated their contribution to instruction. In his defense to the National Assembly, Desault presented himself as 'a man, who has initiated in this hospital a multitude of new modes of instruction . . . a method which in the space of four years has developed more true surgeons than have emerged from the Hôtel Dieu during the previous century' (Desault, 1791, pp. 275–276). Whereas his predecessors had provided scant formal instruction—thirty one-hour lessons per year—he gave 'four hours of practical lessons every day throughout the year' (ibid., p. 278). In addition to the instruction and supervision of young surgeons who worked at the Hôtel Dieu, he admitted outsiders to the lessons for a modest fee. Three hundred students, he claimed, had witnessed his operations and teaching.

Desault sketched a debilitating daily routine, beginning at dawn with three hours of rounds to see hundreds of surgical patients and ending with evening rounds, sometimes as late as ten o'clock. In between he received indigent outpatients, held anatomical lessons, and conducted the clinical surgical lessons. There remained just a few hours in the afternoon for him to visit paying patients on the outside. Desault pointed out that he spent a good deal of his hospital salary on instruments and other surgical necessities. Usually he slept in the hospital. Under his responsibility and profiting from his supervision were about a dozen surgeons who, like their chief, lived in the Hôtel Dieu, and ninety younger outside aides (externs) who performed phlebotomies and wound dressing.

Surgical Contributions

Desault published virtually nothing. His burden of surgical duties left little time for literary pursuits, and he evidently had little inclination or talent for writing. As one of his students commented, his teachings were engraved in the minds of his listeners rather than in books. At first circulated by word of mouth, Desault's lessons ultimately found their way into publications by his senior students, who in 1791 began a *Journal de chirurgie* under his name. The last of four volumes, edited by Xavier Bichat, Desault's devoted assistant in his final years, appeared after the master's death. An *Oeuvres chirurgicales* also appeared posthumously.

From these sources and, more significantly, from the publications of literally dozens of chief hospital surgeons and military surgeons (including Larrey and Percy) of the next generation who had worked under him, Desault's substantial contributions can be gleaned. He was said to have revolutionized surgical technique with his meticulous three-dimensional conception of pertinent anatomical relationships. His new operation for ligating dangerous aneurysms of major arteries (1785) became known just prior to a slightly different method employed by his British rival, John Hunter, with whom Desault was often compared. Although he devised or modified instruments (bandages, canulae, needles, bistouris, and sutures) for interventions in a spectrum of disorders (fractures of the long bones, tumors and polyps of the mouth and throat, urinary bladder cysts, etc.), Desault strove for simplicity. If it were possible, he remarked, he would have preferred to operate with only his fingers and fingernails. Unlike many of his predecessors, he had recourse to amputations only in extremis. He pioneered the use of gum elastic sounds (constructed by Bernard, a skilled Parisian artisan) to intubate the esophagus and the trachea for feeding and breathing in cases of obstruction of these passages.

Revolutionary Torment

Desault's declaration to the National Assembly in defense of his authority over access to his lessons at the Hôtel Dieu tells much about the character of the man. Proud of his achievement, imperious to the point of arrogance, condescending, quick to anger, and violent in rejoinder, the chief surgeon lashed out against the effrontery of those he considered an ignorant rabble, including 'a so-called delegation of surgical students . . . all, or nearly all of them, wigmakers' (Desault, 1791, p. 276). Two of Desault's most devoted followers, Marc-Antoine Petit and Bichat, revered the memory of a mentor robust in build, rapid in his movements, supremely confident, and passionately and completely dedicated to his vocation, but at times severe, even brusque, with students and patients alike.

As the Revolution wore on, Desault ran afoul of the radical Jacobins. In 1792, after the massacre of 10 August, he was

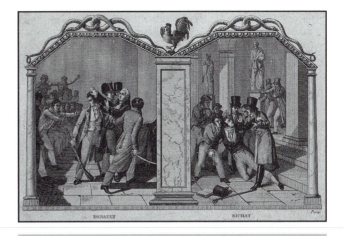

Desault (left) and Xavier Bichat (right) being rescued from the revolutionaries. Line engraving, Iconographic Collection, Wellcome Library, London.

accused, falsely, of not treating the wounded. A petition by hundreds of his hospital patients and students was made in his defense, and Desault escaped with only a reprimand. But the following year, soldiers surrounded the hospital in the midst of Desault's lesson and took him away to prison. This time, the intervention of his influential colleague, Antoine Fourcroy, obtained his release. In 1794 Desault was summoned to treat the young son of the executed Louis XVI in the prison of the Temple. Rumors circulated as to the identity of the child and his fate. Shaken by the political events of the Terror, his own health failing, Desault nonetheless kept up his work for another year before ultimately succumbing at age fifty-seven to fever with delirium. Autopsy revealed nothing to support talk of his being poisoned. The post-Thermidorian government, in recognition of his service, accorded an annual pension to Desault's widow and son. After the dissolution of the medical institutions of the Old Regime and throughout the chaos of the Reign of Terror of 1793–94, Desault's clinical surgical school at the Hôtel Dieu (renamed Hospice d'Humanité for a time) had remained virtually the only site of medical instruction in the capital.

Contemporaries pronounced Desault a 'genius' in two senses. First, in accord with the traditional meaning of the word, he was said to be possessed by the demiurge, or genius, of the surgical art. At the same time, eulogists asserted that Desault personally possessed genius as a surgeon. This new Romantic (and distinctively modern) conceit portrayed Desault as an isolated figure transcending his contemporaries. In fact, he was very much the product of the Enlightenment and its surgical institutions. His greatest achievement was his hospital school, where he trained not only future surgeons but also those who would become the leaders of post-Revolutionary French medicine, including Jean-Nicolas Corvisart and Bichat. Desault reluctantly accepted the chair of surgery in the new *école de santé* (1794). In line with the old guard of Paris surgeons, he considered internal medicine an imprecise and obscure partner for surgery, and he opposed the Revolution's unification of the two professions.

Bibliography

Primary: 1779. (with Chopart, François) *Traité des maladies chirurgicales et des opérations qui leur convient* (Paris); 1791. 'Réclamation de M. Desault, chirurgien en chef de l'Hôtel-Dieu de Paris' (mss) in Archives nationales de France DXXXVIII, 3, 47. Transcription and translation in Gelfand, Toby, 1973. 'A confrontation over clinical instruction the Hôtel-Dieu of Paris during the French revolution.' *Journal of the History of Medicine and Allied Sciences* 28: 268–282; 1791–96. (ed.) *Journal de chirurgie*, 4 vols. (vol. 4 ed. by Bichat, Xavier) (Paris); 1798–1803. *Oeuvres chirurgicales* 3 vols. (ed. by Bichat) (Paris).

Secondary: Gelfand, Toby, 1980. *Professionalizing Modern Medicine. Paris Surgeons and Medical Science and Institutions in the 18th Century* (Westport, C T); Genty, Maurice, 1934. 'Desault (Pierre-Joseph)' in Genty, Maurice, ed., *Les maîtres du passé. Les biographies médicales* (Paris) pp. 1934–1936; Bichat, Xavier, 1798. 'Eloge de P.-J. Desault' in *Œuvres chirurgicales de P.-J. Desault* vol. 1 (Paris) pp. 194–217; Petit, Marc-Antoine, 1795. 'Eloge de Pierre-Joseph Desault' in *Essai sur la médecine du cœur* (Lyon) pp. 73–115.

Toby Gelfand

DESGENETTES, RENÉ-NICOLAS DUFRICHE (b. Alençon, France, 23 May 1762; d. Paris, France, 3 February 1837), *military medicine.*

Desgenettes was descended from a Norman family with a long record of public service; his father was a barrister and royal official. The son was educated first in his native Alençon and then in Paris, where he enrolled in the Faculty of Medicine. He interrupted his studies in 1783 after receiving a modest inheritance and embarked on a grand tour of England and then Italy. In 1789 he returned to France to complete his medical education at Montpellier; he defended his thesis in 1790, on the physiology of the lymphatic vessels.

As the French Revolution turned increasingly radical, Desgenettes's friends encouraged him to join the army, which provided a political haven for young men from privileged backgrounds. In February 1793 he received a commission as a physician for the Army of Italy, commanded by Napoleon Bonaparte. From 1796 to 1798, he served as physician and professor of medical physics at the Val-de-Grâce, a former abbey in Paris that had been converted into a military hospital during the Revolution and charged with training medical personnel for the army. Desgenettes accompanied Bonaparte on his ill-fated invasion of Egypt in 1798, as chief physician of the Army of the Orient. When bubonic plague broke out, he tried to reassure frightened soldiers who feared that they would contract the disease. Two gestures became legendary: he inoculated himself with a lancet dipped in pus from a bubo and shared the drink of a dying plague victim. In Antoine-Jean Gros's celebrated painting *Bonaparte Visiting the Plague-Stricken at Jaffa,* he

appears next to the general. In 1802 Desgenettes returned to Paris. A series of appointments followed: chief physician of the Paris military hospital, inspector general of the army health service, chief physician of the Grande Armée. He was often in the field on Napoleon's campaigns. Captured during the disastrous Russian campaign of 1812–13, he won release only when the Tsar personally intervened.

After the abdication of the Emperor and the restoration of the Bourbon monarchy in the spring of 1814, Desgenettes remained at the Val-de-Grâce, where he was promoted to chief of medicine and head professor. When Napoleon returned from exile in the spring of 1815, Desgenettes rallied to his cause; he was with the Emperor at Waterloo as head physician of the army and the Imperial Guard. After Napoleon's final exile, Desgenettes was stripped of many of his functions. A reprieve came in 1819; he returned to the military health service and was appointed professor of hygiene at the Paris Faculty of Medicine. In 1822, however, he was among the victims of a political purge of professors considered disloyal to the regime. The Revolution of 1830, which overthrew the house of Bourbon and installed a more liberal monarchy, made it possible for Desgenettes to reclaim the chair of hygiene. In 1832 he was named head physician at the Invalides, a home and hospital for sick and elderly soldiers. In 1835 he suffered a stroke, which forced him to curtail his activities.

Desgenettes's long record of service brought him many honors and distinctions, among them officer and then commander of the Legion of Honor; chevalier and then baron of the Empire; founding membership in the Academy of Medicine, created in 1820 by Louis XVIII; and membership in the Academy of Sciences (1832).

Along with the military surgeons Dominique Larrey and Pierre-François Percy, Desgenettes exemplifies the ways in which the wars of the French Revolution and of Napoleon helped to shape French medicine and created career opportunities for ambitious young men of his generation.

Bibliography

Primary: 1802. *Histoire médicale de l'armée d'Orient . . .* (Paris); 1835–36. *Souvenirs de la fin du XVIIIe siècle et du commencement du XIXe . . .* 2 vols. (Paris).

Secondary: Lemaire, Jean-François, 2003. *La médecine napoléonienne* (Paris); Blaessinger, Edmond, 1947. *Quelques grandes figures de la chirurgie et de la médecine militaires* (Paris).

Matthew Ramsey

DESPARS, JACQUES (aka JOHANNES DE PARTIBUS) (b. Tournai, France, *c.* 1380; d. Paris, France, 3 January 1458), *medicine.*

Despars was born the son of a knight in Tournai, France. In 1403 he received the degree of master in arts at the University of Paris and three years later was elected as rector of the university. He enrolled in the Faculty of Medicine of Paris around 1404 and received his bachelor's in medicine there in 1408, having also studied for six months at the University of Montpellier. In 1410 he obtained his master's degree in medicine.

Soon after his graduation, Despars served as regent master of the Faculty of Medicine from 1411 until his departure from Paris in 1419. From 1420 to around 1450, Despars lived alternately in Tournai and Cambrai in northern France, where he held several ecclesiastical benefices. During these years, he carried on his medical practice and was even called upon several times to serve as both physician and adviser at the court of Burgundy. In addition to his medical practice, Despars wrote a number of shorter treatises on medical topics, including a list of remedies found in the works of the Arabic physician Mesue (Ibn Māsawayh). His most influential work was a commentary on the *Canon* of Avicenna (Ibn Sīnā), specifically on Books I and III and *fen* 1 of Book IV, which he wrote between 1432 and 1453. Despars returned to Paris around 1450 to serve as a canon at Notre Dame and resumed work with the Faculty of Medicine.

Despars's commentary on Avicenna's *Canon* reveals his appreciation for the works of the 'illustrious' Greek authors—Hippocrates, Aristotle, and Galen—as well as those of other leading Arabic scholars—Rhazes (Al-Rāzī), Serapion, Mesue, and Avenzoar (Ibn Zuhr). Commenting on the *Canon* allowed Despars to engage a variety of theoretical issues related to teaching (in the form of scholastic questions), as well as topics more directly related to practice. On several occasions, he displayed a concern with the difficulty of applying theoretical rules in practice. For example, when discussing the causes of plague, he raised the possibility of contagious diseases and, following Avicenna, he recognized nine diseases that appeared to be passed from one person to another. However, he carefully explained that the disease itself was not transferred, but rather putrid vapors emanating from the sick person's body could generate a similar disease in those people who were near the patient and were already predisposed to this type of illness. Ultimately, his explanation for the role of contagion in the spread of plague and a general belief that the art of medicine was not capable of defeating it led him to emphasize the use of quarantine measures to isolate infected people and places from healthy people. On the other hand, Despars downplayed the significance of astrological causes of the plague, in part because he saw no direct practical implications for these theories in terms of treatment.

Like other physicians during the fifteenth century, Despars felt the pressure of competition from the growing number of empirical, magical, and astrological healers. In response, he advocated the superiority of rational medicine and discounted the abilities of empirics and magical healers, all of whom he felt lacked necessary theoretical training. He even questioned the efficacy of astrological medicine, which had numerous scholarly advocates, although he advised his readers to pretend to take astral signs into account in order to win the trust of patients who expected astrological advice from their physicians.

Bibliography

Primary: 1498. *Canon Avicenne cum explanatione Jacobi de Partibus* 3 vols. (Lyons).

Secondary: Jacquart, Danielle, 1990. 'Theory, Everyday Practice, and Three Fifteenth-Century Physicians.' *Osiris* (2nd series) 6: 140–160; Jacquart, Danielle, 1980. 'Le regard d'un médecin sur son temps: Jacques Despars (1380?–1458).' *Bibliotheque de l'ecole des Chartes* 138: 35–86; Wickersheimer, Ernest, 1936. *Dictionnaire biograhique des médecins en France au moyen age* (Geneva) pp. 326–327.

William H. York

DEVOTO, LUIGI (b. Borzonasca, Genoa, Italy, 23 August 1864; d. Milan, Italy, 20 July 1936), *medicine, occupational medicine.*

Devoto graduated from medical school in Genoa in 1888 and obtained a specialization in clinical chemistry in Prague. He started his career at the teaching hospital of the University of Genoa under Ettore Maragliano (1849–1940). In 1899 he was appointed professor of medical pathology at the University of Pavia.

In 1901 Devoto founded a special clinic for treating pellagra in Pavia, studied rice field pathology, taught a course on 'Professional diseases' and took other initiatives outside the clinic and hospital confines. Devoto hoped to create and diffuse a special cultural atmosphere, following both the forgotten precepts of Bernardino Ramazzini (1633–1714) and the more modern ones of the Belgian sociologist Hector Denis (1842–1913), who wished to bring social problems within the confines of scientific institutions.

In 1901 Luigi Devoto also started the *Il lavoro, rivista di fisiologia, clinica ed igiene del lavoro* [The Work, Journal of Physiology, Clinic and Hygiene of Work]. This periodical was renamed *La medicina del lavoro* [Occupational Medicine] in 1925 and is still published today. In the first issue Devoto published an article entitled 'Occupational Illnesses in Italy', in which he characterized six groups of work-related diseases and for the first time clearly defined the field of action of the new discipline, 'medicine and clinic of work', or occupational medicine.

Devoto turned his attention to Milan, which was far more industrialized and animated by a wide social and political debate. In Milan he combined private practice in medical hydrology and clinical medicine. Thanks to his intense organizational work the first 'Clinica del Lavoro' ['Work Clinic'] was officially inaugurated in 1910. That 'clinic' still exists today and is named in honor of its founder. In 1906, at the conclusion of the work in the Simplon Tunnel, he organized the first International Convention on Occupational Diseases, which gave birth to the International Commission of Occupational Health (ICOH).

Devoto's initiatives in this period brought him both approval and criticism. The criticism came from a group of 'maximalist' doctors who belonged to a socialist party. These doctors reproached Devoto for focusing on building hospital structures rather than on creating a service of medical inspectors for factories, who would have been able to enforce laws to protect workers' health. These same doctors criticized the politics and scientific attitude of Devoto and his followers, accusing them of accepting a certain degree of exploitation of workers in order to respect the needs of production and to fuel economic development. This ideological approach accepted a rather slow, gradual approach to the solution of the health and safety problems of factory workers.

Among the important research projects done by Devoto, one must single out the studies regarding effects of dust on the respiratory system and the thorough clinical description of all the phases of lead poisoning, even in its earliest phases. These studies bear witness to the diffusion and impact of occupational illnesses in industrial workers, especially in the period between the two world wars when, under fascism, the 'authoritarian development', that is to say, the second and decisive Italian industrial revolution, took place. Under fascism, to which he seems to have adhered for mere convenience, Devoto continued and intensified the peacekeeping role of his clinic, which flourished thanks to an influx of private donations. A new sister clinic was created in Salice, a spa near Pavia, during this period.

In 1934 Luigi Devoto was named Senator of the Kingdom of Italy. Even after retiring, he continued to use his organizational skills, managing the compound of hospitals to which his 'La Clinica del Lavoro' belonged.

Bibliography

Primary: 1902. *Patologia e clinica del lavoro* (Pavia); 1935. *Medicina del lavoro, conferenze, lezioni scritti* (Milan).

Secondary: Carnevale, Francesco, and Alberto Baldasseroni, 1999. *Mal da lavoro: storia della salute dei lavoratori* (Rome and Bari); Carbonini, Anna, 1982. 'Luigi Devoto e la Clinica del Lavoro di Milano' in Betri, Maria Luisa, and Gigli Marchetti Ada, eds., *Salute e Classi Lavoratrici in Italia dall'Unità al Fascismo* (Milan) pp. 489–516.

Franco Carnevale

DHARMENDRA, K. R. (b. Lahore, India, 1 February 1900; d. Delhi?, India, 10 March 1991), *leprology.*

Dharmendra, the son of a government servant, attended several schools in northern India, as his father had a transferable job. Matriculating from Punjab University, he went on to do his intermediate science course at the Government College, Lahore. After two years of botany honors, Dharmendra began his medical studies at the same college. Following Gandhi's call for a boycott after the Jalianwalla Bagh Massacre (1917), Dharmendra joined the movement and gave up his medical studies for a year. The following year, he returned to medical college and completed his MBBS degree.

He worked in two laboratories in Delhi and Simla before joining the School of Tropical Medicine, Calcutta, in 1928 as an assistant research worker. He began by refining the Zondek-Aschem pregnancy test, followed by work on the preparation of antigens to test the sensitivity of asthma patients. He then moved on to research on pneumococcal typing, and worked out a successful method that fell into disuse after the coming of antibiotics.

The influence of Gandhi and the Indian nationalist movement was to remain with him throughout his life. The spirit of nationalism inspired him to turn to leprosy as his field of specialization in 1935. Dharmendra noticed that there were no Indians occupying senior positions in leprosy research in India. He decided to join the leprosy department at the School of Tropical Medicine, Calcutta, despite his family's strong opposition. He became head of department in 1943, a post he occupied until his retirement in 1955.

Dharmendra spent his initial years as a leprologist investigating clinical and epidemiological aspects of the disease. Around that time, although Mitsuda had developed the *in vivo* lepromin test in Japan, the nature of the active principle in the leprosy bacillus responsible for the positive reaction was unknown. In 1941, working with artificially infected armadillos, Dharmendra went on to discover that the active principle was a protein. Consequently, the 'Dharmendra antigen' used a source different from the Japanese one, and has a definite prognostic value even now.

In 1955 he was appointed the first director of the National Leprosy Control Programme. During this period, Dharmendra standardized forms for keeping systematic records in leprosy centers in India. Following this, he was appointed the director of the Central Leprosy Teaching and Research Institute, Chingleput, Tamil Nadu (1958–66), where he initiated a study of Dapsone chemoprophylaxis in contacts of leprosy patients and found that Dapsone gave only 52 percent protection. Several other studies confirmed his findings, but administrative difficulties made the use of his record-keeping methods difficult initially to implement on a large scale. Their later use contributed to the creation of a systematic database about the disease.

Dharmendra also pioneered the clinical study of traditional Indian cures described in the *Sushruta Samhita*. He identified the cure *tuvarka* mentioned in the text as *Hydnocarpus hightiana*, the plant that yields the traditional cure *chaulmogra*, or Hydnocarpus oil. His two-volume book *Leprosy* (1978, 1985) is still used as a textbook, and includes chapters that discuss ancient Indian systems of classification of leprosy.

Dharmendra served as an adviser to, as well as an expert member of, the leprosy panel of the WHO. From 1943 until 1989 he edited the journal *Leprosy in India* (renamed *Indian Journal of Leprosy*). He was awarded the Damien Dutton Award in 1970 and the International Gandhi Award in 1986.

Bibliography

Primary: 1956. (with Chatterjee, K. R.) 'Prognostic Value of the Lepromin Test in Contacts of Leprosy Cases.' *International Journal of Leprosy* 24: 315–318; 1960. *Notes on Leprosy* (New Delhi, 2nd edn., 1967); 1978. *Leprosy Volume I* (Delhi); 1985. *Leprosy Volume II* (Mumbai); 1989. 'An Autobiographical Sketch: Dr Dharmendra' in *Indian Leprologists Speak Out* (Mumbai) pp. 33–41.

Secondary: Desikan, K. V., and B. R. Chatterjee, 1991. 'Dr Dharmendra: Born, 1-2-1900, died, 10-3-1991.' *Indian Journal of Leprosy* 63: 147–152.

Indira Chowdhury

DICKINSON, ROBERT LATOU (b. Jersey City, New Jersey, USA, 21 February 1861; d. Amherst, Massachusetts, USA, 29 November 1950), *gynecology.*

Robert Latou Dickinson was the son of Horace and Jeannette Latou Dickinson. He attended Brooklyn Polytechnic Institute and was schooled in Germany and Switzerland before studying medicine at Long Island College Hospital, later known as Long Island College of Medicine (MD, 1882). After a brief internship, he practiced in obstetrics and gynecology both privately and at Brooklyn Hospital, a specialty to which he devoted the rest of his career. He also taught at Long Island College Hospital. He married Sarah Truslow, and they had three daughters, one of whom died in infancy.

Dickinson's place in American gynecology and obstetrics is secure, a fact helped by his longevity. His various activities included being secretary to (and a founding member of) the National Committee on Maternal Health, 1923–37; senior vice-president of the Planned Parenthood Federation, 1939–50; president of the Euthanasia Society, 1946–50; and president of the American Gynecological Society, 1920.

Well before Alfred Kinsey, Dickinson began collecting sexual histories from his many patients. Each of his patients was usually required to fill out a four-page questionnaire about family and general health as well as particular illnesses and special symptoms. This questionnaire was augmented with Dickinson's own observations, including an explicit discussion of sexual orientation. Many illnesses that were reported to Dickinson, such as insomnia, menstrual irregularities, and generic pain, were believed to have their roots in sexual problems.

A part of Dickinson's hour-long initial consultation included a series of quick anatomical drawings of the sexual organs of the patient. The first set of five or so sketches was drawn while the patient was on the examining table and included depictions of her uterus, cervix, and vulva. In this activity, Dickinson showed particular artistic skill and accuracy (he would later use these works to build wax models of female anatomy for teaching purposes). The initial drawings of each patient were supplemented during ensuing visits, with up to sixty illustrations being made of a woman's genitals throughout her life, showing various changes brought about by sexual activity, childbirth, and aging.

Dickinson's case histories were extensive. The earliest surviving one is from 1890, with forty-six others taken before 1900—making them valuable historical documents of nonpathological cases. By the end of his career, Dickinson had amassed 5,200 cases, 1,200 of which were from unmarried women. These cases formed the basis of his 200 research papers and five books (all of which are from the twilight of his career). Two of these books were based on collaboration with Lura Beam, who collated his vast archive of case records for the purpose of publication. Dickinson also published an atlas of sexual anatomy, based on his sketches of female anatomy, which included chapters on male genital anatomy, the anatomy of coitus, and the anatomy of contraception (particularly barrier methods). His papers are kept in the Countway Medical Library at Harvard University.

Bibliography

Primary: 1932. (with Beam, Lura) *A Thousand Marriages: A Medical Study of Sex Adjustment* (Baltimore); 1933. *Human Sex Anatomy.* (Baltimore) (rev. edn., 1949); 1934. (with Beam, Lura) *The Single Woman: A Medical Study in Sex Education* (Baltimore).

Secondary: Bullough, Vern, 1994. *Science in the Bedroom* (New York); *DAMB*.

Ivan Crozier

DIETL, JOSEF (b. Podbuze, Galizien, Poland, 24 January 1804; d. Krakow, Poland, 18 January 1878), *medicine, therapeutics.*

After his medical training in Vienna, Dietl worked as a police district physician at Vienna-Wieden from 1832, and from 1841 onward he was 'Primararzt' (chief physician) at the hospital there. In 1851 he was called to the chair of the Medical School at Krakow University. Following his election as Rector of the university, he was suspended by the Vienna Ministry of Education. During the years 1866–74 he served as president of the self-governed 'Republic' of Krakow.

The main emphasis of Dietl's research was on pathological anatomy, clinical chemistry, and balneology; in addition he dealt with hygienic matters (such as the regulation of the river Weichsel) and promoted modern hospital structures. His commitment to political action made him speak up for the self-administration of universities and, later on, to support total Polish national autonomy in educational issues. J. Skoda, C. Rokitansky, and Dietl were the leading figures of the New Vienna School. In German-speaking and other countries he was well-known for his advocacy of limited therapeutic intervention. Great doubts about the therapeutic efficiency of many of the drugs of that time made him plead strongly for practicing, as far as possible, a therapeutical abstinence, known in medical history as 'therapeutic nihilism'. Dietl felt that this abstinence should be applied as long as pathological anatomy and chemistry did not deliver adequate scientific results and well-tested drugs along with substantive therapeutic procedures. His programmatic paper, published in 1845, defended the priority of medical science over medical practice. The task of medicine as natural science should not be to strive for universal remedies and miracle cures. It should rather find out why patients get sick, recover, or die.

Guided by these ideas Dietl continued the tradition of therapeutic skepticism, which was also supported by the clinic of Paris. Above all, he rejected heroic therapies, such as the extensive bloodletting or the continuous use of laxatives. At times, he was falsely accused of propagating naturopathy, in the sense of a self-healing effect of nature (*vis medicatrix naturae*). His justified skepticism toward traditional therapy was supported by statistical examinations on the harmfulness of bloodletting in the treatment of pneumonia. Representatives of competing schools, especially C. A. Wunderlich in Germany, used the term 'therapeutic nihilism' as a bullet, fired against the clinic of Vienna. Within the medical community Dietl agitated for the weak group of university professors and against the powerful group of practical surgeons in Vienna, who through their local college of physicians (*Doktorenkollegium*) occupied essential functions of the Vienna Medical Faculty. In the beginning Dietl did not prove very successful in exploiting the methods of natural science as ideological weapons. The traditionally centralistic and authoritarian structures were still established. It was not until 1848 that Dietl's efforts showed effects and the reform movement got the upper hand. Dietl remained a controversial person, particularly in Austria, in the European medical community in the nineteenth and twentieth centuries. Notably, his strong political commitment to the Polish liberation movement at Krakow induced Vienna to mistrust him. In Poland, however, he is still regarded as a fighter for freedom and a national hero.

Bibliography

Primary: 1845. 'Praktische Wahrnehmungen nach den Ergebnissen im Wiedner-Bezirkskrankenhause' *Zeitschrift der Gesellschaft Aerzte Wien* 1–2: 9–26, 99–113, 186–204, 304–329, 431–465; 1849. *Der Anderlass in der Lungenentzündung* (Vienna).

Secondary: Wiesemann, Claudia, 1995. 'Josef Dietl' in Eckart, Wolfgang U., ed., *Ärztelexikon* (Munich) pp. 109–110; Wiesemann, Claudia, 1991. *Josef Dietl und der therapeutische Nihilismus—Zum historischen und politischen Hintergrund einer medizinischen These* (Frankfurt and Berne).

Wolfgang U. Eckart

DING, FUBAO 丁福保 (AKA TING, FU-PAO; ZHONGHU 仲祜) (b. Wuxi, Jiangsu Province, China, [22nd day of the 6th month, Chinese luni-solar calendar] 3 August 1874; d. Shanghai, China, 28 November 1952), *medicine.*

Ding was a Chinese traditional scholar, famous in the early twentieth century for translating and publishing many textbooks of modern medicine into Chinese. He attended the Nanjing Academy in nearby Jiangyin, a prestigious school established with funds from Governor Zuo Zongtang, an advocate of Western sciences in late nineteenth century China. Ding specialized in mathematics and classical studies in Chinese 'evidential research'. In 1901, he studied briefly at Suzhou University, which was run by American Southern Methodists, but left because he contracted tuberculosis. Instead, he went to Shanghai and recuperated before studying medicine and chemistry at the Jiangnan Arsenal Polytechnic Institute, China's leading government-run school for assimilating Western sciences at the time. He also studied Japanese.

In 1909 Manchu Governor-General Duanfang instituted the first licensing examination for physicians in China. The examination paper required familiarity with the classical texts of elite Chinese medicine as well as proficiency in modern (Western) medicine. Ding was ranked first in the examination, and was therefore chosen to go to Japan to study and report on the modern medical reforms instituted there as part of the Meiji Reformation (1868–1910). With the fall of the last imperial dynasty in China in 1911, Ding lost his powerful mentors, and instead turned to publishing and medical practice to earn his living. Between 1909 and 1921, Ding Fubao translated, collated, and published at least eighty-three medical titles, the majority of which were translations from Japanese works on Western medicine. He also contributed to almost all of the medical journals of the time, so that his writings dominated the market for information about Western medicine. Several of these were published as a series, *Ding's Medical Compendium* (*Ding shi yixue congshu*), which he entered in two competitions run by the League of Nations Health Organization in 1913. The *Compendium* won first prize in both Rome and Berlin. Ding had been able to use his knowledge of Japanese and of Western medicine to succeed in meeting the burgeoning demand for the new sciences. His publishing activities had not only enabled him to survive in the absence of his former mentors; they also made him rich. With his increasing capital, Ding was able to build himself new houses in both Shanghai and Wuxi, give generously to charitable works in Wuxi, and employ many people in his publishing enterprise.

Early in his career, Ding held that Chinese medicine was valuable and should be retained as part of modern China's medical heritage. After visiting Japan, he revised this opinion and rejected Chinese medicine as backward and unscientific. He adopted the Japanese attitude that some of the Chinese herbal pharmacopoeia held useful medicines, but that these should be first isolated, purified, and subjected to clinical trials before further use was made of them. All of the theory of Chinese medicine should be rejected. This alienated those of Ding's colleagues with whom he had previously promoted the modernization of Chinese medicine; his status as a physician of Western medicine was also compromised by his lack of a medical degree. Ding practiced for many years in Shanghai, nonetheless, specializing in the treatment of tuberculosis. His two sons took over the publishing house until the Communist takeover in 1949. Ding died in 1952.

Although he was most prolific in the field of medical studies, Ding Fubao is better remembered today for his work in the tradition of evidential research. Three of his publications remain the standard sinological reference works in their fields: his *Encyclopedic Dictionary of Buddhism* (*Fojiao da cidian*), his *Collected Glosses on the Shuowen Dictionary* (*Shuowen jiezi gulin*), and his *Collected Poetry of the Han, Three Kingdoms, Jin, and Northern and Southern Dynasties Period* (*Quan Han, Sanguo, Jin, Nan, Beichao shi*). Taken together with his medical translations, they are a powerful testimony to the ability of traditional scholars and traditional societies to assimilate new knowledge and technologies rapidly and effectively.

Bibliography

Primary: 1948. *Autobiography of the Retired Scholar of Mathematical Mysteries* (*Chouyin jushi zizhuan*) (Shanghai).

Secondary: Minehan, Bridie Andrews, in press. *The Making of Modern Chinese Medicine* (Cambridge).

Bridie Andrews Minehan

DING, GANREN 丁甘仁 (AKA ZEZHOU 澤周) (b. Menghe, Wujin county, Jiangsu province, China, 8 February 1866; d. Shanghai, China, 6 August 1926), *Chinese medicine.*

Ding Ganren belongs to a small group of scholar-physicians from Wujin who decisively shaped the development of Chinese medicine in early Republican China. Ding Ganren began to study medicine at the age of twelve. Over the next seven years, he studied with various physicians in his hometown, a renowned center of medical excellence. In 1895, Ding Ganren established his medical practice in Suzhou. Unable to compete with more famous local physicians, he moved to Shanghai (1890), where eventually he gained employment at a charitable dispensary for the poor. In 1896, when a scarlet fever epidemic swept Shanghai, Ding Ganren gained a reputation for providing the most successful treatment. This allowed him to establish his own medical practice. He was soon treating members of Shanghai's Chinese business elite, and by the early twentieth century he had become one of Shanghai's most successful and wealthy physicians. Besides his clinical practice, Ding Ganren had an interest in the manufacture and distribution of over-the-counter remedies, exploiting and enhancing his reputation by producing a number of patent medicines.

Following the proclamation of the Chinese Republic in 1911, Ding Ganren began using his wealth and influence to modernize and professionalize Chinese medicine in the medical culture of new China. He was instrumental in establishing the Shanghai Technical College of Chinese Medicine 上海中醫專門學校 in 1916, eventually the most influential institution of its kind in Republican China; many of its graduates became leading figures in the modernization of Chinese medicine during the Republican and Maoist eras.

Supported by other scholar-physicians from Wujin, Ding Ganren promoted new-style 'lecture notes' (*jiangyi* 講義) to complement the reading of classical texts and institutionalized clinical training modeled on internships in Western medical hospitals. For this purpose, he convinced members of the Shanghai business community to fund the construction of the Shanghai North and South Guangyi Chinese Medicine Hospitals 瀘北南廣益中醫醫院, which opened in 1918. The college and affiliated teaching hospitals became the center of activity among physicians in Shanghai practicing Chinese medicine, facilitating the transition of their tradition from one organized around family and lineages into a modern professionalized medicine. To this end, Ding Ganren sponsored the foundation of the Shanghai National Medicine Association 上海市國醫學會 (1921), financed the publication of the *Journal of Chinese Medicine* (*Zhongyi zazhi* 中醫雜志), and participated in establishing the Shanghai Technical College of Chinese Medicine for Women 上海女子中醫專門學校 (1925).

In spite of his prominent role in the modernization of Chinese medicine, Ding Ganren was not a radical innovator. His unique gift was that of networker and synthesizer. His clinical practice and outstanding clinical skills integrated the diverse styles of practice he had assimilated during his studies in Menghe, Suzhou, and Shanghai. This integration of a range of traditions prefigured the systematization of Chinese medicine in Maoist China. The same skills underpinned his success as a professional networker. Under the motto 'developing medical learning, preserving the national essence' (Qiu, 1998, p. 24) he brought together diverse groups whose joint interest was to preserve a space for traditional medicine in a rapidly modernizing society.

Ding Ganren died with many new projects yet unaccomplished.

Bibliography

Primary: 1927. *Menghe Dingshi yi'an* 孟河丁氏醫案 [The Case Records of Mr. Ding from Menghe] (Menghe).

Secondary: Qiu Peiran, ed., 1998. *Mingyi yaolan (Shanghai) zhongyi xueyuan (Shanghai zhongyi zhuanmen xuexiao) xiaoshi* [Cradle of Famous Physicians: The History of the Shanghai College of Chinese Medicine and the Shanghai Technical College of Chinese Medicine] (Shanghai); Yang Xinglin 楊杏林 and Lou Shaolai 樓紹來, 1997. 'Ding Ganren nianbiao' 丁甘仁年表 [A chronology of Ding Ganren's life] *Zhongyi wenxian zazhi* 中醫文獻雜誌 [Journal of Chinese Medicine Literature] 1: 37–40; Huang Wendong 黃文東, 1962. 'Dingshi xueshu liupai de xingcheng he fazhan.' 丁氏學術流派的形成和發展 ['The formation and development of Mr. Ding's learning and trend'] *Shanghai zhongyiyao zazhi* 上海中醫藥雜誌 [Shanghai Journal of Chinese Medicine and Pharmacology] 1: 5–9; Cao Yingfu 曹穎甫, ed., 1927. *Ding Ganren xiansheng zuogu jinian* 甘仁先生作古紀念錄 [A Record of the Commemoration [Service] for Mr. Ding Ganren] (Shanghai).

Volker Scheid

DIOCLES OF CARYSTUS (fl. late fourth century BCE), *medicine.*

Son of the physician Archidamus, Diocles of Carystus was called the 'younger Hippocrates' and was placed by later authorities among the best physicians of his time. Nothing is known about his life and his work is almost entirely lost, but the fragments and titles of numerous works display the typical sophistication and comprehensiveness of learned fourth-century BCE medicine. Diocles combined empiricism with philosophical method, while rejecting speculation. His interests ranged from anatomy, on which he wrote the first treatise, to therapy, prognosis, etiology, surgery and bandaging, fevers and critical days, embryology and gynecology, and pharmacology and pharmacy combined with dietetics or hygiene (poisons, plants with medicinal properties, foodstuffs, anointing, exercise).

One longstanding historical problem has been Diocles' relation to Aristotle, with whom he had intellectual affinities (although neither referred explicitly to the other). They were probably independent, contemporary intellectuals each of whose ideas influenced the other, without either of them being the other's teacher.

Diocles' theory of physiology was humoral. Based on four primary elements and four qualities, it considered that there were four humors: blood, phlegm, yellow bile, and black bile. These were alterations of nutriment, produced in the blood vessels under various degrees of innate heat. Like Alcmaeon, Diogenes, and others, he made much of air (*pneuma*) and, although only hints of his views survive, he contributed to the prominence achieved by this entity in the systematic theories of Hellenistic medicine.

In his theories, there was both *pneuma* originating in the heart and *pneuma* breathed in from outside through cutaneous respiration and respiration through nose and mouth. *Pneuma* traveled through the blood vessels and imparted voluntary motion; when blocked, it caused disease. Apoplexy arose when its flow was disrupted by thick phlegm congealed in the aorta. Fevers developed when the skin-breathed *pneuma* was impeded through the boiling or cooling of the blood produced by excessive bile or phlegm. Pleurisy arose from obstruction in the veins around the pleura, etc.

Diocles' theory of pathology was characterized by the increasing attempt at precision that stimulated medical controversy in the fourth century BCE; he distinguished, for example, between pleurisy and pneumonia. He was concerned with crises and critical days, which he reckoned by multiples of seven; with prognosis and diagnosis; and with the discovery of the relevant internal causal chains. So a humoral excess or deficiency was due to the imbalance of primary elements and produced, in turn, local obstructions of *pneuma*, which led to various diseases. Therapy was a restoration of the natural balance specific to each patient.

In discussing properties of foodstuffs Diocles showed reservations about causes, but this attitude, however qualified, did not make him a proto-Skeptic—he did not, for example, reject the possibility of discovering the causes, or their relevance for therapy. He only warned against naive reductivist methodologies in the search for causes, and qualified by certain limitations the areas in which the search is useful or practicable. In anatomy, Diocles gave more accurate descriptions than his predecessors had of the internal organs, including the gall bladder and the ileocecal valve, and of the blood vessels, although he was unaware of the distinction between arteries and veins. Like Aristotle, he regarded the heart as the source of blood. In embryology and gynecology, he believed, like Diogenes, that the semen was drawn from the brain and spinal marrow, and, like Empedocles, that it derived from both parents (Fragment 183). He described the embryo and held that its full development occurred in forty days. In surgery, he is credited with two inventions: a bandage for the head and a spoon for the extraction of arrowheads.

Bibliography

Primary: Van der Eijk, Philip, ed., 2000–2001. *Diocles of Carystus. A Collection of the Fragments with Translation and Commentary* I–II (Leiden); Wellmann, M., ed., 1901. *Fragmentsammlung der griechischen Ärzte*, I: *Die Fragmente der sikelischen Ärzte Akron, Philistion und des Diokles von Karystos* (Berlin) pp. 117–207.

Secondary: Nutton, V., 2004. *Ancient Medicine* (London) pp. 120–124; Staden, Heinrich von, 1992. 'Jaeger's "Skandalon der historischen Vernunft": Diocles, Aristotle, and Theophrastus' in Calder, W. M., ed., *Werner Jaeger Reconsidered* (Atlanta) pp. 227–265; Staden, Heinrich von, 1989. *Herophilus. The Art of Medicine in Early Alexandria* (New Haven, CT); Harris, C. R. S., 1973. *The Heart and Vascular System in Ancient Greek Medicine* (Oxford); Jäger, W., 1938. *Diokles von Karystos* (Berlin).

Manuela Tecusan

DIOGENES OF APOLLONIA (fl. 435–400 BCE), *natural philosophy, medicine.*

Diogenes of Apollonia, a Pre-Socratic doctor and philosopher, was ridiculed for his doctrines in Aristophanes' *Clouds*, whose dramatic date, 423 BCE, provides the basis for our knowledge of Diogenes' period of activity. Diogenes developed a monistic system in which air (*pneuma*) was the principle of life, the primary constituent of things, and the substrate of change. He argued first that the basic stuff was one, because otherwise change was not possible, and second that everything, including sensation and thought, was derived from air, because air permeated all things and was the basis of life. Diogenes was also the author of the famous 'argument from the order of the universe', later developed by Aristotle in support of teleology. Theophrastus presented (in *De sensibus*) his philosophy as an incoherent mixture of ideas from Leucippus and Anaxagoras, but its main ingredients were derived from Anaximenes and Alcmaeon: inspired by Alcmaeon's analysis of sensation, Diogenes produced a physiological extension of Anaximenes' cosmology, in which the primary stuff was air.

Like Alcmaeon, Diogenes was aware of the brain's connection with cognitive and sensory activity, but did not regard any organ in particular as the single locus of intelligence and sensation, as he reserved that role for *pneuma*. However, the topic of the *hegemonikon* (the ruling force or organ of the body) appeared in later Hellenistic medicine, so scholarly dispute over this point is otiose.

Diogenes held that *pneuma* is drawn directly into the brain when we breathe. Sense-impressions, which travel through it, reach the brain and are received by the inner *pneuma* around it. Thought is produced in a similar way. Its quality depends on the dryness and cleanliness of the air; in drunkenness or sleep, *pneuma* is damp and thought muddled. During intense thought one is unaware of external perceptibles because respiration is suspended and sensation blocked.

There was also hot *pneuma* carried through the vascular system, along with the blood—*pneuma* that Diogenes (like Anaximenes) identified with soul. The causal link between life, consciousness, and *pneuma* made him produce one of the two oldest surviving descriptions of the vascular system, quoted by Aristotle in *Historia animalium*. His was the more detailed one, yet 'based almost entirely on what could be deduced from surface anatomy, and possibly from observing sacrificial victims' (Nutton, 2004). Unaware of the difference between veins and arteries (not known before Praxagoras), Diogenes only recognized the distinction between the cava and the aorta, which he represented as each serving one half of the body. He thought that the source of all vessels was the brain, but he included the heart in his picture, observing that 'two very large [branches]' of the 'two biggest vessels' lead to this organ. He also represented the two vessels as being connected with the uterus and the testicles.

Diogenes was the first to propose a hematogenetic view of the origin of sperm, regarding it as a *spuma sanguinis*—a foamy product of blood's concoction or pneumatization in the spermatic vessels, and hence ultimately derived from (surplus) nourishment. This view, modified and elaborated upon by Aristotle, eliminated its rivals and prevailed both in medicine (Erasistratus, Herophilus) and in philosophy (the Stoics). But Diogenes' original thesis grafted the hematogenetic theory onto the old encephalogenetic model: the seed, he claimed, resulted from blood arriving from the spinal marrow. Hence, its trajectory presupposed the existence of a direct physical channel between spinal marrow and testicles, and this idea (with the implicit links suggested between brain, soul, and embryo) lasted in the medical imagination until the Renaissance.

Diogenes also argued for the significance of bodily colors in diagnosis.

Bibliography

Primary: Diels, H., and W. Kranz, eds., 1964. *Die Fragmente der Vorsokratiker* (Zurich–Berlin), II: 51–69; Kirk, G. S., J. E. Raven, and M. Schofield, eds., 1983. *The Presocratic Philosophers* (Cambridge); Laks, A., ed., 1983. *Diogène d'Appolonie. La dernière cosmologie présocratique* (Lille).

Secondary: Nutton, V., 2004. *Ancient Medicine* (London) pp. 48–49; Staden, Heinrich von, 1989. *Herophilus. The Art of Medicine in Early Alexandria* (Yale) pp. 169–170, 290–294; Hanslik, R., 1970. 'Diogenes' (42) in Pauly, A., and G. Wissowa, eds., *Real-Encyclopädie der classischen Altertumswissenschaft* (Stuttgart), Suppl. XII, coll. 233–236.

Manuela Tecusan

DIONIS, PIERRE (b. ?, 1643; d. Paris, France, 11 December 1718), *surgery.*

Dionis gained his education and credentials at the École of Saint Côme, the guild of surgeons under the official jurisdiction of the Faculty of Medicine. He trained as an apprentice in Paris and then on the king's battlefields. Around 1670 Dionis returned to set up his practice in Paris. In an era when surgery was rising in prestige, Dionis worked in a fiercely competitive medical market and operated not only with other surgeons, but also with physicians, bonesetters, dentists, apothecaries, midwives, and empirics.

His diligence and competence and social skills were rewarded in 1673 when he was named as the demonstrator of public anatomies held in the Jardin du Roi. He introduced anatomical dissections and surgical operations on the cadaver. Intended by the king as free public lectures for medical students, these anatomies proved vastly popular. Given the erratic interest of his physician supervisors, Dionis here got his first taste of teaching and lecturing on the surgical art. He was also struck by the lack of any adequate surgical textbook for students.

In 1680 he surrendered the post at the Jardin du Roi to become a court surgeon at Versailles, for reasons unknown. He claimed as clients several noble persons, including the Dauphines and the duchess of Burgundy. Perceiving correctly that his professional superiors had no time or interest in writing about their expertise, Dionis turned to textbook writing to supplement his income and his prestige. By the time of his death he had published five surgical books, three of which went through numerous posthumous editions, including one on anatomy, one a reference work on operations in general, and one on obstetrics and childbirth. He was among the best accoucheurs at Versailles.

Written in French when most medical texts were still in Latin, Dionis's books were practical, hands-on guides giving technical information about surgical procedures and surgical instruments, accompanied by illustrations. His texts also contained much-appreciated advice to young surgeons on how to pursue their careers. His name is associated with no particular surgical innovation or anatomical discovery, but his textbooks provided a lucid exposition of the surgical knowledge of his day. Dionis taught about the circulation of the blood at a time when the Paris Faculty of Medicine still had not recognized William Harvey's work on the circulation of the blood, and he kept abreast of the anatomical discoveries of others.

His services in providing autopsies for the privileged were early examples of forensic medicine. He cautioned surgeons on the risks of undertaking heroic, but usually fatal, operations such as trepanation, but he believed a well-trained surgeon could significantly improve the health of his patients through competent setting of bones, extraction of foreign objects, suturing of wounds, and well-managed bloodlettings. He was an enthusiastic advocate of bloodletting and believed his countrymen, especially the aristocracy, benefited particularly from this simple procedure, since their rich diet, scorn for physical exercise, and excessive consumption of fine wines made their blood thick and sluggish.

Bibliography

Primary: 1690. *Anatomie de l'homme suivant la circulation du sang et les nouvelles découvertes* (Paris) [with subsequent editions in 1698, 1705, 1716, also with translations into English, Latin, and Chinese]; 1707. *Cours d'opérations de chirurgerie démontrées au Jardin Royal* (Paris, 1707), 1714 [posthumous editions edited and annotated by Georges de la Faye (Paris), 1736, 1740, 1746, 1751, 1765, and 1788, with translations into Flemish (1710), German (1712), and English (1733)]; 1718. *Traite Général des Accouchements Qui Instruit de tout ce qu'il faut faire pour être habile Accoucheur* (Paris) [with subsequent translations in English (1719), Dutch, and German].

Secondary: Guerrini, Anita, 2004. 'Duverney's Skeletons.' *Isis* 94: 577–608; Brockliss, Laurence, and Colin Jones, 1997. T*he Medical World of Early Modern France* (Oxford); Gelfand, Toby, 1980. *Professionalizing Modern Medicine: Paris Surgeons and Medical Science in the Eighteenth Century* (Westport, CT).

Martha Baldwin

DIOSCORIDES (aka PEDANIUS DIOSCORIDES of ANAZARBUS) (b. Anazarbus, Cilicia [now Turkey]; fl. c. 40–80), *botany, medicine, pharmacology.*

Dioscorides (Pedanius) grew up in the Greek milieu of southeastern Asia Minor in the Roman province of Cilicia, and flourished in a period of imperial stability. IIe studied in Alexandria and Tarsus, the latter city being known for teachers who specialized in botany and pharmacy. One of his teachers was Areius of Tarsus, who must have exerted a great influence on him, because the preface to Dioscorides' own work is a dedicatory letter to him. Accounts that place him in Egypt during the time of Cleopatra and Mark Antony may be discounted. He traveled widely within the Empire, and sometimes made forays outside it (to Petra, the ancient Arabian city, now in Jordan, for example) in search of plants and drugs: that he did so as a physician in

the legions is disputed. Dioscorides' claim to have led a 'soldier-like life' is best interpreted as a reference to a limited form of military service, perhaps equivalent to a short-service commission.

Dioscorides' *De materia medica* [Materials of Medicine] consisted of five books, and not only reflected a long tradition in pharmaco-botany but also was the product of an innovative approach to the subject. Dioscorides claimed that, unlike his predecessors, his knowledge of plants was gained in the field, not from books. Dioscorides did consult other authors, and he stated that he utilized the works of seventeen of them. Apart from his mentor and teacher Areius, he mentioned, among others, Sextius Niger (fl. 20 BCE), whose own *De materia medica* is now lost, and Philonides of Catana, born during the principate of Tiberius and with whom Dioscorides agreed on the use of white hellebore. The herbal of Crateuas, physician to Mithridates VI of Pontus (famous for having made himself proof against poisoning), was used approvingly by Dioscorides. Like his own, it too was illustrated. He also utilized Nicander of Colophon's work on toxicology, although Dioscorides does not mention him by name. Dioscorides largely refrained from discussing the various disputes among the medical sects within the Roman Empire. An exception was his criticism of those who, like Niger, were followers of Asclepiades of Bithynia. Dioscorides did not comment on Asclepiades' theories directly, restricting his criticism to Asclepiades' followers by stating that their knowledge of drugs was perfunctory.

Dioscorides listed 700 plants, over 1,000 drugs, and 4,740 medicinal uses for them according to 360 types of action. The work is much more than just an impressive set of lists of drug actions augmented and validated by experience. To Dioscorides, pharmacology was not simply an empirical skill in preparing medications, but was also literally 'reasoning about drugs', and a central part of medicine. Dioscorides was more than just an herbalist, root-cutter, or maker or purveyor of medicaments, although he must have been adept in these skills. His aim was a comprehensive synthesis of all pharmaco-botanical knowledge. A further, crucial, refinement lay in Dioscorides' method of organizing this vast amount of data. Unlike his predecessors, who arranged their information either alphabetically or by a set of biological characteristics, Dioscorides ordered his material according to category (type of animal and plant, their parts and products, earths and minerals). In each category, the drugs made from each source were then listed according to the reactions they produced, which were due to the unique property each drug possessed. This has been called arrangement by 'drug affinities', but Dioscorides was never explicit on this point, and later writers found it easier to rearrange the work alphabetically. Nevertheless, even with his originality obscured, Dioscorides' work was widely used until the Renaissance and remains the best work of its kind antiquity produced.

Bibliography

Primary: Wellmann, Max, 1906–14. (reprinted 1958) *Pedanii Dioscuridis Anazarbei De materia medica libri quinque* (Berlin).

Secondary: Riddle, John, 1985. *Dioscorides on Pharmacy and Medicine* (Austin, TX); Scarborough, John, and Vivian Nutton, 1982. 'The *Preface* of Dioscorides' *Materia Medica*: Introduction, Translation, and Commentary.' *Transactions of the College of Physicians of Philadelphia* 5(4): 187–227.

Julius Rocca

DIX, DOROTHEA LYNDE   (b. Hampden, Maine, USA, 4 April 1802; d. Trenton, New Jersey, USA, 17 July 1887), *psychiatric reform.*

Dix, daughter of Joseph Dix and Mary Bigelow, was a layperson who exercised enormous influence on the establishment of lunatic asylums in nineteenth-century America and in the process did much to establish the nascent specialty of psychiatry.

Dix's father was the black sheep of a prosperous Massachusetts merchant family. Exiled to the frontier of Maine, Joseph further disgraced himself in the eyes of his family by becoming an itinerant, impoverished Methodist preacher, his economic circumstances worsened by his persistent intemperance. In the midst of a nightmarish childhood, Dix fled her parents in 1815, taking refuge with her widowed grandmother in the family mansion in Boston. After spending a year there, she then left to care for her siblings in the home of her grandmother's niece in Worcester, Massachusetts. There, she opened a school, which she ran until she returned to Boston in 1820.

An immensely serious and deeply religious woman, Dix now lived for almost two decades with her grandmother in an emotionally deprived and sterile environment. Intermittently depressed and an invalid, she blamed her weak constitution on her parents. In 1821 she had resumed her career as a schoolmistress, establishing a small charity school in her grandmother's house. Dix wrote a common school reader, *Conversations on Common Things* (1824), which enjoyed a considerable commercial success, going through sixty editions before the Civil War, and this was followed by a series of religious books aimed at children.

Influenced by William Ellery Channing, Dix became a Unitarian, adopting the view that it was her Christian duty to assist the poor and the downtrodden. Ultimately, it was this religiously motivated drive that would lead her into a crusade in behalf of the mentally ill, work that dominated her life for two decades in the 1840s and 1850s, and marked her as the most successful female actor in the political arena in nineteenth-century America. The crusade followed a period of depression and mental instability in the late 1830s; a visit to England, where she first encountered reformed lunatic asylums run on moral treatment lines; and the death of her grandmother, which seems to have had a liberating impact on Dix, besides rendering her financially independent.

In 1841 she began an investigation of the condition of lunatics in Massachusetts that two years later led to the publication of her first memorial on the subject to a state legislature, denouncing their neglect and mistreatment and demanding legislative intervention. In subsequent years, this became her life's work, and she traveled the length and breadth of the United States, descending on a state, searching for local scandals, inventing them if necessary, and lobbying state legislatures for funds to establish an asylum run along modern lines. Again and again she proved successful, even in the Deep South, where a Yankee intruder (let alone a woman desiring access to the political arena) would ordinarily have been scorned. It helped that while urging the need to relieve the sufferings of the mentally ill, Dix remained utterly blind to the evils of slavery, increasingly the object of abolitionist agitation in her native New England. Beginning with the State Asylum in New Jersey (an institution she later referred to as her first-born child), Dix enjoyed an almost uninterrupted string of successes, as cynical politicians were worn down by her singlemindedness. Her political influence extended to the power to place particular medical men into jobs as asylum superintendents, and in 1854 she even secured the passage of legislation to provide federal funding for the mentally ill, only to have it vetoed by President Franklin Pierce.

Thereafter, Dix seems to have lost her way. In 1855 she visited Britain and, hearing that Scotland had lagged behind in asylum provision, rushed northward. Dix employed her well-honed political skills, and soon forced Westminster to pass reform legislation, even in the face of widespread opposition from the Scots. It would be her last hurrah. The outbreak of the Civil War in America saw this formidable woman appointed as Superintendent of Women Nurses for the Union Army, self-consciously following in the footsteps of Florence Nightingale (1820–1910). In this role she was a disaster. Impatient, eccentric, authoritarian, and with no talent for administration, she was sidelined by the end of 1863.

The number and size of asylums continued to grow in the post–Civil War era. Dix traveled, and was heaped with honors. By 1881, aged seventy-nine, she was in serious decline, and moved to specially constructed quarters in the New Jersey State Lunatic Asylum at Trenton, where she lived until her death six years later.

Bibliography

Primary: 1971. *On Behalf of the Insane Poor; Selected Reports* (New York).

Secondary: Browne, Thomas J., 1998. *Dorothea Dix: New England Reformer* (Cambridge, MA); Gollaher, David, 1995. *Voice for the Mad: The Life of Dorothea Dix* (New York); *DAMB*.

Andrew Scull

DJORDJEVIĆ, VLADAN GEORGEVIC (b. Belgrade, Serbia, 3 December 1844; d. Baden, Austria, 31 August 1930), *surgery, military surgery, medicine, public health, history of medicine, politics.*

Vladan, the son of Georgios and Maria Djordjević, was descended from a Greek or Armenian family, which was not atypical among the early nineteenth century urban population of Serbia. His father had been an assistant physician at a military hospital. Djordjević attended medical school in Vienna, where he studied with Hyrtl, Bruecke, Skoda, Hebra, and others; Billroth had been his mentor for his surgical specialization. Two years after graduation in 1869, Djordjević became Serbia's first surgeon. In 1871 he volunteered for the Franco-Prussian War, and was appointed a medical lieutenant in the Prussian army reserves. Upon his return, he was assigned as a chief of the surgery ward at Belgrade Military Hospital. Djordjević later established a chair for military hygiene and surgery at the Artillery School, which at the time was only the second such military education institution in Europe.

Djordjević was a founder of the Serbian Medical Society (1872), the oldest such association in the Balkans, and of the Red Cross of Serbia (1876). In 1874 he began publishing Serbia's first medical magazine, *Srpski Arhiv za Celokupno Lekarstvo*. Rising to distinction, Djordjević served as personal physician to the Serbian Prince (later King) Milan, as well as head of the Sanitary Units within the Supreme Command of the Serbian army during wars with Turkey (1876–1878) and Bulgaria (1885).

In 1879, as a head of the Sanitary Department of the Interior Ministry, Djordjević undertook reform of the civilian medical system. He wrote comprehensive draft laws on health care and medicine, for which he campaigned in parliament using his extraordinary rhetorical skills. Most notably, his 'Law of Sanitary Funds' took the unprecedented step of providing an independent operating budget for the health care system. Another of Djordjević's legal initiatives, the 'Law Concerning the Regulation of the Sanitary Profession and Protection of the People's Health' (1881), provided for proportional distribution of physicians throughout the country and introduced a licensing system for physicians as well as regulatory controls over their work. This law emphasized prevention work, and established obligatory vaccinations and revaccinations against smallpox; it also regulated the education of medical assistants, midwives, and the quarantine system. Elected mayor of Belgrade in 1884–85, Djordjević sought to improve medical facilities in the city, but resigned after political quarrels. He later served as minister of education and economy, as envoy to Athens and Istanbul, and later as prime minister (1897–1900).

Djordjević's bibliography of published works contains roughly 170 items, including a book on the history of military medicine in Serbia, a book on folk medicine in Serbia, and several books on history and literature.

Bibliography

Primary: 1872. *Narodna medicina u Srba* [Folk Medicine in Serbia] (Belgrade); 1879, 1880, 1886, 1893. *Istorija srpskog vojnog saniteta* (Belgrade); 1905. 'Das Ende der Obrenowitsch.' *Beitrage zur Geschichte Serbiens 1897–1900* (Leipzig); 1910. *Ministarstvo narodnog zdravlja—prilog za istoriju sanitetske reforme u Srbiji 1879–1910* (Belgrade).

Secondary: Rajić, Suzana, 2005. 'Dr Vladan Đorđević—biografija pouzdanog obrenovićevca.' PhD thesis, Univerzitet U Beogradu, Filozofski Fakultet; Subotić, Vojislav, 1910. *Dr Vladan Đorđević—pedesetogodišnjica književnog rada* (Belgrade).

Jelena Jovanovic Simic and
Predrag J. Markovic

DOBROSLAVIN, ALEKSEI PETROVICH (b. Diad'kovo, Orlov province [now Briansk oblast'], Russia, 29 September [11 October] 1842; Petersburg, 4 December [16 December] 1889), *experimental and military hygiene, public health.*

After finishing Kaluga gymnasium, Dobroslavin was admitted in 1859 to the Medical-Surgical Academy in Petersburg where he stood out as a student of chemistry Professor N. N. Zinin. He graduated in 1865 but remained in the therapeutic clinic for his residency.

From 1866 onward he was occupied exclusively in laboratory-experimental activities, defending his dissertation in 1868, 'Materialy dlia fiziologii metamorfoza (obmen veshchestv)' [Materials for the Physiology of Metamorphosis (exchange of substances)], and simultaneously sent abroad by the academy with the aim of receiving further training in hygiene. He was back in Petersburg as a sessional lecturer from 1871, an adjunct-professor from 1872, and an ordinary professor from 1876 in the department of hygiene of the Medical-Surgical Academy.

He was the first professor in Russia to specialize in hygiene as an independent subject. Dobroslavin began giving lectures for fourth-year students in November 1871, an important date in the development of experimental hygiene in Russia. From 1872 to 1882 he taught hygiene in upper-level women's courses in Petersburg.

He created a hygiene laboratory in 1872, expanding it in 1883 and again in 1888, when it became the first analytical station in Russia for research into foodstuffs (with the purpose of fighting their adulteration).

Dobroslavin created a scientific school of hygienists in Russia, with a series of his students and colleagues later heading their own departments of hygiene. He directed a total of nearly 100 dissertations. He was the author of fundamental leading works on hygiene: *Ocherki osnov sanitarnoi deiatel'nosti* [Studies of bases of sanitary activities] (1874–76) and *Gigiena. Kurs obshchestvennogo zdravookhraneniia* [Hygiene. A course for public health] (1882–84).

The distinctive characteristics of Dobroslavin's scientific creativity were its multisidedness and universality, its erudition on the basis of laboratory experiments, and his energetic attempts to put science in the service of the health and life of the people and to introduce them to everyday medical-sanitary activity.

He joined the staff of the Military Medical Academic Committee in 1884 and headed the commission to rationalize nutrition in the Russian army. Dobroslavin became closely acquainted with the conditions of everyday life for the armed forces, the results of which became the articles 'Kakovy teper' kazarmy i kakimi oni dolzhny byt' [How the barracks are now and how they should be] (1873), 'Lager' i ego gigienicheskie usloviia' [The camp and its hygienic conditions] (1876), and others. In the course of the Russo-Turkish War of 1877–78 he struggled with epidemics in the armed forces, developed a series of sanitary-hygienic requirements, and suggested new disinfection apparatuses. He was the author of the two-volume textbook *Kurs voennoi gigieny* [Course for Military Hygiene] (1885–87).

From 1879 to the end of his life Dobroslavin headed the sanitary section of the main prison of the Ministry of Internal Affairs, publishing a series of articles on the nutrition and transportation of prisoners, and sanitary-prison statistics. In 1883 he completed a visit to Tomsk for the study of the transportation and medical servicing of prisoners.

To familiarize himself with the sanitary institutions and urban economies of the largest cities of Europe, Dobroslavin visited abroad, about which he wrote 'Ob uspekhakh gigieny za granitsei v poslednie gody' [About the successes of hygiene abroad in recent years] (1875), 'Zdravookhranenie Evropy v 1882 g.' [Public health in Europe in 1882], and other works. He visited hygiene exhibitions in Berlin in 1883 and in Warsaw in 1887, then took part in the International Hygiene Congress in Vienna, where he gave a speech on disinfection.

Dobroslavin helped liquidate an outbreak of plague in Vetlianka, province of Astrakhan, generalizing this experience in the article 'Chuma v Vetlianke i nash karantinnyi ustav s medico-politseiskoi tochki zreniia' [The plague in Vetlianka and our quarantine regulations from a medical policing point of view].

One of the founders of the Russian Society for the Protection of Public Health (1877), he chaired the section on the problem of public health, and permanently chaired the sanitary commission of the St Petersburg provincial council. He was one of the organizers and activists of the first three Pirogov congresses of Russian doctors. He worked actively on the St Petersburg municipal council on problems of welfare, water supply, and sanitation of the city; the organization of cemeteries; the organization of disinfection and the struggle with epidemics; sanitary-nutritional observation; and the planning of the construction of schools and hospitals. Through the active participation of Dobroslavin, the 'first normal cafeteria' with a school of culinary arts was opened in Petersburg in 1888.

He was the founder (1874) and editor of *Zdorov'e*, the first journal on popular hygiene in Russia. Persuaded of the impossibility of keeping the profile and orientation of the journal, Dobroslavin in 1884 was compelled to resign from it, paying off significant editorial debts from his personal means.

Bibliography

Primary: 'Letter from A. P. Dobroslavin to K. Saint-Hilaire' in Rossiiskaia gosudarstvennaia biblioteka [The Russian state library] 1879. F. Dost./II, op. 3, d. 31. (Moscow).

Secondary: Anon., 1998. *Professors of the Military-Medical (Medical-Surgical) Academy* (St Petersburg); Belitskaia, E. Ia., 1966. *A. P. Dobroslavin i razvitie eksperimental'noi i obshchestvennoi gigieny v Rossii* [A. P. Dobroslavin and the Development of Experimental and Social Hygiene in Russia] (Leningrad); Anon., 1891. *Biografiia professora A. P. Dobroslavin* [The Biography of Professor A. P. Dobroslavin] (St Petersburg).

Mikhail Poddubnyi

DOCK, GEORGE   (b. New Hope, Pennsylvania, USA, 1 April 1860; d. Pasadena, California, USA, 30 May 1951), *pathology, medicine.*

Dock was the son of Gilliard Dock, owner of a machine shop and superintendent of a coal mine, and Lavinia Lloyd Bombough. He obtained his BA from the University of Pennsylvania (Penn) in 1881. Upon graduation, Dock began his medical studies, completing Penn's three-year medical course in 1884. He honed his clinical and conversational German skills while he interned at St Mary's, a Catholic hospital in Philadelphia. Dock then took an eighteen-month trip to Austria and Germany. He studied bacteriology under Becker, gross and microscopic pathological anatomy under Virchow, and pathology under Paltauf and Weigert. During this trip, Dock incorporated pathological laboratory methods and procedures into his diagnostic armamentarium. Meanwhile, William Osler, professor of clinical medicine at the University of Pennsylvania, and John Herr Musser established a clinical pathology laboratory at Penn. At Osler's request, Dock returned in 1887 to become head of the lab. Throughout his professional career, he sought to apply clinical pathology to medical diagnosis.

In 1888 Dock left Philadelphia to become professor of pathology at the Texas Medical School in Galveston. Three years later, he went to Ann Arbor, where the University of Michigan Medical School was in the midst of curricular reorganization. Dean Victor Vaughan sought to incorporate laboratory science and clinical medicine within the same institution and recruited Dock to be professor of internal medicine.

When Dock arrived, Michigan's teaching hospital was under construction. The hospital had neither classrooms nor laboratories: Dock's first clinical laboratory was in a ten-by-ten-foot bathroom. In 1899 he introduced a program of clinical instruction at Michigan in which medical students provided direct patient care under faculty supervision. The Michigan program was comparable to the clinical clerkship that Osler implemented at Johns Hopkins in 1895. All fourth-year medical students at Michigan were required to attend Dock's clinical demonstrations. Held each Tuesday and Friday afternoon, Dock stressed the importance of recording a patient's medical history and performing a thorough physical examination.

In 1908 Dock left Michigan for Tulane University. Throughout his tenure at Michigan, he had called for a central clinical laboratory for the hospital, to no avail. Vaughan had also attempted to move the clinical years of the program to Detroit, much to the disapproval of Dock and other faculty members. Dock's relationship with Vaughan fractured, and Dock left. Tulane had access to the nine-hundred-bed Charity Hospital, a facility with a capacity seven-fold that of Michigan's. Dock's tenure at Tulane was quite short, and in 1910 he left Tulane to become dean and professor of internal medicine at Washington University in St Louis, Missouri. Although his deanship was short-lived, ending in 1912, Dock maintained a substantial internal medical service. In 1922 Dock resigned from Washington University and entered private practice in Pasadena, California.

Dock was also a noted bibliophile, collecting numerous rare medical texts. In 1892 Vaughan named Dock chairman of the library committee at Michigan. He also played an integral role in organizing the new medical library at Washington University. Dock was a member of the Medical Library Association and served as its president from 1906 until 1909. He left more than 1,500 volumes to the Los Angeles County Medical Society.

Dock married Laura McLemore in 1882 and had two children with her; their marriage ended with her death. Dock remarried in 1927. His second marriage, to Miriam Gould, was childless.

Bibliography

Primary: 1902. *Outlines for Case Taking as Used in the Medical Clinic of the University of Michigan* (Ann Arbor).

Secondary: Davenport, Horace, 1993. 'George Dock at Michigan, 1891–1908' in Howell, Joel, ed., *Medical Lives and Scientific Medicine at Michigan, 1891–1969* (Ann Arbor) pp. 29–44; Davenport, Horace, 1987. *Doctor Dock: Teaching and Learning Medicine at the Turn of the Century* (New Brunswick); Hermann, George, 1924. *Methods in Medicine: The Manual of the Medical Service of George Dock, M.D., D.Sc.* (St Louis); *DAMB*.

Todd M. Olszewski

DOCK, LAVINIA LLOYD (b. Harrisburg, Pennsylvania, USA, 26 January 1858; d. Chambersburg, Pennsylvania, USA, 17 April 1956), *nursing*.

Dock was a leader in forming nursing organizations, a historian of nursing, a settlement house worker, and a suffragist. She was the second of the six children of Gilliard and Lavinia Lloyd Bombaugh Dock who were descendants of early Pennsylvania German settlers. The family was financially comfortable; Lavinia attended a girls' academy in Harrisburg. At age twenty-eight she read, in *Century* magazine, of the Bellevue Hospital Training School for Nurses in New York City. After completing its program in 1886, she went into practice, which ultimately included service during a yellow fever epidemic in Florida.

In 1890 she published her first book, *Materia Medica for Nurses,* which became the standard text on pharmaceuticals for a generation of nurses. That same year she moved to Baltimore, Maryland, to become assistant superintendent of nurses at the Johns Hopkins Training School for Nurses, where she became allied with Isabel Hampton (Robb) and Adelaide Nutting. She left Hopkins in 1893 to become superintendent at the Illinois Training School in Chicago, a position she resigned after two years.

In 1896, after a year at home in Harrisburg, Dock took up residence at the Henry Street Settlement on the Lower East Side in New York City. Here she would remain for almost twenty years. The settlement nurses were independent practitioners and involved themselves in all aspects of health, from direct care to teaching to social advocacy. Dock came to know many Progressives, trade unionists, and radical philosophers, such as Peter Kropotkin. She became an activist in the labor movement and an ally of Leonora O'Reilly, who worked on labor rights for women. Dock also advocated for protection of women from sexual abuse, publishing *Hygiene and Morality* in 1910.

Dock saw organization of women as the route to freedom of thought and action. She was secretary of the Society of Superintendents for its first five years and was instrumental in the founding of the International Council of Nurses (1899), serving as its secretary for twenty-three years. In these capacities she became a main conduit of information within the emerging occupation of nursing. In the *American Journal of Nursing,* her column 'Foreign Department' reported on progress in nursing, public health, suffrage, and social issues around the world.

The four-volume *History of Nursing,* begun in 1907 and completed in 1912, was a deliberate effort on the part of Dock and her colleague Adelaide Nutting to place modern nursing in the best possible historical light. It is a monumental collection of information and photographs depicting nursing and women's work as essential to modern life. Dock wrote all but two chapters.

Dock gave up her nursing practice around 1908 and focused more energy on the suffrage movement. She demonstrated, was jailed three times, and tried to arouse her nursing colleagues to the urgency of the vote. She was a severe critic of war, a supporter of birth control, and, later, an advocate of Roosevelt's 'New Deal'.

In 1922 Dock returned home to live with her four sisters, but she continued writing. Unfortunately, much of her correspondence is lost; she destroyed her papers late in life, believing (correctly) that she was under surveillance by the Federal Bureau of Investigation. Dock was a guest of honor at the International Council of Nurses' first postwar meeting in 1947. At age eighty-nine, her enthusiasm, humor, and resistance to eulogy charmed the audience. Dock fell and broke her hip in 1956 and died soon after of pneumonia.

Bibliography

Primary: 1890. *Materia Medica for Nurses* (New York and London); 1907–12. (with Nutting, Adelaide) *A History of Nursing* 4 vols. (New York and London).

Secondary: Estabrooks, Carole A., 1995. 'Lavinia Lloyd Dock: The Henry Street Years.' *Nursing History Review* 3: 143–172; James, Janet Wilson, ed., 1985. *A Lavinia Dock Reader* (New York and London); *DAMB*.

Joan E. Lynaugh

DODONAEUS, REMBERTUS (aka DODOENS, REMBERT)

(b. Mechlin, Belgium, 29 June 1517; d. Leiden, the Netherlands, 10 March 1585), *botany, medicine, cosmography.*

Descended from a Frisian family, Dodoens was born in Mechlin as the son of Denis Dodoens and Urssula Roelands. In 1530 Rembert matriculated at Leuven University. After studying cosmography, geography, medicine, and botany there, he became a licentiate on 10 September 1535. After that, he sampled the universities of France, Italy, and Germany. On returning to his place of birth, he was appointed town physician. In 1557 Dodonaeus turned down an invitation to become professor of medicine at Leuven University. Between 1568 and 1572, negotiations to become court physician to the Spanish king Philip II—as the successor of Vesalius—led to nothing, as Dodonaeus preferred to continue his research in Mechlin. In 1572 his wife, Katrien de Bruyn, died. In the same year, Dodonaeus lost all his possessions when Mechlin was plundered by Spanish troops. It is perhaps for these reasons that the Habsburg emperor Maximilian II did succeed in appointing Dodonaeus court physician in 1574. After the emperor's death two years later, Dodonaeus continued to serve Maximilian's successor, Rudolph II. In 1580 Dodonaeus left Vienna, his mind set on returning to his place of birth. However, a second plundering of Mechlin made him go into exile in Cologne. In 1581, he decided to settle in Antwerp, presumably to be close to his new publisher, Christoffel Plantijn. The very same year, he accepted an invitation to become professor of medicine and botany at the newly founded Leiden University, where he was to spend only a few years. In 1593 he was succeeded by Carolus Clusius (1526–1609), his friend, colleague, and French translator.

Although Dodonaeus published on cosmography as well as on medical casuistry—and had a fine reputation as a practicing physician—he became famous for his groundbreaking botanical work. It was perhaps the commercial success of *De stirpium historia* by Leonardt Fuchs (published in 1542) that caused the Antwerp publisher Jan Vanderloe to suggest that Dodoens publish a similar book. He accepted the invitation and spent the rest of his life striving for the perfect botanical work. In 1554 his *Cruijdeboeck* was published. In order to give it a wide readership (apart from physicians and apothecaries, he was also aiming for the interested layman), he decided to write it in the vernacular.

It was Dodonaeus's ambition to rely on his own observation rather than on accepted knowledge of classical authors like Dioscorides, Theophrastus, Pliny, and Galen. He wanted to study plants in their own habitat. As a result, he added many native plants to the collection that the classics had provided. Still more important were his attempts to classify plants. Before Dodonaeus, it had been quite common to order plants alphabetically. This could hardly be called a systematic procedure, if only because botanical nomenclature was far from unequivocal. Dodonaeus suggested six plant categories. Of each plant, he described the different varieties, its parts, and its growth and inflorescence. Furthermore, he indicated where they grew, when they blossomed, and what medicinal value they had. Last but certainly not least, Dodonaeus was keen on including as many true-to-life renderings of the plants he described. Therefore, all editions of the book were lavishly illustrated.

The book was very well received, and between 1554 and 1644 many editions and translations (into French, English, and Latin) were published. Each edition was an improved and extended version of the original, textually as well as pictorially. Dodonaeus can be said to have accomplished for botany (together with Carolus Clusius and Mathias Lobelius) what Andreas Vesalius contributed to anatomy, that other descriptive discipline.

Bibliography

Primary: 1554. *Cruijdeboeck, in den welcken die gheheele historie, dat es tgheslacht, tfatsoen, naem, natuere, cracht ende werkinghe, van den cruyden, . . . begrepen ende verclaert es* (Antwerp) [Translated from the French edition by Clusius into English by Henry Lyte in 1578 as *A Nievve Herbal or Historie of Plantes* (London)]; 1581. *Medicinalium observationum exempla rara, recognita et aucta* (Cologne); 1583. *Stirpium historiae pemptades sex* (Antwerp).

Secondary: Sloover, Jean Louis de, 1997. *Hépatiques, mousses et muscinées. Des livres de simples (1554–1644) de Rembert Dodoens* (Namur); Meerbeeck, P. J. van, 1841/1980. *Recherches historiques et critiques sur la vie et les ouvrages de Rembert Dodoens (Dodonæus)* (Mechelen; reprint Utrecht); *DSB*.

Jean Louis De Sloover

DOLL, WILLIAM RICHARD SHABOE (b. Hampton, Middlesex, England, 28 October 1912; d. Oxford, England, 24 July 2005), *epidemiology.*

Born to a father who was a general practitioner, Richard Doll was educated at Westminster School, London (where his contemporaries included the spy Kim Philby). He had intended to become a mathematician, and sat for an open scholarship at Trinity College, Cambridge. The night before his final paper, however, he was treated by some friends to a liter and a half of strong college ale (eight percent alcohol) and was muddleheaded the next morning. He was offered the lesser award of an exhibition to the college, but rejected this out of pique, deciding instead to follow his father's wish and enter medicine. This began a lifelong immersion in medicine, and Doll was subsequently to describe the ale as the best drink of his life.

Qualifying from St Thomas's Hospital Medical School, London, in 1937, Doll became a junior doctor in the hospital's accident and emergency department and subsequently a house physician there. He then undertook an unpaid research post at the Postgraduate Medical School (PMS), London, but became convinced that laboratory research was not for him. In any case he was called up for service in the RAMC. He had earlier abandoned his pacifism, and with strong left-wing views (he had participated in the 1936 Jarrow March of unemployed workers, had become a member of the Communist Party, and to the fury of the dean had helped to start the St Thomas's Socialist Society), he had joined the reserve after the Munich crisis.

Initially Doll served in France, taking part in the Dunkirk evacuation, and then in the Middle East and on a hospital ship in the Mediterranean. In 1944 he was found to have tuberculosis of a kidney, and, though the aircraft to Britain was full, Doll shamed a senior officer into giving up a seat for which he had no priority by threatening to publicize the officer's refusal to yield it. He spent six months in convalescence as a psychiatrist but claimed that this was too arduous for him. Nevertheless, it was not easy to find another job, for John McMichael (1904–93), at the PMS, refused to have Doll back to his old department because he was a Communist. Through an old acquaintance, Joan Faulkner, who was a staff member at the Medical Research Council (MRC) and whom he would marry in 1949, he obtained a research post at the Central Middlesex Hospital, London, with the distinguished gastroenterologist Francis Avery Jones (1910–98). The task was to investigate the etiology of peptic ulcer. Not only was the popular idea of the cause of gastric or duodenal ulcers—overwork or stress—untrue, Doll showed, but the conventional treatment with milk and soft foods was useless, with only three factors important in cure: bed rest, stopping smoking, and licorice preparations. Doll employed his mathematical bent—as a student he had shown statistically that one surgeon's favorite method of treating undescended testes was useless—and in 1947 he attended a brief course on statistical ideas and

methods given by Austin Bradford Hill (1897–1991). Hill was greatly impressed by Doll's work on peptic ulcer, and in 1948 he offered Doll a post in the unit at the London School of Hygiene and Tropical Medicine, specifically to help in investigating the alarming rise in cancer of the lung.

In the earlier part of the twentieth century, cancer of the lung had been a rarity. Nevertheless, by the late 1940s Britain had the highest rate of this tumor in the world, and in 1950 it was for the first time causing more deaths annually (13,000) than tuberculosis. Prompted by Percy Stocks (1889–1974), the chief government statistician, the MRC asked Hill to investigate the cause. Initially, this was thought to be due to atmospheric pollution, such as smuts from burning coal, car exhaust fumes, or tar from road surfaces (Doll's own favorite hypothesis).

The preliminary study, carried out in twenty London hospitals, was based on a questionnaire administered by social workers to 650 patients with suspected cancer of the lung, liver, or bowel. The results were clear-cut: those with lung cancer proved to be heavy cigarette smokers; those with other conditions were not. Though previous anecdotal research in Germany and the United States had hypothesized a link between the two, smoking was such a universal and apparently harmless activity (80 percent of British men were smokers) that the Secretary of the MRC, Sir Harold Himsworth (1905–93), urged caution on Doll and Hill, suggesting that before they published their unexpected results they should replicate them in provincial cities, lest the phenomenon be restricted to London. Not that such urging was needed: throughout their lives both men were instinctively cautious, and Doll often waited for further results before coming down on one side of a fence or the other.

Thus other, similar studies were set up in Bristol, Cambridge, Leeds, and Newcastle. Nevertheless, while this was under way Doll and Hill's priority was snatched from them by the publication in the *Journal of the American Medical Association* of a less rigorous study that had similar findings. Doll and Hill therefore persuaded the *British Medical Journal* to publish their original paper quickly, which it did in 1950. Another initiative was to set up in the following year a rigorous survey—a prospective study of 34,439 male British doctors. Not only were these doctors willing to document their smoking habits, but, given their need to stay on the *Medical Register* to qualify as practitioners, the group was easy to keep track of, and in those who died the cause could be established fairly easily.

Although in the first twenty-nine months of the study there were only thirty-six lung cancer deaths, after four years there had been 200, all but three in heavy smokers. Importantly also, several other conditions were found to be linked with heavy smoking—among them emphysema, coronary disease, and cancer of the kidney and urinary bladder. Given that follow-up of the doctors was so easy, the 1951 study continued for much longer than originally anticipated, with the doctors providing information about any changes in smoking habits in 1957, 1966, 1971, 1978, 1991, and 2001, when the study concluded. The respective findings were published after each survey, with the final ones presented at a celebratory meeting at the RCP London (June 2004) near the fiftieth anniversary of the first publication by a sprightly Richard Doll (who had had a cardiac pacemaker inserted only a few months previously). The conclusions were that men born between 1900 and 1930 who smoked only cigarettes and continued smoking throughout their lives, died on average about ten years younger than lifelong nonsmokers. The excess mortality chiefly involved vascular, neoplastic, and respiratory diseases that could be caused by smoking. Those who gave up smoking at age sixty, fifty, forty, and thirty improved their life expectancy by, respectively, about three, six, nine, or ten years.

At first Doll was reluctant to crusade on the basis of these findings, agreeing with Hill that the epidemiologist's task was to present rigorously analyzed data and to let society and individuals draw their own conclusions and actions. Similarly, epidemiologists had to choose their language very carefully in the discussion sections of their articles. Later, however, Doll was less reluctant to speak out about smoking, and in the 1990s was prominent in the campaign for a government ban on tobacco advertising. And in any case, apart from continuing to work at the Central Middlesex Hospital, Doll—who in 1961 had been appointed to succeed Hill as director of the MRC's statistical unit—branched out into other research topics. An important initial study was into the effects of radiation, whether from the atomic bomb, on babies whose mothers who had had diagnostic radiation during pregnancy, or in patients with ankylosing spondylitis who had been given radiotherapy. He refuted conclusively the concept of a threshold for radiation dosage below which it had no effect: there was, in fact, a linear relationship between damage and the most minimum of levels. Other studies tackled the side-effects of the contraceptive pill, with its increased risk of venous thrombosis; the link between blue asbestos and mesothelioma in asbestos workers, for which Doll devised a new man-years method of calculating expected numbers; and, later, the damage caused by contaminated rapeseed cooking oil in Spain.

These and other projects were continued when in 1969 Doll became Regius professor of medicine at Oxford. Here he helped develop the burgeoning undergraduate medical school and the clinical trials service, while he was much in demand as an expert witness in legal cases and as a member, and often chairman, of expert committees. Among the latter was one that provided reassurance against the fear that living near strong electromagnetic fields (for example, under power lines) caused leukemia.

Retiring from the chair in 1979, Doll set up a new Oxford college, becoming its first warden. Named after its main benefactor, Cecil Green (1900–2003, a British-born chairman of Texas Instruments), this aimed at providing a base for the many senior health personnel who lacked a college or university appointment. At first the undergraduate members of Green College were mostly medical students—a feature attracting much local criticism—but later the college became more broadly based and an acknowledged success. In particular, many praised the hard work of Doll, and especially his wife, in restoring the old Radcliffe Observatory to its original elegance and creating a garden to match it, complementing this with their warm approach to students, fellows, and visitors.

Doll retired from the college in 1983 but continued to work, preaching the necessity for the over-sixty-fives to 'live dangerously'. Having been knighted in 1971, he became a Companion of Honour in 1997, while The Richard Doll Building, housing several related units, was opened at the end of 2005. He was the recipient of many honors and awards and was nominated several times for the Nobel Prize. The obituary tributes to Doll concentrated on the tens of millions of deaths his work must have prevented when people either stopped smoking or never started. Thus his contributions, as the Nobel laureate Sir Paul Nurse (b. 1949) commented, 'transcended the boundaries of professional medicine into the general community of mankind'. And Doll may be seen to have occupied two pivotal positions. As a chief player in the modern medico-statistical movement—which had started with Karl Pearson (1857–1936) only in 1910 and continued with Major Greenwood (1880–1949) in the 1920s and 1930s and with Hill in the 1940s and 1950s—Doll was the first to apply its discoveries to the wholesale prevention of human disease. Hence he exemplifies the tradition that each Regius professor at Oxford contributes an important but different light on medical progress. His predecessor, Sir George Pickering (1904–80), had overseen the quintessential culmination of clinical science in the human being; his successor, Sir David Weatherall (b. 1933), was no less important in demonstrating the future medical benefits of molecular biology. In between, Doll also took medical progress largely out of the laboratory and showed how society could improve its own health by action against common threats, whether in the home or factory. Allied to this was a strong social conscience, which had surfaced earlier, for instance, when in helping to establish the National Blood Transfusion Service, he had insisted that blood donations should not be paid for, but should be seen as a contribution from an individual to the rest of society. His discoveries, then, may have been different in character but were no less fundamental or important than those before or since his time, and they helped to reignite a way of thinking about disease and its causation.

Bibliography

Primary: 1950. (with Hill, A. B.) 'A Study of 1,465 Cases of Lung Cancer and 1,465 Matched Controls, Which Confirmed and Extended the Studies of Wynder and Graham, and Others.' *British*

Medical Journal ii: 739–748; 1990. 'Dunkirk Diary.' *British Medical Journal* 300: 1183–1186, 1256–1259, 1324–1328, 1385–1387, 1449–1452; 1991. 'Conversation with Sir Richard Doll.' *British Journal of Addiction* 86: 365–377; 2004. (with Peto, R., J. Borcham, and I. Sutherland) 'Mortality in Relation to Smoking: 50 Years' Observations on Male British Doctors.' *British Medical Journal* 328: 1519–1543.

Secondary: Tucker, A., 25 July 2005. *The Guardian*; Beckett, C., 2002. 'An Epidemiologist at Work: The Personal Papers of Sir Richard Doll.' *Medical History* 46: 403–421.

Stephen Lock

DOMAGK, GERHARD   (b. Lagow, Brandenburg, Germany, 30 October 1895; d. Münster, Germany, 24 April 1964), *pharmacology*.

Domagk was the son of a teacher. After completing school in 1914 he was sent to war, first as grenadier, then as a medical soldier. There he witnessed wounded soldiers dying of gas gangrene, septic infections, traumatic fever, and other conditions. Thus, an interest in bacteria was aroused that would direct his medical studies, which started at Kiel at the age of nineteen, toward pathology and bacteriology. Later in life, at Münster University, these two disciplines also dominated his lecturing activities. During those days each fifth clinical casualty resulted from infection, and Domagk searched for a way to fight acute bacteriological infections by means of chemotherapy. After his medical training (at Kiel), he received his MD with the thesis *Beeinflussung der Kreatininausscheidung durch Muskelarbeit* in 1921.

In 1924 Domagk was habilitated under W. Gross at Greifswald University for pathological anatomy, handing in a study entitled *Untersuchungen über die Bedeutung des Retikulo-endothelialen Systems für die Vernichtung von Infektionserregern und für die Entstehung des Amyloids.* In 1925 he left for Münster University, where he was appointed associate professor in 1928; in 1927 he was called to the institute for chemotherapeutics of IG Farben at Elberfeld. After the death of its director, Wilhelm Roehl (1881–1929), the institute was divided and Domagk was made the head of the department for experimental pathology and bacteriology. In 1932 he there furnished proof that 4-sulfonamide-2',4'diaminoazobenzol hydrochloride—called Prontosil thereafter—showed chemotherapeutical and antibacterial effects. Domagk had observed that bacteria in an organism tend to be phagocytized more rapidly the more they had been impaired by other substances beforehand. It would therefore be sufficient to damage the bacteria in an organism by an appropriate preparation, and thus to deliver them to a more rapid phagocytosis, and not necessary to speculate on an 'inner disinfection' from the start. Bacteriostatics, rather than bactericides, were the new objective.

Domagk started with the dyes that Paul Ehrlich had used during the initial phase of his chemotherapeutical experiments. The addition of sulfonamide components to such dyes in animal experiments was successful for the first time in 1931. One year later the specific chemotherapeutical intervention in an experimental streptococcus infection in mice and rabbits proved to be successful. The efficiency of the new preparation was proved by clinical experiments on patients. The drug, developed by Domagk, was used until the 1960s. The results of those and other experiments were not published until 1935. In 1939 Domagk was awarded the Nobel Prize for Physiology or Medicine for the discovery of the antibacterial effect of Prontosil. Due to the Nazi prohibition, though, he could not accept it until 1947.

The discovery of the first sulfonamides and their bacteriostatic development by Domagk and his team was followed soon by hectic pharmacological research activities worldwide during the 1930s. Multiple new sulfonamide derivatives were produced and applied in clinical tests. Thus, extremely specific chemotherapeutical agents were developed to fight a variety of different infectious diseases. The progress of that research was further accelerated by the needs of the war. In particular, groups in England and the United States were trying to improve local surgical dressing by using sulfonamides, the efforts to treat gas gangrene resulting from clostridia being the primary challenge. In addition, the scientists furnished proof of the therapeutical effect of Uliron (1938), yet another sulfonamide, the derivates of which were effective against anaerobic infections and led to the development of Supronal. The discovery of the antitubercular effect of both thiosemicarbazone (Conteben, 1947), and $C_6H_7N_3O$ (Neoteben, 1952) were important contributions to the chemotherapy of tuberculosis. Later in life Domagk left industrial research for his former university. There, at Münster, where he had been appointed full professor in 1958, he died on 24 April 1964.

Bibliography

Primary: 1935. 'Ein Beitrag zur Chemotherapie der bakteriellen Infektionen.' *Deutsche Medizinische Wochenschrift* 61: 250–253; 1950. *Chemotherapie der Tuberkulose mit den Thiosemicarbazonen* (Stuttgart).

Secondary: Grundmann, Ekkehard, 2001. *Gerhard Domagk—der erste Sieger über die Infektionskrankheiten* (Münster and Hamburg) [English edn., 2004]; Alstaedter, Rosemarie, 1990. *Ein Pionier, der Medizingeschichte machte—eine Dokumentation über Prof. Dr. med. Gerhard Domagk zum 50. Jahrestag der Verleihung des Nobelpreises für Medizin* (Leverkusen); DSB.

Wolfgang U. Eckart

DONALD, IAN   (b. Liskeard, Cornwall, England, 27 December 1910; d. Paglesham, Essex, England, 19 June 1987), *obstetrics, gynecology, ultrasound*.

Donald was the eldest of four children of John Donald, a general practitioner, and Helen Wilson. Despite its location, his birth added to an extended family of Scottish doctors. Donald attended Fettes College, Edinburgh. In 1925 his family moved to South Africa, and Donald enrolled at Diocesan College, Rondebosch. Dr and Mrs Donald both died in 1926. Supported by money from a trust fund, the Donald children effectively brought themselves up. Ian graduated in Arts from the University of Cape Town in 1930, after which the siblings moved to London. Donald qualified from St Thomas's Medical School in 1937.

From boyhood Donald had been fascinated with inventions and, while a house physician at St Thomas's, he devised an automatic bladder irrigator. From 1942 onward, Donald served as a medical officer in the RAF, receiving the military MBE and being mentioned in dispatches for bravery. He also gained a working knowledge of the pulse-echo principles of radar and sonar.

In 1946 Donald returned to St Thomas's, where he developed an interest in neonatal respiratory distress, inventing a new mechanical ventilator. Moving to the Royal Postgraduate Medical School in 1952, he began a study of hyaline membrane disease, which led to his first venture into medical imaging. With Robert Steiner, he conducted the first radiological study of the condition. In 1954 Donald was appointed Regius professor of midwifery, University of Glasgow.

In the industrial yards of the Clyde, ultrasonic pulse-echo flaw detectors were used to check for cracks in metal. Donald knew that several investigators had attempted, with limited success, to adapt this technology for diagnostic purposes. In 1956, at the Research Department of Babcocks and Wilcox in Renfrew, near the river Clyde, he conducted a series of tests at the end of which he was able to distinguish a cystic from a solid tumor by their distinctive ultrasonic echo patterns.

Donald was fortunate in securing the services of the brilliant young engineer, Tom Brown, who built the first contact B-scanner, which produced clinically useful two-dimensional images. Donald's researches with Brown and with his clinical colleague John MacVicar were first published in *Lancet* (1958). Over the next decade, working with intense energy and enthusiasm despite a chronic cardiac condition, Donald led the team of clinicians and engineers who were to establish ultrasound imaging as an essential diagnostic tool in obstetrics and gynecology. The first commercially available scanner, the Diasonograph, designed and built in Glasgow, appeared in 1963.

The new imaging modality produced many insights into the development of the fetus and transformed the monitoring of pregnancy. Gestational age could be determined accurately, multiple pregnancies easily recognized, and fetal abnormalities detected. The ability to localize the placenta greatly improved the management of placenta previa.

Donald was a committed Anglican. He believed that ultrasound images of the fetus confirmed its individuality and humanity, a view that was endorsed by Pope John Paul II. Few abortions were performed in the units under Donald's control and he was active in the campaign against the 1967 Abortion Act. Donald was, however, saddened by the realization that 'my researches into early intrauterine life may yet be misused towards its more accurate destruction'. Ultrasound scanning has led to an ever more detailed scrutiny of fetal structure for abnormality, with abortion often the only feasible intervention if pathology is detected.

Donald was made CBE (1973) and received many other honors. His opposition to the 1967 Act deprived him of a knighthood. Married, with four daughters, he was also an accomplished pianist and watercolorist and, into old age, an enthusiastic yachtsman.

Bibliography

Primary: 1958. (with MacVicar, J., and T. G. Brown) 'Investigation of Abdominal Masses by Pulsed Ultrasound.' *Lancet* i: 1188–1195.

Secondary: Willocks, J., and W. Barr, 2004. *Ian Donald: A Memoir* (London); Nicolson, M., 2004. 'Ian Donald, Diagnostician and Moralist.' *Website publication* (Edinburgh): http://www.rcpe.ac.uk/library/history/donald/donald1.php; *Oxford DNB*.

Malcolm Nicolson

DONDERS, FRANCISCUS CORNELIS (b. Tilburg, the Netherlands, 27 May 1818; d. Utrecht, the Netherlands, 24 March 1889), *physiology, ophthalmology.*

Donders was born into a middle-class Roman Catholic family. In 1835 he entered Utrecht Military Medical School to become a health officer. In the early 1840s, he served in the garrisons of Vlissingen and the Hague as a health officer. Meanwhile, he obtained his MD and PhD at Leiden University. In 1845 Donders married Ernestine Zimmerman. Their daughter married Th. W. Engelmann, who eventually succeeded Donders as professor of physiology in 1888. After Ernestine died in 1887, Donders married his second wife, the painter Bramine Hubrecht.

Donders became a teacher at the Utrecht Military School in 1842. He joined the scientific circle of Gerrit Jan Mulder, professor of chemistry at Utrecht University, and made a name for himself as a proponent of scientific medicine. In 1847 Donders obtained a professorship, choosing ophthalmology as his special field. In 1859 he established the 'National Eye Clinic for the Poor', which was to gain an international reputation, both as an outpatient clinic and as an institution for teaching and research. In 1862 Donders succeeded J. L. C. Schroeder van der Kolk as professor of physiology.

Donders's research focused on the physiology of the senses. For instance, he found regularities in the orientation of the eyes during eye movements ('Donders' law'), and was the first to measure 'thinking time', the reaction time of the mind. The centerpiece of his research was a large-scale and systematic investigation of the anomalies of refraction and accommodation of the eye, i.e., of the deviations of eyesight that can be corrected by lenses. His research findings on myopia were based on the examination of more than 2,500 patients. These data enabled him to show the development of myopia with age. He also clarified the anatomical foundations of myopia and other vision anomalies, and established a clear difference between errors of refraction and errors of accommodation. Donders's results attracted wide interest and he became the internationally acknowledged expert in the field.

The eyesight deviations that Donders studied could not be healed. What he did was explain them. His explanations were of a scientific nature and did not change the practice of lens prescription in any fundamental way. Therapy consisted in finding the correct lenses to restore normal eyesight, and this was—and has remained—a matter of trial and error. Still, Donders could claim to be able to help his patients better than the nonacademic opticians and 'eyedoctors' of his time could. He had a library and a whole array of instruments at his disposal, of which the average optician could only dream, and his scientific network kept him abreast of developments in ophthalmology elsewhere. Combined with his research data, these resources enabled him to help patients who had been treated unsuccessfully by others. One example is his finding that astigmatism was far more widespread than was generally assumed. Thanks to the many different cylindrical lenses that he had at his disposal, Donders could help many patients whose astigmatism had until then been overlooked.

Thus, even though Donders' physiological insights did not change the practice of lens prescription, his activities did mark the beginning of a major change in the field. What had always been a craft and a trade performed by lens grinders and opticians was to become a scientific activity for which academic training was required. Donders' scientific approach and academic resources enabled him to begin the medicalization of the field of eyesight anomalies. In many Western countries, the prescription of lenses ultimately became the monopoly of academically trained ophthalmologists.

Bibliography

Primary: 1864. *On the Anomalies of Accommodation and Refraction of the Eye* (London).

Secondary: Draaisma, Douwe, 2002. *The Age of Precision. F. C. Donders and the Measurement of Mind* (Nijmegen); Theunissen, B., 2000. 'Turning Refracting into a Science. F. C. Donders and the Medicalisation of Lens Prescription.' *Studies in History and Philosophy of Biological and Biomedical Sciences* 31: 557–578; Fischer, F. P., and G. ten Doesschate, 1958. *Franciscus Cornelis Donders* (Assen); *DSB*.

Bert Theunissen

DONIACH, DEBORAH (b. Geneva, Switzerland, 6 April 1912; d. London, England, 1 January 2004), *medicine, immunology.*

After a peripatetic early childhood, Doniach, the eldest of three daughters, was brought up in Paris, where her father was a concert pianist and her Ukrainian mother ran a school of therapeutic movement. She did not start school until age nine but did her baccalaureate at the Lycée Molière before studying medicine at the Sorbonne. In 1934 she moved to London to marry Israel ('Sonny') Doniach, later professor of pathology at the London Hospital, whom she had met in Palestine (1925). Deborah qualified from the Royal Free Medical School (1944) and, after considering a career in endocrinology, opted for chemical pathology, which was an easier field for a woman to get into. In the early 1950s, she became clinical assistant to the thyroid surgeon at the Middlesex Hospital. Here she noticed that patients with Hashimoto's disease had raised levels of immune proteins and that the excised glands contained large numbers of antibody-producing plasma cells. Doniach made the intuitive leap that these cells were producing anti-thyroid antibodies. This was against accepted dogma that the body never produced antibodies against its own tissues (*horror autotoxicus*). The catalyst for the discovery of organ-specific autoimmunity was a 1956 experiment by the Americans Ernest Witebsky and N. R. Rose, who ground up one lobe of a rabbit's thyroid with Freund's adjuvant, injected it back, and found that the thyroid remnant was attacked by inflammatory cells. When Ivan Roitt showed Deborah the picture in Rose and Witebsky's paper, she recognized the similarity to Hashimoto's thyroiditis—Witebsky, a hematologist, had apparently never heard of it. Doniach, Roitt, and Peter Campbell did experiments in a test tube in which they layered thyroid extract on serum from a Hashimoto's patient and found precipitins at the interface. *Lancet* accepted the paper within a week of submission in October 1956. Doniach and Roitt's work led to the concept of a spectrum of autoimmune disorders, from organ-specific diseases to rheumatological disorders that involve antibodies against widely distributed body components. Within a few more years they found an autoantibody to gastric parietal cells in patients with pernicious anemia and antimicrosomal antibodies in primary biliary cirrhosis.

Type 1 or insulin-dependent diabetes (IDDM), often associated with hypothyroidism, Addison's disease, and pernicious anemia, was another putative autoimmune disease. In 1968 Doniach looked for an autoantibody but her 100 cases were a mixture of type 1 and type 2, and she never published her negative findings. Better fluorescent reagents and the introduction of epi-illumination in the fluorescence microscope paved the way for the first description of islet cell antibodies in 1974, simultaneously from the laboratories of Doniach and James Irvine in Edinburgh. Doniach and her young coworker Franco Bottazzo studied 171 patients with adrenal or thyroid autoimmunity and with or without diabetes. Strong staining reactions were seen in thirteen, of whom eight had diabetes at the time the sample was taken. Two others subsequently developed it. In retrospect the choice of polyendocrine patients was fortunate because in 1976 Richard Lendrum, encouraged by Doniach, showed that ICA (Islet cell antibodies) disappeared in 'ordinary' patients with IDDM within a year.

Deborah was a modest and unassuming person but was interested in everyone and everything. Many young research workers (myself included) were interviewed by her after a presentation and greatly encouraged when she said 'how fascinating'. She was multilingual and in retirement reread the whole of Proust, and studied Spinoza, Freud, and Molière.

Bibliography

Primary: 1956. (with Roitt, I. M., P. N. Campbell, and R. V. Hudson) 'Autoantibodies in Hashimoto's Disease (Lymphadenoid Goitre)' *Lancet* ii: 820–821; 1974. (with Bottazzo, G. F., and A. Florin-Christensen) 'Diabetes Islet Cell Antibodies in Diabetes Mellitus with Autoimmune Polyendocrine Deficiencies.' *Lancet* ii: 1279–1283.

Secondary: Tansey, E. M., et al., eds., 1997. 'Self and Non-Self: A History of Autoimmunity' in *Wellcome Witnesses to Twentieth Century Medicine* vol. 1 (London) pp. 39–66.

Robert Tattersall

DOWN, JOHN LANGDON HAYDON   (b. Torpoint, Cornwall, England, 18 November 1828; d. Hampton Wick, England, 7 October 1896), *medicine, psychiatry.*

Down, the youngest child of Thomas Joseph Almond Down, a Cornish grocer and apothecary of Irish descent, and his wife Hanna Haydon, was educated in Torpoint, Cornwall, but left school at the age of thirteen to help in his father's business. Five years later, he moved to London to work as an assistant surgeon before enrolling as a student at the Royal Pharmaceutical Society in 1847. Although he completed his examinations and worked for a period as research assistant to Michael Faraday (1791–1867), Down did not register as a member of the Society and in 1850 a period of illness forced him to return to the West Country to recuperate. When his father died in 1853, Down entered London Hospital's medical school, where he won many prizes and medals before graduating in 1858. That year, he was appointed resident physician and medical superintendent at the Earlswood Asylum for Idiots in Surrey, a post that he combined with his position as assistant physician to the London Hospital. In 1868 Down established his own institution for mentally defective children from the wealthier classes at Teddington, Middlesex, naming it Normansfield after one of his close friends and managing it with his wife, Mary. Down became FRCP in 1869. In 1884 he was also appointed as a magistrate for London, Westminster, and Middlesex, and five years later became an alderman of Middlesex County Council.

Influenced by contemporary ethnology and anthropology and concerned to improve the classification of idiots and imbeciles in asylums, Down began to investigate the structure and function of various organs amongst mentally defective children in his care. In an initial speculative paper published in *Lancet* in 1862, Down argued not only that anomalies of the mouth could facilitate the diagnosis of idiocy but also that improvements in physical condition might ameliorate mental ability. In addition, Down identified a particular group of patients whose shared features suggested 'that they might readily be taken for members of the same family'.

Four years later, in his 'Observations on an Ethnic Classification of Idiots', Down extended these observations by attempting to classify his patients on the basis of their resemblance to certain ethnic groups. In particular, he argued that many idiots shared the physical features and behavioral characteristics of Mongols, referring to this group as 'mongolian idiots'. According to Down, the ethnic features of 'mongolian idiots' were largely the result of tuberculous degeneration and provided further support for monogenist 'arguments in favour of the unity of the human species'. Down later expanded his account of 'mongolian idiocy' in his 1887 monograph *On the Mental Affections of Childhood and Youth.*

Down was not the only late–nineteenth-century physician to link features of mental deficiency to the appearance of certain racial groups. In 1876, for example, John Fraser and Arthur Mitchell introduced the term 'Kalmuc idiocy' to describe asylum inmates with features similar to those of Down's 'mongolian idiots'. In addition, many writers challenged Down's understanding of the etiology and pathology of 'mongolian idiocy'. Nevertheless, subsequent medical authorities generally reinforced the stereotypical ethnological bias evident in Down's work and routinely adopted the term 'mongolism' or 'mongolian idiot' to describe this group of mental defectives well into the twentieth century.

In the 1950s and 1960s, in the wake of evidence that 'mongolism' was the product of an extra chromosome 21 and in the context of growing sensitivity to the racial implications of Down's initial classification, many physicians and scientists fought to reject the words 'mongolism', 'mongoloid', and 'mongolian idiocy', suggesting that Down syndrome, or trisomy 21, constituted more objective and less objectionable descriptive terms.

On Down's death in 1896, his wife and two of his sons, Reginald and Percival, took over the management of his private institution at Normansfield.

Bibliography

Primary: 1862. 'On the Condition of the Mouth in Idiocy.' *Lancet* i: 65–66; 1866. 'Observations on an Ethnic Classification of Idiots.' *Lectures and Reports from the London Hospital for 1866* 3: 259–262; 1876. *On the Education and Training of the Feeble in Mind*

(London); 1887. *On the Mental Affections of Childhood and Youth* (London).

Secondary: Wright, David, 2001. *Mental Disability in Victorian England: The Earlswood Asylum 1847–1901* (Oxford); Jackson, Mark, 1999. 'Changing Depictions of Disease: Race, Representation and the History of Mongolism' in Ernst, Waltraud, and Bernard Harris, eds., *Race, Science and Medicine 1700–1960* (London) pp. 167–188; Zihni, Lilian, 1989. 'The History of the Relationship between the Concept and Treatment of People with Down's Syndrome in Britain and America from 1866 to 1967.' PhD thesis, University of London; *Oxford DNB*.

Mark Jackson

DRAKE, DANIEL (b. Plainfield, New Jersey, USA, 20 October 1785; d. Cincinnati, Ohio, USA, 6 November 1852), *medicine, medical education, medical geography.*

Physician, professor, and medical author Drake was the oldest surviving child of poor farmers Elizabeth Shotwell (1761–1831) and Isaac Drake (1756–1832). The Drakes and several relations emigrated in the spring of 1788 from Essex County, New Jersey, to Mason County, Kentucky, where they settled at Mayslick. Because young Daniel had to labor on the family homestead, he received little formal schooling; romantically-minded biographers have opined that Nature inculcated in him the skills of observation and description that would serve him so well in compiling his *magnum opus*, a two-volume treatise on the medical geography of the Mississippi basin.

At the age of fifteen, Drake was apprenticed for $400 a year to William Goforth, a physician related to the Drakes by marriage who had traveled west with them and was then living in Cincinnati. Although apprenticeship was the most common medical education a would-be doctor received in early–nineteenth-century America, Drake has been hailed as Cincinnati's first medical student. After four years of compounding his preceptor's drugs and committing to memory classics by such venerable authors as Herman Boerhaave and William Cheselden, Drake is supposed to have received the first medical degree issued west of the Allegheny Mountains, although it was simply Goforth's testament that Drake had studied with him and was qualified to practice medicine.

'Diploma' notwithstanding, Drake scraped together enough money to spend one winter semester (1805–06) attending medical lectures at the University of Pennsylvania. From Benjamin Smith Barton, Drake acquired a reverence for the systematic collection of facts and Baconian induction, and from Benjamin Rush he adopted such heroic therapies as bloodletting and calomel. Drake matured into a careful, detail-oriented practitioner, generous with his time and advice, whose consulting practice eventually extended as far as a letter could reach.

In 1806 Drake returned from Philadelphia to Mayslick as an independent physician. The next year he took over Goforth's practice in Cincinnati and married Harriet Sisson (1787–1825). Drake cherished Harriet's company at home and on patient calls, and after she died of a 'bilious remittent fever' he faithfully observed her death date by fasting and composing elegies. Three of their five children survived to adulthood: Charles Daniel (1811–92), a rebellious youth who became a lawyer and successful state and federal public official; Elizabeth Mansfield (1817–64); and Harriet Echo (1819–64). Drake's autobiographical letters to his grown children, published as *Pioneer Life in Kentucky* (1870), offer rich accounts not only of his early life but also of conditions on the American frontier.

Drake came to love his adopted home, soon to become the 'Queen City of the West' thanks to the commerce fostered by its river port. The good doctor even garnered this center of hog and whiskey trade a European reputation among immigrants, speculators, and readers of travel literature with his *Picture of Cincinnati* (1815), an expanded version of his privately-printed *Notices Concerning Cincinnati* (1810). Warming to his 'booster' role, Cincinnati's 'first' citizen contributed to the town's social and cultural growth by supporting the establishment of a number of institutions, among them a School of Literature and Arts (1813) and Cincinnati College (1819). Drake encouraged the formation of libraries and museums, and he campaigned for a Commercial Hospital, a Poor House, and an Asylum for the Insane (1821). From his work in the first eye clinic in the Mississippi Valley (1827), Drake developed not only respectable ophthalmologic skills but also a sensibility for the education of blind children; he was instrumental in the founding of schools for the blind in Columbus, Ohio, and Louisville, Kentucky.

Drake's greatest ambition in life was to found and teach at the most progressive medical college in the West, but to do so he needed a medical degree. Thus, in 1815 Drake moved his family to Philadelphia in order to attend the lectures at the University of Pennsylvania again. Degree in hand, Drake set about organizing a group of Cincinnati physicians to offer medical classes. Upon learning of the plans of their potential rival, however, the medical faculty at nearby Transylvania University in Lexington, Kentucky, hired him as professor of materia medica and botany (1817–18). But Drake's dream drew him back to Cincinnati, and in 1819 the state legislature granted a charter to the Medical College of Ohio. Drake was its first president and professor of medicine.

A medical school at that time was as much a business venture as a teaching enterprise, and the physicians in Cincinnati accused Drake of profiteering. Unable to bear criticism or to compromise, Drake made many enemies at the Medical College and was ultimately voted out of his positions. He returned to his former chair at Transylvania University (1823–25), where he was elected dean and professor of medicine (1825–27). Squabbling among the faculty eventually drove Drake back to his practice in Cincinnati.

In 1830 Drake returned to teaching, this time as professor of medicine at Jefferson Medical College in Philadelphia. After only one term, he had persuaded several other physicians to join him in attempting to set up a medical department at Miami University (Oxford, Ohio). No classes were ever held, however, as the nascent faculty merged with their competitors at the Medical College of Ohio. Drake resigned the next year (1832). In 1835 he again organized a rival medical department, at Cincinnati College, but lacking the public funds the Medical College enjoyed, the new faculty dissolved in 1839.

Drake's peripatetic faculty-hopping ceased for the decade following his acceptance of a special eighth chair of clinical medicine and pathological anatomy at the Louisville Medical Institute (1839–44); he later moved to the chair of medicine (1844–49). During almost every summer recess, Drake traveled from the Gulf of Mexico to Lake Superior and from the Allegheny Mountains to the Mississippi River, collecting data for his treatise on the physical and disease geography of the interior of the North American continent.

In 1849 Drake resigned from his professorship and returned to Cincinnati, where he hoped to devote more time to writing and to enjoying his daughters' families. The Medical College of Ohio was in the process of yet another reorganization, and Drake—ever the optimist when it came to the school he had originally chartered—agreed to teach clinical medicine and special pathology. Nevertheless, the next year internal dissension drove him again to the Louisville Medical Institute, where he spent two more years (1850–52). Finally, in 1852, Drake retired from the Institute. He accepted a final position at the Medical College of Ohio, but he did not live to the end of the year, instead succumbing to pneumonia.

Because of his passionate oration and his devotion to training the next generation of healers, Drake was a popular lecturer wherever he taught. He was constantly attentive to both the moral and the physical well-being of his students. Ironically, for all the intrigues he instigated at the Medical College of Ohio, fellow professors at other schools turned to Drake as a mediator of their own disputes.

A prolific writer, Drake published around 700 lectures, essays, and pamphlets on topics ranging from cholera, milk sickness, and cancer to temperance, democracy, and slavery. His thoughts on medical education are among his better known and most eloquent. Despite his own relatively meager schooling, Drake wished for his students a grasp of French, Greek, and Latin in order to enhance their access to the medical literature and to give them an appropriately gentlemanly demeanor. He was also of the opinion that the term of lectures should be lengthened to five or six months, that a young man should study medicine for four instead of two years, and that students should study basic sciences such as anatomy and chemistry before attempting to master pathology and obstetrics. Better-trained doctors would improve both professional medicine's image and the actual practice of medicine, in his view.

Drake also served as co-editor of three different publications: *The Western Medical and Physical Journal* (Cincinnati, 1827–1828), with Guy W. Wright; its competitor, *The Western Journal of the Medical and Physical Sciences* (Cincinnati, 1828–1838); and *The Western Journal of Medicine and Surgery* (Louisville, 1840–1849). For the second of these Drake adopted the emblem of a dogwood blossom overlaid with the motto *e sylvis nuncius* ('a voice from the woods'), suggesting his affinity for nature. Until his teaching duties increased in the 1830s, Drake frequently demonstrated his versatility in the multiple pieces he contributed to each volume.

Above all, Drake is best known for his *A Systematic Treatise, Historical, Etiological, and Practical, on the Principal Diseases of the Interior Valley of North America* (1850, 1854). Drake intended his extensive observations of the Mississippi Basin, its people, and their diseases to help physicians promote the healthy and moral development of what he perceived to be the great democratic civilization arising in the West among the last new race on Earth, a social and biological hybrid of the Caucasian, African, and Aboriginal peoples. This combination of geography and anthropology complemented Drake's belief that 'medicine is a physical science, but a social profession.'

So social an undertaking was Drake's medicine that in the late 1820s he became a temperance man, lecturing on the medical and moral dangers of alcohol to medical and lay audiences alike. Well before the rise of bacteriology, Drake used military metaphors to describe individual and social physiology; he led the 'Army of the Temperate'. The other social cause Drake attacked was abolitionism. He believed the state of the slave was gradually improving toward more palatable serfdom; in the meantime, however, forcing the hand of their masters not only unnecessarily disrupted the social order but would surely lead to civil war and the dissolution of his beloved Union.

In politics Drake was a Whig, a friend of Henry Clay, and a campaigner for William Henry Harrison. Never very religious, he came from a long line of Baptists, but in 1840 joined his late wife's Episcopalian sect, though he disdained the formality of High Church. Drake never made a fortune in his lifetime; neither an optimistic business venture undertaken in the 1810s, a drug and grocery store, nor any of his publications brought him profit.

Drake has been called the Benjamin Franklin of the West, but the comparison is perhaps overly enthusiastic, as the reputation of the good doctor is today more or less confined to his boosterism for formal medical education and for the Midwest. One of Cincinnati's first citizens many times over, he should be remembered for his obstinacy and ambitions as well as for his social and medical accomplishments. As one of the discipline's most devoted professors, he cared enough about his patients and his profession to insist on standards for the teaching and practice of medicine. And as one of the foremost natural historians of his day, Daniel Drake thought holistically, connecting body, natural environment, and society, advocating that by considering physical and moral factors together, the properly trained physician could aid the healthy development of citizen and democracy.

Bibliography

Primary: 1970. (Shapiro, Henry D., and Zane L. Miller, eds.) *Physician to the West: Selected Writings of Daniel Drake on Science and Society* (Lexington); 1832. *Practical Essays on Medical Education and the Medical Profession in the United States* (Cincinnati); 1842. *The Northern Lakes: A Summer Residence for Invalids of the South* (Louisville); 1850–54. *A Systematic Treatise, Historical, Etiological, and Practical, on the Principal Diseases of the Interior Valley of North America* 2 vols. (Cincinnati).

Secondary: Dorn, Michael Leverett, 2002. 'Climate, Alcohol, and the American Body Politic: The Medical and Moral Geographies of Daniel Drake (1785–1852).' PhD thesis, University of Kentucky; Horine, Emmet Field, 1961. *Daniel Drake (1785–1852): Pioneer Physician of the Midwest* (Philadelphia); Mansfield, Edward Deering, 1855. *Memoirs of the Life and Services of Daniel Drake, M.D. Mid-American Frontier* (New York); *ANB*; *DAMB*.

Kristen Ann Ehrenberger

DREW, CHARLES EDWIN   (b. Lambeth, London, England, 15 December 1916; d. London, 31 May 1987), *surgery.*

Drew went to King's College, London, as an undergraduate and qualified in medicine in 1941 from Westminster Hospital, where he later made his career. After his first resident appointments he joined the navy. During the war, his ship was sunk in the Mediterranean and he survived by swimming from a porthole. He served throughout the war. Apart from time as a resident at the Brompton Hospital, his career was all at the Westminster and at St George's hospitals, near to Parliament, Buckingham Palace, and the center of government. In 1952 King George VI was operated on by Clement Price Thomas (1893–1973) for lung cancer, during which Drew assisted.

These were small hospitals without any room to grow and Drew probably had the disadvantage of being allowed to plow a solitary furrow. This was a feature of the British system throughout that era, which permitted and encouraged each of the many London teaching hospitals to do a little of everything through the years when heart surgery was developing. Both St George's and Westminster had virtually single-handed staffs of cardiothoracic surgeons throughout the 1960s and 1970s.

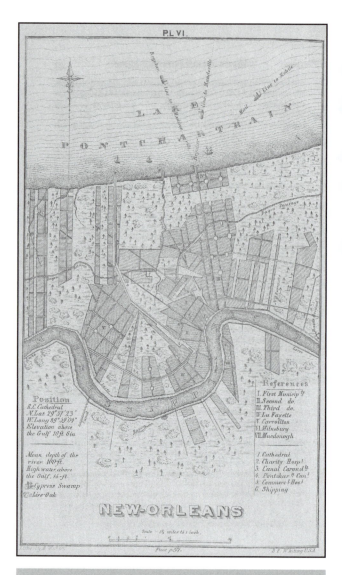

Map of New Orleans showing the city surrounded by lakes and bays, a habitat for yellow fever and malaria. Lithograph from . . . *on the Principal Diseases of the Interior Valley of North America* . . . Cincinnati, 1850. Rare Books, Wellcome Library, London.

Drew's own contribution was in developing an original and unique method of performing heart surgery. To set this accomplishment in context, simple operations to open the mitral and pulmonary valves were being performed with reproducibly good results from 1948 onward, but attempts at performing more complex repairs within the heart had met with little success. The competing methods being actively pursued were clever tricks and devices to work within the still-beating heart, while externally supporting the circulation with cross-circulation from, for example, the mother of sick child or the use of a heart-lung machine. Yet another approach was the use of profound cooling to create a state of suspended animation. Drew devised his own method, using pumps on the right and left side of the heart until the temperature of the body was twelve degrees Celsius and then arresting the circulation for up to an hour. He achieved success, and his results were as good as others at the time, but as expertise developed and heart-lung machines improved he was left behind. He persevered with his own method, 'the Drew technique', until the 1970s. The culture of the time was that colleagues were not openly criticized, and it was not until later that surgeons with results less than expected were called to account.

When the subject of profound hypothermia was reviewed in a Hunterian lecture at the College in 1983 (Treasure, 1984), Charles Drew attended. His obituary has a characteristically euphemistic tone: 'Charles Drew was a highly original thinker who was occasionally out of step with his less enterprising fellows' (Lyle et al., p. 99).

Bibliography

Primary: 1959. (with Keen, G., and D. B. Benazon) 'Profound Hypothermia.' *Lancet* i: 745–747; 1959. (with Anderson, I. M.) 'Profound Hypothermia in Cardiac Surgery: Report of Three Cases.' *Lancet* i: 748–750.

Secondary: Treasure, T., 2000. 'Cardiac Surgery' in Silverman, M. E., et al., eds., *British Cardiology in the 20th Century* (London) pp. 192–213; Treasure, T., 1998. 'Lessons from the Bristol Case. More Openness on Risks and on Individual Surgeons' Performance.' *British Medical Journal* 316: 1685–1686; Hollman, A., and T. Treasure, 1998. 'Pulmonary Valvotomy—50 Years Ago.' *Lancet* 352: 1956; Westaby, S., 1997. *Landmarks in Cardiac Surgery* (Oxford); Treasure, T., and A. Hollman, 1995. 'The Surgery of Mitral Stenosis 1898–1948: Why Did It Take 50 Years to Establish Mitral Valvotomy?' *Annals Royal College Surgeons England* 77: 145–151; Treasure, T., 1984. 'The Safe Duration of Total Circulatory Arrest with Profound Hypothermia.' *Annals Royal College Surgeons England* 66: 35–40; *Plarr's Lives.*

Tom Treasure

DREW, CHARLES RICHARD   (b. Washington, DC, USA, 3 June 1904; d. Burlington, North Carolina, USA, 1 April 1950), *surgery, blood transfusion.*

Drew was the eldest of the five children of Richard T. Drew (a carpet layer) and his wife Nora (Burrell) Drew (a school teacher). His prowess in athletics earned him a scholarship to Amherst College, Massachusetts. After graduation (1926) he took a job as professor of chemistry and biology at Morgan State College in Baltimore and began saving for medical school. He graduated in medicine and surgery from McGill University, Montreal, Quebec (1933), his interest in blood transfusion having been stimulated by the visiting British surgeon John Beattie (1902–33). Drew was appointed instructor in pathology (1935) at Howard University and an assistant in surgery (1936). He continued his studies at Columbia University (1938) with a two-year Rockefeller Fellowship, writing his MD thesis on 'Banked Blood': he was the first African American to receive this degree. Working with John Scudder and Edward H. L. Corwin, he demonstrated that liquid plasma lasted longer than whole blood and could be used as a blood substitute. Furthermore, its lack of red blood cells prevented problems of matching blood type. If correctly processed and preserved, plasma could also be stored and shipped over long distances.

In 1940 Drew was asked to work on blood bank improvement in New York by administering the Blood Transfusion Betterment Association of New York. This supplied blood products for U.S. forces and civilians who were wounded in Britain during the German bombing raids. He developed a system to produce plasma, separating it from red cells, and used 'bloodmobiles', refrigerated trucks, to meet the enormous demand. It is recorded that in the six months between August 1940 and February 1941, about 10,500 units of liquid plasma were shipped to London to support the 'Plasma for Britain Project'. Methods were also developed to produce dried plasma that could be preserved longer than the liquid plasma. The British military used his process extensively during World War II, establishing mobile blood banks to aid in the treatment of wounded soldiers at the front lines.

In February 1941 Drew became the medical director of the American Red Cross Blood Bank program and, as assistant director for blood procurement for the National Research Council, organized the world's first blood bank drive, nicknamed 'Blood for Britain'. The Red Cross established blood donor stations to collect plasma for the U.S. armed forces but to Drew's disgust, the military issued a directive to the Red Cross, which they accepted, asking for blood to be sorted on racial lines and for the rejection of the donations of African Americans. Drew's insistence that this was an unscientific policy (later vindicated by others) apparently led to his resignation from the blood bank. He was appointed professor of surgery at Howard University, Washington, D.C. (1941). A popular teacher with high standards, Drew became an examiner to the American Board of Surgery two years later (1943) another first for an African American. In 1949 Drew toured hospital facilities in occupied Europe as part of a team working for the Surgeon General's office.

He died in 1950 from injuries suffered in a car accident in North Carolina after falling asleep at the wheel. He married (Minnie) Lenore Robbins (1939); they had four children.

Bibliography

Primary: 1940. 'Banked Blood: A Study in Blood Preservation.' MD thesis, Columbia University.

Secondary: Love, Spencie, 1996. *One Blood: The Death and Resurrection of Charles R. Drew* (Chapel Hill, NC); Wynes, Charles, 1988. *Charles Richard Drew: The Man and the Myth* (Champaign, IL).

Tom Treasure

DU COUDRAY, ANGELIQUE MARGUERITE LE BOURSIER (b. Paris? 1715?; d. Bordeaux, France, 1794), *midwifery, obstetrics*.

Mme du Ouray was the most important midwife of the French Enlightenment, commissioned by Louis XV and then Louis XVI to travel throughout the realm teaching the art of childbirth to illiterate peasant women in an effort to reduce infant mortality. France feared its population was shrinking, so this midwife was given the task of single-handedly bringing about the obstetrical mobilization of the nation by training a new cadre of skilled professionals.

She taught in nearly forty cities and reached (with the help of a network of disciple-demonstrators coached in her method) an estimated 10,000 students. She wrote a textbook on birthing, *Abrégé de l'art des accouchements* (1759), and invented a life-size obstetrical mannequin, which she proudly called her 'machine', on which her students practiced maneuvers. Because hers was an official royal mission, the king's provincial administrators were obliged to facilitate her teaching in their regions. But the fact that these men had never before been ordered around by a powerful woman created many problems for her. During her more than three decades of itinerant teaching, from the Seven Years' War to her death during the Revolution, she developed creative strategies for success, ingratiating herself with finance ministers like Turgot, Necker, and Calonne, dazzling local officials, even soothing the tender vanities of the male medical practitioners.

Though a celebrity, Mme du Ouray was maddeningly private, revealing next to nothing about her feelings. The record is rich in detail about her work but empty of any personal revelations. That she was herself childless is fascinating. Her portrait, showing a plump bourgeoise in an imposing regal frame, announced that she was 'pensioned and sent by the king' to teach throughout the realm. How had she been given this enormous responsibility? Why did she, already in her forties, decide to undertake such a huge and exhausting task?

During the time before her fame she was just one of about 200 midwives practicing in Paris in the 1740s. She befriended Frère Côme, the famous medical monk, and then suddenly departed for Auvergne, where she saw for the first time the blood and gore of rural delivery practices and began to teach her art for free to the local peasant girls. From there she traveled and taught in Moulins, Chalons-sur-Saône, Tulle, Angoulême, Bourdeilles, Poitiers, Rochefort-sur-Mer, Montargis, Bourges, Issoudun, Perigueux, and Agen. During this time she published the second edition of her textbook, this one with twenty-six very costly and beautiful color engravings, and her entourage grew to include a teenage apprentice, whom she adopted as her 'niece' and designated as heir of her pension and her mission.

Forging further afield, Mme du Ouray traveled from the Bordeaux area toward the outskirts of the country and even across the Flemish border, from Auch to Montauban, Grenoble, Besançon, Chalons-sur-Marne, Verdun, Neufchâteau, Nancy, Amiens, Lille, Ypres, Caen, Rennes, Nantes, Evreux, Le Mans, and Angers. A trusted young surgeon-assistant, Coutanceau, joined her traveling team and married her 'niece'. Although there were by now rival mannequins and textbooks by male accoucheurs, the midwife negotiated an advantageous retirement pension for herself (on a par with military generals). Always the loyal patriot, she did the king's bidding and even taught childbirth to veterinarians at the Royal School of Alfort. During the Revolution Mme du Ouray revealed that she had saved Lafayette's life at his birth, but she and Mme Coutanceau, now living in Bordeaux, still had to plead for continued support from the National Assembly in an effort to keep their clinic going.

Mme du Coudray's mission, the obstetrical enlightenment of France, while of course not solely responsible for the dramatic demographic upswing after 1750, surely played a significant role therein.

Bibliography

Primary: 1759. *Abrégé de l'art des accouchements* (Paris) [and many subsequent editions].

Secondary: Gelbart, Nina Rattner, 1998. *The King's Midwife: A History and Mystery of Mme du Ouray* (Berkeley); Gels, Jacques, 1988. *La sage-femme our le medicine* (Paris).

Nina Rattner Gelbart

DUBINI, ANGELO (b. Milan, Italy, 8 December 1813; d. Milan, 28 March 1902), *medicine, anatomy, hygiene, parasitology*.

After receiving his MD at the University of Pavia in 1837, Dubini began working in the Ospedale Maggiore in Milan, where he was to spend almost his entire working life. He returned to Pavia for the academic biennium 1839–1841 as an assistant at the Medical Clinics, where he gave a free course in auscultation and fostered the clinical method based on anatomo-pathological observation, as elaborated by Giovanni Battista Morgagni (1682–1771) and developed by the Paris School of Jean-Nicolas Corvisart (1755–1821) and René Laennec (1781–1826).

From November 1841 to the end of 1842, Dubini traveled to France, England, and Germany, and then returned to Milan, resuming his work as an assistant physician at the Ospedale Maggiore. In 1865 he was nominated as head physician and director of a new department of dermatology.

Dubini's most important discovery was made at the Ospedale Maggiore in May 1838, during an autopsy, as a result of his anatomo-pathological practice. Observing the intestines of a peasant woman who had 'died of "croupous pneumonia"', Dubini noted a large number of a 'new human intestinal worm', new in the sense that there was no description of it in the medical literature. He confirmed his observations in other autopsies and published his description in April 1843, naming the new worm *Ankylostoma duodenale*, a name derived from the hooked mouth of the organism and from its presence in the human intestine. Dubini's helminthological description is highly accurate and was further developed in his *Entozoografia* (1850). This hookworm is the agent causing ankylostomiasis—hookworm disease—which is endemic in tropical areas and was then present in the humid regions of Northern Italy.

Dubini noted the very high frequency of occurrence of the worm, 'which, although it had not yet been seen by others, nor described, is nevertheless found in twenty out of one hundred corpses that are dissected with the aim of finding it'. However, he did not consider the ankylostoma as a specific pathogenic cause.

The specific pathogenicity of ankylostoma was eventually confirmed in the course of studies on Egyptian chlorosis made by F. Pruner (1808–82), W. Griesinger (1817–68), and T. M. Bilharz (1825–62) and in O. E. H. Wucherer's (1820–73) work on tropical chlorosis. A direct confirmation of Dubini's anatomo-pathological and epidemiological observations came from the study of the serious epidemics of miner's cachexia that spread among the miners of the St Gotthard tunnel (1872–80). Many of the miners came from the plains of Northern Italy and brought the worm to the tunnel, where the special conditions of work created in the heart of the Alps a tropical microclimate in which the ankylostomiasis could become epidemic. The research by G. B. Grassi (1854–1925), C. and E. Parona, E. Perroncito (1847–1936), C. Bozzolo (1845–1920), and L. Pagliani (1847–1932) confirmed the nature of the epidemic and the causative role of the ankylostoma.

In 1846 Dubini published the first description of an acute, fatal disease, due to acute infection of the central nervous system; now called 'Dubini's chorea' or electric chorea.

Bibliography

Primary: 1843. 'Nuovo verme intestinale umano (*Anchylostoma duodenale*), costituente un sesto genere dei Nematoidei proprii dell'uomo.' *Annali universali di medicina* 106: 5–13; 1843. 'Primi cenni sulla corea elettrica.' *Annali universali di medicina* 117: 5–50; 1850. *Entozoografia umana per servire di complemento agli studi d'anatomica patologica* (Milan); 1859. *Indices nosologici ordine alphabetico adnotationibus therapeuticis accomodati* (Milan).

Secondary: Belloni, L., 1962. 'La scoperta dell'Ankylostoma duodenale.' *Gesnerus* 19: 101–118; Bertarelli, A., 1902. 'Angelo Dubini.' *Bollettino dell'Associazione sanitaria milanese* 4: 115–119; DSB.

Bernardino Fantini

DUBOIS, JACQUES (aka SYLVIUS, JACOBUS)

(b. Amiens, France, 1478; d. Paris, France, 13 January 1555), *anatomy, medicine.*

A late starter from a poor background, Sylvius went to Paris at the age of thirty-six (1514) to assist his older brother François, principal of the Collège de Tournai, and evidently began to learn Latin, Greek, and Hebrew at that time. He studied Galen's works while acquiring practical knowledge of anatomy by working with barber surgeons. He matriculated at Montpellier in 1527, took the bachelor's degree in 1529, and the MD the following year. In 1531 he dedicated an introductory French grammar to Queen Eleanor (1498–1558), the new wife of Francis I (1494–1547) whose French was poor. Perhaps this was instrumental in enabling him to return to Paris and to begin teaching at the Collège de Tréguier in 1532.

By 1536 his classes were so popular that he was recognized by the Faculty of Medicine as an extramural lecturer and allowed to charge students for attendance. Sylvius began to reform the teaching of anatomy at Paris, placing greater emphasis not only upon Galen's anatomical writings, but also upon public dissections. Having incorporated his Montpellier degrees at Paris only as bachelor of medicine, he had avoided the doctor's oath against manual craft, and would frequently anatomize parts of animals in his lectures to illustrate details. Among his admiring students were Charles Estienne (1505–64), Michael Servetus (1511–53), and Andreas Vesalius (1514–64). He also began to publish a succession of commentaries and textbooks expounding Galen's system. His combination of Galenic detail, based on the latest medical humanist scrutiny of Galen in Greek, and personal observation, derived from performing dissections, ensured that Sylvius was seen by his contemporaries as a medical teacher with a very progressive outlook. It is an unfortunate irony of history, therefore, that he has come to be seen as a hidebound defender of ancient authority against the innovations of Vesalius.

Certainly Sylvius's response to Vesalius's criticisms of Galen in his *Rejection of the Calumnies of a Certain Madman on Hippocratic and Galenic Anatomy* (1551) was aggressive and intemperate. Learned contemporaries would have spotted the punning use of Vesanus (madman) as a substitute for Vesalius. Sylvius's defensive suggestion that human anatomy may have changed since Galen's day is often held up for ridicule, but at least it does not deny the observational evidence. Furthermore, Sylvius even supported this view by comparing humans with domestic animals, which were known to have changed (albeit as a result of selection by breeders). There was clearly a professional dimension to Sylvius's defense of Galen and the system of medicine that depended upon him, and possibly even a religious dimension at a time when the traditional authority of the Roman Church was also under attack—for Sylvius, Hippocrates was 'divine' and Galen 'pious' and 'sacred', while Vesalius was 'impious' and 'sacrilegious'.

Sylvius's reputation has also been tarnished by accusations of avarice and the love of money. Evidence suggests this is the result of willful misinterpretation (by enemies) of attitudes and traits deriving from his poverty-stricken background. His sympathy for the poor is shown in his *Regimen for Poor Scholars* (*Victus ratio, scholasticis pauperibus paratu facilis et salubris,* 1542), and in his *Useful Advice against Famine and the Lack of Nourishment* (*Consilium perutile adversus famem et victuum penuriam,* 1545), a sadly moving attempt to deal with the rigors brought about by extreme hunger simply as aspects of humoral pathology. At his own request he was buried in a graveyard reserved for poor students, but not without a large attendance from former students and colleagues.

Bibliography

Primary: 1634. (Moreau, René, ed.) *Opera medica* (Geneva); 1962. 'Advice for Poor Medical Students' [1542]. trans. O'Malley, C. D., *Journal of the History of Medicine* 17: 141–151.

Secondary: Carlino, Andrea, 1999. *Books of the Body: Anatomical Ritual and Renaissance Learning* (Chicago); Baader, G., 1985. 'Jacques Dubois as a Practitioner' in Wear, Andrew, Roger K. French, and I. M. Lonie, eds., *The Medical Renaissance of the Sixteenth Century* (Cambridge) pp. 146–154; Kellet, C. E., 1961. 'Sylvius and the Reform of Anatomy.' *Medical History* 5: 101–116.

John Henry

DUCHENNE DE BOULOGNE, GUILLAUME (b. Boulogne-sur-Mer, France, 17 September 1806; d. Paris, France, 17 September 1875), *neurophysiology, neurology.*

The son of a buccaneer captain, Duchenne received a classical education. In 1825 he began medical studies in Paris. Upon receiving his degree, he returned to Boulogne in 1831 to become a general practitioner. On his return to Paris in 1842, he eked out a modest living in private practice. A chance success using electrotherapy opened up to him the possibilities of a technique of investigation to which he would passionately devote the rest of his career. Immersing himself in the works of Galvani, Volta, Faraday, and Magendie, Duchenne designed an ingenious electrical machine for medical use. His *De l'art de limiter l'action électrique dans les organs sans piquer ni inciser la peau, nouvelle méthode d'électrisation localisée* (1847) represented a major innovation.

By 1847 Duchenne had already published extensively. Although he had no hospital or other official positions and lacked influential connections, Duchenne managed to attend the lessons of leading hospital physicians. Trousseau in particular appreciated his talent and gave him an opportunity to apply his techniques to patients, with the most notable result being Duchenne's collaboration with Aran. He performed the electroclinical examinations for Aran's *De l'atrophie musculaire progressive* (1850).

This work inaugurated a long series of investigations of disorders of motion. By combining clinical study with the electrical exploration of muscle physiology, Duchenne was able to classify both new and already known but poorly defined pathologies. His description in 1854 of infantile paralysis in children and, in 1872, of an adult form completed the nosography of poliomyelitis. In 1860 he described progressive paralysis of the tongue, palate, and lips (later incorporated by Charcot into the definition of amyotrophic lateral sclerosis). In 1868 his elucidation of a pseudohypertrophic muscular paralysis, later known as Duchenne muscular dystrophy, marked a breakthrough in knowledge of muscle pathology. Here he used a 'histological punch' to perform muscle biopsy.

Duchenne's famous clinical account of progressive locomotor ataxia (1858–59) went beyond the associated muscular atrophies. Duchenne clearly distinguished this 'disturbance of equilibrium and coordination' from Romberg's description (1851) of tabes dorsalis—a consequence of syphilis—and characterized it by preservation of muscular strength (he had invented a dynamometer by which this could be measured) and electrical contractility. His description of the associated pains and ocular and sphincter disorders would later be confirmed and elaborated by Charcot.

The study of paralyses necessitated understanding the action of each muscle, a veritable 'living anatomy', which Duchenne described in *Physiologie des mouvements* (1867). Here he corrected the 'mechanical' methods used by anatomists and gave priority to *muscular synergy* and the function of antagonists. His study of the hand and fingers exemplified his subtle physiological method. Duchenne's earlier *Mécanisme de la physionomie humaine ou analyse electro-physiologique de l'expression des passions* (1862), dealing with the facial muscles, had already displayed his interest in philosophical and aesthetic questions. His system of 'psychological classification', accompanied by photographs, noted 'flaws' in a few famous sculptures from antiquity. Charles Darwin's book on the emotions referred to Duchenne's work. Darwin annotated his personal copy and he corresponded with his French colleague.

Duchenne's masterpiece, *L'electrisation localisée* (1855) with its *Album de photographies pathologique* was a compilation of his earlier pioneering publications. New results enriched subsequent editions, of which the third (1872), a volume of 1,100 pages of minute and repetitive text, makes for difficult reading. Nonetheless, the clinical description and classification of new disease entities established a framework for neurology which would be filled in by subsequent pathological studies.

Bibliography

Primary: 1855. *L'electrisation localisée* [2nd edn. 1861, 3rd edn. 1872] (Paris); 1862. *Mécanisme de la physionomie humaine ou analyse electro-physiologique de l'expression des passions* (Paris); 1867. *Physiologie des mouvements* (Paris).

Secondary: Cuthbertson, R. A., 1990. *The Mechanism of Human Facial Expression* (Cambridge); Guilly, P., 1936. *Duchenne de Boulogne* (Paris) [reprint 1977, Marseille].

Michel Bonduelle

DUHRING, LOUIS ADOLPHUS (b. Philadelphia, Pennsylvania, USA, 23 December 1845; d. Philadelphia, 8 May 1913), *dermatology.*

Duhring was the son of Heinrich Dühring, a prosperous businessman and German immigrant, and Caroline Oberteuffer, of Swiss ancestry. After private school at the Delancey School (now part of Episcopal Academy), he matriculated at the University of Pennsylvania, Philadelphia (1861–64) with a short interruption to serve in the American Civil War. From 1864 to 1867 he was a student at the University of Pennsylvania School of Medicine, following which he interned at the Philadelphia (Blockley) Hospital. His dermatology training was taken in Europe (1868–70) under the masters of the new specialty, not only in London (Jonathan Hutchinson, Tilbury Fox, Erasmus Wilson), Paris (Alfred Hardy, Ernest Bazin), and Vienna (Ferdinand von Hebra, Moritz Kaposi [Kohn]), but also in Berlin, Breslau (Wroclaw) (Heinrich Koebner), Christiania (Oslo) (Caesar Boeck), and Constantinople (Istanbul).

Returning to Philadelphia in 1870, he began the private practice of dermatology, a specialty that had only recently appeared in American medicine. He opened the Dispensary for Skin Diseases (1871–90) and began his long association with the University of Pennsylvania School of Medicine, first as lecturer (1871–76), then becoming the school's first professor of skin diseases (clinical professor, 1876–90; professor, 1890–1910; emeritus professor, 1910–13). From 1870 to 1872 he edited, with Francis Fontaine Maury, a surgeon at Jefferson Medical College, the *Photographic Review of Medicine and Surgery*, an innovative periodical focusing on pictures rather than on text.

Duhring became the pathfinder for American dermatology. He delineated three skin diseases: pruritus hiemalis (winter itch) (1874), emphasizing a common problem in nineteenth-century Philadelphia; seborrhea corporis (1874), showing that seborrheic dermatitis could be found on many parts of the body; and dermatitis herpetiformis (Duhring's disease) (1884), synthesizing a disparate collection of observations into one vesicular-bullous entity. His books demonstrate both his pioneering skills and his international recognition in dermatology: *An Atlas of Skin Diseases* (1876), *A Practical Treatise on Skin Diseases* (translated into Chinese, French, German, Italian, and Russian) (1877, 1881, 1882), *Epitome of Diseases of the Skin* (with Henry Wile) (1885), and *Cutaneous Medicine* (of which only two of five projected volumes appeared) (1895, 1898). He was also one of the editors of the *International Atlas of Rare Skin Disease* (1891).

He was a founder (1876) and later president (1878, 1879) of the American Dermatological Association, the oldest national dermatology society in the world. Duhring participated in the First International Congress of Dermatology and Syphilography (Paris, 1889). The Philadelphia Dermatological Society was initially called the Duhring Dermatology Club after its founding in 1900. Duhring was elected to the Berliner Dermatologische Gesellschaft (corresponding), Sociedad Dermatologica Argentina (corresponding), Société Française Dermatologie et de Syphiligraphie (corresponding), Società Italiana di Dermatologia e Sifilografia (honorary), and Wiener Dermatologische Gesellschaft (corresponding).

During his later years, Duhring became increasingly eccentric and parsimonious; he lived for several years with his maiden sister, Julia. At the time of his death, he was immensely wealthy, leaving an estate in excess of $1,600,000 to several institutions. His endowment to the College of Physicians of Philadelphia meant that the library could subscribe to almost every dermatology journal extant for many years. The monies given to the University of Pennsylvania Department of Dermatology were to maintain the wax model collection and other academic activities; the research building was called the Duhring Laboratories while it was still extant. The Department of Archeology and Paleontology recognized his generosity by naming the stacks of the original, main library in his memory.

Duhring's legacy to American dermatology would also continue through his students: Henry Stelwagon (first professor of dermatology at Jefferson Medical College), Milton B. Hartzell (his successor at the University of Pennsylvania), Arthur Van Harlingen, and Jay Frank Schamberg.

Bibliography

Primary: 1877. *A Practical Treatise on Diseases of the Skin* (Philadelphia).

Secondary: Crissey, John Thorne, and Lawrence Charles Parish, 1981. *The Dermatology and Syphilology of the Nineteenth Century* (New York); Friedman, Rueben, 1955. *A History of Dermatology in Philadelphia* (Fort Pierce Beech, FL); *DAMB*.

Lawrence Charles Parish

DUKA, THEODORE [TIVADAR] (b. Dukafalu, Sáros, Hungary, 22 June 1825; d. Bournemouth, England, 5 May 1908), *medicine, surgery, medical scholarship.*

Duka, Hungarian-born, was a man of diverse interests and international outlook. He became a naturalized British citizen and spent more than two decades in India as medical officer to Her Majesty's Bengal Army, seeing active duty during the mutiny at Monghyr and serving at Simla, Patna, and Darjeeling. While in India, Duka—already fluent in Hungarian, German, and English—gained proficiency in several Asian languages.

Following his early education at the Lutheran college in Eperjes (now Presov, Slovakia), Duka studied law at the University of Pest, passing his examination with honors. Appointed in 1848 to a government post in the finance department, he quickly joined other Hungarians in the national forces fighting against the Hapsburgs. He was made aide-de-camp to General Arthur Görgey, and received the Order of Valor and was promoted to the rank of captain for his role at the battle of Komárom. Taken prisoner when the Hungarians capitulated at Világos in 1849, he escaped and made his way via Paris to London in 1850.

There Duka taught German and studied English at the Birkbeck Institute. He undertook medical studies, first at St George's Hospital and then at the University of St Andrews, where he earned his MD in 1853. He married Anna Jane Taylor, daughter of an English clergyman, in 1855, and was made a Fellow of the Royal College of Surgeons in 1866.

In India, Duka published notes in medical journals on varied subjects: emasculation as practiced by Mohamedans in East India (1864–65), Simla and Darjeeling as sanitaria (1870, 1874), dry gangrene in the lower extremities (1874–75). He retired in 1877 with the rank of lieutenant colonel and returned to England, where he became a member of the Bible Society and the council of the Royal Asiatic Society.

A loyal Hungarian at heart, Duka was eager to spread word about Hungarian contributions to knowledge. He wrote an admiring biography of his countryman Alexander Csoma de Körös, the earliest serious Western student of Tibetan languages, and he also did everything he could to make sure the work of Ignác Semmelweis was recognized. (Many credit Duka with having alerted Joseph Lister to Semmelweis.) As soon as Duka learned about Semmelweis's hand-washing theory, from notes in the Hungarian medical weekly *Orvosi Hetilap*, he discussed it in the *Indian Lancet* in 1860, and in 1888 he published a 'Life' of Semmelweis (based on Jakob Bruck's 1887 work). He attended the meeting in London (1892) where plans were laid to establish an internationally funded memorial to Semmelweis (a statue was erected in 1906 in Budapest). When an elaborate tombstone for Semmelweis was unveiled in Budapest, in 1894, Duka was one of the speakers.

At the Eighth International Congress of Hygiene and Demography, held in Budapest in 1894, Duka—first president of the section on tropical medicine—gave an address in which he helped lay the basis for future work in tropical medicine. Carefully reviewing climatological and geographical conditions in India, he used observations on three diseases prevalent there to show that studying hygiene and demography could 'lead to practical solutions of many hitherto obscure problems' (Duka, 1894, p. 23).

Duka received many honors. He was a corresponding member of the Hungarian Academy of Sciences from 1863 and was made an 'honored member' in 1900. In 1883 King-Emperor Francis Joseph conferred on him the Order of the Iron Crown, and in 1899 the University of Budapest awarded him an honorary MD.

Bibliography

Primary: 1885. *Life and Works of Alexander Csoma de Körös* (London); 1888. *Childbed Fever; Its Causes and Prevention: A Life's History* (Hertford, England); 1894. *An Address on Tropical Medicine* (Hertford, England).

Secondary: Gortvay, György and Imre Zoltán, 1968. (trans. Róna, Éva) *Semmelweis: His Life and Work* (Budapest) pp. 222, 247, 282–283; Stein, Aurél, 1913. *Duka Tivadar emlékezete* [In Memoriam Theodor Duka] (Budapest); [Obituary], 1908. 'Theodore Duka.' *Lancet* i: 1520–1521.

Constance Putnam

DUNGLISON, ROBLEY (b. Keswick, Cumberland, England, 4 January 1798; d. Philadelphia, Pennsylvania, USA, 1 April 1869), *physiology, medical education.*

Dunglison was the son of William Dunglison and Elizabeth Jackson. His father died when he was young, and he chose medicine to support himself. His medical studies began with an apprenticeship in Keswick, and then one in London with the surgeon Charles Haden. He also spent time in Edinburgh and Paris taking courses and, on returning to London, became a licentiate of the Society of Apothecaries (LSA). He practiced medicine in London from 1819 onward, and in 1823 obtained an MD by written examination from the University of Erlangen with a dissertation on neuralgia. He became accoucheur at the Eastern Dispensary in London and began teaching obstetrics. Even at this early stage Dunglison was making a reputation as a medical writer, translating works of François Magendie and Dominique Larrey from the French and publishing medical articles in at least half a dozen journals, including the *London Medical Repository* and the *London Medical Intelligencer*. Such literary activities were to continue throughout his career.

A turning point in his life was the invitation he received from Francis Gilmer, Thomas Jefferson's envoy, who had been sent to England to recruit professors for the University of Virginia. Dunglison agreed to become the first professor of medicine at the new university. Part of the agreement was that he would have only a consultation practice. In October 1824, with his new wife, Harriet Leadam, he embarked for America. He established himself in Charlottesville and had close contacts with Jefferson, whose personal physician he became, and with James Madison. He later was a medical consultant for two other American presidents, James Monroe and Andrew Jackson. While at Virginia he had time to prepare works on physiology and hygiene and the first edition of his celebrated *Dictionary of Medicine*. His only venture into research came in 1832 and 1833 when he helped William Beaumont with some of the famous experiments on Alexis St Martin investigating the physiological action of the stomach. Beaumont did not fully acknowledge Dunglison's assistance in his written account.

In 1833 Dunglison answered the call to a professorship in materia medica, therapeutics, hygiene, and medical jurisprudence at the University of Maryland in Baltimore, which had a medical faculty. This position he held for three years before accepting, in 1836, a professorship in the institutes of medicine and medical jurisprudence at Jefferson Medical College in Philadelphia. Dunglison believed this city to be the center of medical education in America and he lived there for the rest of his life, resisting all offers of other positions. Dunglison is noted for his efforts to reorganize the teaching at Jefferson, enhance the College's reputation, and increase the number of students. He was named Dean in 1854, a position he held until his retirement in 1868, although he disliked administration.

His literary activities continued unabated. He edited a new journal, the *American Medical Intelligencer*, from 1837 to 1842, as well as publishing further editions of his *Dictionary* and books on human physiology, elements of hygiene, and general therapeutics. Other topics for books were new remedies, guidance for medical students, and the practice of medicine. In his time, Dunglison was America's most prolific medical author; he sold thousands of copies of his books. Dunglison also played an active role in many Philadelphia institutions, including the American Philosophical Society, of which he became Vice-President; the Pennsylvania Institution for the Instruction of the Blind; and the Musical Fund Society. He was a member of numerous scientific and literary societies in the United States, England, and Europe. He died soon after his retirement in 1869.

Bibliography

Primary: 1832. *Human Physiology* (Philadelphia) [eight editions]; 1833. *A New Dictionary of Medical Science and Literature* (Boston) [nine editions]; 1836. *General Therapeutics, or Principles of Medical Practice* (Philadelphia) [six editions]; 1839. *New Remedies: The Method of Preparing and Administering Them* (Philadelphia) [seven editions].

Secondary: Bylebyl, Jerome J. 1970. 'William Beaumont, Robley Dunglison, and the "Philadelphia Physiologists."' *Journal of the History of Medicine and Allied Sciences* 25: 3–21; Radbill, Samuel X., ed., 1963. *The Autobiographical Ana of Robley Dunglison, M.D. Transactions of the American Philosophical Society* (ns) 53(8); *DAMB.*

Caroline Hannaway

DUNLOP, ERNEST EDWARD (b. Major Plains, Victoria, Australia, 12 July 1907; d. Melbourne, Victoria, Australia, 2 July 1993), *surgery.*

Dunlop, the son of James Dunlop and Alice Emily Maude Walpole, was educated at Benalla High School in Victoria, Australia, and later at Ormond College, University of Melbourne. During this period he was given the nickname 'Weary' after a famous brand of car tire (thus the play on the word). The cognomen stuck with him for the rest of his life. A well-built man standing 1.93 m (6 feet, 4 inches), Dunlop was a keen and accomplished sportsman.

He graduated MB BS in December 1934, then worked variously as a resident and in other appointments in the Children's, Austin, and Melbourne Hospitals. He was awarded his Master of Surgery in 1937 and his FRCS in 1938. In London he worked at St Bartholomew's Hospital under such luminaries as Sir Thomas Dunhill.

After the outbreak of World War II, Dunlop enlisted in the Australian Army Medical Corps on 13 November 1939. He was posted to Jerusalem and on 18 April 1940 was appointed acting assistant deputy of the Army Medical Service under his former anesthesia teacher, Clive Disher. In March 1941 he was sent to Greece to act as a liaison officer with the British Headquarters in that ill-fated campaign. After escaping the advancing German army he served with the 2/2nd Australian Casualty Clearing Station at Tobruk, and later became its commanding officer. His unit subsequently accompanied the 1st Australian Corps when it was redeployed to the Far East and then to Sumatra, just prior to its capture by Japanese forces in early 1942. Dunlop was fearless in standing up for the rights of his patients and staff in the face of his captors, who showed no regard for the protocols under the Geneva Convention.

Along with most of his staff and thousands of Australian and Allied prisoners of war, Dunlop spent the rest of the war in captivity, being moved first to Singapore, then in 1943 to Thailand. Dunlop and other medical staff attended to their fellow captives who, in the most primitive conditions, were ravaged by disease and the brutal privations of the Japanese. With only crude instruments and homegrown pharmacopoeia they endured until the Japanese surrender. He returned to Australia in October 1945 after helping supervise first the acute care, then the evacuation of his fellow prisoners.

The decades after the war's end saw Dunlop return to surgery to become a leader in laryngectomy, but against the prejudices of several prominent Australian doctors who doubted his surgical skills. Failing eyesight did not help him, nor was he widely published. Later, in the 1960s, he went on to pioneer ileostomies and esophageal surgery.

After he retired in 1967, Dunlop continued to lead a busy life focused on humanitarian works. In 1969 he led a medical team to South Vietnam during that country's conflict with the Communist North. He remained a passionate champion of POWs' rights and consistently fought the Australian rehabilitation system for what he saw as the hard-won rights of his fellow wartime captives.

Dunlop's postwar honors included the OBE and CMG and a knighthood in 1969; and later still, in 1987, he was made a Companion of the Order of Australia. He was also the recipient of several honorary fellowships and a number of foreign decorations.

An iconic Australian to those of his generation, Dunlop is rightly held up as an example of self-sacrifice and heroic humanitarian endeavor during the horrors of Japanese captivity during World War II. He might perhaps be more properly remembered as a representative of the many army medical colleagues who shared his labors and altruism.

Bibliography

Secondary: Tyquin, Michael, 2003. *Little by Little: A Centenary History of the Royal Australian Medical Corps* (Sydney); Geddes, Margaret, 1996. *Remembering Weary: Sir Edward Dunlop* (Ringwood, Victoria); Ebury, Sue, 1994. *Weary: The Life of Sir Edward Dunlop* (Ringwood, Victoria); Dunlop, E. E., 1986. *The War Diaries of Weary Dunlop* (Melbourne).

Michael Tyquin

DUPUYTREN, GUILLAUME (b. Pierre-Buffière, Haute Vienne, France, 5 October 1777; d. Paris, France, 8 February 1835), *surgery, pathological anatomy.*

Dupuytren was the son of Jean-Baptiste Dupuytren, a small-town lawyer of modest means, and Marguerite Faure. He was educated locally until age twelve, when he went to Paris as a scholarship student from the Limoges district and was enrolled in the Jesuit Collège de la Marche in 1789. His studies there came to an early end when the college was closed in 1793 during the Revolution. Dupuytren's first career choice was to join the military, but it is said that he acceded to his father's wish that he become a surgeon, as his grandfather had been before him. Michel Thouret was a patron of his Parisian medical studies, and Dupuytren's early teachers included Alexis Boyer for anatomy at the Charité hospital, and Nicolas Vauquelin and Edmé-Jean Bouillon-Lagrange for chemistry at the École de Pharmacie. Success in the career that lay ahead of him—as the leading French surgeon of his time and important proponent of the study of pathological anatomy—was obtained by both patronage and his ability to win in the competitive examinations for positions that were a prominent feature of French medical professional life.

In 1795 Dupuytren gained his first post after a competitive examination, that of prosecutor at the new École de Santé. In the post-Revolutionary reorganization of medical education in France, anatomy had been incorporated into the teaching of the medical school. Dupuytren threw himself into the study of the subject, dissecting hundreds of cadavers, making anatomical preparations for use in teaching, and learning to identify morbid appearances in the organs of the deceased. This work laid the foundation for his life-long devotion to pathological anatomy. In 1801 he was appointed to the position of chief of anatomical investigations at the medical school, following Honoré Fragonard, and he set about reorganizing the anatomy teaching. He began giving his own courses on both normal and abnormal anatomy, initially with Gaspard Bayle and René Laennec as assistants. Early on, Xavier Bichat's courses were rivals to those of Dupuytren, but the death of Bichat in 1802 removed this competition. In company with Bayle and Laennec, Dupuytren founded the Société anatomique in 1803, which had the principal goal of fostering the study of anatomy, physiology, and pathological anatomy. Also in that year, he defended his doctoral dissertation, which was on several propositions related to these subjects. Shortly afterward, Dupuytren became estranged from Laennec in a public dispute over who had first proposed a classification system for organic lesions in the human body, which Laennec believed was original to himself. The two men were professional rivals thereafter.

Dupuytren's surgical career began in earnest in 1802 when, after a competitive examination, he was named adjunct surgeon at the Hôtel Dieu of Paris. The thousands of patients who came to this hospital and the variety of ailments with which they presented gave Dupuytren the opportunity to develop his surgical skills in many areas. He treated wounds and burns, set fractures, restored dislocated joints and bones, and amputated limbs when necessary. He operated to drain cysts, remove tumors and polyps, and treat fistulas and hernias. His ambition was to work his way up the surgical hierarchy of the Hôtel Dieu, and in September 1808 he was named adjunct chief surgeon. His academic triumph in the surgical area came in February 1812, when he was awarded the chair of operative medicine at the Faculty of Medicine of Paris following one of the most notable *concours* of the period. This was a contest in which an applicant demonstrated surgical skill by performing a particular operation on a cadaver chosen by the examiners as well as by offering lectures and a written thesis. Dupuytren beat out three other contenders. In September 1815, he became chief surgeon of the Hôtel Dieu, following the forced retirement of Philippe Pelletan from the post, and achieved his ambition of twenty years standing.

Once in charge of surgery at the Hôtel Dieu, Dupuytren established a routine that he followed for the rest of his career. He arrived at the hospital early in the morning and made ward rounds, accompanied by his staff and other visitors, during which he examined new patients, taking detailed histories and making physical examinations, and checked on those recently operated on. After rounds, he gave a clinical lecture on surgery to large numbers of students and colleagues. Operations and treatments were conducted after the lecture, with Dupuytren continuing his teaching in the operating room, explaining what each case was, what he proposed to do, and what the outcome was likely to be. He was noted for his ability to remain calm even in the face of the patients' suffering and of unexpected complications in operations. Next, he read the postmortem results of all those who had died in order to increase his knowledge of morbid anatomy; he then gave advice on treatment in surgical cases at the Hôtel Dieu's free clinic for the poor. In the afternoon he went home and saw patients in what became a very extensive and lucrative private practice, or attended meetings of the Faculty of Medicine and learned societies. He returned to the Hôtel Dieu in the early evening to see how the patients he had operated on were faring. Dupuytren became known as the 'eagle' of French surgery. His disputatious personality, inability to suffer fools gladly, and jealousy of potential rivals meant that he was not a popular man or an easy man to deal with, but his reputation was such that young surgeons, both French and foreign, wanted to study with him, despite his overbearing treatment of them, and patients likewise flocked to him.

Dupuytren was noted for his wide-ranging knowledge of anatomy and surgery, his powers of elocution, and his diagnostic prowess. For instance, he reportedly could often detect abscesses within the body for which there were no visible signs externally. He modified or improved many surgical procedures, including control of hemorrhages, extraction of stones from the bladder, removal of tumors and polyps, treatment of burns, cataract operations, repair of strangulated hernias and fistulas, resection of the elbow, and resetting of improperly treated fractures. Dupuytren's most recognized surgical accomplishments were the excision of the mandible in a case of tumor of the jaw, the introduction of compression of the subclavian artery, and the development of a new method of constructing an artificial anus.

Dupuytren also played a part in the larger medical and scientific world of Paris. In addition to helping found the Société anatomique early in his career, Dupuytren was a member of the Société de l'École de Médecine, founded in 1803, and published some of his youthful observations in its journal. The most notable of these was a detailed investigation on the cause of death of three workers who were asphyxiated in a cesspool. Dupuytren was a founding member of the Académie Royale de Médecine in 1820 and became a member of the Académie Royale des Sciences in 1825. After the monarchy was restored in 1815, he became a consultant surgeon to Louis XVIII, and the king conferred a hereditary baronetcy on him on 17 April 1821 for his services to his nephew, the Duc du Berry, after the assassination attempt in February 1820 that led to the duke's death. This event and the recognition enhanced Dupuytren's public reputation. When Charles X ascended the throne in 1824, Dupuytren became the First Surgeon to the King. During the political turmoil in Paris late in June 1830, which resulted in the overthrow of Charles X, the Hôtel Dieu was inundated with hundreds of casualties with gunshot and other wounds. Dupuytren distinguished himself in the organization and quick treatment of the wounded.

In 1833 Dupuytren suffered a stroke while teaching. He took time off and traveled to Italy to recover, but, after his return, a continuing series of strokes led to his death in February 1835. According to his wishes, his body was

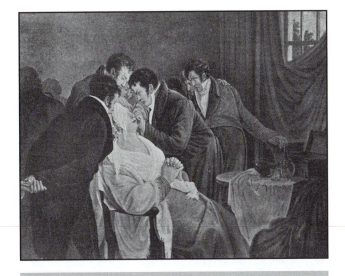

Guillaume Dupuytren operating on a cataract. Wellcome Library, London.

autopsied to determine the causes of his demise. By the time of his death, Dupuytren was an enormously wealthy man, a far cry from the impoverished youth who features prominently in the accounts of his early studies and career. Accounts vary as to how large his fortune (at least several million francs) actually was, but there is agreement that he initially proposed to give in his will 200,000 francs to the Faculty of Medicine of Paris to endow a chair in pathological anatomy and give formal recognition to the status of the new discipline in medicine. The dean of the medical school, Mathieu Orfila, persuaded the government to support the establishment of the chair and, with Dupuytren's agreement, the money was willed for the building of a museum of pathological anatomy to be named in honor of the donor. Jean Cruveilhier, Dupuytren's student, was appointed to the new chair in 1836.

Dupuytren did not publish very much, and his works consist primarily of his theses and articles on surgical procedures in medical and society journals. His long-planned treatise on pathological anatomy never reached fruition. Students put together volumes of his teachings at the surgical clinics of the Hôtel Dieu and of his views on treating war wounds. His name lives on in Dupuytren's contracture, a condition of the hand in which the contracture of the tissue of the palm causes the fingers to be deformed. Dupuytren devised an operation to relieve this condition. He appears in Balzac's *La comédie humaine* under the thinly veiled disguise of the surgeon, 'Desplein'.

Bibliography

Primary: 1812. *Lithotomie. Thèse soutenue publiquement dans l'amphithéâtre de la Faculté de Médecine de Paris; en présence des juges concours, le 1812* (Paris); 1832. *Leçons orales de clinique chir-urgicale, faites à l'Hôtel-Dieu de Paris par M. le Baron Dupuytren, recueillies et publiées par les docteurs [Alexandre] Brière de Boismont et [Edmond] Marx* 4 vols. (Paris); 1834. *Traité, théorique et pratique, des blessures par armes de guerre, rédigés d'après les leçons cliniques de M. le Baron Dupuytren, et publié sous sa direction par MM. les docteurs [Alexandre] Paillard and [Edmond] Marx* 2 vols. (Paris).

Secondary: Mondor, Henri, 1945. *Guillaume Dupuytren, 1777–1835* (Paris); Pariset, Etienne, 1850. 'Eloge du Baron G. Dupuytren' in *Histoire des membres de l'Académie Royale de Médecine ou recueil des éloges lus dans les séances publiques* vol. 2 (Paris) pp. 103–148; Vidal, Auguste-Théodore, 1835. *Essai historique sur Dupuytren, suivie des discours prononcés par MM. Orfila, Larrey, Bouillaud, H. Royer Collard, Teissier; du procès-verbal de l'ouverture du corps du Dupuytren* (Paris).

Caroline Hannaway

DURÁN CARTÍN, CARLOS   (b. San José, Costa Rica, 12 November 1852; d. San José, 23 November 1924), *surgery, parasitology, public health.*

Durán was the son of a Salvadoran immigrant to Costa Rica who had prospered with the coffee boom of the mid–nineteenth century. Along with a score of other children of prosperous coffee growers and merchants, he was part of the first wave of young nationals to study medicine abroad in the 1860s (Costa Rica was then without a medical school). Durán enrolled in the medical school at Guy's Hospital, London, in 1871, apprenticing under the eminent surgeon, Henry Howse. He witnessed the dramatic transformation in nursing, hospital design, and asepsis that marked the era (Guy's was an early convert to Listerism, as was Howse), and received his credentials from Guy's and from the Royal Colleges of Physicians and Surgeons in 1874.

For four decades following his return to Costa Rica in 1875, Durán was at the heart of efforts to organize the medical profession and promote scientific culture among a small but cosmopolitan community of practitioners. In 1880–81 he was the driving force behind the country's first medical publication and promoted its first clinical society. Durán was also an indefatigable hospital reformer, overseeing the redesign and reconstruction of the Hospital San Juan de Dios, the country's principal charity hospital, and installing in it a bacteriological laboratory and up-to-date operating theaters. He also instituted a modern hospital regime and began to train midwives and a nursing corps. In 1895 Durán helped to establish the country's first professional association of physicians and surgeons, the Facultad de Medicina (despite the promise contained in its name, it did not found a medical school) and was its president on two occasions.

Growing political influence helped Durán push through his reforms. He was the medical luminary in the circle of young positivists who controlled the government in the 1880s, serving as minister of the interior in 1886–87 and as interim president in 1889–90. Subsequent attempts to recapture the presidency were unsuccessful, but Durán was a perpetual congressional deputy and a central figure in the political class through to World War I.

Durán's most significant scientific contributions were in the area of parasitology and public health. He was among the earliest medical researchers in the Americas to discover that the peculiar, and often acute, tropical anemia suffered by large proportions of Costa Rica's rural population was actually hookworm disease. This 1894 discovery, reported to a Guatemalan medical journal in 1895, won him regional acclaim, and anticipated by six years the so-called American discovery of hookworm disease by Bailey Ashford and Charles Wardell Stiles. More importantly, Durán continued researching the nature of hookworm infection and disease and in 1907, while head of the Facultad de Medicina, organized a national treatment program for sufferers of hookworm disease that received funding from the government. This was the first such national initiative in the world, and preceded by two years the Rockefeller Sanitary Commission's extensive hookworm program in the U.S. South. The Costa Rican hookworm campaign was also ahead of its time in Latin America in that it targeted a disease afflicting rural populations during a period when states in the region were focused on questions of urban sanitation and rarely extended health services into the countryside. Durán's research and promotion of reform can be seen as crucial early steps in the development of Costa Rica's highly successful model of state-supported medicine and public health.

Bibliography

Secondary: Palmer, Steven, 2003. *From Popular Medicine to Medical Populism: Doctors, Healers and Public Power in Costa Rica, 1800–1940* (Durham, NC); Palmer, Steven, 1998. 'Central American Encounters with Rockefeller Public Health, 1914–1921' in Joseph, Gilbert M., et al., eds., *Close Encounters of Empire: Writing the History of U.S.-Latin American Relations* (Durham, NC); González Pacheco, Carlos Eduardo, 1995. *Hospital San Juan de Dios: 150 años de historia* (San José).

Steven Palmer

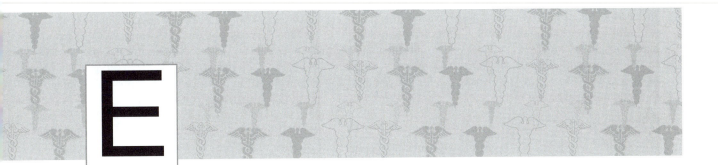

E

EARLE, PLINY (b, Leicester, Massachusetts, USA, 31 December 1809; d. Northampton, Massachusetts, USA, 17 May 1892), *psychiatry.*

Earle, son of Quaker manufacturer and farmer Pliny Earle and Patience Buffum, was educated at Leicester Academy and a Quaker boarding school in Rhode Island, where he subsequently taught for six years. He left there in 1835 to seek an MD at the University of Pennsylvania. He had visited the Worcester State Lunatic Asylum under its then superintendent, Samuel Woodward, and this led him to write his MD thesis on the treatment of insanity. On a subsequent trip to England, he became personally acquainted with Samuel Tuke (1784–1857) and with the York Retreat, a Quaker-run institution which had pioneered the approach to the therapeutics of insanity known as 'moral treatment'.

Earle subsequently visited a number of reformed asylums elsewhere in Europe, and returned to the United States in 1839 aiming for a career treating the mentally ill. The following year, after a stint in general practice, he served as physician to the Friends' Asylum in Frankford (what is now northeast Philadelphia), moving from there to the superintendency of the Bloomingdale Asylum in New York in 1844. Like many of the first generation of American asylum superintendents, Earle voiced great optimism about prospects for successfully treating insanity, and enthusiastically promoted a mix of moral and medical treatment for his charges. In keeping with Tuke's emphasis on the therapeutic value of labor, he encouraged his patients to work; but here he ran into difficulties because the families of his richer patients objected to their being employed at manual tasks. Arrogant and sure of his ground, Earle resisted such pressures. The asylum's board of managers, however, proved more pliable, and to assuage their moneyed clientele, dismissed Earle in 1849.

Earle promptly left for another inspection tour of European asylums, this time in Prussia and Austria, and briefly reentered private practice in New York before returning to Leicester. Having now published three books on the treatment of insanity, in a period where many new asylums were being built, resulting in a shortage of experienced alienists, Earle expected that he would soon be summoned to another superintendency. However, his hopes were repeatedly disappointed, and even when the State of Massachusetts opened a second state asylum in neighboring Northampton, his candidacy was passed over. Only the administrative incompetence and swift dismissal of the first superintendent allowed Earle to escape his long years in the wilderness.

Appointed as superintendent at Northampton in 1864, Earle remained in that post until 1885, despite periodic bouts of depression. If his early work in asylums had coincided with a brief burst of optimism associated with what subsequent generations referred to as 'the cult of curability', now the asylum sector was dominated by an increasing therapeutic pessimism. Reluctant to spend 'extravagant' sums on chronic patients, states sought to cut costs. Earle's popularity soared with the State Board of Charity, which oversaw the Massachusetts asylums, because he proved adept at pinching pennies.

He also used his annual reports to reexamine the curability of insanity, collecting and publishing these essays as a book in 1883. A better title for this work would have been *The Incurability of Insanity*, for Earle now alleged that the early optimism exhibited by American alienists had been based on mistaken, if not fraudulent, statistics, and that insanity was all too frequently an incurable condition. Elected president of the Association of Medical Superintendents of American Institutions for the Insane in 1884 (a society he had helped to found forty years earlier), he helped spread the notion that mental illness was a hopeless, hereditary disease. After his resignation as superintendent in 1885, apparently content to live in a warehouse for the unwanted, Earle spent the last years of his life boarding at the asylum he had once directed.

Bibliography

Primary: 1841. *A Visit to Thirteen Asylums for the Insane in Europe* (Philadelphia); 1853. *Institutions for the Insane in Prussia, Austria, and Germany* (New York); 1887. *Curability of Insanity; A Series of Studies* (Philadelphia); 1898. *The Memoirs of Pliny Earle* (Boston).

Secondary: McGovern, Constance, 1985. *Masters of Madness: Social Origins of the American Psychiatric Profession* (Hanover, NH); *DAMB*.

Andrew Scull

EASMON, CHARLES ODAMTTEN (b. Adawaso, Eastern Province, British Gold Coast (now Ghana), 22 February 1913; d. Accra, Ghana, 19 May 1994), *surgery.*

Easmon was the first Ghanaian to qualify as a medical surgeon and worked throughout his lifetime to extend the privilege of medical education to ensuing generations. He was a cofounder of both the Ghana Medical School and the Noguchi Memorial Institute for Medical Research.

Although his parents were not engaged in medical work (his father, Victor Farrell Easmon, was an accountant based in Nigeria and his mother, Kate Salomey Odamtten, lived in the Gold Coast, where her family had coffee estates), Easmon was descended from an illustrious medical family. His grandfather, John Farrell Easmon, originally from Sierra Leone, was the first African medical officer in the Gold Coast during the 1880s. Easmon received his primary school education in the Ga ethnic township of Osu, near the seat of colonial government, under the sponsorship of his grandaunt, Betty Lokko.

Easmon continued his training at the Prince of Wales College (presently Achimota School) from 1927 to 1929, where he qualified for the Intermediate BS. In 1935, Easmon was the third student (after Oku Ampofo and Eustace Akwei) to receive the new Gold Coast Medical Scholarship to study medicine in Edinburgh. He earned certification in Tropical Medicine. Upon his return, he was accepted into the ranks of the Junior African Medical Officers along with Akwei.

Easmon was one of the pioneers of Africanization, and subsequently witnessed the ironies of racial discrimination present in the higher ranks of Gold Coast Society. His wife, Genevieve Dove, regularly played tennis with the governor's wife during the 1940s. Yet when a British administrator, delighted to find an African surgeon in the country, convinced him to spend several years working in the Northern Territories, Easmon was not accepted to the local Tamale Social Club.

During the tenure of Ghana's first president, Kwame Nkrumah, Easmon was appointed director of Ghana's Medical Services (1960–62). Easmon worked to establish the first Ghana Medical School at the Korle Bu Hospital, where he served as academic dean (1964–71) until he retired to private practice in his home community at Osu. Easmon's initiation of medical professionalization processes in Africa extended to his co-founding of the Ghana Medical Association and to serving as the first Ghanaian president of the West African Organization of Surgeons. He also served as the first chairman of the Ghana Medical and Dental Council (1972–80) and as president of the Ghana Academy of Arts and Sciences (1977–81).

Together with his surgical activities benefiting a generation of Ghanaians, Easmon paved the road for medical research in the new country. He crafted a proposal to develop a medical research center honoring the Japanese scientist, Hideyo Noguchi, who died tragically in the Gold Coast from complications of his yellow fever experiments in 1928. The Noguchi Memorial Medical Research Institute, with primary funding from the Japanese government, established a critical laboratory research site for Ghanaian scientists (1979). Additionally, Easmon chaired the original Council for Scientific Research into Plant Medicine. The resulting Centre for Scientific Research into Plant Medicine (CSRPM), founded by the physician Oku Ampofo in 1972, connected indigenous therapies and biochemical analysis in the town of Mampong-Akuapem and became a World Health Organization collaborating institution. Easmon remained one of the few physicians sympathetic to plant-based therapies, staying active with CSRPM through the 1990s.

Easmon actively mentored many younger Ghanaian physicians and students. He also provided strong leadership within his extended family, and was very involved with the Masonic Lodge. With other physicians in the Osu area of Accra, Ghana, Easmon established the Osu Medical Foundation to support community health care for poorer residents.

Bibliography

Secondary: Ashitey, Gilford A., 2001. *Charles Odamtten Easmon: The Beacon* (Accra); Vieta, Kojo, 1999. *The Flagbearers of Ghana* (Accra); Addae, Steven, 1996. *The Evolution of Modern Medicine in a Developing Country: Ghana 1880–1960* (Durham, NC); Patton, Adell Jr., 1996. *Physicians, Colonial Racism, and Diaspora in West Africa* (Gainesville, FL).

Abena Dove Osseo-Asare

EASMON, JOHN FARRELL (b. Freetown, Sierra Leone, 30 June 1856; d. Cape Coast, Gold Coast (now Ghana), 9 June 1900), *medicine, bacteriology.*

Easmon was born into a Nova Scotian settler family in Freetown, Sierra Leone, West Africa. His maternal grandfather, John McCormack, from a well-known Irish medical family, became wealthy in the Sierra Leone Crown Colony. Easmon inherited £400 from McCormack's estate, and in 1876 departed Freetown for medical study at University College, London. He earned the MRCS (1879), then the LM and LKQCP (Ireland), and the MD with distinction from the University of Brussels. Upon returning to Freetown as a medical practitioner, he was recruited in 1880 into the Colonial Medical Service as assistant colonial surgeon in the Gold Coast at a standard salary of £400 per annum, with increments and rights to private practice. In spite of intra-professional conflicts, his medical achievements prompted promotions to higher posts than previously achieved by any other African doctor in the locally organized Colonial Medical Service of nineteenth-century sub-Saharan Africa.

Easmon headed the Medical Department of the Gold Coast, where he made his most important contribution to medical knowledge. He was the first to describe blackwater fever (later known as hemoglobinuric fever) by writing the first clinical analysis of the symptoms of the disease in English in 1884. This was a significant publication because hemoglobinuric fever was a very poorly defined complication of falciparum malaria, and yet the most severe form in West Africa. Although rare in indigenous people thanks to their genetic adaptations to malaria, and recognized as a unique fever only in 1864 by the medical establishment, Europeans in West Africa suffered mortality as high as 50 percent from the disorder. Easmon's findings revealed its most significant symptoms as severe anemia and massive hemoglobin levels in the urine. In 1888 the Gold Coast governor sent Easmon's report to the Colonial Office, which recommended forwarding it to medical officers elsewhere in the Empire as part of systematic efforts to reduce mortality. In *Tropical Medicine* (2nd edition, 1913), Castellani and Chambers belatedly acknowledged Easmon's first description of 'blackwater fever'.

Easmon became Chief Medical Officer of the Gold Coast in 1893. The European population had increased significantly and Easmon served as a private physician to many colonial families. The nature of his practice is evidenced in part by the survival of his 'Private Prescription Book (1894–1896)'. During this time, Easmon treated a number of patients from the Basel Mission, which played a role in African education. Another group of patients came from well-known people involved in the development of The Gold Coast: the Bannerman, Musgrave, and Vanderpuye families; Thomas Hutton Mills; and Peter Awooner-Renner. Typical of the times, Easmon's treatments included morphine derivatives and alcohol.

Easmon died at Cape Coast at the age of forty-three. Despite his brief lifespan, he received many honors. After successful academic studies during which he earned six gold and silver medals, Easmon was offered a position as House Surgeon at St. George's Hospital in London by his cousin, Senior Surgeon Sir William McCormick, president of the Royal College of Surgeons and surgeon to Queen Victoria. But Easmon declined the first such appointment ever offered to a West African, returning instead to Sierra Leone.

Bibliography

Primary: 1884. *The Nature and Treatment of Blackwater Fever, with Bibliographical notes and temperature charts of cases treated* (London).

Secondary: Patton, Adell Jr., 1996. *Physicians, Colonial Racism, and Diaspora in West Africa* (Gainesville, FL); Patton, Adell Jr., 1989. 'Dr. John Farrell Easmon: Medical Professionalism and Colonial Racism in the Gold Coast, 1856–1900.' *The International Journal of African Historical Studies* 22(4): 601–636; Patterson, K. David, 1974. 'Disease and Medicine in African History: A Bibliographical Essay.' *History in Africa Journal* 1: 141–148.

Adell Patton Jr.

EDDY, MARY BAKER (b. Bow, New Hampshire, USA, 21 July 1821; d. Chestnut Hill, Massachusetts, USA, 3 December 1910), *Christian Science.*

The daughter of Mark Baker and Abigail Ambroise, Mary Baker was educated privately. In 1843 she married George Glover, who died the following year; the marriage produced a son. She married Daniel Patterson in 1853, then after an 1873 divorce wed Asa Gilbert Eddy in 1877.

Mary Baker Eddy experienced poor health throughout her life. In 1862, while still Mary Patterson, the semi-invalid journeyed to Portland, Maine, to seek help from Phineas Parkhurst Quimby, a noted practitioner of mind cure. Quimby believed that physical disease was the product of a negative mental state, and he healed by instilling a positive outlook and faith in recovery in the patient's mind. Patterson not only improved under Quimby's care; she also embraced his belief in the mental origin of sickness and developed it into a distinctive approach to healing she would call Christian Science.

There is a long-running controversy between the defenders of Quimby and representatives of the Christian Science Church over the question of Patterson's debt to Quimby. The former assert she borrowed freely but without attribution from Quimby's teachings and unpublished writings; the latter maintain she received inspiration from no one but God. Be that as it may, by 1868 she was taking on students for initiation into a new theological analysis of disease. Since God comprises all of existence and is an entirely spiritual being, she argued, matter does not exist. Hence there is no body to be affected by disease. 'Disease', rather, is an imagined condition, an erroneous belief in the reality of a mortal body and physical suffering, and can be relieved by purging the victim's mind of that mistaken notion through instruction and prayer. Such, she maintained, was the healing method used by Christ.

Mary Baker taught and practiced her system for seven years until publishing, in 1875, the founding document of Christian Science: *Science and Health with Key to the Scriptures* (the book would go through numerous editions, and its author become wealthy from royalties). The following year, she organized students into The Christian Scientists' Association, which in 1879 received a charter from the state of Massachusetts as the Church of Christ, Scientist. A more formal program for training Christian Science practitioners in the art of correcting patients' mental errors began in 1881 with the opening of the Massachusetts Metaphysical College in Boston; Mary Baker Eddy was the only instructor. In 1883 she established the *Journal of Christian Science*, which featured a 'Healing Department' whose reports of extraordinary cures were instrumental in attracting members to the Church. By the early 1900s Christian Science was the fastest-growing denomination in the United States, its ranks of 40,000 swelling to more than 200,000 by 1925.

From its beginnings, Christian Science came under constant attack from the orthodox medical profession both as an unscientific theory and as a danger to seriously ill people denied conventional treatment. Eventually, to avoid negative publicity and legal conflict, Eddy decreed that church members should accept vaccinations and standard medical care for seriously ill children. She also determined that it was permissible for adults to seek conventional therapy in situations in which Christian Science practitioners were failing to provide relief, though they were to return to Church practitioners as soon as their pains subsided. She herself wore eyeglasses and used a dental plate, and over the last decade of her life took morphine for relief from gallstones. Eddy became a recluse during her last years, but in 1908 she founded *The Christian Science Monitor*, which would develop into one of America's leading newspapers.

Bibliography

Primary: 1875. *Science and Health, with Key to the Scriptures* (Boston); 1891. *Retrospection and Introspection* (Boston).

Secondary: Gill, Gillian, 1998. *Mary Baker Eddy* (Reading, MA); Peel, Robert, 1977. *Mary Baker Eddy, The Years of Authority* (New York); Peel, Robert, 1966. *Mary Baker Eddy, The Years of Discovery* (New York); Dakin, Edward, 1929. *Mrs. Eddy* (New York); *DAMB*.

James Whorton

EDSALL, DAVID LINN (b. Hamburg, New Jersey, USA, 6 July 1869; d. Cambridge, Massachusetts, USA, 12 August 1945), *medicine, industrial medicine, occupational medicine.*

Edsall was a leader in American academic medicine in the early twentieth century, spending much of his career at Harvard University, where he served overlapping terms as Dean of the medical school from 1918 to 1935, and Dean of the school of public health from 1921 to 1935. Edsall achieved national prominence as a researcher, a clinician, and an academic administrator among a generation of American physicians who helped establish full-time careers in academic clinical medicine.

Edsall began his studies as an undergraduate at Princeton University. After an early trial in the Department of Classics, he turned to the sciences, taking courses in zoology, botany, chemistry, physics, and histology, ultimately deciding on a career in medicine. Upon graduating in 1890, he was accepted to the University of Pennsylvania and completed his medical degree there in the requisite three years. In 1893 he took a one-year internship at Mercy Hospital in Pittsburgh, where his brother, Frank, was already in medical practice. Following the completion of the internship, Edsall traveled for a year, visiting medical centers in London, Vienna, and Graz. He returned to Pittsburgh and briefly attempted to set up in practice, but soon followed his strong connections back to the University of Pennsylvania. There, he followed a rising path through the academic hierarchy, beginning as a clinical associate in the William Pepper Laboratory in 1895, and attaining an appointment in 1907 to succeed H. C. Wood in the professorship in therapeutics and pharmacology.

Edsall's family life started off on an equally favorable path. He was born the sixth of seven boys to a prosperous couple, Richard Edsall and Emma Everett (Linn) Edsall. Emma's family included several physicians who may have influenced Edsall's decision to enter medicine. Richard Edsall had a successful political career, beginning as sheriff and postmaster of Hamburg, and eventually becoming a state senator before David's birth.

In 1899, after his return to Philadelphia, Edsall married Margaret Harding Tileston. The couple had three children, but Margaret died suddenly in Boston of pneumonia in 1912. Edsall remarried in 1915, but ended that troubled marriage to Elizabeth Pendleton Kennedy in 1929. Following his divorce, he married a final time in 1930 to Louisa Cabot Richardson.

Edsall would eventually achieve academic prominence in the field of industrial medicine, but he met with important early recognition for his research in metabolism and nutrition. His first efforts were encouraged through his involvement with an emerging network of university-affiliated, academic physicians. Edsall contributed to the establishment of a series of cosmopolitan academic medical associations that would form the backbone of his professional life. In 1905 he became one of the inaugural members of William Osler's influential Interurban Clinical Club, which drew together a rising generation of academically affiliated physicians along the Atlantic axis from Baltimore and Philadelphia to New York and Boston. That same year he joined the new Society for Experimental Biology and Medicine, and in 1907 he helped found the influential American Society for Clinical Investigation. This tight-knit group, which promoted itself as the 'Young Turks' of academic clinical medicine, included Samuel Meltzer of New York, Warfield Longcope of Philadelphia, Joseph Pratt of Boston, and Henry Christian of Baltimore.

The possibility of full-time academic clinical medical careers took root with the efforts of this network of affiliated colleagues. Clinical professors from a generation before Edsall were expected to occupy a good part of their time in private medical practice and to derive significant income from this work. Edsall and his colleagues helped shift the balance of academic clinical medicine into the medical school.

With the support of his professional network, Edsall parlayed an early interest and expertise in the clinical use of chemical analysis into a set of researches on metabolism. One of his first publications after his return to the University of Pennsylvania concerned the measurement of hydrochloric acid in stomach contents, a technique that was thought at the time to help in distinguishing stomach cancer from gastric ulcer. Edsall also began to review and extend the existing applications of chemical analysis of the urine. In his eclectic research during the early 1900s, Edsall published on urinary carbohydrates and benzoyl esters in diabetes, urinary sulfates in pancreatic disease, urinary potassium in periodic familial paralysis, and uric acid in the urine in gout.

His skill in chemical analysis also lent itself to clinical questions of the day about nutrition. Edsall studied the proper composition of artificial infant feeding formula, and the nutritional effects of rectal feeding—both vital concerns of clinicians in the early twentieth century. Specific questions about the chemistry of excretions and feedings easily broadened into general questions about the nature of metabolism in disease states. Edsall studied the changes in metabolism created during the x-ray treatment of leukemia and wrote on the metabolic derangements of diabetes.

Through this period Edsall also published individual case reports of patients seen during routine clinical duties, a form of publication representing the largest single item in the medical literature of the day. One of Edsall's important early cases represented a bridge between his work on metabolism and his later, more widely known research in industrial medicine. In 1904 Edsall published a brief paper describing severe muscle cramping in two men he saw at Episcopal Hospital in Philadelphia. One of the men had been a locomotive fireman in the city. Edsall drew no general conclusions from these cases. But when he later

encountered similar cases in patients with extended exposure to hot conditions, it triggered his renewed interest.

He performed a variety of chemical and metabolic assays to determine the excretion of nitrogen, uric acid, creatinin, and related substances in these individuals. In addition, he surveyed his colleagues searching for additional cases that might shed more light on the condition. The metabolic studies proved to be less revealing than his survey. He found a strong association of this condition with occupations that required work near high heat, such as ships' stokers. He also discovered that previous descriptions of the adverse effects of heat had not mentioned muscle spasms. Edsall speculated that the problem might represent a distinct, but previously unrecognized, syndrome, closely related to occupational hazard. Edsall gradually left behind his metabolic studies as he increasingly turned his attention to the medical consequences of industrial and occupational exposures.

One well-known and substantive contribution from this phase of Edsall's career was his work on manganese poisoning. The problem came to attention in a plant of the New Jersey Zinc Company, where workers who had spent considerable time exposed to dust with significant levels of manganese developed a set of striking and disturbing impairments (Edsall, 1919). Edsall, F. P. Wilbur, and Cecil Drinker conducted a study that settled some existing questions about the clinical condition. More importantly, their work helped in clarifying and emphasizing the need to reduce exposure to manganese dust in industrial applications in order to prevent the condition.

Although he established a substantial reputation as a researcher, Edsall made his most lasting contributions through his administrative leadership in academic medicine. The growth of Harvard Medical School during Edsall's period as Dean drew considerable praise, and moved the school from a being a local leader in New England to become a national model for medical education (Ludmerer, 1999, pp. 55–56). With Edsall's vigorous efforts at recruitment, the size of the medical faculty doubled during his tenure. The budget of the school nearly quadrupled during Edsall's first decade, although when he arrived in 1918, the school was running a budgetary deficit. In the first years of the twentieth century prior to Edsall's arrival in Boston, more than 90 percent of Harvard's medical students were drawn from New England. By the time Edsall retired in 1935, nearly 70 percent of the students came from outside the region.

Edsall was especially influential on developments in public and occupational medicine, expanding their institutional base in academic medicine. He served as the first American editor of the *Journal of Industrial Hygiene*. He took an important role in securing the support of the Rockefeller Foundation that led to its initial gift of $1,785,000 for the creation of the Harvard School of Public Health. In 1921 he agreed to serve as the school's first dean, while continuing to serve as dean of the medical school. Edsall was equally successful at the helm of the School of Public Health. During the first decade of his stewardship, the school's endowment grew to over $3,000,000.

Closely linked to his efforts to establish public health at the university were Edsall's negotiations with one of the nation's early leaders in the field of industrial medicine, Alice Hamilton. Edsall worked hard to bring her to the school of medicine as its first woman professor. When Hamilton joined the school in 1919, Edsall described this accomplishment as more than a local advance in building expertise in industrial toxicology. He wrote to Hamilton, 'Aside from my very great desire that we may be able to secure you for this work, I desire it also for the reason that I think it would be a large step forward in the proper attitude toward women in this University and in some other Universities' (Aub and Hapgood, 1970, p. 251). Hamilton's work on industrial lead poisoning that she continued in Boston apparently gained local support based in part on Edsall's established record of collaborative research on manganese. Hamilton retired from Harvard and the School of Public Health in 1935, the same year that Edsall stepped down as Dean.

Bibliography

Primary: 1905. 'A case of acute leukemia, with some striking observations on metabolism in this case.' *American Journal of the Medical Sciences* 130: 589–600; 1908. 'A disorder due to exposure to intense heat.' *JAMA* 51(23): 1969–71; 1919. (with Wilbur, F. P., and Cecil K. Drinker) 'The occurrence, course, and prevention of chronic manganese poisoning.' *Journal of Industrial Hygiene* 1: 183–193.

Secondary: Ludmerer, Kenneth M., 1999. *Time to Heal: American Medical Education from the Turn of the Century to the Era of Managed Care* (New York); Aub, Joseph C., and Ruth K. Hapgood, 1970. *Pioneer in Medicine: David Linn Edsall of Harvard* (Boston); *DAMB.*

Christopher Crenner

EDWARDS-PILLIET, BLANCHE (b. Milly-La-Forêt, Seine et Marne, France, 24 November 1858; d. Paris, France, January 1941), *medicine, nursing education.*

Edwards-Pilliet was the daughter of an English-born, French-educated physician, George Hugh Edwards, and Amanda née Froc, a French woman. She adopted her father's Protestant religion. As a young girl, she accompanied her father on his medical rounds and he prepared her in general studies and sciences which enabled her to pass the Baccalaureat in letters (1877) and the Baccalaureat in sciences (1878). From 1878 to 1882, she studied at the Paris Faculté de Médecine.

Far more protected as a middle-class French girl than were English or American women of her generation, initially she was accompanied to her medical school classes by her father. After graduation, she joined the service of the distinguished neurologist, Jean-Martin Charcot, at Salpêtrière Hospital. After two years under Charcot, both Edwards and an American woman, Augusta Klumpke, became the first women permitted to compete in *l'externat*, the examination for the Paris hospital internship. Edwards petitioned Paul Bert, then Minster of Education, who overruled the objections of the medical faculty. When both young women passed with excellent marks, conservative members of the faculty and a group of medical students protested in front of the medical school and in the medical press. As a Frenchwoman, Edwards came in for most of the abuse, which included a figure burned in effigy.

Edwards was made a 'provisional intern' to Dr Labadie-Lagrave at a Paris children's hospital, l'Hôpital des Enfants Assistés (1886–89). She reported to a Paris newspaper that her experience at the interns' dining room, the *salle de garde*, was made bearable only by the presence of Alexandre-Henri Pilliet, a fellow intern and her fiancé.

In 1889 Edwards successfully defended her medical thesis on hemiplegia that emanated from her work with Charcot. She began private medical practice, which she continued until 1941. In 1891 she married Pilliet; he died in 1898, leaving her with three children. She took over his position as Professor of Nursing Instruction at Salpêtrière Hospital (1898–1927). During this period she developed health and hygiene programs for schoolgirls as consulting physician to two distinguished Paris girls' schools, Lycée Lamartine and Lycée Victor-Duruy.

Edwards-Pilliet served as chairman of the medical division for the Conference on Women's Work in Paris, at which she urged women to insist on the expansion of girls' secondary education. Since at the time no women physicians in France held important positions in hospitals or medical schools, she urged wealthy French women to support women's medical schools and hospitals similar to the one run by Elizabeth Garrett Anderson in London. Her suggestion went unheeded in the highly centralized French medical world.

Edwards-Pilliet was a founding member of the Ligue des Mères that provided health instruction and medical assistance to working women. During World War I she participated as a Red Cross instructor (1914–17) and as physician to female personnel at the Puteaux Arsenal (1917–19). She was a strong supporter of middle-class feminism, serving as vice president of the Ligue pour les Droits des Femmes, and worked much of her life on behalf of women's suffrage. In her sixties she was made a Chevalier of the Legion of Honor. Edwards-Pilliet died in Paris during the Nazi occupation.

Bibliography

Primary: 1889. *De l'hemiplégie dans quelques affections nerveuses.* Thesis (Paris); 1889. Discussions. *Congrès des Oeuvres et Institutions Feminines. passim* (Paris); 1902. Discussion as president of 'Arts, Lettres, Sciences' June 22, 1900. (Madame Pegaud, ed.) *Con-*

grès des Oeuvres et Institutions Feminines vol 4 *passim*. (Paris); 1906–1911. Series of feminist articles, *La Française*.

Secondary: Leguay, Françoise, and Claude Barbizet, 1988. *Blanche Edwards-Pilliet: Femme et médecin 1858–1941* (Paris); Lipinska, Mélanie, 1930. *Les femmes et le progrès des sciences médicales* (Paris); Lipinska, Mélanie, 1900. *Les femmes médecins depuis l'antiquité jusqu'à nos jours* (Paris).

Joy Harvey

EGAS MONIZ, ANTÓNIO CAETANO DE ABREU FREIRE

(b. Avanca, Portugal, 29 November 1874; d. Lisbon, Portugal, 13 December 1955), *neurology*.

Born into an old, decadent, and noble country family, Moniz had his youth marked by the death of his sister (1887) and the emigration of his father to Mozambique in an effort to ameliorate the family's difficult economic condition. Moniz had the support of his uncle, an abbot who funded and abetted his studies, first in a Jesuit Catholic school, *S. Fiel*, near Castelo–Branco, and afterwards in the ancient University of Coimbra, where he studied medicine (1894–99). During this period he suffered the death of his father, brother, mother, and finally his uncle, evidencing psychological strength and the capacity to deal with loss. He also suffered the onset of gout, an affliction that would progressively cripple his hands.

In 1901 Moniz became a Doctor in Medicine, and in 1902 a professor with two theses about sexual life that created a sensation. Together they became a bestseller published under the title, *A vida sexual (fisiologia e patalogia)* [Physiology and Pathology of the Sexual Life]. In 1911 Moniz moved to Lisbon University, and was appointed to the Chair of Clinical Neurology, newly created after the 1910 Republican Revolution.

By this time Moniz already had a strong career in politics, begun while he was still a student. He became a member of Parliament, the founder of a political party, Ambassador to Madrid, and Minister of Foreign Affairs. In the latter capacity he led the Portuguese delegation to the 1919 Versailles Peace Conference. Immediately afterwards, disenchanted with Portuguese politics, he devoted full attention to his scientific career.

Moniz became director of the neurology service at the *Santa Marta* Hospital in Lisbon. There, from the 1920s through the 1940s, he developed his research, continuing to teach and practice neurology at the Lisbon Medical School. He had begun his neurological training in 1902 in Bordeaux, France, under Jean-Albert Pitres (1848–1928) and Joseph Abadie (1873–1934), and studied psychiatry with Emmanuel Régis (1855–1918), developing a special interest in toxic psychoses. Afterwards, he moved to Paris where he worked with Fulgence Raymond (1844–1910), Pierre Marie (1853–1940), Jules Dejérine (1849–1917), Joseph Babinski (1857–1932), and Jean-Athanase Sicard (1872–1929).

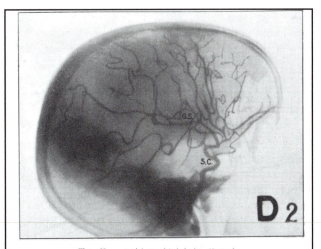

Fig. 163. — Artériographie à droite. Normale. Forte circulation de l'hémisphère cérébral (obs. XXVIII).

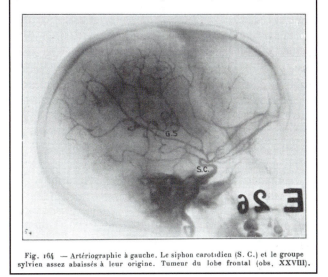

Fig. 164 — Artériographie à gauche. Le siphon carotidien (S. C.) et le groupe sylvien assez abaissés à leur origine. Tumeur du lobe frontal (obs. XXVIII).

Arteriographs showing normal circulation of the right cerebral hemisphere (top) and displacement of the vessels (bottom), indicating a frontal lobe tumor. Halftone reproduction from *Diagnostic des tumeurs cérébrales . . .* Paris, 1931. Wellcome Library, London.

Moniz contributed materially to the spread of psychoanalytic ideas in Portugal. In 1915, within his course on neurology, he dedicated a lecture to the basis of psychoanalysis which was subsequently published. This was the first known scientific work on the subject in Portugal, and highlighted the enormous value of the discipline to the etiologic and symptomatic interpretation of neuroses and their treatment.

From Arterial Encephalography to Angiography

'To obtain by contrast methods, a better visualization of the brain, always has been a concern of neurologists . . . we have then thought about researching new processes of brain visibility' (Moniz, 1931, p. 233).

After 1924 Moniz understood that neurology should progress through the deepening of basic sciences and by the development of new diagnostic techniques, especially by the use of radiography. By then, neurosurgeons were beginning to operate on cerebral tumors. One of the most difficult problems for neurologists and neurosurgeons was the precise localization of brain tumors. Moniz's working hypothesis was that it should be possible to produce opacity in brain tissue by injecting a radiopaque substance, thus making available information on what neurologists called 'the silent part of the brain'. Step by step, he developed the first experimental phase: searching for a substance neither toxic nor painful, radiopaque, and able to give good contrast to the arterial cerebral vessels. He first experimented on cadavers (1925) with bromides and iodides, and made some attempts with dogs to discover the optimal concentration of the product, finally choosing sodium iodide at a concentration of 25 percent for injecting into the carotid artery.

After trying in the cadaver to determine the amount of radiopaque substance necessary, and deciding about the precise technique for injecting the carotid, the first human trials were carried out in epileptic patients, patients with suspected brain tumors and in Parkinsonian post-encephalitic patients. On 28 June 1927, in the old *Santa Marta* Hospital, Moniz and his closest assistant, Almeida Lima, made the first arterial encephalography in a patient suspected of a sellar tumor.

Soon afterward, Moniz published his first monograph, *Diagnostic des Tumeurs Cerebrales et Epreuve de l' Encephalographie Arterielle* (1931), with a preface by Babinski, who judged it a 'magisterial exposition of the classic notions about cerebral tumors'. For Moniz, arterial encephalography helped indicate the height, position and, more importantly, the nature of tumors. However, it was not easy to convince neurologists about the potentials of the method. During the 1940s, a British neurosurgeon stated of arterial encephalography that 'the trouble for a small gain remains disproportionately great' (Imaginário, 1956, p. 656).

Also in 1931, Moniz began to employ a new radiopaque substance: thorium dioxide (thorotrast), which was easier to use, apparently safer, and which remained visible to X-rays long after the injection, allowing (by happy accident) the visualization of the brain's venous system—the first phlebography.

'It was by using this new substance that we succeeded in transforming arteriography into angiography' (Moniz, 1934, p. 20). Afterwards, the technique interested not only neurologists and neurosurgeons, but also general surgeons, physiologists, and anatomists.

Some researchers maintain that 'if till 1931, Moniz was interested in giving use and meaning to arteriographic images, after 1934–35 he was involved in the work of establishing a "vision of the brain"; such a vision was not about a theory of how the brain works but about a way of seeing the brain work. The visualization technique Moniz was proposing made new symptoms, new anatomical and physiological knowledge and methods emerge' (Moreira, 1997, p. 30).

In 1935 Moniz gave a talk at London's International Neurology Congress about 'Angiography in the Diagnosis of Brain Aneurisms and Angiomas'. Thus angiography turned into a method of diagnosing vascular problems, Moniz later admitted, with greater benefit than in any other kind of disorders.

In 1928 and 1933 Moniz was nominated for the Nobel Prize for the discovery of this new technique—angiography.

The Intervention in Psychiatric Therapeutics—Prefrontal Leucotomy

In 1935, skeptical about all nonorganicist models of mental disease, Moniz, in collaboration with the neurosurgeon Almeida Lima (with whom he had discussed the subject for more than two and a half years), decided to carry out a surgical procedure to treat mental disease.

He based his ideas on a naturalist 'neuronism'. For him, psychic life was founded on the activity of cerebral cells and their reciprocal connections (nervous circuitry). As some of those circuits could become fixed by conditioning, it followed that patients with delusions or obsessive-compulsive traits of behavior might suffer from a wrong fixation of some of those synaptic circuits. That would cause continuous obsessive, morbid ideas, completely resistant to verbal and pharmacological therapy—'the fixed connection principle' (Moniz, 1936, p. 46). The partial destruction of flawed circuitry might lead to improvement; disrupting aberrant circuits could change the deviant behavior.

Why in the frontal lobe? In his Birmingham lectures of 1948, John F. Fulton commented that 'in the thoughtful prefatory chapters of Moniz's monograph on lobotomy he indicates that for some years prior to 1935 he had entertained the thought of interrupting frontal lobe projections as a possible therapeutic weapon for dealing with some of the more severe psychoses. He cites the work of Henri Claude on the functions of the frontal lobe, and also the observations of the late Clovis Vincent . . . he directs attention to the report which I made with Jacobsen on the behavior changes observed in chimpanzees, following bilateral removal of frontal areas' (Fulton, 1949, p. 62).

First, alcohol injections were used for the destruction of pre-frontal white matter pathways, until Moniz and Lima made a special instrument—the cerebral leucotome—that sectioned the subcortical pathways with a small lesion over the related cortex. The first leucotomy was performed on 27 December 1935.

In 1936 Moniz published a report in Paris on the first twenty patients operated on, concluding that 35 percent (seven patients) showed great improvement, 35 percent (seven patients) mild improvement, and 30 percent (six patients) no change. Subsequently, 'he and his close associates were carried away by this new opportunity of actually determining some therapeutic benefit to otherwise condemned patients' (Damasio, 2000, p.107).

In 1939 Moniz was shot by one of his patients, but survived and partially recovered. He retired in 1944. In 1945 he was awarded the Oslo Prize for cerebral angiography which, until the end of Second World War, was practically ignored. In 1948 the International Congress of Neurology took place in Lisbon, where Moniz read his paper, 'How I came to perform prefrontal leucotomy'. He was proposed for a Nobel Prize for Medicine that was awarded to him the following year, with a citation referring to 'his invention of a surgical treatment for mental illness and to his elaboration of the psychophysiological concepts that make it possible'.

But this assessment was not completely accepted by the scientific community, and fueled controversy: 'Leucotomy . . . whose scientific foundation was somewhat fragile and might even have questioned religious and philosophical beliefs' (Damasio, 2000, p.107). As late as 1954, Moniz had to defend leucotomy from its critics with the paper, '*A leucotomia está em causa*'.

Other Activities

Moniz was a prominent medical writer. He also published several books and articles about literary, historical, and artistic matters, specifically many articles about Portuguese writers and painters, and also about scientists he admired, such as Ramon y Cajal.

Bibliography

Primary: 1915. 'As bases da psicanálise.' *A Medicina Contemporánea* 33(47): 377–383; 1931. *Diagnostique des tumeurs cérébrales et épreuve de l'encéphalographie artérielle* (Paris); 1934. *L'Angiographie Cérébrale. Ses applications et résultats en Anatomie, Physiologie et Clinique* (Paris); 1936. *Tentatives opératoires dans le traitement de certaines psychoses* (Paris); 1949. *Confidências de um investigador científico* (Lisbon).

Secondary: Damasio, António R., 2000. 'Egas Moniz, Pioneer of Angiography and Leucotomy' in Pereira, Ana Leonor, and João Rui Pita, eds., *Egas Moniz em livre exame* (Coimbra) pp. 97–109; Pressman, Jack D., 1998. *Last Resort: Psychosurgery and the Limits of Medicine* (Cambridge); Moreira, Tiago, 1997. 'Large Gain for Small Trouble: The Construction of Cerebral Angiography.' Unpublished MSc. thesis, University of Edinburgh; Fernandes, Barahona, 1983. *Egas Moniz, pioneiro de descobrimentos medicos* (Lisbon); Comissão Executiva das Comemorações do Centenário do nascimento do Professor Egas Moniz, 1977–78. *Egas Moniz centenary: Scientific Reports* 2 vols. (Lisbon); Imaginário, Joaquim G., 1956. 'Contribuição para a História da Angiografia Cerebral. A expansão da angiografia em Inglaterra.' *Gazeta Médica Portuguesa* 9: 655–658; Fulton, John F., 1949. *Functional Localization in the Frontal Lobes and Cerebellum* (Oxford); *DSB*.

José Morgado Pereira

EHRLICH, PAUL   (b. Strehlen, Upper Silesia, Germany [now Poland], 14 March 1854; d. Bad Homburg, Germany, 20 August 1915), *immunology, bacteriology, chemotherapy.*

Ehrlich was the son of a merchant. Between 1872 and 1878 he studied medicine in Breslau, Strasbourg, Freiburg im Breisgau, and Leipzig (MD, 1878). He worked as a physician and scientist at the First Medical Clinic of the Charité Hospital in Berlin (1878–85) under the well-known specialist of internal medicine, Theodor Frerichs (1819–85). Ehrlich got his teaching license (*Habilitation*) and also the title professor in 1885. After the sudden death of Frerichs that same year, Ehrlich became an assistant to Carl Gerhardt (1833–1902) at the Second Medical Clinic of the Charité Hospital.

In 1888 Ehrlich became infected with tuberculosis at work. He resigned and went to Egypt for one year to recover. In 1889, he came back to Berlin and performed immunological research work in a small laboratory, which he set up with the help of his father-in-law. In 1890 the well-known bacteriologist, Robert Koch (1843–1910), hired Ehrlich, his helping hand in former years, as clinical supervisor for studies on tuberculosis at the city hospital, Berlin-Moabit. The following year, Koch gave Ehrlich a laboratory in Berlin's newly founded Institute for Infectious Diseases (*Institut für Infektionskrankheiten*), where Ehrlich continued his immunological studies.

In 1896 Ehrlich became director of the newly-founded Institute for Serum Research and Serum Testing (*Institut für Serumforschung und Serumprüfung*) in Berlin Steglitz. This institute, still headed by Ehrlich, moved to Frankfurt/ Main in 1899 and was renamed the 'Institute for Experimental Therapy' (*Institut für experimentelle Therapie*). In 1914, Ehrlich became regular professor (*Ordinarius*) at the newly-inaugurated University of Frankfurt/Main. In 1915 Ehrlich died from the aftermath of a stroke.

Ehrlich received many honors in his life, among them the 1908 Nobel Prize for Medicine or Physiology, which he received together with Elie Mechnikov (1845–1916) for his immunological research. Paul Ehrlich's work was decisive for the development of modern scientific medicine. He introduced microscopic examinations based on dyes into medical research and practice, making contemporary knowledge in chemistry accessible for scientific medicine. Thereby, he promoted diagnostics and therapy of many diseases, and laid the path for the examination of human metabolism. Ehrlich accomplished this through important studies on immunology and chemotherapy.

Ehrlich aimed at applying advances in chemistry to medicine, especially methods of staining which he had already considered as a student. In his years in Strasbourg under the anatomist Wilhelm Waldeyer (1836–1921), Ehrlich stained histological specimens (cuttings through human tissue). The staining of cells enabled Ehrlich to undertake a much more detailed investigation of their functions. In 1875–76 Ehrlich first described 'mast cells'

(*Mastzellen*), which are important for the defense system of the human body. Ehrlich soon became convinced that cells and dyes would bind chemically, and that the metabolism of the cell obeyed chemical laws. He summarized these views on the theory and practice of histological staining in his thesis of 1878.

Ehrlich's studies on dyes while a student in Breslau were mainly promoted by the pathologists Carl Weigert (1845–1904), Ehrlich's cousin, and Julius Cohnheim (1839–1884). Cohnheim especially was eager to foster and to perform animal experimentation, thereby complementing static morphological enquiries in the morgue. The ultimate aim was to uncover pathological processes and to set up a pathological physiology. For Cohnheim, this also meant research in close collaboration with practical medicine. Ehrlich and Cohnheim became pioneers of 'clinical pathology', which rested on a connection between ward and lab and was introduced first in England after 1900.

Therefore, it was not by chance that Ehrlich started his career in medical practice. From the beginning, the clinical application of results achieved in the laboratory had great importance for him. Under Frerichs, a pioneer of scientific clinical work, Ehrlich had both his own laboratory and access to the wards at the Berlin Charité Hospital. He examined tissues from the morgue with the help of dyes, as well as tissue samples and body fluids from the living. The results he obtained helped elaborate diagnostic and therapeutic measures. A landmark of Ehrlich's research under Frerichs was his hematological work, dealing with pathological conditions of blood. With the help of staining, Ehrlich detected different kinds of red and white blood cells, thereby contributing decisively to diagnostics and therapy of blood diseases. Ehrlich became a pioneer of modern hematology.

Work in the wards (also human experimentation) and staining methods in the lab could be combined with animal experimentation. One of the most important results of merging these different approaches was Ehrlich's study on the oxygen-utilization of mammalian cells. In his *Habilitation* thesis of 1885, based primarily on animal experimentation, he determined the oxygen-consumption of the mammalian organism. The tissues' absorption of dyes indicated their differing ability to absorb oxygen. According to his theory about the chemical binding of substances to cells, Ehrlich speculated that the cell would absorb oxygen through so-called 'side-chains' at its surface, which would bind specifically to oxygen. But in those years such theories had no impact on Ehrlich's practical work.

Frerich's death produced a decisive break in Ehrlich's career. Carl Gerhardt, his new superior, had little interest in Ehrlich's laboratory work and integrated him into the daily clinical routine, which was clearly a setback for him. Also, his disease intruded, imposing an inevitable one-year work break. When Ehrlich opened his small private lab in Berlin in 1889, he first focused solely on laboratory research and ven-

tured into the field of immunology. Robert Koch's bacteriological work was very inspiring, particularly since Ehrlich had already developed a new staining method for tubercle bacilli for Koch in 1882. In his private enterprise, Ehrlich was successful in immunizing mice against the plant poisons abrin and ricin. He found evidence that offspring from immunized mice had received a passive immunity, and this passive immunity was also transferred via breastfeeding.

When Koch gave Ehrlich a new job, he proceeded with his immunological studies, supported by the inspiring and motivating group in Koch's institute. Koch's pupil, Emil von Behring (1854–1917), and von Behring's assistant, Shibasaburo Kitasato (1852–1931), had discovered in 1890 in cases of diphtheria and tetanus, that the respective organism had produced antibodies against these microbes. Thereafter, the idea to immunize the human body against diseases with the respective sera fascinated Ehrlich. His work in this field could rely on his studies on the plant poisons. The plan was to develop antitoxins, but he tried to duplicate the working conditions he had in former years under Frerichs: laboratory experiments were combined with human experimentation and the practical application of the substances to be tested. Together with a colleague, for example, Ehrlich tested diphtheria serum on 220 children. Also, staining investigations were continued.

Although busy with interesting and demanding research, Ehrlich's situation was difficult. As a Jew, he had no tenured post at Koch's institute, and his academic survival was not guaranteed. Two circumstances ameliorated his situation. First, Koch's group needed Ehrlich in 1894 more than ever. Von Behring and the pharmaceutical company Farbwerke Hoechst had difficulties producing diphtheria serum in reliable concentrations with a calculable effect on patients. Von Behring asked Ehrlich for help, and Ehrlich now had access to a field occupied firmly by von Behring, namely the standardization of therapeutic sera.

But Ehrlich still had no secure position, and a second circumstance was important for his rescue. One of his friends and supporters, the ministry councilor in the Prussian Ministry of Science and Education (*Ministerialrat im preußischen Kultusministerium*), Friedrich Althoff (1839–1908), arranged the formation of an Institute for serum standardization, which was opened in 1896 in Steglitz, then in the Berlin suburbs. Ehrlich became head of this institute. It was also Althoff who organized a new institute for Ehrlich in Frankfurt/Main in 1899.

At Steglitz, Ehrlich concentrated mainly on theoretical laboratory work to solve problems with diphtheria sera. In 1897, he developed and broadened his old idea of side-chains into a side-chain theory. Based on a large number of intricate experiments with guinea pigs, he detected that toxin (poison released by microbes) was neutralized by antitoxin (antibodies). But both fractions did not remain in constant relationship. Ehrlich continuously performed experiments to investigate the immunological effects of toxins and antitoxin.

In the end, his side-chain theory offered an elegant explanation. Certain side-chains of the cell were able to bind certain toxins. Because these occupied side-chains would then become unable to fulfill their physiological functions, the cell would overcompensate by producing a lot of additional side-chains. These side-chains would be released into the blood stream, where they acted as antibodies or antitoxins.

In the ensuing years Ehrlich investigated the side-chain theory in detail with his assistant, the bacteriologist Julius Morgenroth (1871–1924). In 1900, Ehrlich and Morgenroth renamed the side-chains 'receptors'. By about 1905 Ehrlich had developed a microcosm of different interacting immunological substances and broadened his side-chain theory into a 'receptor theory'. The latter was hotly debated and needed to be defended by Ehrlich. Although partly refuted, the receptor theory opened the door for modern immunology and pharmacology, and led to Ehrlich's 1908 Nobel Prize.

After an unsuccessful pursuit of a branch of his immunological research, namely research on cancer, Ehrlich began in 1906 to seek a practical application of his receptor theory through research on chemotherapy. That same year, a wealthy sponsor gave Ehrlich an additional new research institute to be devoted to chemotherapy, referred to as the 'Georg-Speyer House'. Even in earlier years, Ehrlich had used his dyes for therapeutic purposes, e.g. in 1890, when he tried to combat neural pain (neuralgia) with methylene blue (*Methylenblau*). But it remained unclear whether drugs could specifically bind to cells.

Ehrlich had questioned this and thought his side-chain theory to be true only for toxins and nutritive substances, but he performed further experiments with his dyes to clarify the effect of drugs on cells. The elimination of microbes with chemical and synthetic substances, essentially chemotherapy, fascinated him. In 1904, with his assistant Kiyoshi Shiga (1870–1957), he could detect the deleterious effect of trypan red (*Trypanrot*) on trypanosomes, a specific parasite. When in 1905 the spirochete Treponema pallidum was identified as the cause for syphilis, many scientists tried to find a new therapeutic agent to combat the threat. In 1907 Ehrlich changed the theoretical basis of his experiments when he admitted that drugs, also, could bind to microbes via specific receptors, so-called 'chemoreceptors'.

In 1909 Ehrlich tested arsenical substances that he had examined and formerly applied to patients in a different context, on the syphilis bacilli. One of his assistants, Sahachiro Hata (1873–1938), discovered the positive effects of the substance No. 606 on the microbes. After clinical testing, Ehrlich announced in 1910 the development of No. 606, then called Salvarsan. His discovery created a sensation, and Ehrlich had to deal with the consequences. On the one hand he became a world-famous scientist; on the other hand he became responsible for all queries and criticism. He was haunted even by anti-Semitic denigrations. Furthermore, problems of the application of the substance, as well as unwanted side effects, made further research

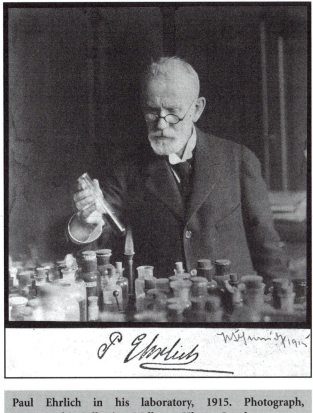

Paul Ehrlich in his laboratory, 1915. Photograph, Iconographic Collection, Wellcome Library, London.

indispensable. In 1912 these efforts lead to the introduction of an improved drug called Neosalvarsan, without solving the basic problems.

Ehrlich slowed down; his health had deteriorated over many years of sorrows and hard work. The outbreak of World War I and the loss of his international scientific contacts made things worse. In 1915, during a stay at a spa, Ehrlich died. Although Ehrlich's work contributed significantly to the development of scientific medicine after 1900, its reception and historical analysis was neglected after his death. The main reason was Nazi Germany's efforts (and their lingering effects) to eradicate his name and his achievements. Ehrlich's wife and daughters emigrated to the United States. After 1945 the full impact of Ehrlich's work upon modern medicine gradually began to be recognized. This process continues.

Bibliography

Primary: 1956, 1957, 1960. (Himmelweit, Fred, ed.) *The Collected Papers of Paul Ehrlich in Four Volumes Including a Complete Bibliography:* Vol. I, *Histology, Biochemistry and Pathology* (London/New York); Vol. II, *Immunology and Cancer Research* (London/New York/Paris); Vol. III, *Chemotherapy* (London/Oxford/New York/Paris).

Secondary: Prüll, Cay-Rüdiger, 2003. 'Part of a Scientific Masterplan?—Paul Ehrlich (1854–1915) and the Origins of his

Receptor Concept.' *Medical History* 47: 332–356; Silverstein, Arthur M., 2002. *Paul Ehrlich's Receptor Immunology. The Magnificent Obsession* (San Diego and London); Bäumler, Ernst, 1997. *Paul Ehrlich. Forscher für das Leben* (Frankfurt am Main)[1984. *Paul Ehrlich, Scientist for Life* (New York)]; *DSB*.

Cay-Ruediger Pruell

EIJKMAN, CHRISTIAAN   (b. Nijkerk, the Netherlands, 11 August 1858; d. Utrecht, the Netherlands, 5 November 1930), *physiology, bacteriology, nutrition.*

Eijkman was the seventh child of Christiaan Eijkman, headmaster of a local school, and Johanna Alida Pool. In 1875 he joined the Military Medical School in Amsterdam, where he was trained as a medical officer for the Netherlands Indies Army. In 1883 he earned his doctorate (with his thesis, *On Polarization of the Nerves*), married Aaltje Wigeri van Edema (who died three years later), and left for the Dutch East Indies. Severe bouts of malaria forced him to return to the Netherlands in 1885.

Back in Europe, Eijkman specialized in bacteriological research, first with Joseph Forster in Amsterdam and then in Robert Koch's laboratory in Berlin. In 1886, he was invited to assist a commission appointed by the Dutch government to study beriberi, a progressive paralytic disease that had become a serious problem throughout East Asia in the late nineteenth century. In 1887, Eijkman was appointed director of the new laboratory in the military hospital in Batavia, Indonesia, and also of the Javanese Medical School. His research was wide ranging, but he is best known for his work on beriberi.

Beriberi is generally presented as the first rigorously demonstrated case of a vitamin deficiency disease, and Eijkman is credited with this achievement. In 1929, he shared the Nobel Prize for Physiology or Medicine with Cambridge biochemist Frederick Gowland Hopkins for 'the discovery of vitamins'. In feeding experiments conducted in Batavia in the 1890s, Eijkman found a link between diets of polished white rice and an animal analogue of beriberi in hens (fowl polyneuritis), and showed that this disease could be prevented and cured by the husk surrounding the unpolished rice grain. Furthermore, epidemiological research carried out in prisons at Eijkman's request showed a persuasive correlation between beriberi and staple diets of polished rice. Retrospectively, this work was interpreted as establishing that beriberi is caused by a dietary deficiency of a substance in the husks of rice—a substance later taken to be a 'vitamin' (a term coined by Casimir Funk in 1912). Although Eijkman stressed the importance of the preventive and curative role of such a substance, he did not conclude that polyneuritis is caused by its dietary absence. At least until the late 1910s, Eijkman thought that a bacterial pathogen was the primary cause of both fowl polyneuritis and beriberi.

After ill health forced Eijkman to return to the Netherlands in 1897, he was appointed to the Chair in the Institute of Hygiene in Utrecht (1898). In Batavia, his colleague Gerrit Grijns (1865–1944) continued the investigations of fowl polyneuritis and was appointed Eijkman's successor in 1901. Grijns showed that the disease is prevented also by eating certain beans and pulses. This wider distribution of some protective substance made Grijns think in terms of a dietary deficiency, or 'partial hunger', as he called it in 1901. By 1910, Grijns concluded that beriberi is caused by a lack of a particular 'food for the nerves'.

Eijkman remained cautious about the cause of beriberi, but gradually shifted his position and presented a retrospective account of his beriberi research from the point of view of the vitamin theory in his Nobel lecture. By then, the active substance had been isolated from rice (in 1926) by colleagues in Batavia. One of them, B. C. P. Jansen, aptly called Eijkman a 'reluctant father of the vitamin theory'.

Bibliography

Primary: 1897. 'Eine Beri-beri-ähnliche Krankheit der Hühner.' *Virchows Archiv für pathologische Anatomie* cxlviii: 523–532; 1897. 'Ein Versuch zur Bekämpfung der Beri-beri.' *Virchows Archiv für pathologische Anatomie* cxlix: 187–194; 1929. 'Antineuritic Vitamin and Beri-beri.' Reprinted (1965) in *Nobel Lectures in Physiology or Medicine* vol. 2 (Amsterdam) pp. 199–210.

Secondary: Carpenter, Kenneth, 2000. *Beri-beri, White Rice, and Vitamin B. A Disease, a Cause and a Cure* (Berkeley); Kamminga, Harmke, 1998. 'Credit and Resistance: Eijkman and the Transformation of Beri-beri into a Vitamin Deficiency Disease' in Bayertz, Kurt, and Roy Porter, eds., *From Physico-Theology to Bio-Technology: Essays in the Social and Cultural History of Biosciences* (Amsterdam) pp. 232–254; Jansen, B. C. P., 1959. *Het levenswerk van Christiaan Eijkman, 1858–1930* (Haarlem).

Harmke Kamminga

EINTHOVEN, WILLEM   (b. Semarang, Indonesia, 21 May 1860; d. Leiden, the Netherlands, 28 September 1927), *physiology, cardiology.*

Willem was the son of the town physician of Semarang, Jacob Einthoven (who had gone to the Dutch East Indies as a military physician) and Louise M. M. C. de Vogel. His father died when Willem was six years old. In 1870 his mother returned to the Netherlands with her six children. They settled in Utrecht, where Einthoven started his medical studies in 1878. He had set his mind on specializing in ophthalmology, hoping to become a colonial military physician like his father. He became an assistant in the Eye Clinic for the Poor of Franciscus C. Donders, who supervised his thesis (*Stereoscopie door kleurverschil* [Stereoscopy through color difference]), on which he graduated *cum laude* on 4 July 1885. A few months later Einthoven was offered a professorship in physiology and histology in Leiden, which changed his career plans. He resigned from the military and accepted the invitation (in 1905 histology was transferred to the anatomist J. Boeke). In 1886 Einthoven delivered his inaugural address, entitled *De leer der specifieke energieën* [The theory of specific energies] and married his cousin, Frédérique J. L. de Vogel, with whom he would have four children.

Until the late 1880s, Einthoven had mainly engaged in the fields of optics and respiration. From the early 1890s, his research interests gradually shifted to electrical physiological phenomena, especially those related to the heart. He reorganized the physiological laboratory of Leiden (established in 1867), turning it into a laboratory for electrophysiology. Keen on measuring and registering the heart action, Einthoven started off by using the mercury capillary electrometer. It had been designed by Gabriel Lippmann in the early 1870s, although its possibilities for recording human cardiac currents from the body surface had been shown by the British physiologist Augustus D. Waller in 1887. However, since the instrument could not be put to practical clinical use, Einthoven decided to develop his own. His string galvanometer consisted of a thin, short wire in a strong magnetic field, capable of registering the heartbeat of both humans and animals, and producing 'electrocardiograms'—a concept that Einthoven used for the first time in 1893. The vibration of the string was enhanced using a microscope, after which it was registered on photographic paper.

Einthoven tried to establish a meaningful correlation between the shape of the cardiogram and cardiac activity. Although he had developed a very sensitive device, he realized the necessity of developing standardized measuring procedures in order to produce meaningful clinical data. In 1903 he published on the system for electrocardiographic standardization that he had developed during the previous years. Because he had succeeded in establishing uniformity of the recording process, he greatly contributed to the acceptance and introduction of his electrocardiograph in clinics and laboratories around the world, facilitating international exchange and comparison of measuring results. Throughout his life, Einthoven kept working on the galvanometer, improving its sensitivity in collaboration with his son, also Willem (1893–1944), who was an electrical engineer.

Einthoven had a keen eye for both the clinical significance and the commercial potential of his instrument. In 1906, the year in which he delivered a rectorial address on the meaning of electrophysiology, thus presenting and explaining his research to the wider academic community, he succeeded in making 'telecardiograms'. Using a mile-long cable, cardiac patients in the hospital were connected to the string galvanometer in Einthoven's laboratory. Through this connection he was able to collect much information on the many different conditions of the heart without having to transport the patients or his immobile equipment. Apart from putting his research findings to clinical use, Einthoven may be called a 'scientific entrepre-

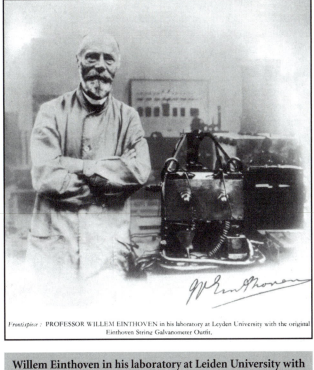

Frontispiece : PROFESSOR WILLEM EINTHOVEN in his laboratory at Leyden University with the original Einthoven String Galvanometer Outfit.

Willem Einthoven in his laboratory at Leiden University with the original Einthoven String Galvanometer. Half-tone reproduction from Seth Lee Barron, *The development of the electrocardiograph* . . . London, 1952. Wellcome Library, London. Reproduced with permission of D.J. Unwin Archive.

neur' (Wyers, Grob). Soon after he had published on his newly developed string galvanometer, he tried to persuade instrument manufacturers in the Netherlands, Germany, and Great Britain to develop the prototype into a standardized instrument and take it into serial production. Eventually he reached agreement with the Cambridge Scientific Instrument Company. After some changes in the design, production was started in 1905.

In 1908 Einthoven received a letter from London physician Thomas Lewis, who took great interest in his work. This led to a lively correspondence that would last nearly two decades. Because their expertise was complementary, their cooperation in developing clinical electrocardiography proved to be highly productive. Einthoven—who was a physician but had the mind of a theoretical physicist—greatly welcomed Lewis's clinical ingenuity and creativity in devising experiments, and Lewis valued Einthoven's input. In his cardiological research at University College Hospital, Lewis was using the Einthoven string galvanometer produced by the Cambridge Company. When Einthoven was awarded the Nobel Prize in 1924, he gratefully acknowledged Lewis's contribution.

Bibliography

Primary: 1901. 'Un nouveau galvanometer.' *Archives néerlandaises des sciences exactes et naturelles* 2nd series 6: 625–633; 1903. 'Die galvanometrische Registrierung des menschlichen Elektrokardiogramms.' *Pflüger's Archiv für die gesamte Physiologie des Menschen und der Tiere* 99: 472–480; 1906. 'Le télécardiogramme.' *Archives internationales de physiologie* 4: 132–164.

Secondary: Grob, B. W. J., 2004. 'The Laboratory Equipment of Willem Einthoven' in *Museum Boerhaave Communication 305* (Leiden) pp. 157–183; Wyers, P. J. H., 1996. 'De snaar van de snaargalvanometer van Einthoven.' *Gewina. Tijdschrift voor de geschiedenis der geneeskunde, natuurwetenschappen, wiskunde en techniek* 19: 80–94; Snellen, H. A., 1995. *Willem Einthoven (1860–1927). Father of Electrocardiography* (Dordrecht); Waart, A. de, 1957. *Het levenswerk van Willem Einthoven 1860–1927* (Haarlem); DSB.

Frank Huisman

ELLIOTSON, JOHN (b. Southwark, London, England, 24 October 1791; d. London, 29 July 1868), *medicine, mesmerism.*

Elliotson was the son of John Elliotson, a successful apothecary, and Elizabeth. He received an MD from Edinburgh University (1810). From Jesus College, Cambridge, he received an MB (1816) and an MD (1821). Despite a testy relationship with hospital authorities over his enthusiastic lectures, he was appointed assistant physician at St Thomas's Hospital, London (1817).

Early in his career, Elliotson displayed a penchant for pushing the boundaries of acceptable behavior. He was one of the first London physicians not to wear the traditional knickers, and one of the first to display a beard. In 1823 he founded the Phrenological Society of London. When he took a position as professor of medicine at the new University College London (1832), and thereafter at University College London Hospital (1834), he joined the company of a diverse group who had founded the institution based on democratic, Scottish ideals, and did not attempt to emulate the more staid worlds of Oxford and Cambridge. Elliotson belonged as a nonconformist, and as a progressive physician. He introduced England to a new, continental device for listening to the heart and lungs—the stethoscope—and followed up on this new technology by teaching the new ideas of physical diagnosis. He became widely acknowledged as an expert in the diagnosis of heart disease. He also used quinine to treat malaria, and iodine to treat goiter. He believed medicine needed to improve its therapeutic armamentarium, and was known for pushing drug dosages higher than did most physicians. Nonetheless, he was highly regarded; his lectures were well attended and regularly published in *Lancet.*

It was in his enthusiasm for mesmerism that Elliotson went too far, at least too far for the medical establishment to countenance his continued presence at the center. In 1837 a Frenchman calling himself the Baron J. Dupotet (1796–1881) asked if he could attempt to treat some patients with mesmerism. Elliotson agreed, and was

impressed. He then tried to use this new remedy for a pair of eighteen-year-old twins with epilepsy—Elizabeth and Jane O'Key. They claimed to go into a trance with mesmerism, and while in that state to be able to prescribe for others and to give medical prognoses.

At the time, mesmerism was quite in vogue. The writer Charles Dickens (1812–70) was a friend of Elliotson, and witnessed a demonstration of the O'Key twins. Dickens also tried mesmerism on his wife. The novelist William Thackeray (1811–63) was also a friend of Elliotson, and used him as the model for Dr Goodenough in *Pendennis* (1848–50, and dedicated to Elliotson) and in *The Adventures of Philip* (1861).

The O'Keys were presented in public demonstrations in the hospital that drew crowds of distinguished visitors. But then Elliotson carried on some demonstrations in the home of Thomas Wakley (1795–1862), founder and editor of *Lancet.* Wakley was a radical Member of Parliament who took great delight in attacking the London medical establishment. Unfortunately for Elliotson, Wakley concluded that the O'Keys demonstrations were a fraud. The following public outrage caused Elliotson to resign his post at the hospital in 1839.

Elliotson was not dissuaded in his beliefs, and continued to use mesmerism in his private practice. In 1843 he founded a mesmerist magazine, *The Zoist,* which lasted for thirteen volumes, and in 1849 he founded a mesmeric hospital. He claimed that mesmerism allowed painless surgery, a claim that probably attracted less attention after the introduction of chemical anesthesia.

Elliotson continued to be well regarded. His textbooks were said to be the 'favorites' in American medical schools, although editors took care to disassociate Elliotson's mesmerist views from his lessons on clinical medicine. In 1846 Elliotson gave the Harveian Oration to the RCP. Near the end of his life he converted to a belief in spiritualism.

Bibliography

Primary: 1839. *Lectures on the Theory and Practice of Medicine* (London); 1843. *Numerous Cases of Surgical Operations Without Pain in the Mesmeric State* (Philadelphia); 1982. (Kaplan, Fred, ed.) *John Elliotson on Mesmerism* (New York).

Secondary: Ridgway, Elizabeth S., 1993. 'John Elliotson (1791–1868): A Bitter Enemy of Legitimate Medicine? Part1: Earlier Years and the Introduction to Mesmerism.' *Journal of Medical Biography* 1: 191–198; Ridgway, Elizabeth S., 1993. 'John Elliotson (1791–1868): A Bitter Enemy of Legitimate Medicine? Part II: The Mesmeric Scandal and Later Years.' *Journal of Medical Biography* 2: 1–7; Williams, Harley, 1946. *Doctors Differ* (London); Rosen, George, 1936. 'John Elliotson: Physician and Hypnotist.' *Bulletin of the History of Medicine* 4: 600–603; *Munk's Roll; Oxford DNB.*

Joel D. Howell

ELLIS, (HENRY) HAVELOCK (b. Croydon, England, 2 February 1859; d. Hintlesham, Suffolk, England, 8 July 1939), *sex psychology, social philosophy.*

Ellis was the first son of a captain in the Merchant Navy, whose long periods of absence left Ellis very close to his mother and to one of his four sisters. He was educated at various schools, including a boarding school in Merton where he excelled at languages. At seven and again at sixteen, he traveled around the world with his father, although on the latter trip Ellis fell ill and was quarantined in Sydney, New South Wales, until his father returned four years later. During this time, Ellis taught at a number of schools, but mostly in the rural area of Sparkes Creek (fictionalized in his novel, *Kanga Creek*, 1922). While in Australia, Ellis read voraciously in politics, science, and literature, and was profoundly influenced by James Hinton's *Life in Nature* (1862) which, combined with his already strong interest in sexuality, led him to study medicine at St Thomas's Hospital upon his return to England (1880–1889). His aim, encouraged by Hinton, was to solve 'the problem of sex'.

Ellis began writing while at St Thomas's—at first works of literary criticism, but also scientific and ethical works. He also became politically active, and was a founding member of the Fellowship of the New Life, an organization that emphasized social change through education. Other members included Edward Carpenter (1844–1919); Edith Lees (1861–1916), a lesbian whom Ellis married; Olive Schreiner (1855–1920), with whom Ellis had an affair; Karl Pearson (1857–1936); and George Bernard Shaw (1856–1950). Some members required more revolutionary action, and split away to found the Fabian Society. Contemporaneously, Ellis associated with poets such as Arthur Symons (1865–1945) and W. B. Yeats (1865–1939); these three indulged in psychedelic experiments with mescaline, the results of which Ellis published. He traveled to Paris and met with the *literati*, and translated Emile Zola's *Germinal*.

Ellis is most remembered for his copious writings on sexual topics. In the 1890s he began work on his multi-volume *Studies in the Psychology of Sex* (1896–1928), of which the initial volume—*Sexual Inversion*—was coauthored with historian John Addington Symonds (1840–93). Symonds died before publication, and Ellis had his name removed from later, expanded editions. This was the first English medical text on homosexuality, and presented an argument that Ellis used in all of his sexual writings: that sexual desire is biologically grounded, but is shaped through events in an individual's life. Because various desires, be they homosexual, masochistic, fetishistic, etc., were biologically rooted, they should not treated as legal issues. Indeed, Ellis argued, homosexuality should be decriminalized, as it was natural. Evidence for the naturalness of various 'perversions' was drawn from ecology, history, and ethnology. The fact that various 'perversions' could be seen in nature, or in Morocco, supported Ellis's argument that they were not simply cases of moral turpitude. He maintained that individuals should find their own pleasures, provided they did not harm others and interacted with consenting adults. He was especially insistent on women's rights to sexual pleasure. This radical secular program relied upon sexual education.

Specifically, Ellis made a number of important psychological advances. He refined the theory of autoerotism (a term he coined) to include daydreams and psychological events as well as masturbation. He introduced the concept of narcissism, and developed Albert Moll's (1862–1939) ideas of the sexual impulse to explain sexual desire as a process of tumescence (arousal) and detumescence (orgasm). All sexual proclivities could be explained through such a schema. Many of these ideas were later rearticulated by psychoanalysts, with whom Ellis had an ambivalent relationship (although he enjoyed a friendly correspondence with Sigmund Freud).

Ellis was famously reclusive. Although joint president of the World League for Sexual Reform (with Magnus Hirschfeld, 1868–1935, and August Forel 1848–1931), he did not attend any of the Congresses—even that in London in 1929. Nor did he attend meetings of the British Society for the Study of Sex Psychology, although he had his papers read there regularly. He lived with Edith Lees, and after her death with Françoise Lafitte (1886–1974), who changed her name to Delisle, an anagram of 'of Ellis'. He also had numerous sexual relationships with women. These often satisfied his desire for watching women urinate, which he detailed in his autobiography.

Increasingly, he spent time away from his Brixton flat, preferring life in Suffolk and Surrey, although he occasionally traveled in Europe. Ellis is famed for his correspondence, which took many hours of his days, but left an enormous international archive. Some of his interlocutors turned up as case histories in his *Studies*. Others he simply helped in coming to terms with their sexual troubles. Ellis died in 1939 after a long bout of illness.

Bibliography

Primary: 1899–1928. *Studies in the Psychology of Sex* 7 vols. (Philadelphia); 1939. *My Life: Autobiography of Havelock Ellis* (London).

Secondary: Crozier, Ivan, 2000. 'Taking Prisoners: Havelock Ellis, Sigmund Freud, and the Politics of Constructing the Homosexual, 1897–1951.' *Social History of Medicine* 13: 447–466; Grosskurth, Phyllis, 1980. *Havelock Ellis: A Biography* (New York); *Oxford DNB*.

Ivan Crozier

EMERSON, HAVEN (b. New York, New York, USA, 19 October 1874; d. Greenport, New York, USA, 21 May 1957), *epidemiology, public health.*

Emerson, son of a physician and grandnephew of Ralph Waldo Emerson (1803–82), received a bachelor's degree from Harvard University (1896) and a medical degree from

Columbia University, College of Physicians and Surgeons (1899). From 1899 until 1913 he conducted a general medical practice while teaching physical diagnosis, physiology, and clinical medicine at Columbia. In 1914 he joined the New York City Health Department, first as Sanitary Superintendent, then (1915–17) as Commissioner of Health. During his tenure as Commissioner, Emerson dealt with the worst epidemic of poliomyelitis ever to affect the City—more than 8,000 cases. In 1918 he joined the U.S. Army, where he served as chief epidemiologist to the expeditionary force in France. From 1920 until his retirement in 1941, Emerson taught public health practice to students of medicine and public health at Columbia. During this period and after retirement until his death, he was engaged in a variety of other activities.

He served on innumerable committees concerned with the control of both acute and chronic disease, and with the organization of public health services. Perhaps the most important was the Committee on the Costs of Medical Care (CCMC) that, between 1928 and 1932, with funding from eight philanthropic foundations and with a staff of fifty investigators, carried out twenty-six studies of disease prevalence, intervention strategies, and medical care facilities nationwide. These studies resulted in several far-reaching recommendations: medical services, both preventive and therapeutic, should be provided on a group basis and be paid for by group insurance or taxation; basic public health services should be made available to the entire population according to need; evaluation and coordination of medical and public health services should be functions of state and local health agencies; and professional training should be extended to encompass prevention and social aspects of practice. The CCMC recommendations generated considerable controversy; nevertheless, they have ever since provided the framework for the evolution of medical and public health organization in the United States.

Emerson was a strong advocate for the establishment of local health departments, arguing that preventive medicine and environmental sanitation are more important than medical care in determining the level of community health. His experience in public health administration led to his concern about the accuracy and standardization of medical statistics available for the guidance of public health policy. He proposed corrective procedures, namely separating statistics based on postmortem examinations from those based on clinical diagnosis. Emerson opposed the use of alcoholic beverages, and recommended that health departments should mount education programs to discourage drinking. During these years he carried out or supervised a number of surveys of public health programs and facilities, in cities throughout the country and as far away as Athens, Greece. Emerson published 158 articles, and left unpublished the results of fifteen surveys (Emerson, 1949).

Among the many positions of leadership Emerson held, three are preeminent. In 1927, with Edward S. Godfrey, Jr., he convened and organized the American Epidemiological Society, an elite group with limited membership that has met annually ever since to discuss new research in the field. Subsequently, in 1930, Emerson and Godfrey led the establishment of the Epidemiology Section of the American Public Health Association (APHA), with open membership. The Section became the major venue for the presentation of epidemiological research in the United States until after World War II (Paul, 1973). In 1934, in the depths of the worldwide economic depression, Emerson served as President of the APHA.

Emerson received many awards, including the Sedgwick Medal for distinguished service in public health (1935), and the Lasker Award for his achievement in promoting local health services (1949). John Rodman Paul described him in this way: 'In action and in appearance Haven Emerson's tall and almost ascetic figure has epitomized the title which has been bestowed upon him, namely "the last of the great Puritans"' (Paul, 1958, p. 23).

Bibliography

Primary: 1949. *Selected Papers of Haven Emerson* (Battle Creek, MI).

Secondary: Paul, J. R., 1973. *An Account of the American Epidemiological Society* (New York and London); Paul, J. R., 1958. [Obituary] *Transactions of the Association of American Physicians* 71: 23–24; *DAMB*.

Warren Winkelstein, Jr.

EMPEDOCLES OF ACRAGAS

(b. Acragas [now Agrigento, Sicily], c. 492 BCE; d. c. 432 BCE), *embryology, medicine, natural philosophy.*

Empedocles, an aristocrat from the Hellenic city of Acragas in Sicily, lived in the fifth century BCE, traveled widely in Greece and was at Olympia for the games where he recited his poetry. Beyond this, the sources must be treated circumspectly. He is said to have won great fame in his lifetime as a poet and philosopher who could attract vast crowds with promises of healing (perhaps incorporating magicoreligious practices). The various accounts of his death, including his leap into Mt. Etna to prove his divinity, are fanciful. It is open to question whether Empedocles should be considered a doctor, a profession at odds with his aristocratic background. That he had broad philosophical interests is more in keeping with one of his class; in the context of the wide-ranging nature of philosophical enquiry during this period, these interests would include medical matters. Empedocles was mentioned by the author of the Hippocratic text, *On Ancient Medicine,* as an example of a deplorable trend of philosophic speculation in medicine. We may discount accounts that he cured the plague in the city of Selinus (Sicily); these are similar to stories told about Hippocrates and Athens.

Empedocles' surviving writings consist of two poems, *On Nature* and *Purifications*, which survive as approximately150 fragments. These may well be one and the same work with two different titles. It is claimed that he also wrote specific medical works, but this should be discounted. Some of the extant fragments deal with theories concerning the structure and function of the body. According to Empedocles, matter consisted of four elements, earth, water, fire, and air (or *ether*). These forms were unchangeable and may possibly have been originally postulated as particulate in nature. The varying combinations of these elements, under the twin governing principles of Love and Strife, accounted for everything in nature, including our bodies, the flesh of which was composed of equal proportions of the four elements.

Empedocles also examined sense perception. According to him, every substance gave off 'effluences' or emanations that passed through pores in the sense organs. The pores were constructed in such a way as to receive only the appropriate effluences. Although criticized by Aristotle, this general theory of sense perception was not really bettered in antiquity. Empedocles seems to have adumbrated a theory of cognition, according to which the blood about the heart is responsible for thought. In terms of pharmacology, Empedocles stated that, from him, it would be possible to 'learn all the drugs that are a defense against ills and old age'.

Empedocles postulated a pangenic theory of human development, where the seed from both parents contained miniature copies of themselves and, when mixed in the womb, accounted for individual characteristics. Empedocles has also been credited with formulating the earliest known account of the development of living creatures, initially coming from a melding of individual limbs and body parts formed from the earth. Most of these monstrosities would die out, with the exception of present day life forms (allied to this was the developmental account of human development in which 'shoots' of men and women arose from the earth and developed and unfurled as does a plant bud). To consider Empedocles a proto-Lamarckian (inheritance of acquired characteristics) or proto-Darwinian (survival of the fittest) is to read back into concepts whose full nuances cannot be determined. What is beyond dispute is the influence Empedocles exerted on those who came after him.

Bibliography

Primary: Inwood, Brad, 1992. *The Poem of Empedocles. A Text and Translation with an Introduction* (Toronto); Wright, M. R., 1995. *Empedocles, the Extant Fragments* (Bristol).

Secondary: Kingsley, Peter, 1995. *Ancient Philosophy, Mystery and Magic: Empedocles and Pythagorean Tradition* (Oxford); Osborne, Catherine, 1987. 'Empedocles Recycled.' *Classical Quarterly* 37: 24–50; *DSB*.

Julius Rocca

ERASISTRATUS OF CEOS **(see under HEROPHILUS OF CHALCEDON).**

ERISMAN, HULDREICH FRIEDRICH (b. Gontanschwill, Switzerland, 24 November 1842; d. Zurich, Switzerland, 30 October 1915), *hygiene.*

Erisman (Russian name Fedor Fedorovich), son of pastor Johann Friedrich Erisman and Wilhelmina Benker, attended the gymnasium of Aarau, then the universities of Zurich, Würzburg, and Prague (1861–65). In 1865 he started work at a Zurich ophthalmological clinic and graduated with his MD in 1867. At the same time he made the acquaintance of Russian revolutionary emigrés and, under their influence, moved to Russia in 1869 and entered the ranks of the International Workingmen's Association (IWA), also known as the First International (1870–74). From 1868 to 1878 he was married to Nadezhda Prokofievna Suslova, one of the first Russian women physicians.

In St Petersburg, Erisman started work as an ophthalmologist, but soon became captivated by hygiene. Having examined the vision of gymnasium students, he concluded that the physical classroom itself fostered the development of myopia in children. His interest in school hygiene expanded into research of communal, alimentary, and occupational hygiene. In 1871 he inspected the sanitary state of working-class housing in Petersburg and published his results, which brought him general popularity among Russian intellectuals.

In 1872–73 he completed graduate work at Zurich University, then studied physiology with Carl Voit and hygiene with Max von Pettenkofer in Munich (1873–74). The latter became a scientific authority for him. Erisman believed hygiene to be the main part of preventive medicine, and closely interconnected with the natural and social sciences.

During the Russian-Turkish war (1877–78), Erisman worked in the Red Cross Sanitary Commission on the territory of Romania, Bulgaria, and Turkey, where he fought spreading typhoid epidemics. In 1879 the Moscow Province *Zemstvo* (elective district council) invited Erisman to work as a sanitary physician. For seven years (1879–85) he performed sanitary inspections of industrial establishments in Moscow Province with his assistants, Alexander Vasil'evich Pogozhev and Evstaphi Mikhailovich Dement'ev. They examined the physical development of workers, the quality of their foods, and conditions of life and labor. They reported their findings at the meetings of Moscow *Zemstvo* physicians and published in the statistical accounts of Moscow Province.

In 1882 Erisman was invited to Moscow University to give lectures on hygiene. In the same year the university awarded him an MD 'honoris causa'. From 1884 he was chair of the department of hygiene and established a laboratory there. From 1887 at Devich'e field in Moscow new clinics and an Institute for Hygiene were built. In 1891 the Moscow Sanitary Station (in 1921 renamed the F. F. Erisman Moscow

Research Institute of Hygiene) was established on this base. The quality of produce from city markets and the condition of water from Moscow's rivers and wells were all examined there.

Erisman wrote widely on Russian medical and popular issues (in *Arkhiv sudebnoi meditsiny i obshchestvennoi gigieny, Vrach, Zemskii vrach, Moskovskaia meditsinskaia gazeta, Novoe slovo, Otechestvennye zapiski, Pedagogicheskii sbornik, Russkaia mysl'* and many others), and also for *The Brockhaus and Ephron Encyclopedia*. A number of his papers were published in Germany and Switzerland.

He participated in a number of Pirogov Society meetings (1887–96). At its second meeting (1887) he criticized the adherents of bacteriology and pointed out the auxiliary role of this science to hygiene. He was a regular member of the organizing committee for society meetings and presented the principal reports. In 1889 he was elected chairman of the third meeting of the Pirogov Society and, in the same year, also headed the Moscow Hygiene Society.

Erisman was an expert on the construction of waterworks and sewerage in Moscow, and advised the builders of waterworks in Nikolaev, Samara, St Petersburg, and Tula. He also researched the problems of the influence of the classroom milieu on the vision of students, and constructed rational school furniture ('the Erisman desk'). He advocated vigorous child play in fresh air. Erisman demanded that child labor in factories be prohibited and that adolescents younger than fourteen not be employed.

In 1896 Erisman was dismissed from his positions at Moscow University under pressure from Minister of Education Count Ivan Davidovich Delianov. With his second wife (since 1885), Sophia Iakovlevna Gasse, and three children, he settled in Switzerland. There he entered the Swiss Social Democratic party, was elected a magistrate in Zurich, and reformed hygiene in his native country. He also advocated the ideas of Russian *Zemstvo* medicine, and maintained correspondence with his Russian colleagues.

Bibliography

Primary: 1959. *Izbrannye proizvedeniia* [Collected Works] 2 vols. (Moscow). 1872–77. *Rukovodstvo k gigiene* [Guide to Hygiene] 3 vols. (St Petersburg); 1878. *Obshchedostupnaia gigiena* [Popular Hygiene] (St Petersburg); 1887–88. *Kurs gigieny* [Course of Hygiene] 3 vols. (Moscow).

Secondary: Petrov, Boris Dmitrievich, 1970. *F.F. Erisman* (Moscow); Bazanov, Victor Alekseevich, 1966. *F.F. Erisman (1842–1915)* (Leningrad).

Dmitry Mikhel

ERXLEBEN, DOROTHEA CHRISTIANA (NÉE LEPORIN)

(b. Quedlinburg, Germany, 13 November 1715; d. Quedlinburg, 13 June 1762), *medicine*.

Erxleben was the second of four children of the physician Christian Polycarp Leporin (1689–1747) and Anna Sophia Meineke (1680–1757), a pastor's daughter. She attended neither school nor university, but was a product of home schooling, educated mainly by her father, who taught both her and her brother about the theory and practice of medical science. Along with other standard works of the day, she became familiar with the writings of Friedrich Hoffmann (1660–1742) and Georg Ernst Stahl (1660–1734), medical professors at the University of Halle. Erxleben acquired practical experience by accompanying her father on his medical rounds visiting patients. In this way, she obtained an education far in excess of the normal education for girls in the eighteenth century. In subsequent years, she ran the medical practice together with her father, even substituting for him in his absence.

When Frederick II (1712–1786) took the Prussian throne in 1740, Erxleben asked the king for permission to take the medical examinations at a university together with her brother. The king approved her request in 1741, yet Erxleben initially did not take advantage of this concession. In Quedlinburg, the medical edict of 1725, which stipulated that only licensed physicians were permitted to treat internal diseases, had not been implemented in practical terms. Thus, she was able to pursue a medical practice without state licensing.

In 1742 she married the widowed deacon, Johann Christian Erxleben (1697–1759), who had five children by a previous marriage. The couple had four more children of their own. As the wife of a pastor, and supported by the social network of her family in the town, she was able to continue her medical practice. Only in 1753, after three physicians in Quedlinburg complained, accusing her of 'quackery', did she seek a medical doctorate. In 1754 Erxleben submitted a thesis at the Medical Faculty of the University of Halle and was granted the doctorate that same year. She was licensed after the Medical Faculty had gained assurances from the king regarding the legality of the procedure. After this and until her death, Erxleben practiced medicine as a legally recognized and licensed physician.

In her dissertation, *Quod nimis cito ac iucunde curare saepius fiat causa minus tutae curationis*, which was published a year later in German, Erxleben espoused the view that the causes of a disease should be treated, not the symptoms. The various medications (of which she described the effects) should be applied with restraint, she reasoned, to avoid endangering the patient. Given the state of knowledge in the middle of the eighteenth century, this was an innovative study. Twelve years prior to attaining her doctoral degree, Erxleben had written a treatise for the declared purpose of gaining practice in argumentation. In this work she dealt with the question of 'the causes which keep the female gender from studying at university', examining the prejudices against women and concluding that gender alone should not be a reason to deny anyone the chance to study. This work was read in a small circle of educated contemporaries, but caused no broader echo.

Dorothea Christiana Erxleben did not achieve fame through her scientific writings. Her works are known today primarily because she was the first woman to earn a doctorate at a German university, as well as a license to practice. For a long period, she was the only academically trained female doctor in Germany. Not until some 150 years later did the implementation of regular training of female physicians at the universities become possible.

Bibliography

Primary: 1742. *Gründliche Untersuchung der Ursachen, die das weibliche Geschlecht vom Studiren abhalten . . .* (Berlin); 1755. *Academische Abhandlung von der gar zu geschwinden und angenehmen, aber deswegen öfters unsichern Heilung der Krankheiten . . .* (Halle).

Secondary: Riha, Ortrun, 2006. 'Die wissenschaftlichen Schriften von Dorothea Christiane Erxleben, geb. Leporin' in Brinkschulte, Eva, and Eva Labouvie, eds., *Dorothea Christiane Erxleben—Weibliche Gelehrsamkeit und medizinische Profession seit dem 18. Jahrhundert* (Halle); Schmiedgen, Ursula, 2006. 'Dorothea Leporin, verh. Erxleben (1715–1762). Pfarrfrau und streitbare Ärztin in Quedlinburg' in Brinkschulte, Eva, and Eva Labouvie, eds., *Dorothea Christiane Erxleben—Weibliche Gelehrsamkeit und medizinische Profession seit dem 18. Jahrhundert* (Halle); Fulda, Annette, 2004. 'Da dergleichen Exempel bey dem weiblichen Geschlechte insonderheit in Deutschland etwas rar sind: Gelehrtes Wissen, ärztliche Praxis und akademische Promotion Dorothea Christiana Erxlebens (1715–1762)' in Hohkamp, Michaela, and Gabriele Jancke, eds., *Nonne, Königin und Kurtisane: Wissen, Bildung und Gelehrsamkeit von Frauen in der Frühen Neuzeit* (Königstein im Taunus) pp. 60–82; Meixner, Brigitte, 1999. *Dr. Dorothea Christiana Erxleben. Erste deutsche promovierte Ärztin* (Halle).

Jürgen Helm and Karin Stukenbrock

ESPEJO, FRANCISCO JAVIER EUGENIO DE SANTA CRUZ (b. Quito, Ecuador, 21 February 1747; d. Quito, 27 December 1795), *public health, medical education.*

Espejo was the son of Luis de la Cruz Espejo, a surgeon, and Catalina Aldaz y Larraincar. His father being the surgeon of the Hospital de la Misericordia, the most important health center in Quito, Eugenio Espejo became acquainted with medical issues from childhood. He attended the Jesuit School of San Luis, the Dominican Seminary College and the University of Santo Tomás, in Quito, where he obtained a degree in medicine (1767). He also studied law and canon law.

In 1785 Espejo wrote his most celebrated medical treatise on how to prevent smallpox: *Reflexiones acerca de un método seguro para preservar a los pueblos de las Viruelas.* Espejo's medical ideas are particularly interesting because he emphasized the need for further microscopic research to reveal the invisible pathogens causing the spread of fevers and smallpox epidemics. He thereby set a Latin American precedent predating by a century the emergence of bacteriology. In this book, Espejo exposed the conta-

gious nature of smallpox and the need for isolating patients immediately after epidemic outbreaks. However, in his *Reflexiones*, Espejo also put emphasis on the relation between public hygiene, poverty, malnutrition, and disease. He identified the poor living conditions of the population as a primary health problem and the principal cause for the spread of diseases. He also encouraged the reform of medical education, demanding more practical instruction and closer links between medical studies and hospital practice.

Espejo was also concerned with the properties and commercial uses of local medicinal plants. He argued against the attempts of the Spanish Crown to monopolize the commercialization of quinine. In a report entitled *Voto de un Ministro Togado de las Audiencias de Quito* (1792), Espejo intertwined his defense of a free commercial system for quinine with demands for a reform in the political administration of the Spanish American colonies. The report also included an analysis of the medical properties of quinine for the treatment of intermittent fevers. Thanks to his combination of original political and scientific ideas, and his promotion of the latest European scientific novelties, Espejo is considered the main representative of the Enlightenment in Ecuador, and one of the first South American physicians to embrace the Enlightenment. He was the founder and first director of the National Library of Ecuador, established on the basis of the collections left by the Jesuit order after its expulsion from the Spanish territories.

Espejo had a very active political life. In 1787 he was arrested and exiled to Colombia for the publication of a pamphlet against Charles III, King of Spain. In 1791 Espejo returned to Quito, and as a member of the Sociedad Patriótica de Amigos del Pais, initiated a campaign to promote reforms in the administration of the Hispanic American territories. He also established relations with revolutionary leaders from other Hispanic American territories. In January 1792 Espejo began the publication of *Primicias de la Cultura de Quito*, the first newspaper published in Quito. This paper was devoted to promoting political reforms. He had recurrent conflicts with the Spanish authorities and was arrested on several occasions. During one of these arrests, Espejo's health deteriorated dramatically, leading to his death. He is considered a precursor of Hispanic American independence.

Bibliography

Primary: 1785. *Reflexiones acerca de un método seguro para preservar a los pueblos de las Viruelas* (Quito); 1792. *Voto de un Ministro Togado de las Audiencias de Quito* (Quito).

Secondary: Fierro Benítez, Rodrigo, 2003. 'Eugenio Espejo, Médico Quiteño de la Ilustración: Pionero de la Bacteriología en las Américas.' *Anales de la Real Academia Nacional de Medicina*, 120(1): 79–93; Breilh, Jaime, 2001. *Eugenio Espejo: La Otra Memoria* (Cuenca, Ecuador); Estrella, Eduardo, 1993. *Apuntes para una discusión sobre el Pensamiento Médico de Eugenio Espejo* (Quito); Astuto, Phillip, 1969. *Eugenio Espejo* (Mexico City).

Jorge Lossio

ESQUIROL, JEAN ETIENNE DOMINIQUE (b. Toulouse, France, 3 February 1772; d. Paris, France, 12 December 1840), *psychiatry, medical legislation.*

Born into a family of merchants and municipal administrators (*capitouls*), Esquirol was destined for a career in the Church. He studied the humanities at the Collège de l'Esquille in Toulouse and theology with the Sulpicians at Issy near Paris where he received the tonsure. The Revolution made him return to Languedoc. He began to study medicine in Toulouse, then enlisted in the army; he worked at the hospital in Narbonne, then studied more medicine at Montpellier where he served as secretary to the famous Paul Joseph Barthez. In 1798 he returned to Paris and received his medical degree in 1805.

In Paris, Esquirol studied under Philippe Pinel, professor of internal medicine at the Paris l'École de Santé and physician-in-chief of the Salpêtrière Hospice. Although Pinel was much older, the two men, both from the same region of France, got along well. Esquirol became Pinel's disciple, and eventually his rival. In 1811 he joined the Salpêtrière staff, replacing Jean-Baptiste Pussin as supervisor of mentally ill women; in 1812 he served as a physician at the hospice and Pinel's assistant; and in 1826 he became director of Charenton asylum. He had by then accumulated considerable experience at the private *maison de santé* he established in 1799 with Pinel's sponsorship on rue Buffon, across the street from the Salpêtrière. Esquirol then became the first French physician to be trained exclusively in mental medicine or psychiatry.

Esquirol collaborated closely with Pinel during medical rounds in the General Infirmary at the Salpêtrière: the professor asked him to write up the case history after each patient had been examined. In his way, Esquirol contributed substantially to Pinel's *La médecine clinique* (1802, 1804).

At rue Buffon, Esquirol treated his patients with respect and kindness, applying 'moral treatment'. This was easier for him in his private asylum, which usually housed only about twenty patients (all of whom paid for their stay and many of whom brought their personal servant), than for Pinel who was responsible for hundreds of mental patients, all of them destitute, and had a paucity of staff. (Some insight into Esquirol's asylum practice can be gained from his patient register housed in the History and Special Collections Division of the Louise Darling Biomedical Library at UCLA.)

Another important technique Esquirol learned from his teacher was the use of medical statistics. In the second edition of his *Traité medico-philosophique de l'aliénation mentale* (1809), Pinel had experimented with the 'calculus of probability' to predict the likelihood of cures. Esquirol went much further, in his statistical memoirs on Charenton and on the asylum at Aversa in Italy.

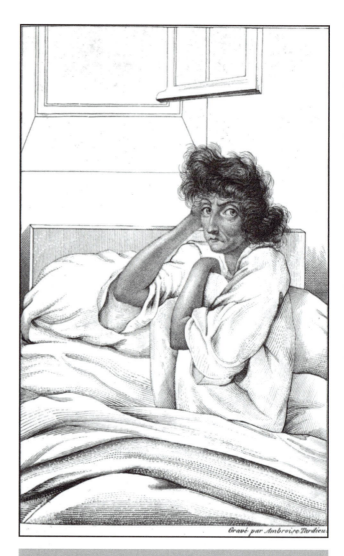

Gravé par Ambroise Tardieu

Insane patient in an asylum. Engraving by Ambroise Tardieu from *Des maladies mentales* . . . Paris, 1838. Rare Books, Wellcome Library, London.

Besides clinical talents Esquirol had essential administrative skills. He toured French asylums several times, at his own expense, according to his American biographer, but surely not without official backing from the Restoration government. His report of 1818, on '*Des établissements des aliénés en France*', inspired widespread concern for conditions in asylums and, eventually, reforms. Almost single-handedly, Esquirol elaborated, promoted, and implemented the Law of 30 June 1838 that—somewhat modified in 1968 and 1990—still regulates the internment of the mentally ill in France.

This was the first law in any country to go beyond incarcerating the insane on the basis of complaints and vague diagnoses by the family, neighbors, or the authorities. It assigned responsibility for institutionalization to two physicians versed in the 'special science', under supervision of the government and in accordance with the law. And the 'special science', psychiatry, followed Pinel's dictum of treating the insane as medical patients.

Esquirol had prepared for the implementation of the Law of 1838 in two crucial ways: at the Salpêtrière and at Charenton, he trained a whole circle of specialists in psychiatric diagnosis and therapy, among them the well-known alienists Jules Baillarger, Jean-Pierre Falret, François Leuret, and Félix Voisin. Esquirol placed his students as future administrators at provincial asylums. At the same time he modernized and beautified Charenton, making it a model institution. He also transferred his private asylum from rue Buffon to Ivry, near Paris, where he frequently received his circle of students.

Esquirol broadened the influence of his specialty through his writings on forensic psychiatry. These focused on an illness he named and defined: monomania. If a crime is committed by a person totally fixated on a specific aim, Esquirol argued, that person may be suffering from homicidal monomania: only a psychiatrist could make the diagnosis protecting the mentally ill from criminal prosecution. The *Code Napoleon* had already stipulated: 'There is no crime or transgression, if the accused was demented at the time of the act, or if compelled by an irresistible force.' (Article 64) Criminal responsibility was thus debated in France years before the McNaghten Rules were elaborated in England.

Another of Esquirol's diagnostic innovations enjoyed only a brief vogue: he proposed that melancholic depression be called 'lypemania', while the term 'melancholy' should be left to everyday language and to literature. While 'monomania' endured, 'lypemania' was soon abandoned. Perhaps his most telling contribution to psychiatric vocabulary was 'asylum' as the appropriate term for the institution where the mentally ill would find refuge.

Esquirol's prolific writings ranged over all of mental illness. His most original work was his MD thesis, presided over by Pinel, on *Des passions considérés comme causes, symptoms, et moyens curatifs de l'aliénation mentale* (1805). Alerted by the work of the Scotsman, Alexander Crichton, Esquirol came to consider the passions not only as aspects of human behavior that the psychiatrist could observe and explain, but as instruments of therapy. Another memorable contribution was Esquirol's memoir on hallucinations, read to the Academy of Sciences in 1817.

Esquirol contributed fourteen important articles to the *Dictionnaire des sciences médicale* on the following: suicide, delirium, dementia, demonomania, hallucinations, imbecility, mania, and melancholia. They form a major part of his comprehensive published work, *Des maladies mentales, considérées sous les rapports medicaux, hygiénique et médico-légal* (1838, English trans., 1845). In contrast to most of his compatriots, Esquirol paid heed to foreign developments: he traveled in Italy, Switzerland, Germany, Belgium, Holland, and Russia, and wrote about his opinions of their asylums.

In the 1820s Esquirol's rivalry with Pinel became more evident. Beginning in 1817 he lectured on psychiatry at the Salpêtrière. Pinel was not involved in these lessons, but Esquirol awarded the best students a copy of Pinel's *Traité* and 300 francs. In 1822 the reactionary Corbière ministry closed the Medical Faculty and purged it of eleven of its senior professors, Pinel among them. Esquirol became inspector-general of public instruction in reward for his monarchist and conservative loyalties.

Late in life Esquirol became a corresponding member of the Academy of Moral and Political Sciences and joined the Public Health Council of Paris. In 1829 he helped found the *Annales d'hygiène publique et de médecine légale*, a long-lasting and very influential journal.

Esquirol spread the famous 'Pinel myth' fabricated by young Scipion Pinel, Pinel's son. According to this story, Pinel's major claim to fame was the liberation of the madmen at Bicêtre from their chains in 1794, at the time of the Terror. His writings, teaching, and thirty years of care for the mentally ill women at the Salpêtrière tended to disappear behind this 'gesture'. Esquirol helped popularize this myth in his writings, thus advancing his own claims to originality. Nonetheless, he was a fine clinician, the architect of the Law of 1838, the creator of asylums throughout France and the teacher of their administrators—in short, the organizer of the psychiatric profession in France.

Bibliography

Primary: 1805. *Des passions considérés comme causes, symptômes, et moyens curatifs de l'aliénation mentale* (Paris); 1819. *Des établissements des aliénés en France et des moyens d'améliorer le sort de ces infortunés* (Paris); 1829. 'Mémoire historique et statistique sur la maison royale de Charenton.' *Annales d'hygiène publique et de médecine légale* 13: 5–192; 1838. *Des maladies mentales, considérées sous les rapports médicaux, hygiénique et médico-légal* 2 vols. (Paris).

Secondary: Weiner, Dora B., 1999. *Comprendre et soigner: Philippe Pinel (1745-1826) et la médecine de l'esprit* (Paris), English tr. forthcoming (Aldershot); Weiner, Dora B., 1989. 'Esquirol's Patient Register: The First Private Psychiatric Hospital in Paris, 1802-1808.' *Bulletin of the History of Medicine* 63: 110–120; Goldstein, Jan, 1987. *Console and Classify: The French Psychiatric Profession in the Nineteenth Century* (Cambridge and New York); Mora, George, 1972. 'On the Bicentenary of the Birth of Esquirol (1772–1840), the First Complete Psychiatrist.' *American Journal of Psychiatry* 129: 74–79; Légée, Georgette, 1971. 'Evolution de l'étude clinique, sociale et juridique de l'aliénation mentale sous l'impulsion de Jean Etienne Dominique Esquirol, médecin aliéniste d'origine toulousaine.' *Comptes-rendus du 96ème Congrès national des sociétés savantes* (section sciences) 1: 63–81.

Dora B. Weiner

EUSTACHI, BARTOLOMEO   (b. San Severino Marche, Macerata, Italy, *c.* 1500–1510; d. on the Via Flaminia near Fossato di Vico, Perugia, Italy, 27 August 1574), *medicine, anatomy.*

Eustachi was the second son of Mariano, a physician, and Francesca Benvenuti. He received a sound education in the humanities, acquiring an excellent knowledge not only of Latin, but also of Greek, Hebrew, and Arabic. He published a Latin version of Erotian's Hippocratic glossary (1556), and it seems that he also translated some writings of Avicenna (Ibn Sīnā) from Arabic. He studied medicine at the Archiginnasio della Sapienza in Rome, but it is not known precisely when. On 20 December 1539 he was appointed as physician in his native town, but soon he became physician to the Duke of Urbino, and then, in 1547, to the duke's brother, Giulio Della Rovere, nominated Cardinal, whom Eustachi followed to Rome in 1549. A few years later he was appointed to the Sapienza, where he taught practical medicine and anatomy from 1555 to 1568, obtaining cadavers for dissection from all the hospitals of Rome. With advancing years, Eustachi was so severely afflicted by gout that he was compelled to resign his chair. He continued, however, to serve Cardinal Della Rovere, and it was in response to the Cardinal's summons to Fossombrone in 1574 that he set forth, only to die on the way.

Eustachi's first work, *Examen ossium et de motu capitis*, was written in 1561 against Vesalius's anti-Galenism. In 1562 he published *De auditus organis* on the auditory organ, and in 1563 he followed this with three more treatises: on the kidney (*De renibus*); on the venous system (*De vena quae azygos Graecis dicitur*); and on teeth (*De dentibus*). All these works were published in *Opuscula anatomica* (1563). The *Opuscula anatomica* contained eight large octavo plates which illustrated aspects of the kidneys, the azygous vein and its ramifications, the veins of the arm and heart, and Eustachian valve, i.e., the valve situated at the outlet of the vena cava inferior in the right auricle.

The *De renibus* was the first work specifically dedicated to that organ, and here he described and portrayed the suprarenal glands for the first time. In his *De auditus organis* he provided a correct account of the auditory tube, which still bears his name (Eustachian tube); moreover, he was also the first to describe the tensor tympani and stapedius muscles. He also described in detail the ossicular chain, including the stapes, recognized by Giovanni Filippo Ingrassia (1510–80) in 1546. In *De dentibus* Eustachi was the first to make a careful study of the teeth, describing also the first and second dentitions. In his work on the azygous vein, Eustachi described the thoracic duct in the horse, revealing a good knowledge of the heart's structure.

In 1552 Eustachi, with the help of his pupil Pier Matteo Pini, prepared a series of forty-seven anatomical copperplate engravings for a book entitled *De dissensionibus ac controversiis anatomicis*, which was, however, never published. The first eight plates were used in the *Opuscula anatomica*, the remainder apparently lost after his death. The missing thirty-nine plates (in folio size) were discovered in the early eighteenth century in the possession of a descendant of Pini. In 1714 Giovanni Maria Lancisi (1654–1720) published the plates, together with the eight smaller ones that had already appeared, under the title *Tabulae anatomicae*, assuring Eustachi a distinguished position in the history of anatomy.

Bibliography

Primary: 1563. *Opuscula anatomica* (Venice); 1566. *Erotiani . . . vocum, quae apud Hippocratem sunt, collectio . . . Libellus de moltitudine* (Venice); 1714. *Tabulae anatomicae . . . quas a tenebris tandem vindicata . . . praefatione notisque illustravit . . .* Jo. Maria Lancisius (Rome) [1944. Reprinted, Pazzini, Adalberto (Rome)].

Secondary: Belloni, Luigi, 1979. 'Bartolomeo Eustachi, anatomico del Cinquecento, al lume di recenti ricerche.' *Archives internationales d'histoire des sciences* 29: 5–10; Belloni, Luigi, 1974. 'Bartolomeo Eustachi (nel IV centenario della morte).' *Simposi clinici* 11: ix–xvi; Bilancioni, Guglielmo, 1913. *Bartolomeo Eustachi* (Florence); *DSB*.

Giuseppe Ongaro

EVANG, KARL INGOLF

EVANG, KARL INGOLF (b. Oslo, Norway, 19 October 1902; d. Oslo, 3 January 1981), *public health*.

Evang, son of civil servant Jens Ingolf Evang and Anna Beata Wexelsen, graduated MD at the University of Oslo in 1928. His career as a professional pointed early toward public health. In 1926 he joined Mot Dag [Dawn], a radical organization of intellectuals, and was the initiator and first chair of The Socialist Medical Association, founded in 1931. In 1936 he became a member of the more moderate Labor Party. He was inspired by Sigmund Freud's psychoanalysis and by Alfred Grotjahn's *Soziale Pathologie* (1912), the latter providing a guide to the principles of social medicine. He married MD Gerda Sophie Landmark Moe in 1929; they had four children.

In the 1930s he took interest in eugenics, nutrition, mental health, occupational medicine, venereal diseases, and women's health, and he advocated public sexuality education. In the same decade he campaigned for reorganizing the national health services, calling for a centrally organized and financed service, universal in its distribution and with extended power to the medical profession.

In 1938 Evang was appointed Director General of Health. In June 1940, after the German occupation of Norway, he fled to London. Here he joined the Norwegian exile government until May 1945, but spent long periods in the United States. During his years abroad—stimulated not least by *The Beveridge Report* and American public health education—he worked on a scheme for rebuilding the health care system in a free country. He made international contacts and contributed to defining the missions for two of the UN's organizations, the Food and Agriculture Organization (FAO) and the World Health Organization (WHO).

Once home in Norway, he started building what was later called 'the Evang Model' as part of the Norwegian welfare state. His premise was that people's health and work capacity is an absolute condition for rebuilding society, materially and economically. Ideologically he had a strong belief in rationalism, and was convinced that the planning of societal life should be based on scientific results. Under the auspices of the Labor Party he had a free hand in modeling a comprehensive and strongly centralized health care system. The aim

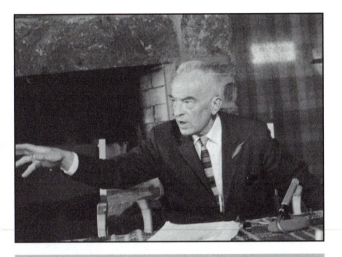

Karl Evang. Photograph, National Archives of Norway.

was to produce health services of the highest quality, financed from the national insurance scheme, and equally distributed, socially and geographically. In an organization modeled after a military hierarchy, he placed his 'own' people in central positions on all levels, many of them physicians whom he had encouraged to study public health in Britain or in the United States. The Directorate of Health, which expanded considerably, moved physically into the Ministry of Social Affairs. It was a controversial organization accused of mixing administration with politics.

Evang was highly respected but also criticized, mostly because of his radicalism and dominating leadership. His work increasingly became more devoted to international affairs. He was instrumental in framing the constitution of the WHO and in formulating the organization's concept of health, a concept that has been disputed for being too encompassing and 'imperialistic'. Through the WHO—which came into force on 7 April 1948—and other international organizations, Evang devoted special attention to nutrition and family planning among the poor.

Retiring as Director General of Health in 1972, Evang was rather pessimistic. His leadership model had lost its legitimacy. His dreams of social medicine as an embracing ideology in medicine were broken. Besides, increased urbanization around the world created 'inhuman cities'—places for extensive and insuperable health problems. As early as the 1960s, Evang foresaw mental illness and the abuse of narcotics as the greatest challenges in the years to come.

Bibliography

Primary: 1960. *Health Services in Norway* (Oslo); 1972. *Narkotika, generasjonene og samfunnet* (Oslo); 1975. *Helse og samfunn* (Oslo).

Secondary: Berg, Siv Frøydis, 2002. *Den unge Karl Evang og utvidelsen av helsebegrepet* (Oslo); Nordby, Trond, 1987. *Karl Evang. En biografi* (Oslo).

Aina Schiøtz

EWING, JAMES (b. Pittsburgh, Pennsylvania, USA, 25 December 1866; d. New York, New York, USA, 16 May 1943), *pathology, oncology.*

Ewing was the third of five children. As a youngster, he suffered a sports injury resulting in a broken femur and osteomyelitis. While confined to bed, he won a microscope in a contest; this instrument would have a major influence on his subsequent interest in medicine. Ewing earned undergraduate and masters degrees from Amherst College. In 1891 he received his MD from the College of Physicians and Surgeons of New York (Columbia). His mentors at Columbia included Frances Delafield and Theophil Mitchell Prudent. He interned at Roosevelt and Sloan Maternity in New York City. During this period he developed his interest in pathology.

After returning to Columbia, he served as tutor in histology from 1893 to 1897, and as instructor in clinical pathology the following year. In 1898 Ewing volunteered as a contract surgeon with the U.S. Army treating soldiers evacuated from Cuba and Manila. This experience led to his publication of several papers on malaria. At age thirty-three, Ewing was appointed in 1899 as the first professor in clinical pathology at Cornell. Research activity in experimental cancer followed. Ewing was married to Catherine Halsted in 1900. She died during pregnancy in the third year of their marriage. Ewing never fully recovered from this blow and thereafter became somewhat reclusive.

By 1910 Ewing had decided that the best hope for progress in cancer was to study the disease in humans. He met a wealthy mining engineer, James Douglas, whose daughter had died of breast cancer. Together they concluded that cancer research should be carried out at a special hospital, and selected the Memorial Hospital (originally the New York Cancer Hospital).

Ewing became one of the most influential authorities on cancer in the world. His major treatise, *Neoplastic Diseases* (1919), became the leading textbook on the pathology of cancer. Ewing was critical of surgery and became a strong proponent of radiation therapy. His paper on what is now known as Ewing's sarcoma was published in 1921. Ewing emphasized that this tumor occurred mainly in young people and was radiosensitive, although it tended to recur after treatment. He was strongly critical of his Memorial Hospital colleague, William B. Coley, who treated sarcomas with bacterial filtrates (Coley's toxins).

Ewing was one of the founders of the American Society for the Control of Cancer (later the American Cancer Society) and the American Association for Cancer Research. Identified as the 'Cancer Man', he was on the cover of *Time Magazine* in January 1931. Ewing served as Director of Memorial Hospital from 1931 until 1939. He was eccentric, cynical, blunt, and contemptuous of pretension. Despite a permanent limp from his childhood osteomyelitis, he became an excellent tennis player. He had longstanding trigeminal neuralgia for which he ultimately underwent an unsuccessful surgical procedure by Harvey Cushing. In his later years Ewing developed urinary stones. He diagnosed his own incurable bladder cancer in 1943 and was resuscitated after a cardiac arrest. After voicing his displeasure about the resuscitation, he was allowed to die peacefully several days later.

The James Ewing Society was founded in 1939 for alumni who had trained at Memorial Hospital. In 1975 the name of the organization was changed to The Society of Surgical Oncology (founded as the James Ewing Society). Its annual meeting is among the leading scientific gatherings for cancer surgeons.

Bibliography

Primary: 1919. *Neoplastic Diseases* (Philadelphia); 1921. 'Diffuse Endothelioma of Bone.' *New York Pathological Society* 21: 17–24; 1931. *Causation, Diagnosis and Treatment of Cancer* (Baltimore).

Secondary: Huvos, A. G., 1998. 'James Ewing: Cancer Man.' *Annals of Diagnostic Pathology* 2: 146–148; Leffall, L. D., 1987. 'James Ewing, MD: Contemporary Oncologist Exemplar. The James Ewing Lecture.' *Archives of Surgery* 122: 1240–1243; *DAMB*.

Marvin J. Stone

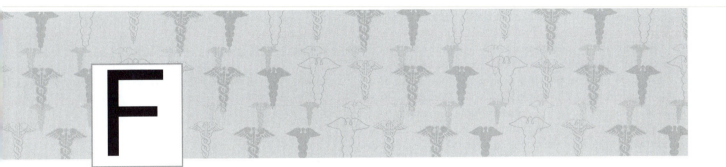

F

FABRICIUS, WILHELM (aka WILHELM FABRY or FABRICIUS HILDANUS) (b. Hilden, Germany, 25 June 1560; d. Bern, Switzerland, 15 February 1634), *surgery.*

Fabricius was the son of the local court scribe Peter Drees (Dreyß, Dreß, or Dresen) and his wife, Margarethe auf dem Sand. The name Fabry or Fabricius probably resulted from a Latinization of their house name, 'Schmidt', 'Schmitz', or 'In der Schmitten'. Fabricius initially enjoyed a good education, which he was able to continue after his father's early death and his mother's second marriage. At age thirteen, however, he had to leave school because of the outbreak of the Dutch civil war. In 1576 he was apprenticed to Johann Dümgens, a barber surgeon in nearby Neuß. Beginning in 1580 he worked for several years with the renowned Düsseldorf surgeon Cosmas Slot. Fabricius accompanied Slot on his travels as court surgeon of the Duke of Cleve and became acquainted with some of the leading learned physicians of the time when Slot was called to consult about one of their patients. His acquaintance with Reiner Solenander, among others, probably goes back to that period. After Slot's death in 1585, Fabricius traveled to Metz and then continued to Geneva and Lausanne, where he became friendly with the well-known surgeon Jean Griffon and began to work with him.

Griffon inspired Fabricius's future work and influenced his approach as a surgeon. Griffon was not only an accomplished surgeon who performed very complicated operations; he also stressed the value and importance of the surgeon's understanding of detailed anatomical knowledge. Together they dissected corpses, and it was from Griffon that Fabricius got into the habit of practicing difficult operations first on a corpse.

In 1587 Fabricius married Marie Colinet, the daughter of a local printer. In time she also acquired extensive surgical skills. She greatly supported Fabricius, especially in obstetrical and gynecological cases, and she sometimes substituted for him during his prolonged periods of absence. Marie is remembered for suggesting the use of a lodestone to extract metallic foreign bodies from the eye. The couple had eight children, among them Peter, who also became physician but died in 1630 at an early age.

For unknown reasons, Fabricius and his family left Geneva in 1588, returning to Hilden and practicing there. From 1593 he lived and worked predominantly in Cologne, interrupted by various journeys and extended sojourns in Lausanne. In 1593 he published his first treatise, *De gangraena et sphacelo* (which roughly translates as 'gangrene and wound infection'), which proved highly successful, going through at least twelve editions. In Cologne, Fabricius also began to attend medical lectures at the university, making himself familiar with the learned medicine of his time. From 1602 until 1611 he worked as a town surgeon in Peterlingen (Payerne), a small town under Bernese rule. Since he continued his extensive traveling, his long absences from Peterlingen proved a source of serious conflict with the town officials, and in the end he asked for his dismissal. From 1611 to 1614 he worked predominantly in the Rhineland, where he lost two daughters to the plague. He continued to travel extensively, visiting Amsterdam and Leiden, among others. In 1615 he accepted the post of town surgeon in Bern and acquired citizen rights there in 1616. For the following years until his death in 1634, he lived and worked in Bern but continued to treat many patients in other places. Only toward the end of his life did his increasingly ailing body force him to limit his activities largely to consulting by letter.

From being an apprenticed barber surgeon, Fabricius rose to become the greatest surgical authority in contemporary Germany, more renowned even than his famous contemporaries Georg Bartisch and Felix Würz. Although he was not endowed with any formal academic degree, he corresponded on equal terms with some of the best-known academic physicians and anatomists of his time, including Gregor Horst, Johannes Vesling, Johannes Wier, Michael Döring, and Sebastian Schobinger. He combined erudite knowledge with unusually extensive personal experience. This experience he emphasized in his publications by referring to countless case histories and observations, most from his own practice. He published on a wide range of subjects, some of them surgical, such as his treatise on gangrene and sphacelus (moist gangrene) or his work on burns, others touching on topics, such as dysentery, that were commonly considered the prerogative of learned physicians.

Fabricius's principal publication was *Observationes*, which he began to publish in 1606 and numbered six hundred before his death. Many of them were written in the style of letters directed to leading physicians of his time; others contained case histories and observations these eminent men had communicated to him. Thus the work reflected Fabricius's intensive epistolary networking and underlined his status in the world of learned medicine. The collection combined two popular medical genres of the period. Some observations referred to highly unusual, if not unique, pathological phenomena, satisfying a widespread scientific interest in the rare and monstrous. Others—indeed the majority—consisted of difficult cases occurring in ordinary practice, most of them from Fabricius's own experience. They presented Fabricius as a highly skilled and knowledgeable surgeon and were designed, at the same time, to provide a model for other surgeons dealing with similar cases. Repeatedly Fabricius applied new techniques and surgical tools that he himself had conceived. Drug therapy also played a considerable role, in preoperative preparation and in the nonsurgical treatment of various internal diseases.

Like Scultetus, Bartisch, and other contemporary surgeons striving to raise surgery to the status of a scientific discipline, Fabricius vehemently attacked uneducated barber surgeons and, above all, itinerant empirics offering a

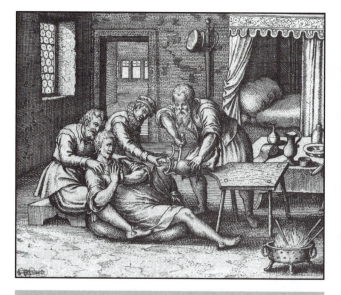

Method of amputating a leg. Woodcut from *De gangraena et sphacelo, tractatus methodicus*, 1620. Rare Books, Wellcome Library, London.

quick surgical fix. Again and again he stressed the value of extensive anatomical knowledge in surgery and illustrated the often fatal consequences of anatomical ignorance. His treatise on the eminence, use, and necessity of anatomy was explicitly devoted to that topic. He also seems to have performed repeated public anatomical demonstrations. He considered anatomy a highly fruitful way to explore the causes and effects of diseases, and he demanded that patients should be dissected in cases of a fatal outcome. During his time in Lausanne, he successfully sought permission to dissect patients who had died in the local hospital, and even his own seven-year-old son was submitted to an autopsy. He also recommended that those responsible for criminal justice should be acquainted with human anatomy, pointing out that common torture practices such as tying the hands of suspects behind their backs and lifting them up with ropes could cause fractures and other irreversible damage and risked making them confess to crimes which they had never committed.

Bibliography

Primary: 1646. *Opera omnia quae extant* (Frankfurt); 1593. *De gangraena et sphacelo. Das ist: von dem heissen vnd kalten Brandt* (Cologne); 1606–1641. *Observationum et curationum chirurgicarum centuriae* (Basel et al.); 1624. *Anatomiae praestantia et utilitas. Das ist kurtze Beschreibung der Fürtrefflichkeit/Nutz/und Nothwendigkeit der Anatomy oder kunstreichen Zerschneitung/vnd Zerlegung menschliches Leibs* (Bern).

Secondary: Olivier, Eugène, 1965. 'Drei Lausanner Chirurgen. Franco–Griffon–Fabry,' in Wennig, W., ed., *Fabrystudien II* (Hilden) pp. 13–145; Jones, Ellis W. P., 1960. 'The Life and Works of Guilhelmus Fabricius Hildanus.' *Medical History* 4: 112–134,

196–209; Becker, Georg, 1957. 'Wilhelm Fabricius von Hilden. Ein Lebensbild unter Berücksichtigung seiner Beziehungen zum Bergischen Lande' in Strangmeier, H., ed., *Wilhelm Fabry von Hilden. Leben–Gestalt–Wirken* (Wuppertal-Elberfeld) pp. 9–53.

Michael Stolberg

FABRIZI DA ACQUAPENDENTE, GIROLAMO (aka FRABRICIUS AB ACQUAPENDENTE)

(b. Acquapendente, Italy, c. 1533; d. at his villa, La Montagnola, outside Padua, Italy, 21 May 1619), *medicine, anatomy, embryology, orthopedics, surgery.*

Fabrizi was born at Acquapendente, a small village north of Rome. His father was Fabrico Fabrici. The family is said to have been noble and once wealthy, but was in decline at the time of Fabrizi's youth. He studied Latin, logic, and philosophy, and then medicine in Padua for nine years, and took his degree in medicine and philosophy in about 1559. He studied with the great anatomist Gabriele Falloppia (1523–62) and succeeded him at his death in teaching anatomy. In 1565 he was nominated professor of anatomy and surgery at the Padua Medical School, retiring in 1613, aged eighty.

In 1594 Fabrizi was able to convince the faculty to build a permanent anatomical theater (still extant) designed for public anatomical dissections. The theater was a wonderful construction with six concentric galleries, with a capacity of about 300 people, all standing not farther than thirty feet from the dissecting table.

Fabrizi enjoyed wide respect and could command high remuneration as a physician. He treated famous people, including the Duke of Mantua; some members of the Medici family; and his colleague in Padua, Galileo Galilei, but he also often treated poor people without charge, according to the testimonies. The King of Poland sought Fabrizi's advice (by correspondence) and rewarded him with a gold chain and medal. He was made knight of St Mark by the Republic of Venice for his treatment of Paolo Sarpi.

Although he was a good teacher, Fabrizi had a difficult character, and because of this and of his worries about the printing of his books he was often in bitter disagreements with his relatives and his students, including Caspar Bartholin (1585–1629), O. Worm (1588–1654), Caspar Bahuin (1560–1624), Pieter Paaw (1564–1617), and especially William Harvey (1578–1657).

Almost all of Fabrizi's treatises were published toward the end of his life, first around 1600 and then another portion in his late years. Many of his treatises were meant as part of an unfinished *Totius animalis fabricae theatrum.*

Fabrizi's famous surgical works are collected in the *Pentateuchos cheirurgicum* (1592; new edition with the addendum of *Operationes chirurgicae*, 1619). This was the most complete surgical treatise of its time and contained many plates illustrating the instruments. Of particular interest are two plates illustrating an orthopedic device, which was apparently actually used to correct injuries and deformities. In the field of surgery, however, Fabrizi's diagnostic and therapeutics method conformed to the Hippocratic and Galenic tradition.

Fabrizi's importance for the history of medicine and the scientific revolution rests on his anatomical and embryological works and on his role as William Harvey's teacher, who referred often to his theories and observations.

The famous treatise *De venarum ostiolis* (1603) reported the observation made by Fabrizi in 1574 of the valves of the veins, in particular the valves at the opening of collateral branches of the veins, which he called *ostiola*. Fabrizi proposed a teleological and Galenic explanation, suggesting that the function of the valves was to slow down the centrifugal flux of blood, in order to obtain its even distribution in the various parts of the body. In addition, he suggested that the valves have a static function, reinforcing the walls of the veins and preventing the stretching of the blood vessels. Fabrizi described an experiment he performed, ligating the veins and observing the valves in action, through the pressure of a finger. This treatise was used by William Harvey as the starting point of his study on the circulation of blood.

Fabrizi's anatomical observations were centered on three aspects of each organ structure: anatomy, action, and utility. He devoted several treatises to the anatomy of different sensory organs and their functions: *De visione, voce, audito* (1600), *De locutione et ejus instrumentis* (1601), *De musculi artificio* (1614), and *De gula, ventriculo, intestinis* (1618). In these books, he gave much attention to the relation between structure and function of the organs of the body and in this context, in the dedication of the *De musculi artificio*, he wrote of his reluctant obligation to disagree with Aristotle and Galen, as a result of his daily observations.

Fabrizi's primary research field involved the study of fetal anatomy. He hoped to determine the purpose of the different organs, their teleological basis, as a way of reconciling his observations with traditional Galenic concepts. His embryological book *De formatione ovi et pulli* (not published until 1621) and his last treatise on the subject, *De formato foetu* (1603), both contained many plates. In the first treatise, Fabrizi discussed the causes and conditions of generation, the role of the egg and the sperm, and the order in which the various parts of the embryo were formed during development. On the last question, he refuted both the Aristotelian theory that gave priority to the heart, and the Galenic one, which suggested that the liver was formed first, giving priority to the blood. The *De formato foetu* concentrated on the organs required to provide for the necessities of the fetus during intrauterine life and included comparative studies of the placenta, umbilical vessels, fetal membranes, etc., in different animals. For this reason, Fabrizi is considered as a 'comparative anatomist', even if he did not analyze the affinities and homologies of function and structure. His study of the placenta and its significance is the most original part of this treatise, limiting the use of the term, first introduced by Realdo Colombo (1510–59), to the type found in humans and other animals.

Many of the embryological and anatomical illustrations made by Fabrizi, who concentrated on the technical details without attention to the artistic dimension, remained unpublished. Some of the three hundred color plates that Fabrizi produced in 1600—consisting of 167 *Tabulae anatomicae*—are preserved in the St Mark's Library, Venice (these *Tabulae Anatomicae* have now been restored and exhibited).

In the last years of his life, Fabrizi published several physiological treatises, including *De respiratione et ejus instrumentis libri duo* (1615, Padua) and *De motu locali animalium secundum totum* (1618, Padua), which were probably influenced by his contacts with the new generation of scientists (particularly Galileo, who had left Padua in 1610). The new scientific style aimed at formulating general laws based on empirical evidence, and Fabrizi wished to study movement 'in general' in the same way, trying to explain animal movement by simple physical laws. He seems to have been the first to apply physical laws to the study of the movements of the body, establishing in particular the muscular progression needed to overcome a resistance, anticipating the analogous researches by Galileo (1638) and Giovanni Borelli (1680). Because of this new approach, Fabrizi's last treatises have been considered as the weakest part of his scientific work. But they are also an effort to overcome the limits of purely anatomical description and to establish a close relationship between the study of form and the explanation of a function.

Bibliography

Primary: 1592. (Beyeri, Johannis Hartamanni, ed., 1604) *Pentateuchos cheirurgicum* (Frankfurt); 1617. *Opera chirurgica* (Padua) [subsequent edns: 1619 (Venice) 1620 (Frankfurt), 1623 (Leiden)]; 1625. *Opera anatomica* (Padua); 1687. *Opera omnia anatomica et physiologica* (Leipzig).

Secondary: Fossati, Pier Maria, ed., 1988. *Girolamo Fabrizi da Acquapendente, Medico e anatomista—La vita e le opere.* (Acquapendente); Scipio, Rosario, ed., 1978. *Girolamo Fabrici, l'Acquapendente* (Viterbo); Favaro, Giuseppe, 1978. 'L'insegnamento anatomico di Girolamo Fabrici d'Acquapendente' in Scipio, Rosario, ed., *Girolamo Fabrici, l'Acquapendente* (Viterbo) pp. 69–93; Stefanutti, Ugo, 1975. 'Girolamo Fabrici d'Acquapendente' in *Scienziati e tecnologi, dalle origini al 1875* (Milan); Adelmann, Howard Bernhardt, 1942. *The Embryological Treatises of Hieronymus Fabricius of Acquapendente.* (A facsimile edition with introduction, translation, and commentary) (Ithaca) [new edn., 2 vols. 1967]; Costantini, Nazareno, 1888. *Biografia di Girolamo Fabrizio* (Acquapendente); *DSB*.

Bernardino Fantini

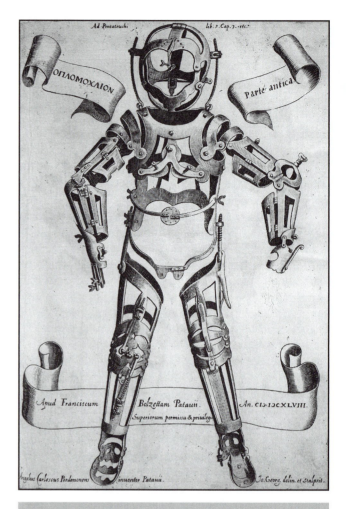

Manikin demonstrating the mechanical principles to be observed in making and fitting artificial limbs. Engraving from *L'opere chirugiche . . .* Bologna, 1678. Rare Books, Wellcome Library, London.

FAIRLEY, NEIL HAMILTON (b. Inglewood, Victoria, Australia, 15 July 1891; d. Sonning, England, 19 April 1966), *military medicine, tropical medicine, medical research.*

Fairley, son of Margaret Louisa Jones and her husband James Fairley, a bank manager, was educated at Scots College in Melbourne and graduated with first class honors in medicine from the University of Melbourne in 1915. In 1916 he enlisted in the Australian Army Medical Corps and was posted as medical officer to 14 AGH in the Middle East. He served in Egypt and Palestine, undertook research on typhus, dysentery, and schistosomiasis, and in 1919 was appointed as research officer to the Lister Institute in London, under Sir Charles Martin.

In 1920 Fairley was appointed Tata Professor of Clinical Tropical Medicine in Bombay and worked for the ensuing five years on schistosomiasis, tropical sprue, and dracunculiasis. In a two-year period of intense research (1927–28) conducted at the Walter and Eliza Hall Institute in Melbourne, he worked on snake envenomation and hydatid disease. In 1929 he returned to London, where he undertook part-time research at the London School of Tropical Medicine and Hygiene (LSHTM), principally working on the complications of malaria.

At the outbreak of World War II, he was promoted to colonel, and in April 1942 he was appointed director of medicine at the Land Headquarters of the Australian Defence Force, based in Melbourne. His work and influence on malaria prophylaxis was immense. The conquest of malaria, with Fairley at the pivot, was one of the most significant factors in the outcome of the Pacific War. Prior to the bombing of Pearl Harbor on 7 December 1941, oral quinine was the mainstay of malaria management in hyperendemic areas. In the Buna and Gona campaigns of 1942, the malaria rate for Australian troops was 2,900 cases per 1,000 troops per year. In 1942 the U.S. 32nd Infantry Division at Buna consisted of 10,000 officers and men, 8,000 of whom became ill from tropical diseases.

In January 1942 Major General Burston (DGMS) recalled Fairley to establish the Medical Research Unit within the Australian Army Land Headquarters. Between 1943 and 1946 he supervised research that defined with great accuracy the life cycle of the *Anopheles* mosquito and outlined the effects of atebrin (mepacrine) in the suppression of malaria. One thousand Australian soldiers volunteered as research subjects for this work. It was found that a daily dose of 0.2 grams of atebrin (or 1.2 grams weekly) suppressed all forms of malaria, and that conditions of extreme heat and humidity, exhaustion, and hypoxia did not modify atebrin's suppressive effects. This impeccable research and the demonstration of the effectiveness of atebrin (1944) and paludrine (1945) resulted in a major paradigm shift in military health. It led to General Sir Thomas Blamey's General Routine Order of September 1944 (further promulgated by Lord Mountbatten in 1945), which held the view that the occurrence of malaria was not primarily a medical responsibility but instead one of command and discipline. Fairley's research forever changed the responsibility for the maintenance of soldier's health from that of a reactive one by doctors and medics to one where responsibility was rightfully placed on individual servicemen and women and those who commanded them. At the conclusion of World War II, Fairley returned to London as foundation Wellcome Professor of Clinical Tropical Medicine at the LSHTM.

Fairley received many honors, including the Fellowship of the Royal Society (1942), the Manson Medal of the Royal Society of Tropical Medicine and Hygiene (1950), and the Neil Hamilton Fairley Medal (1968), bestowed jointly by the Royal Australasian College of Physicians and the Royal College of Physicians of London. He was knighted in 1950.

Bibliography

Secondary: Pearn, John, 2004. 'Medicine at War: "The Pivot Years" of 1943 and 1944 in the New Guinea Campaign' in Dennis, Peter, and Jeffrey Grey, eds., *The Foundations of Victory: The Pacific War* (Canberra); Boyd, John, 1966. 'Neil Hamilton Fairley, 1891–1966' *Biographical Memoirs of Fellows of the Royal Society* 12: 123–145; *Oxford DNB.*

John Pearn

FALLOPPIA, GABRIELE (aka FALLOPPIO, GABRIEL; FALLOPIUS) (b. Modena, Italy, 1523; d. Padua, Italy, 9 October 1562), *anatomy.*

The son of Girolamo Falloppia and Caterina Bergomozzi, Falloppia entered the Church after the death of his father. He later studied medicine in Modena, and in December 1544 he dissected a body for the Collegio dei Medici. He continued his medical studies at the University of Ferrara, where he was Antonio Musa Brasavola's pupil. Toward the end of 1547 he graduated in medicine and became lecturer of simples (medicinal herbs). In October 1548 he obtained the chair of anatomy at the University of Pisa, where he was later wrongfully accused of practicing human vivisection. In September 1551 he was appointed professor of surgery and lecturer of simples at the University of Padua. He gained fame not only as a teacher but also as a practicing physician, and many famous people used his services.

Of the many works that bear his name, only *Observationes anatomicae* (1561), written in Padua in 1557, was published during his lifetime. His students, who had collected his lectures and perhaps sometimes used his own notes, published the rest of his books posthumously. The *Observationes anatomicae* is not a systematic anatomical treatise; it is a series of observations without illustrations in which Falloppia sought to correct errors committed by Andreas Vesalius and to present new material that had hitherto been overlooked. Falloppia's investigations were the result of dissecting not only male and female (some pregnant) adult bodies, but also children of different ages, fetuses in various stages of development, and animals. Thus Falloppia introduced two new methods of study—embryology and comparative anatomy—which were further developed by his pupils Girolamo Fabrizi d'Aquapendente (1533–1619) and Volcher Coiter (1534–76).

The most famous of Falloppia's many contributions to anatomical knowledge was his accurate description of the uterine tubes, which now bear his name (Fallopian tubes). In addition, he described the clitoris and coined the word 'vagina' for what had previously been called the cervix or neck of the uterus.

Many of Falloppia's observations concerned osteology and myology. He described with precision the bones of the cranial base, and particularly the cavities of the auditory organ inside the petrous pyramid, as well as the facial canal

(Fallopian canal, or aqueduct) and its opening (Fallopian hiatus). He also described the vestibule with its canals, the cochlea, and the round and oval windows. He first employed the words 'tympanum', 'labyrinth', and 'cochlea', all of which are still in use today. With his important observations on primary and secondary centers of ossification and on the development of teeth, he was the initiator of embryological studies.

No less important were Falloppia's contributions to myology: of the many observations first made by him, one must remember that of the elevator of the upper eyelid muscle (*levator palpebrae*) and the external pterygoid muscle. He described the occipital muscles, the extrinsic muscles of the ear, several muscles of the pharynx and the soft palate, and the pyramidal muscles of the abdomen; his account of the arrangement and functions of the orbital muscles was also very important. He improved the knowledge of the cranial nerves, and provided a good description of the nervous cardiac plexus. Vesalius replied to Falloppia's work in *Anatomicarum Gabrielis Falloppi observationum examen* (1564).

De partibus similaribus humani corporis (1575) contains lessons dealing with anatomy, in which Falloppia considers the similar constitutive elements, which correspond to our 'tissues', that are found in various parts of the body. Additional works explored syphilis, medical hydrology, surgery, botany, and the composition of drugs.

Bibliography

Primary: 1584. *Opera omnia* (Venice); 1561. *Observationes anatomicae* (Venice) [1964. Italian trans. Righi Riva, Gabriella, and Pericle Di Pietro, 2 vols. (Modena)].

Secondary: Di Pietro, Pericle, ed., 1970. *Epistolario di Gabriele Falloppia* (Ferrara); Favaro, Giuseppe, 1928. *Gabrielle Falloppia modenese (MDXXIII–MDLXII)* (Modena); Montalenti, Giuseppe, 1923. 'Gabriele Falloppia' in Mieli, Aldo, ed., *Gli scienziati italiani dall'inizio del Medio Evo ai nostri giorni*, II (Rome) pp. 43–59; *DSB*.

Giuseppe Ongaro

FANON, FRANTZ OMAR   (b. Fort-de-France, Martinique, 20 July 1925; d. Washington, D.C., USA, 6 December 1961), *psychiatry, psychoanalysis.*

Fanon, the youngest of four sons of customs officer Casimir Fanon (1891–1947) and his wife Eléonore, received a baccalaureate from Lycée Schoelcher in Martinique and an MD from the University of Lyons, France (1946–51). Before attending Lyons, he joined the Free French Forces during World War II, serving in Morocco, Algeria, and France.

In 1952 Fanon worked briefly at Saint-Albin clinic in France, where he met and was influenced by Francesc Tosquelles, a famous Catalan psychiatrist. Tosquelles was developing institutional psychotherapy, or group therapy, which allowed patients to contribute actively to their own

rehabilitation. After passing examinations that qualified him to be a *médicin chef* in June 1953, Fanon accepted an appointment with the French colonial government's psychiatric department at the hospital at Blida-Joinville in Algeria.

Fanon reformed patient care at Blida-Joinville. He eschewed what he saw to be unnecessary restraint and confinement of patients, which he felt worsened their condition. Instead, Fanon instituted a balanced regime of drugs and individual and group psychotherapy. Female European patients responded successfully to his new approach, organizing group sessions and a newsletter as well as participating in movie sessions, knitting, and basket making. The new techniques, however, had no effect on Algerian patients, who remained passive and wedded to their usual routine.

The apparent failure of his reform among Algerian patients forced Fanon to critically examine European approaches to psychiatry among colonized Africans and Arabs. He investigated the role of culture in shaping Arab understanding of psychiatric illnesses and responses to European therapies. He also considered the relationship between colonialism and mental illnesses among colonized peoples. Between 1953 and 1959, Fanon coauthored a number of clinical papers that provided profiles of psychiatric care in Algeria, including hospital conditions, management of mentally ill patients, and experiments conducted at Blida-Joinville. Using a sociocentric approach to psychiatry, Fanon emphasized that it was essential that the diagnosis of patients include consideration of their work, social, and political circumstances as important elements in the etiology of their maladies.

With the onset of the Algerian war of independence (1954–1962), Fanon became horrified by the torture stories of his Algerian patients and their French torturers. He increasingly devoted his medical expertise and the resources of the Blida-Joinville hospital to the Algerian freedom fighters. In 1956 he resigned his position and began to work for the Algerian independence movement.

Fanon relocated to Tunis, where he worked as a psychiatrist at the Manouba Clinic. He also set up a psychiatric day clinic (the first in Africa) at the Hôpital Charles-Nicolle based on his conviction that psychotherapy should not completely isolate mentally ill patients from family, friends, work, and community, and that hospitalization and confinement tends to exacerbate their condition. Fanon's clinical practice gradually took second place to his political activities, journalism, and analysis of colonialism in Africa.

Despite the setbacks at Blida-Joinville, Fanon was a pioneering psychiatrist who applied revolutionary therapeutic techniques that were emerging in Europe in the 1950s to the treatment of patients in African contexts. He highlighted the limits of clinical psychiatry in the face of extreme political oppression and promoted social psychiatry, which did not completely divorce the patients from their political and social realities. He maintained that psychiatrists should endeavor to understand the relationship between culture and the diagnosis and treatment of psychiatric illnesses. Fanon also contributed profoundly to understanding how racism, colonialism, and violence produce harmful psychological effects in the people that they are directed against.

Bibliography

Primary: 1954. (with Azoulay, J.) 'La sociothérapie dans un service d'hommes mussulmans: Difficultés méthodogiques.' *L'Information Pyschiatrique* (4th series) 9: 349; 1959. (with Geromin, Charles) 'L'Hospitalisation du jour en pyschiatrie, valeurs et limites: introduction générale; consideration doctrinales.' *La Tunise Medicale* 38(10): 713–722; 1965. *The Wretched of the Earth* (New York).

Secondary: Cherki, Alice, 2000. *Frantz Fanon, Portrait* (Paris); Macey, David, 2000. *Frantz Fanon: A Biography* (New York); McCulloch, Jock, 1983. *Black Soul, White Artifact: Fanon's Clinical Psychology and Social Theory* (Cambridge).

Ismail Rashid

FARBER, SIDNEY (b. Buffalo, New York, USA, 30 September 1903; d. Boston, Massachusetts, USA, 20 March 1973), *pathology, pediatrics.*

Farber was the third of fourteen children. Four of his siblings became distinguished teachers (three professors of medicine and one a philosopher). Sidney also was exceptional. Even as a youngster, he demonstrated a prodigious capacity for work. As a premedical student at the University of Buffalo, he took part in football, played the violin in a movie theater, and taught high school calculus. After his father's health failed, Sidney and his older brother helped raise their younger brothers and sisters. It was thus not surprising that he was later attracted to pediatrics.

After graduating from college in 1923, Farber went to Europe to study medicine on the advice of his philosopher brother. In Germany, first in Heidelberg and then in Freiberg, he was exposed to Pick and Aschoff. On returning to the United States, he entered Harvard as a second-year medical student. At Harvard, Farber was influenced greatly by S. Burt Wolbach, professor of pathology. Farber received his MD in 1927 and took additional training under Wolbach. Except for the years 1928–29 at the University of Munich and 1935–36 at the University of Ghent, Farber's whole career was at the Boston Children's Hospital, where he was the first full-time pathologist. Farber has been called the founder of pediatric pathology in the United States. He and his colleagues made substantial impact on understanding many diseases seen in infants and children. These included hyaline membrane disease of the newborn, cystic fibrosis, transposition of the great vessels, the histiocytoses, and neuroblastoma and other pediatric tumors. Farber was appointed pathologist-in-chief of Harvard Medical School in 1947 and professor of pathology in 1948.

He was named the first S. Burt Wolbach Professor of Pathology in 1967.

Farber's role in the development of cancer chemotherapy was a milestone for the specialty. The vitamin folic acid was known to be a growth factor for blood cells. Farber asserted that administration of folic acid might accelerate leukemia. Although this was not clearly shown to be the case in humans, scientists at Lederle Laboratories were stimulated to synthesize a folic acid antagonist, aminopterin. In 1948 Farber's group reported that of sixteen infants and children with acute leukemia treated with aminopterin, ten showed clinical, hematologic, and pathologic evidence of improvement. Although the remissions were only temporary, the authors concluded that a promising new area of research had been identified. Their landmark article was the first step in the eventual development of curative therapy for acute leukemia and the first evidence that scientists could create chemical compounds that interfered with the growth of malignant cells. Within a year, another folic acid antagonist, methotrexate, was synthesized. This antimetabolite is still employed in the treatment of a variety of neoplasms.

In 1949 Farber reported a complete remission in a child with acute leukemia after treatment with ACTH. Subsequently, corticosteroid hormones were shown to have significant activity in childhood acute lymphocytic leukemia and continue to have a key role in therapy of this disease.

Farber also pioneered the use of actinomycin D, the first antibiotic demonstrated to cause shrinkage of malignant human tumors. The agent was shown to have major activity in two pediatric cancers—Wilms's tumor and rhabdomyosarcoma—and was the first drug shown to have beneficial effects on either of these malignancies. Farber also employed chemotherapy with actinomycin D following surgical tumor resection. This was the beginning of 'adjuvant' chemotherapy, an approach that has been widely adopted in the treatment of breast and colon cancers as well as of other solid tumors.

A tall man with commanding presence, Farber was characterized as 'formal, but kind'. He was an articulate medical statesman and politician. He focused national attention on the fight against cancer and was one of its most effective spokespersons. Together with Mary Lasker and Dr Cornelius Rhodes, Farber influenced Congress to appropriate funds for leukemia research and for clinical facilities at the National Institutes of Health. Through the Childrens' Cancer Research Foundation and the 'Jimmy Fund', he secured donations to study and care for children with neoplastic disease in the Boston area. He vigorously supported the multidisciplinary approach and emphasized 'total care', with utilization of all medical and social resources to assist the patient and family. Farber had no tolerance for people with negative attitudes or who felt that treatment of malignant disease was hopeless. At times

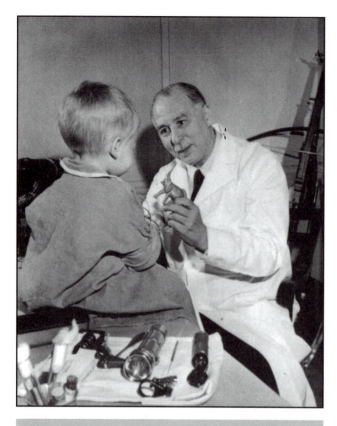

Sidney Farber with young patient. Photograph. Courtesy of The Harvard Medical Library in the Francis A. Countway Library of Medicine.

he was aggressive and quite ruthless. In 1974 he succeeded in extending his program to adults through the establishment of the Charles A. Dana Center, now the Dana-Farber Cancer Institute.

Sidney Farber was a man of action, whose work laid the foundation for development of curative chemotherapy for human leukemia and other malignancies.

Bibliography

Primary: 1947. 'Action of Pteroylglutamine Conjugates in Man.' *Science* 106: 619–621; 1948. (with Diamond, Louis K., R. D. Mercer, R. F. Sylvester, and V. A. Wolff) 'Temporary Remissions in Acute Leukemia in Children Produced by Folic Acid Antagonist 4-aminopteroyl-glutamic Acid (aminopterin).' *New England Journal of Medicine* 238: 787–793; 1956. (with Toch, R., and E. M. Sears) 'Advances in Chemotherapy of Cancer in Man.' *Adv. Cancer Research* 4: 1–71; 1960. (with D'Angio, G., and A. Evans) 'Clinical Studies of Actinomycin D with Special Reference to Wilms' Tumor in Children.' *Ann. NY Acad. Sciences* 89: 421–425.

Secondary: Laszlo, John, 1995. *The Cure of Childhood Leukemia: Into the Age of Miracles* (New Brunswick, NJ); Freireich, E. J., and N. A. Lemak, 1991. *Milestones in Leukemia Research and Therapy* (Baltimore); Wintrobe, Maxwell M., 1985. *Hematology, the Blossoming of a Science* (Philadelphia) pp. 512–514; Gunz, F. W., 1980.

'The Dread Leukemias and the Lymphomas: Their Nature and Their Prospects' in Wintrobe, M. M., ed., *Blood, Pure and Eloquent* (New York) pp. 535–536.

Marvin J. Stone

FARR, WILLIAM (b. Kenley, Shropshire, England, 30 November 1807; d. London, England, 14 April 1883), *vital statistics.*

Although he was born into a farm-laboring family, the support of a local squire enabled Farr to receive a good education. Through a formal apprenticeship he gained medical experience working for a local physician, as a dresser at Shrewsbury Infirmary, and also with an apothecary. A legacy from his patron, John Pryce, in 1828 permitted him to study medicine in Paris and Switzerland for two years. He then studied at University College, London, and gained his license from the Society of Apothecaries (the only medical qualification he obtained by study). After a short period working as house surgeon in Shrewsbury Infirmary, in 1833, he set up as an apothecary in Bloomsbury, London, and supplemented his income by writing articles for *Lancet*. His early contributions were on hygiene (1835), quack medicine (1836), life insurance, and cholera (1838). He also contributed a chapter on vital statistics to J. R. McCulloch's *A Statistical Account of the British Empire* (1837), which was to establish his new reputation as a medical statistician.

Farr secured a temporary position at the new General Register Office in 1837, and through his friendship with Sir James Clark (1788–1870, Queen's Physician, FRS) and Edwin Chadwick (1800–90, Poor Law and sanitary reformer), he was appointed as Compiler of Abstracts in 1839. He had already exhibited an aptitude for medical statistics during his studies, and he quickly proved his worth in this new role. As a result, his title was changed to superintendent of the statistical department in 1842. This new post required him to devise a statistical nosology, comprising twenty-seven fatal disease categories. Farr's list was to be used by local registrars and doctors in the compulsory completion of death certificates. The categories he developed (especially that of 'zymotics'—diseases that were caused by poisons in the body) were influenced by the work of Justus von Liebig (1803–73), a professor of organic chemistry at the University of Giessen, and significantly enhanced the quality of mortality statistics produced in Britain.

Farr's pioneering work in Britain was complemented by similar studies conducted in Geneva by Marc d'Espine (1806–60). They were only nineteen months apart in age, and had both studied in Paris in the early 1830s. Their careers subsequently followed similar trajectories, both deciding to develop nosologies and classifications to enhance their statistical analyses. They provided mutual support through their publications in the quest for the creation of international nosology and classification systems.

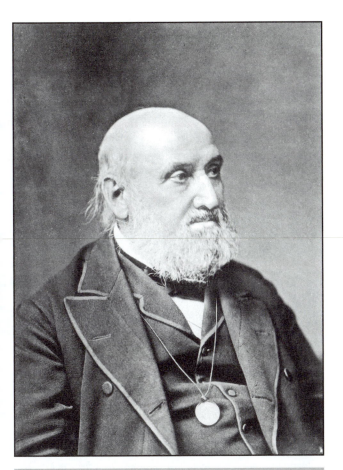

William Farr. Halftone reproduction from Noel A. Humphreys (ed), *Vital Statistics . . .* London, 1885. Wellcome Library, London.

Farr and d'Espine met at the first session of the International Statistical Congress in Brussels (1853), where they were tasked with preparing an agreed-upon 'nomenclature' of causes of death. This proved a difficult exercise, and also attracted the criticism of some doctors who believed that statisticians should not dictate to them on such matters. By the time of the last International Statistical Congress (1878), there was still no agreement, with individual countries developing their preferred nosologies based either on the Farr or the d'Espine models. Farr revised his nosology on several occasions, in response to developments in medical knowledge and the practicalities of coding some 300,000 deaths per year by the 1870s. His last substantial revision was assisted by the RCP, perhaps indicative of the medical profession's recent acceptance of the usefulness of such nosologies.

The issue of classification as separate from nosology was equally contentious, but Farr and d'Espine together made progress and agreed relatively quickly on five of the eight primary groupings that d'Espine proposed. Although they disagreed on elements of each other's classification systems (d'Espine preferring 'acute' and 'chronic' to Farr's 'epidemic' and 'sporadic'), Farr had modified his nosology (1842) to bring all tubercular diseases together in one category, irrespective of their site—undoubtedly influenced by d'Espine's Paris education in pathological anatomy. However, Farr was insistent on maintaining his group of 'zymotics'—those diseases that he considered as providing an 'index of salubrity' for the insanitary urban areas. His classification was essentially a tool for the new public health practitioners, such as the Medical Officers of Health; d'Espine's was in essence a pathological 'research instrument'. When L. A. and J. Bertillon (1821–93, 1851–1919) renewed the quest for an international classification in 1893 at the new International Statistical Institute, their preferred model was Farr's.

The statistics generated through such nosologies and classifications was further analyzed by Farr to produce annual and decennial reports, in which mortality was disaggregated for the first time by disease, parish, age, sex, and occupation. He also exploited the data to produce detailed reports on the sanitary condition of London and thirteen other large towns. Although there had been local attempts at demographic analysis before Farr, and limited national studies conducted by John Graunt (1620–74) and William Petty (1623–87) into the size of the population in the seventeenth century, Farr was the first person to develop a systematic approach to the subject. He also developed a series of life tables illustrating the impact of place and date of birth on a number of factors.

Because of his statistical skills, Farr became enormously influential in the development of public health in Britain at a time of considerable uncertainty and scientific debate over how diseases were transmitted. His clear and easily understood reports allowed him to advocate sanitary reforms based on the miasmatic theory of disease—the principle that disease could be generated from bad gases (miasmas) produced by rotting matter, such as the piles of sewage lying in urban streets. He was able to show a correlation between cholera cases and elevation, which led him (erroneously) to believe that the disease must be airborne. He therefore supported Chadwick in his program of integrated sewer and water systems to reduce the filth in the urban environment.

Despite John Snow's (1813–58) investigations during the 1848–49 and 1854–55 cholera epidemics, Farr refused to accept that cholera could be transmitted by infected water. Although there are some inklings of doubt in the appendix to the 1854 report of the Registrar-General, it was not until he undertook his own investigations during the 1866 epidemic that he was finally persuaded that Snow's theory was correct. His report on cholera, which was published as a supplement to the 1866 Registrar-General's annual report did much to advance the understanding of disease causation. He also supported Florence Nightingale (1820–1910) in her work to reform hospital and army sanitary conditions, and was often called upon to give evidence to parliamentary enquiries.

Farr's achievements in demographic analysis and sanitary reform were recognized in Britain and abroad. Between 1851 and 1876 he attended international statistical congresses in nine European capitals. In 1851 he was adviser to the census commissioners, and served as a census commissioner himself in 1861 and 1871. In 1855 he was elected FRS, and he became President of the Royal Statistical Society in 1871. When the second Registrar-General, George Graham, retired in 1879, Farr applied for the post and colleagues expected him to be appointed. He was not, possibly because of his recent ill health, and he retired in 1880, after which he was made a Companion of the Bath. He also received the Gold Medal from the British Medical Association, and a testimonial fund was established to support his three unmarried daughters. His pioneering statistical work, coupled with his easily accessible writing style, made his contributions to the development of public health some of the most significant of the nineteenth century.

Bibliography

Primary: 1885. *Vital Statistics, a Memorial Volume of Selections from the Reports and Writings of William Farr* (London; reprinted 1975, New York).

Secondary: Halliday, Stephen, 2000. 'William Farr: Campaigning Statistician.' *Journal of Medical Biography* 8: 220–227; Goldman, Lawrence, 1991. 'Statistics, and the Science of Society in Early Victorian Britain: An Intellectual Context for the General Register Office.' *Social History of Medicine* 4: 414–434; Szreter, Simon, 1991. 'The GRO and the Public Health Movement in Britain, 1837–1914.' *Social History of Medicine* 4: 435–463; Lewes, F. M. M., 1988. 'Dr Marc D'Espine's Statistical Nosology.' *Medical History* 32: 301–313; Eyler, John M., 1979. *Victorian Social Medicine: The Ideas and Methods of William Farr* (Baltimore); *Oxford DNB.*

Sally Sheard

FAVALORO, RENE GERÓNIMO (b. La Plata, Argentina, 14 July 1923; d. Buenos Aires, Argentina, 29 July 2000), *cardiac surgery.*

Favaloro is deservedly known as the surgeon who introduced coronary-artery bypass grafting into practice at the Cleveland Clinic. His father was a carpenter and his mother a seamstress, and he attended a neighborhood elementary school. After finishing high school, he enrolled in the Faculty of Medical Sciences of the National University of La Plata. He graduated in 1949 from La Plata University and worked for twelve years as a country doctor, but while doing so established a mobile blood bank and built his own operating room. He described this period in his life in *Memoirs of a Country Doctor.* During the years that he, along with his brother, worked in La Pampa, they created a welfare center and raised the social and educational level of the region. Working with his brother, he brought about a change of attitude in the community, and greatly reduced infant mortality, birth infections, and malnutrition.

He became interested in the newly developing cardiac surgical interventions and wanted to go to the United States to get a master's degree. He chose the Cleveland Clinic, where he went as a resident at the age of forty. He worked with Mason Sones, Willem Kolff, and Donald Effler. Favaloro studied the thousands of cineangiograms that Sones had performed. At the time they were performing Vineberg operations, which involved burying a chest wall artery in the heart muscle in the hope that it would make some anastamoses. He became interested in direct grafting of the coronary arteries. At the beginning of 1967 he began to think about the possibility of using the saphenous vein from the patient's leg as a convenient and expendable graft material. The first successful operation was in May 1967.

Recognition of the importance of the operation was very rapid and in 1970 Favoloro presented his results to the World Congress of Cardiology in London and also performed demonstration operations there.

He returned to Argentina in 1971 and founded the Favaloro Foundation. In 1980 Favaloro created a basic science facility, which became the University Institute of Biomedical Sciences and then in August of 1998 led to the creation of the Favaloro University. In 1992 the Institute of Cardiology and Cardiovascular Surgery of the Favaloro Foundation was inaugurated. With his foundation heavily in debt, he committed suicide in 2000.

Bibliography

Primary: 1969. (with Effler, D. B., L. K. Groves, W. C. Sheldon, and M. Riahi) 'Direct Myocardial Revascularization with Saphenous Vein Autograft. Clinical Experience in 100 Cases.' *Dis. Chest* 56: 279–283; 1970. *Surgical Treatment of Coronary Arteriosclerosis* (Baltimore); 1994. *The Challenging Dream of Heart Surgery: From Pampas to Cleveland* (Boston); 1998. 'Landmarks in the Development of Coronary Artery Bypass Surgery.' *Circulation* 98(5): 466–478.

Secondary: Captur, Gabriella, 2004. 'Memento for René Favaloro.' *Texas Heart Institute Journal* 31: 47–60.

Tom Treasure

FAYRER, JOSEPH (b. Plymouth, England, 6 December 1824; d. Falmouth, Devon, England, 21 May 1907), *surgery, medicine.*

Fayrer was the second of six sons of Commander Robert Fayrer, RN, and his wife Agnes. His childhood was spent in Westmorland and Liverpool, from which his father commanded steam packets to New York. Fayrer showed an early interest in the physical sciences and navigation, and in 1840 he served as a midshipman in the West Indian mail packet service. He became interested in medicine only after accompanying his father on a voyage to Bermuda, where he witnessed an outbreak of yellow fever.

In 1844 Fayrer entered Charing Cross Hospital and was appointed house surgeon of the Westminster Ophthalmic Hospital two years later. In 1847 he was admitted MRCS and received a commission in the Naval Medical Service, which he resigned soon afterwards in order to travel in

Europe. He witnessed the Sicilian revolution and attended the University of Rome, where he was awarded an MD (1848).

In 1850 Fayrer joined the East India Company as an assistant surgeon. Although based mainly in Calcutta, he distinguished himself in several campaigns, including the Burma war of 1852. His valor led the governor-general Lord Dalhousie (1812–60) to appoint Fayrer residency surgeon in city of Lucknow, where he married Bethia Mary Spens, daughter of the commander of the British garrison. Lucknow was at the heart of the Mutiny and Rebellion of 1857, and Fayrer played an important part in the defense of the residency, which was besieged from 30 June to 17 November.

He left India the following year and obtained an MD from Edinburgh University (1859), returning to India to become professor of surgery at the Calcutta Medical College. Soon afterwards, Fayrer joined the Asiatic Society of Bengal, having a keen interest in the languages and natural history of the region, especially its venomous reptiles. He became president of the Society in 1867, and it was largely through his initiative that zoological gardens were established in Calcutta in 1875. In 1868 Fayrer was made CSI and, the following year, was appointed personal surgeon to Lord Mayo (1822–72), the new viceroy. At this time, he also wrote on various aspects of surgery, his principal works being *Clinical Observations in Surgery* (1863) and *Clinical Surgery in India* (1866).

Fayrer's career in India was cut short by illness and he returned to England in 1872, where he practiced as a physician, having being elected FRCP the same year. In London, he researched the properties of snake venom, resulting in the publication of *The Thanatophidia of India* in 1872. In February 1873 Fayrer was appointed to the medical board of the India Office and became its president in December, continuing in that role until January 1895. He returned to India as personal physician to the Prince of Wales in 1875 and was made KCSI in 1876. After his return to Britain, Fayrer was elected FRS in 1877 and received honorary doctorates at Edinburgh and St Andrews.

The remainder of Fayrer's career was spent in the practice of medicine, as consulting physician at Charing Cross Hospital. From 1879 he was also president of the Epidemiological Society and developed a keen interest in the environmental factors—particularly climate—that seemed to have a bearing on disease. His opposition to theories of strict contagion and quarantine led to his being chosen by the government of India as its delegate for a number of international conferences, most notably the sanitary conference at Rome in 1885. He was made a baronet on 7 February 1896.

Fayrer spent his last years at Falmouth, where he enjoyed deep-sea fishing and yachting. He died at home, leaving two sons.

Bibliography

Primary: 1882. *On the Climate and Fevers of India* (London); 1888. *The Natural History and Epidemiology of Cholera* (London); 1890. *Recollections of My Life* (Edinburgh).

Secondary: Harrison, Mark, 1999. *Climates and Constitutions* (Delhi); Harrison, Mark, 1994. *Public Health in British India* (Cambridge); *Munk's Roll*; *Oxford DNB*.

Mark Harrison

FEDOROV, SVIATOSLAV NIKOLAEVICH (b. Proskurov, Ukraine, 8 August 1927; d. Moscow, Russia, 2 June 2000), *ophthalmology, eye surgery.*

Fedorov was born in 1927 to the family of a cavalry officer in Soviet Ukraine. A sickly child, he developed a determined character and strong penchant for physical toughening in his teen years. The family lived in Rostov-on-Don at the time, and Fedorov entered the Medical Institute there by default, as there were then no other institutes of higher education in the city. Influenced by his hobby of photography, he soon specialized in ophthalmology.

Fedorov was already challenging existing methods of eye surgery within a year of graduating in 1952. His more radical cataract surgery, which removed the lens capsule as well as the lens nucleus, achieved early success. After defending his candidate's (graduate) thesis he was appointed as section head at the Cheboksary Branch of the Institute of Eye Surgery. Here he swiftly began the work that would later bring him worldwide fame: the implantation of artificial lenses. The use of plastic lenses in eye surgery ran against the conventional wisdom that the eye was too sensitive an organ to accept prostheses. The British surgeon Harold Ridley had initial successes in 1949 with the implanting of plastic lenses, but the lenses of the time were crude and led to complications after further operations.

Fedorov's early work met deep resistance from the medical community but his record of success brought him a transfer to the Institute of Eye Surgery in Moscow in 1965. He rapidly developed his work in keratoprosthesis, the insertion of plastic discs or lenses into the cornea, summarizing his discoveries in a monograph published in 1987. New moves were taken in the surgical fight against glaucoma, myopia, and astigmatism. Again flying very much against conventional medical opinion, Fedorov experimented with the replacement of the vitreous body of the eye.

Much of Fedorov's research refined already existing scholarship, but he was also renowned for the flamboyance and scale of his surgery. The hospital gowns used by Fedorov's team of surgeons were specially designed by top Soviet fashion designer Slava Zaitsev to afford a maximum of comfort and a modicum of style. One of the controversies surrounding Fedorov's technique was his use of a conveyor belt in the operating room. Large numbers of patients were physically moved between one surgical point and the next as each of

Fedorov's doctors was made responsible for one particular stage of the operation. Not surprisingly, this assembly line method was severely criticized for being dehumanizing, but Fedorov retorted that the lengthy waiting lists for conventional eye surgery were far worse. Up to 150 patients could be treated every day at his surgery. By the late 1980s, his clinic had operated on over 25,000 patients, with a restoration of 70 percent to 100 percent of sight in almost all cases. As his international reputation grew, entire planeloads of eye-swathed patients flew to Moscow for treatment at his clinic.

Fedorov exemplified the flamboyance of those members of the Soviet elite who broke away from socialist strictures in the 1980s and became increasingly preoccupied with money and prestige. His particular 'cult of personality' culminated in his campaign for the Russian presidency in 1996, during which he relied on his fame and the use of his medical staff as campaign workers. Probably reflecting his youthful desire to be a pilot, but certainly reflecting his attraction to the most modern technology, Fedorov liked to fly often and far, both for medical and political purposes. He died this way, on 2 June 2000, in a helicopter crash in Moscow.

Bibliography

Primary: Fedorov, Sviatoslav, Z. I. Moroz, and V. K. Zuev. 1987. *Keratoprostheses* trans. Nicholas Bobrov (Edinburgh); 1990. *Otrazhenie. Svoimi slovami.* [Reflections. By his own words.] (Moscow).

Secondary: 1997. 'Sviatoslav Nikolaevich Fedorov (k 70-letiiu so dnia rozhendiia).' ['Sviatoslav Nikolaevich Fedorov (on his seventieth birthday).'] *Vestnik Rossiiskoi Akademii meditsinskikh nauk* 8: 63–64; Vlasov, Sergei, 1988. *Svyatoslav Fyodorov. Just a Magician Who Gives Back Sight.* (Moscow); 1985. 'Doctor in Moscow,' Frontline Series: Comrades. Video.

Chris Burton

FEI, BOXIONG 費伯姓 (b. Menghe, Wujin county, Jiangsu province, China, February 1800; d. Menghe, China, 16 July 1879), *Chinese medicine.*

'Of all . . . physicians at the end of the Qing, Boxiong was the most outstanding' is how the editors of the semiofficial *Draft History of the Qing (Qingshi gao* 清史搞, 1927) summed up the reputation and achievements of Fei Boxiong. A century later, his medical style continued to attract prominent followers, such as Zou Yunxiang 鄒云翔, (1897–1988), vice president of the influential Nanjing University of TCM and vice secretary of the China Chinese Medicine Association, who 'never stopped admiring the prescriptions authored by [Fei Boxiong]'.

Fei Boxiong was born into a lineage of successful scholar physicians from the small town of Menghe. He gained the *xiu cai* 秀才 [flourishing talents] degree in the provincial examinations but failed to advance further up the civil service ladder. While taking part in the provincial examinations of 1832, Fei was introduced to Lin Zexu 林則徐 (1785–1850), the provincial governor, and apparently treated a

member of his family with great success. His reputation established, Fei subsequently treated some of the most powerful dignitaries of the empire including, according to some accounts, the Daoguang Emperor (r. 1821–50) and his mother. He was famous for a gentle treatment style that relied on mild formulas. They could be taken over long periods and were particularly suitable for the treatment of the chronic disorders associated with the lifestyles of his elite clientele. Fei Boxiong's life coincided with a period of great political and cultural instability. The Taiping Rebellion of 1854–65 almost brought the Qing dynasty to its knees and caused enormous devastation throughout southern China. It was also a period when intellectuals questioned the very foundations of traditional political and moral discourse, a soul-searching reflected in contemporary medical discourse. Fei Boxiong's solution was to ground medical practice in a small number of basic principles that he traced to the oldest sources of tradition, while simultaneously creating space for continued innovation. He labeled these principles 'harmonization' (*he* 和) and 'gentleness' (*huan* 緩): physicians should seek to harmonize disordered body processes with the help of the gentlest treatments possible. Through wide reading and comprehensive practice, a physician would grasp these principles and distill the 'refined essence' (*chun* 醇) of the entire medical tradition. In practice a physician could identify the fundamental principles of physiological process manifest in each unique pattern of disease, rendering all innovation merely a continuation of tradition.

The principles and practice of Fei Boxiong's 'medicine of the refined' are laid out in his two major works, *The Refined in Medicine Remembered (Yichun shengyi* 醫醇勝義) and *Treatise on Medical Formulas (Yifang lun* 醫方論), published in 1863 and 1865, respectively. In addition, he wrote a volume on dietary therapy and another on bizarre and strange illnesses and their treatment in historical sources. He was also an accomplished poet and essayist whose literary esthetics were characterized by a similar search for the 'refined'. His writings reveal a conservative scholar concerned with reconstituting the unity of a fracturing tradition. His was not a static conservatism, however, but one seeking to render tradition useful for the solution of contemporary problems. In this he prefigured the modernization of Chinese medicine in Maoist China.

Bibliography

Primary: 1863. *Feishi quanshu* 費氏全書 [Complete Works of Mr. Fei] (Menghe).

Secondary: Cheng Choufu 程丑夫, 1992. 'Fei Boxiong zhifang qianyao fangfa luetan' 費伯雄制方遣藥方法略談 [A brief account of Fei Boxiong's method of composing formulas and deploying drugs]. *Hunan zhongyi xueyuan xueba o* 湖南中醫學院學報 [Hunan College of Chinese Medicine Journal] 3: 6–8; Wang Yinsan 王荫三, 1987. 'Fei Boxiong linzheng tedian tanwei' 費伯雄臨証特點探微 [A subtle inquiry into the characteristics of Fei Boxiong's (treatment of) clinical patterns]. *Jiangsu zhongyi zazhi* 江蘇中醫雜誌

[Jiangsu Journal of Chinese Medicine] 2: 33–35; Xu Xiangren 徐相任, 1933. 'Menghe Feishi yixue zhi jiepou' 孟河費氏醫學解剖 [A dissection of the medical scholarship of the Fei family from Menghe]. *Shenzhou guoyi xuebao* 神州國醫學報 [China National Medicine Journal) 11: 15–18.

Volker Scheid

FENWICK, ETHEL GORDON (NÉE MANSON)   (b.

Elgin, Morayshire, Scotland, 26 January 1857; d. London, England, 13 March 1947), *nursing*.

Fenwick, third child of Dr David Davidson Manson, a farmer, and Harriette Palmer, grew up in the Vale of Belvoir, Nottinghamshire, at the country house of her stepfather George Storer, MP. Educated privately, she started her nurse training at the Children's Hospital, Nottingham, at the age of twenty-one. She worked at the Royal Infirmary, Manchester, and the London Hospital before being appointed matron of St Bartholomew's Hospital, London, at the age of twenty-four. She spent six years as the matron, reforming the nurses' working conditions and improving the standard of the nurses' training. At the age of thirty she married Dr Bedford Fenwick (1855–1939), a successful London physician, and they had one son, Christian Bedford Fenwick (1888–1969).

As Mrs Bedford Fenwick she turned her attention to the professional development of nurses and this became her life's work. She realized that nurses needed a professional association and founded the British Nurses' Association (BNA) in 1887. Granted a royal charter in 1891, the RBNA became the battleground for the campaign for state registration of nurses, an issue that provoked strong opposition from sections of the British establishment and gave rise to a thirty-year campaign known as the 'battle of the nurses'.

Fenwick was an active supporter of the campaign for women's rights and traveled to the United States several times to attend the meetings of the International Council of Women (ICW), and there she met the leaders in American nursing. When the ICW met in London in 1899, Fenwick seized the opportunity to establish a sister organization, the International Council of Nurses (ICN). Through the ICN and the *British Journal of Nursing*, which Fenwick owned and edited for over fifty years, she disseminated ideas about the professional status of nurses.

During World War I Fenwick was very active and worked particularly for the French Red Cross, for which she received a medal. The war highlighted the lack of organization among British nurses and, as the government urged all women to take up nursing, trained nurses felt increasingly vulnerable. A group of matrons, led by Sarah Swift (1854–1937), the matron-in-chief of the British Red Cross, formed the College of Nursing in 1916, to provide a central body responsible for nurses' educational

standards and registration. Fenwick was completely opposed to the College, seeing it as an unacceptable alternative to state registration. After the war she resumed her campaign and in 1919 legislation was finally passed for the state registration of nurses. Fenwick was appointed to the new statutory body, the General Nursing Council for England and Wales (GNC), and her name was entered as number one on the nurses' register. Always a leader, Fenwick was not good at committee work, and her intransigence forced the Minister of Health to intervene to remove her from the position of chairman of the registration committee. When elections for the GNC were held, she lost her seat and thereafter her hostility to the Royal College of Nursing became fanatical. With her loyal group of supporters she formed the alternative British College of Nurses in 1926.

Fenwick inspired a generation of nurses to regard themselves as part of an international profession of nursing, independent of medicine and governments. Her international status as a nursing leader is celebrated by the ICN, which is the most enduring professional organization founded by women and today represents nurses in 120 countries.

Bibliography

Primary: 1888–1947. *British Journal of Nursing* (absorbed by *Nursing Record*); 1930. (with Breay, Margaret) *The History of the International Council of Nurses*.

Secondary: Brush, Barbara, and Joan Lynaugh, et al., 1999. *Nurses of All Nations, A History of the International Council of Nurses 1899–1999* (Philadelphia); McGann, Susan, 1992. *The Battle of the Nurses* (London); Hector, Winifred, 1973. *The Work of Mrs Bedford Fenwick and the Rise of Professional Nursing* (London); *Oxford DNB*.

Susan McGann

FERNÁNDEZ Y HERNÁNDEZ, JUAN SANTOS   (b.

Alacranes, Cuba, 22 July 1847; d. Havana, Cuba, 6 August 1922), *ophthalmology, tropical medicine*.

Born on his family's *ingenio* (sugar estate) in Matanzas province, Fernández grew up in the heart of colonial Cuba's booming slave-based sugar complex. He began medical studies at the Universidad de la Habana in 1868, but his family sent him abroad after the outbreak of the first war of independence in that year. At the Universidad Central de Madrid the prominent eye surgeon Delgado Jugo encouraged Fernández to specialize in ophthalmology, and he completed his training at the Desmarres clinic in Paris under Xavier Galezowski. Fernández returned to Havana in 1875 and quickly established himself as an elite specialist. His stature was raised further when he married an aristocratic patient, Teresa González Aguilar, daughter of the Countess of San Ignacio.

Fernández was at the center of an illustrious community of scientifically oriented physicians who made up a majority in the Real Academia de Ciencias de la Habana, the leading *criollo* (Cuban-born white) institution in late Spanish colonial Cuba. A member of the academy from 1875, Fernández was the final president of the institution during its colonial incarnation. He retained the presidency following the U.S. overthrow of Spanish rule in 1898, when the academy dropped its 'Royal' designation, and he held the office until his death in 1922. He was a cofounder of the influential Anthropological Society (1877) and publisher of the important medical periodical *Crónica Médico-Quirúrgica* (1875–1940). Fernández was also owner and director of the *Laboratorio Histo-Bacteriológico y de vacunación antirrábica*, one of the earlier bacteriological laboratories in the Americas (and the first in Cuba). It was established in 1887 on the model of Pasteur's laboratories and staffed by Cuban doctors who Fernández had sent to train there following the French scientist's momentous discovery of a rabies vaccine.

Fernández combined private practice, research, and publication with medical entrepreneurship and associationism. Fernández organized the First Cuban Medical Congress in 1890, and following independence he remained Cuba's leading organizer of the national and international medical gatherings that made the young country a showcase for medicine and hygiene in the Americas. In 1901, along with Manuel Menacho Peirón of Barcelona, Fernández founded the journal *Archivos de Oftalmología Hispanoamericanos*, which led to the Society of Hispanoamerican Ophthalmology, founded in 1904.

A devoted clinician, Fernández registered his cases in 142 volumes and used the data for his contributions to tropical ophthalmology. His early postulation that different races had distinct optical pathologies was not borne out by his clinical evidence, and he accepted this in a paper given in 1900 to the XIII International Medical Congress in Paris. He nevertheless maintained that Africans and their descendants were racially inferior, and remained a strong advocate of European immigration. The long personal, professional, and scientific rivalry that Fernández had with another Havana ophthalmologist and member of the Real Academia, Carlos Finlay, ensured that the Academy would deny early recognition of Finlay's theory of yellow fever transmission (first presented to the academy in 1881). Fernández's control over the most sophisticated laboratory in Havana also meant that his rival did not have access to optimal facilities for yellow fever experiments in the late 1880s and 1890s. Like many Cuban physicians, Fernández made amends after 1898 by championing Finlay's pioneering yellow fever work, and fighting to have him receive recognition for his crucial role in the breakthrough 1901 inoculation trials conducted by U.S. military physicians in Havana under the command of Walter Reed.

Bibliography

Primary: 1875–1916. 'Libros clínicos' and 'Libros de operaciones', Museo Finlay (Havana); 1901. *Las enfermedades de los ojos en los negros y mulatos* (Havana); 1918. *Recuerdos de mi vida* 2 vols. (Havana).

Secondary: Funes Monzote, Reinaldo, 2004. *El despertar del asociacionismo científico en Cuba (1876–1920)* (Madrid); Pruna Goodgall, Pedro M., 2002. *La Real Academia de Ciencias de la Habana, 1861–1898* (Madrid); López Sánchez, José, 1999. *Carlos J. Finlay: His Life and Work* (Havana).

Steven Palmer

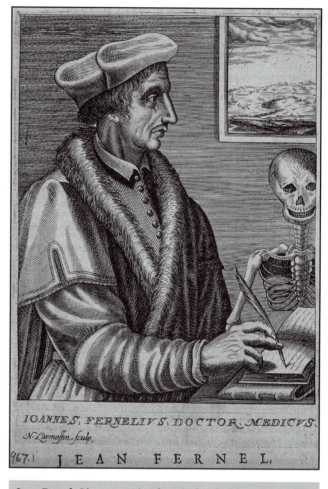

Jean Fernel. Line engraving by Nicolas de Larmessin, 1682. Iconographic Collection, Wellcome Library, London.

FERNEL, JEAN (b. Montdidier, France, *c.* 1497; d. Fontainebleau, France, 26 April 1558), *medicine, natural philosophy, astrology, alchemy.*

Fernel was one of the leading physicians and medical writers of his age. He not only set out compendious synoptic accounts of Galenic theory for the first time, but also offered his own major reforms of medical theory in order to deal with contagious and other infectious diseases (which were not adequately dealt with in ancient medicine). He stands, therefore, alongside Paracelsus (1493/4–1541) and Girolamo Fracastoro (1483–1553) as the only would-be medical reformers of the sixteenth century.

Early Life and Interest in Mathematics

Fernel's first biographer, Guillaume Plancy (1514–c. 1568) never provided a date for Fernel's birth, but he said that Fernel was 'about sixty years of age' when the king's physician, Louis De Bourges (1482–1556), died and Fernel took over as royal physician. This would mean that Fernel was born around 1496. The most commonly accepted date, 1497, derives from the conclusions of a later biographer, Jean Goulin (1728–99), and this was endorsed by Sir Charles Sherrington (1857–1952), Fernel's most recent biographer.

Fernel, son of a substantial furrier and innkeeper, was born at Montdidier in the diocese of Amiens, and although he moved with his family to Clermont, near Paris, when he was twelve years old, he always designated himself as 'of Amiens' (*Ambianus*). Becoming aware of an aptitude for, and love of, learning at the local grammar school, Fernel eventually persuaded his parents to allow him to enroll at the Collège de Ste Barbe, of the University of Paris, to study rhetoric and philosophy. After taking his master's degree in 1519, he turned down the immediate offer to teach dialectic there, and embarked instead on a rigorous course of autodidacticism. As Plancy said, 'He thought every hour lost which was not spent in reading and studying good authors.' Chief among those authors was Plato, recently made available in Latin by the translations of Marsilio Ficino (1433–99), and this led Fernel to a profound interest in mathematics.

When a long and severe illness, perhaps exacerbated by overwork, led Fernel to think about a future career, mathematics was considered as a possibility alongside divinity and jurisprudence. He decided upon a career in medicine, however, because his love of solitude made him unsuited to the public performance required in law and in the church. Fernel was now about twenty-nine years old and his father announced that he could no longer continue to support him. Accordingly, Fernel taught philosophy at the Collège de Ste Barbe while pursuing his MD. It was during this period, however, that Fernel also published his first works: three short mathematical treatises. *Monalosphaerium* (1527) was a description of a new mathematical instrument (based on the astrolabe) devised by Fernel, *Cosmotheoria* (1528) included Fernel's description of how he measured the distance on the ground of a degree of latitude (accurate to within 0.8 percent of today's value), and *De proportionibus libri duo* (1528) was a simple instructor on proportions.

Fernel achieved his doctorate in 1530, but he remained dissatisfied with institutionalized scholasticism and continued his autodidactic course, particularly in mathematics. Fernel's devotion to mathematics, especially geodesy and astronomy, absorbed much of his time and money, to the detriment not only of his medical studies, but also his recent marriage. Fernel not only spent much of his wife's dowry on mathematical instruments of his own design, but he even employed instrument makers and engravers who lived in the family home. Fernel's wife and his father-in-law, a senator of Paris, finally prevailed upon him to abandon these studies which, as they saw it, 'made no contribution to the public weal', and to devote himself to medicine, 'the worthiest of all the arts'.

It is clear that Fernel was very serious about mathematical studies, but it would be a mistake to suppose that in changing his focus to medicine Fernel would have had to exercise a great mental wrench. On the contrary, medicine and mathematics were closely affiliated, and much of the most advanced work in mathematics at this time was conducted in university medical faculties. An obvious association occurred through the juxtaposition of astronomy and astrology, which in Fernel's day were so intimately related that they were hardly distinguished from one another. It was a taken-for-granted assumption that astrology was useful in diagnosis and prognosis. The *Monalosphaerium* included material on 'critical days' in fevers, and the effect of the lunar cycle and the motions of the Zodiac on medical matters. It also gave instruction in casting horoscopes. In the *Cosmotheoria* Fernel suggested that even the sphere of the *primum mobile*, which he agreed was starless, exerted an occult influence on earth. Given these interests, it is hardly surprising that Fernel's first medical work should also have drawn heavily upon astrological theory. It was a major premise of the *De abditis rerum causis* (1548, but written over ten years earlier) that many of the phenomena of life derive from a nature in things that corresponds in some way to the nature of the stars, or the nature of heaven, and that there is a 'celebrated heavenly power, diffused into the whole universe, [which] makes its way right into the remotest recesses of the earth, penetrating the most close-knit and solid bodies' (Book I, Ch. 8).

Medical Career and a New Theory of Medicine

Fernel now embarked on his chosen career in earnest. In addition to developing his skills as a practitioner, he began to lecture on Hippocrates and Galen at the Collège de Cornouailles, and he soon acquired a formidable reputation well beyond those who heard him lecture.

After six years of teaching he was forced to concentrate on his burgeoning practice, but rather than abandon the theoretical part of medicine he decided to write a major study on the nature of contagious and pestilential (by which he meant other infectious) diseases that seemed anomalous according to ancient theory. Fernel's new theory moved closer to what historians of medicine, following Owsei Temkin (1977), call an *ontological*, rather than a *physiological*, concept of disease. Hippocratic and Galenic theory saw all disease in terms of a disturbance of the four humors such that the normal healthy temperament (the balance of the humors in the body) was disrupted. It follows from this that diseases do not have a separate existence in their own right. It was recognized, of course, that diseases can be characterized and can be seen to have their own specific natures: scabies is different from rabies. But for the Hippocratic or Galenic physician, the nature of disease is rooted in the general nature of mankind. In the end, all diseases are the result of a severe imbalance in the four humors. Such a physician, therefore, must always take into account 'the peculiar nature of each individual', effectively his or her unique physiology, when dealing with a patient. The difficulty with the individualistic physiological approach to sickness—seeing every illness as the special problem of one patient—is that it cannot easily explain apparently infectious conditions. Why should one patient's physiological disruption be capable in some cases of being passed on to others with different constitutions or temperaments? The difficulty is especially severe for Galenic theory in the case of epidemic diseases, such as plague. Infectious diseases, especially epidemic ones, seem to strongly suggest that diseases have a kind of life of their own; they are real, distinct entities, which can pass from one person to another—whence the ontological theory of disease.

Fernel did not reject humoral pathology but saw his own theory as an extension of ancient theory, specifically for dealing with infectious and pestilential conditions, as well as what he called 'poisonous diseases' (by which he meant those bodily disturbances brought about by poisons that evidently do not operate by upsetting the balance of the humors). This was written up in the form of a Ciceronian dialogue in *De abditis rerum causis* [On the Hidden Causes of Things], and was already finished by 1538, but withheld from the press.

Fernel decided that before publishing his refinement of, or addition to, the standard medical theory, he should clarify what he took to be the full extent of that theory. By 1538, therefore, he had already embarked upon what he called *De naturali parte medicina* [On the Natural Part of Medicine], which was published in 1542 and which Fernel said was concerned with 'the nature of the wholly healthy human being, all the powers and functions' (Preface to his *Medicina*, 1554). Fernel subsequently appropriated the term *physiologia* (which then signified the study of nature in general) as the title of this work, and so gave rise to the modern usage of physiology as the study of living systems.

The *Physiologia* was extremely useful and made Fernel one of the most renowned medical writers of the day. Its importance lay in the fact that it was the first serious attempt to present the prevailing assumptions about the nature of the human body, which underlay the Renaissance system of medical theory, in a comprehensively synoptic way. The medical theory of Fernel's day was based mostly on the eclectic system of medicine propounded by the Hellenistic physician and philosopher Galen of Pergamum (129–c. 210). Galen's own accounts of the normal function-

ing of the human body were to be found chiefly in his *De usu partium* (*On the Usefulness of the Parts of the Body*) and *De naturalibus facultatibus* (*On the Natural Faculties*). These ideas typically were taught to medical students, however, through the summary and commentary on Galen provided in the *Canon* of Avicenna (980–1037). There was no systematic treatment of physiology until Fernel's. Accordingly, the *Physiologia* is probably the fullest and most clearly organized exposition of Renaissance Galenism that was ever written. Since it would not be long before Galenic physiology was to be superseded by new systems of medicine, Fernel's *Physiologia* represents the high-water mark of European Galenism. Its appearance coincided with changes in demand for published works. During the Renaissance the systematic textbook came to be seen as a more useful commodity than the commentaries on ancient authorities and the compilations of *Quaestiones* that had been more typical in the medieval period. One way or another, the *Physiologia* was a book that made its author's reputation.

Fernel followed this up with would-be comprehensive surveys of pathology (*Pathologia*) and therapeutics (*Therapeutice*), and gathered all three together in the compendious *Medicina* (1554). It seems likely that Fernel intended to withhold the *De abditis rerum causis* until after the appearance of this full survey of ancient medicine, but in the event he published it after the *De naturali parte medicina*, in 1548. It is possible that he decided to publish at this time as a result of the publication of Girolamo Fracastoro's *De contagione* in 1546, which also offered a new theoretical understanding of contagious diseases. After Fernel's death, the three surveys of standard medicine were included together with his additional refinements on infectious and epidemic diseases, in *Universa medicina* (1567).

The appearance of the *De naturali parte medicina* caused such a stir among medical students that Fernel felt obliged, against the protests of his patients and his wife, to return to teaching. Plancy implied that Fernel undertook this teaching without fee and referred to it as Fernel's 'School', from which 'there went forth skilled physicians more numerous than soldiers from the Trojan horse, and spread over all regions and quarters of Europe.'

During this time he also wrote a treatise on bloodletting, *De vacuandi ratione* (1545), and began lecturing upon this important therapeutic method. It seems likely that this was the time, mentioned by Plancy, when Fernel was publicly attacked by a rival physician, known as Flexelle (or de Flesselles, d. 1562?). Fernel was opposed to the overuse of bloodletting, seeing it as a threat to the patient's strength, and used it only sparingly, even in cases judged to result from plethora. Flexelle, by contrast, recommended bloodletting copiously and frequently. Plancy used the controversy with Flexelle as an example of the opposition, even 'hatred', of other medical practitioners toward Fernel. We are also told that he often prepared his own medicaments, thereby raising the resentment of the apothecaries. Fernel's success in practice may well have attracted jealous enmity from other physicians. Plancy tells us that during the ten years in which he lived in Fernel's household, Fernel's annual income often exceeded twelve thousand French pounds, and rarely fell below ten.

On the Hidden Causes of Things (1548)

De abditis rerum causis is concerned with three sorts of 'hidden disease', which is to say, diseases with hidden causes: 'poisonous, contagious, and pestilent'. All three present the standard physiological concept of disease of the Galenic tradition with severe difficulties. The unvarying pattern of such diseases, so that all patients irrespective of type or temperament respond in essentially the same way, seemed to offer evidence that the physiological view of disease, based on an individual's humoral imbalance, was misconceived. Consequently, Fernel offered his own alternative account. Diseases of these types were held to act not on the humors but on the substantial form of the body, which Fernel called the 'total substance' of the body. Furthermore, they acted by means of some occult power. The model for all of them was essentially disease caused by poison. A substance entering the body from outside, either through a bite or a wound, or simply through contact with the skin (and the ability to soak through), or by ingestion or inhalation (sometimes in the *De abditis causis*, explicitly in the form of seeds), could wreak havoc in the healthy body and could work with such immediacy that it was impossible to believe that it acted through an accumulation of corrupt humor, which would have been required by the precepts of humoral pathology.

The problem with this theory, of course, was that its recourse to occult qualities and powers would have been dissatisfying to many of his readers—no better than a confession of ignorance (the position later satirized by Molière when he made a doctor in one of his plays pompously intone that opium puts patients to sleep because of its occult 'dormitive virtue'). Accordingly, Fernel devoted much of the *De abditis causis* to explaining as fully as he could what these particular occult qualities or powers were, where they come from, where they reside, and what they could do. It is evident, however, that Fernel did not believe that his arguments about these matters were sufficient to persuade all his contemporaries, and as a consequence another major effort of the book is directed at justifying in more general terms recourse to occult powers and trying to throw doubt on the validity of the distinction between so-called manifest qualities (hot, cold, dry, and wet) and occult qualities. In this regard he drew extensively upon two influential aspects of the occult tradition: astrology and alchemy. Interestingly, Fernel's use of alchemy to help make his case was taken up by contemporary alchemists who used his views to bolster alchemical theory. It is these nonmedical aspects of the book that made it a major con-

tribution not just to medical theory but also to current natural philosophy.

Fernel's theory of occult diseases has no easy association with modern ideas and for that reason, perhaps, it has failed to attract the kind of attention from historians of medicine accorded to Fracastoro's seeds of disease (which can easily be likened to 'germs'). On the contrary, because Fernel's ideas were bound up with Renaissance theories of the occult they have been treated by his modern commentators, until very recently, with some embarrassment. It is important, however, to judge Fernel's theories according to the standards of his own time. Fernel's explanations, drawing heavily upon supposed occult properties, were controversial, but they were not regarded as in any way absurd or ridiculous. Indeed, the Renaissance was a time of reassessment of the validity of the notion of occult qualities, and Fernel's claims about occult diseases, and occult qualities more generally, undoubtedly fed into that wider debate, helping many to accept them as essential for a proper understanding of the natural world, by enabling the natural philosopher to go beyond what was allowable in scholastic Aristotelianism, or traditional Galenic medicine.

Fernel should be acknowledged as one of the prime movers in the development of theories suggesting an ontological, as opposed to a physiological view of disease. It seems likely, therefore, that his works would have encouraged others to take a more critical view of traditional Galenic medicine. History does not allow counterfactual speculations, and it is impossible to know precisely what difference Fernel's work made in the decline and fall of Galenism. It seems hard to deny, however, that his influence upon his contemporaries was at least as great as Fracastoro's, and may even have rivaled that of Paracelsus, particularly among more conservative thinkers.

Fernal and the Royal House of Angoulême

Fernel's reputation was so great after 1542 that he was summoned by Prince Henri (1519–99) to treat the serious illness of his mistress, Diane de Poitiers (1499–1566). Believing that Fernel saved his beloved mistress's life, Henri wanted to appoint Fernel his physician-in-chief. Fernel evidently saw this as a threat to his studies—including the empirical studies that he derived from his widespread medical practice—and pleaded to be allowed to return to Paris to continue his research. When these pleas failed to sway Henri, Fernel feigned pleurisy and persuaded one of the dauphin's surgeons to suggest to him that Fernel might succumb if he was not allowed to return home. Henri relented and excused Fernel from residing at court, and from all irksome duties, but magnanimously insisted on paying him the annual stipend as chief physician.

Whether Fernel really did save Diane's life remains unproven, since we do not know what ailed her. We do know, however, that Fernel failed to save the life of Henri's father, Francis I (1494–1547), when he was called upon to treat the king's venereal disease. Fernel disapproved of the standard use of mercury inunctions for what later became known as syphilis, but which he always called *lues venerea*. Mercury ointments had been used in the treatment of skin disease for a long time, and since lesions of the skin were a prominent symptom of this new disease, mercury became the standard treatment. Fernel knew of the destructiveness of mercury, however, and believed that, even when seemingly effective, it merely assuaged the symptoms but did not attack the cause. Fernel regarded *lues venerea* as an occult disease, that is to say, a disease that did not result from an imbalance of the humors. Like rabies, which was caused by a poison in the saliva of a mad dog, venereal disease resulted from a poison, which entered the body through broken skin (even a tiny scratch, abrasion, or the like), and could then spread itself through the whole body. The only way to cure it, accordingly, was to develop an antidote or antagonist to the poison. Fernel developed his own herbal concoction as an antidote, which not only included the famous antidotes theriac and mithridatium, but also guaiac bark from the recently discovered New World tree. It is not known when Fernel confidently wrote his short treatise *De luis venereae curatione perfectissima liber* [On the best cure of lues venereal], but it may well have been the death of Francis I that dented his confidence and caused him to withhold it from the press, to await a posthumous publication (1579). It was while Fernel was urging the use of his antidote to treat the king that another royal physician, Antonio Gallus, famously declared, 'He got it the same way as his subjects, and, as with them, mercury will take it away.'

After the death of Francis I in 1547, Henri's faith in Fernel's prowess as a doctor remained undimmed and he wanted Fernel to be his royal physician. Again Fernel managed to escape this obligation; this time by suggesting it was the hereditary right of Louis De Bourges, royal physician to his father, to continue in the post. By the time Louis died in 1556, Fernel had evidently run out of excuses and he became royal physician for the last years of his life. At first, Fernel believed this post would allow him more time to pursue his studies, away from his crowding patients, but war with Spain and England rudely intervened, and Fernel in his sixties had to march with the army. Fernel was with his king in January 1557, for example, when he took Calais, which had been occupied by the English for over two centuries. Even so, Fernel managed to compose a short treatise on the treatment of fevers during these times (*Febrium curandarum methodus generalis*, published posthumously, 1577).

When he returned to court at Fontainebleau, Fernel fetched his wife from Paris but after a few days there she developed a fatal illness. Plancy said that Fernel was overwhelmed by the death of his wife and was himself taken ill with a severe continued fever. Although Fernel at first con-

tributed to his own diagnosis and treatment, he could not heal himself, and he soon followed his wife to the grave. On his deathbed he regretted only that he had not lived long enough 'for the sake of learning and medicine', and in particular that he had never finished the therapeutic part of his *Universa medicina*. Plancy's judgment that Fernel overworked himself seems hard to deny. His daily regime, for over thirty years, was to rise at 4:00 AM and study until daybreak. He would then either give lectures or visit patients, or both, until it was time for his midday meal. He had so many patients, according to Plancy, that throughout the summers he often had to take his meal without sitting down. If he could, he would retire to the library while the meal was being prepared, and return to it after eating, until it was time to make more visits to patients. He resumed his studies again while his supper was being prepared and then continued to work until bedtime at 11:00 PM. Allowing himself only the bare minimum of sleep, whenever he was advised to take more rest he used to reply, 'Fate will grant us a long time to repose' (*Longa quiescendi tempora fata dabunt*).

Bibliography

Primary: 1567. *Universa medicina, tribus et viginti libris absoluta* (Paris); 1579. *De luis venereae curatione perfectissima liber* (Antwerp); 2003. (translated and annotated by Forrester, J. M.) *Physiologia (1567)*. Transactions of the American Philosophical Society 93 (Philadelphia); 2005. (Forrester, John, and John Henry, eds.) *Jean Fernel's On the Hidden Causes of Things: Forms, Souls and Occult Diseases in Renaissance Medicine* (Leiden); 1598. Riolan, Jean [the elder]. *Ad Libros Fernelii de Abditis Rerum Causis Commentarius* (Paris).

Secondary: Matton, Sylvain, 2002. 'Fernel et les alchimistes.' *Corpus* 41: 135–97; Brockliss, Laurence, 1993. 'Seeing and Believing: Contrasting Attitudes towards Observational Autonomy among French Galenists in the First Half of the Seventeenth Century' in Bynum, W. F., and Roy Porter, eds., *Medicine and the Five Senses* (Cambridge) pp. 69–84; Temkin, Owsei, 1977. 'The Scientific Approach to Disease: Specific Entity and Individual Sickness' in Temkin, Owsei, *The Double Face of Janus and Other Essays in the History of Medicine* (Baltimore and London) pp. 441–455; Plancy, Guillaume, 1946. 'Life' of Fernel (first printed in 1607)' in Sherrington, Sir Charles, *The Endeavour of Jean Fernel, with a List of the Editions of His Writings* (Cambridge) [reprinted Folkestone, 1974] pp. 150–70; Sherrington, Sir Charles, 1946. *The Endeavour of Jean Fernel, with a List of the Editions of His Writings* (Cambridge) [reprinted Folkestone, 1974]; Figard, Leon, 1903. *Un médecin philosophe au XVIe siècle: étude sur la psychologie de Jean Fernel* (Geneva) [reprinted, 1970]; *DSB*.

John Henry

FERRÁN Y CLÚA, JAIME   (b. Corbera d'Ebre, Tarragona, Spain, 2 February 1851; d. Barcelona, Spain, 22 November 1929), *medicine, bacteriology, immunology.*

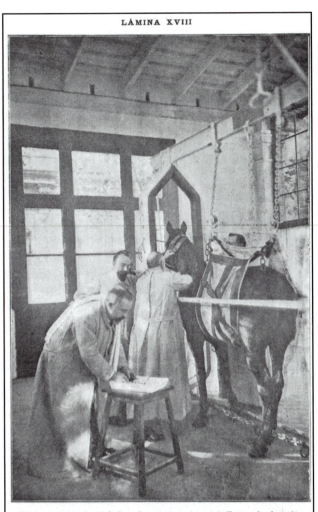

LÁMINA XVIII

Laboratorio Municipal de Barcelona: sangría de un caballo para la obtención de suero antiloímico.

Bleeding a horse to obtain antiplague serum, Municipal Laboratory, Barcelona. Half-tone reproduction from *La peste bubónica*... Barcelona, 1907. Wellcome Library, London.

Ferrán belongs to the pioneer generation of medical bacteriology and immunology. Following Louis Pasteur's trail, he realized the vast therapeutic and prophylactic implications of the germ theory. Consequently, he devoted his life to the production and marketing of sera and vaccines, boldly mixing his research and entrepreneurial activities. He is best remembered for the first use of a human vaccine against Asiatic cholera (1885), the modification of the Pasteurian antirabies vaccine (1887), and the preparation of a tuberculosis vaccine that rivaled BCG, particularly in Spain and some Latin American countries, such as Argentina in the early 1920s.

Ferrán was the son of a rural physician from the southeast region of Catalonia. At school he showed skill in drawing. He studied medicine at the University of Barcelona (1868–73) and was among the first students to be introduced to the microscope as a diagnostic tool. He established friendly relations with

José de Letamendi, a theoretically minded professor who was extraordinarily popular at the time. In 1874 Ferrán began a short and successful career as medical practitioner in his native county until his arrival in Tortosa, the county capital, in 1875, where he became director of the municipal hospital, among other official commitments. He enriched his private practice by offering the most updated facilities, including electrotherapy, hydrotherapy, and ophthalmology. During the decade of his residence in Tortosa, he and his chemist friend Inocente Paulí revealed notable inventive capacities in a wide range of domains, including telephony and photography. The two friends closely studied the experiments of Pasteur by reading the *Comptes Rendus* of the French Academy of Sciences. After the purchase of a microscope, they became highly familiar with the new techniques, which they reproduced and tested in Ferrán's home laboratory, equipped since 1880 with original devices of their own design. They were the first in Spain to produce vaccines against cattle anthrax and swine erysipelas, and in 1884 Ferrán was awarded a prize by the Academy of Medicine of Madrid for a paper on the new etiological hypothesis. Interestingly, he understood bacteria to be a vegetal species.

Experiments with Cholera

In 1885 Ferrán's career underwent an abrupt change after the outbreak of a cholera epidemic. Using guinea pigs, Ferrán and Paulí were the first to determine that the subcutaneous injection of a limited quantity of a pure culture of cholera bacilli defended the animals against death from further intraperitoneal injections of larger amounts of the same. Working with material taken from Marseille's cholera hospital after a stay in September 1884, during which they learned from Koch, Rietsch, and Nicatti how to deal with the comma bacillus, Ferrán made a public announcement of their achievement in December 1884. He then tested the same injection in human beings—starting with himself—demonstrating that human cholera would not develop as a result and that the transient pathological effects were negligible. At this time, he became acquainted with Amalio Gimeno, professor of therapeutics at the University of Valencia, who would become a key character in subsequent events. In support of those who believed that pathological bacteria were plants and especially in opposition to Robert Koch, he defended an evolutionary morphology for the cholera bacillus whereby the comma form was one stage of a complex life cycle that included sporification of what he designated *Peronospora barcinonis*. In March 1885, backed by the official approval of the Academy of Medicine of Barcelona, Ferrán presented his findings to the Paris Academy of Sciences.

A few days later, cholera again broke out in some villages in the province of Valencia, and Ferrán was officially summoned after the active intermediation of Gimeno. Starting in the provincial capital, Ferrán made massive use of his immunization cultures—at times praised and at times derided or opposed by local authorities. By early August 1885, about 30,000 people had been inoculated with the vaccine. Recent calculations (Bornside, 1981) show that it was effective in protecting from death on a population scale, even though only the first dose was applied in most cases, despite Ferrán's claim (following limited experiments on his family and friends) that only a second injection given five days after the first would confer full immunity against cholera.

A combination of concerns fueled the major scandal generated by these practices. Some opposed the speed of implementation in humans after only limited trials in animals. Others criticized the lack of appropriate means to evaluate the effects of the inoculations and stressed the unsafe nature of the materials employed. Finally, a large number of physicians and educated people considered that the bacterial etiology was not the full-fledged science asserted by the microbiologists, and they feared that acceptance of vaccination could undermine the defense against cholera by quarantines and disinfection (called 'little hygiene' by Ferrán). No definitive conclusion, either for or against the vaccination program, was produced by the more than twenty scientific commissions received during the summer of that year. However, the influential French Commission led by Brouardel and the negative official report of the Spanish government combined to create a somber image of the undertaking. Amid a controversy that was heavily tainted by politics (conservatives against, liberals in favor), Ferrán was finally ordered on 24 July to restrict the use of the vaccine to his own patients, and he abandoned any further efforts to improve it. He acknowledged technical shortcomings, such as the lack of a standardized procedure, and presented proposals to the French Academy of Sciences that were only definitively accepted by the scientific community many years later, such as the use of an oral vaccine and the power of a dead culture to generate immunity.

Subsequent international events led Ferrán to return to the defense of the vaccine policy. By 1903, as shown by private correspondence in the archives of the Catalonian Museum of History of Medicine, he had the support of several international leaders of the field, such as Roux and Ehrlich. In 1907 he was jointly awarded the Bréant Prize for his experiments with the cholera vaccine, and he won further support at the first meeting of the *Bureau International d'Hygiène Publique* in 1919. The awards he received during his trips to Germany in 1925 and Argentina in 1926 may have compensated for the hardships caused by the controversy that surrounded his scientific work.

A Microbiological Institute

Ferrán was also the leading figure in establishing this new field's first Spanish public institution, the Microbiological Institute of the city of Barcelona, created in 1886 and inaugurated under his direction in 1887. It was a similar initiative to many others in different parts of the world, based on produc-

tion of the antirabies vaccine developed by Pasteur. From the outset, however, its plans included the full range of activities linked to the emerging science of immunology: the production and selling of biological products, laboratory analysis, research, and even training (although there is no proof that this last activity was ever carried out in Ferrán's times). The antirabies vaccine did not escape the ingenuity of Ferrán, who changed the Pasteurian production and administration method, transforming it into a 'supraintensive method' (1887, with further safety improvements in 1890) that was applied throughout Spain and, according to some witnesses, used in 1925 at the Koch Institute in Berlin. Between 1887 and 1900, he also produced a series of ill-fated vaccines against yellow fever, diphtheria, typhoid fever, and plague (the antiplague vaccine was favorably tested at the Porto outbreak of 1899), as well as antitetanic and antidiphtheric sera.

By the end of the century, criticism of Ferrán's eagerness for human experimentation culminated in the overt questioning of his expertise and methods by such influential figures as Santiago Ramón y Cajal. Indeed, when the majority on Barcelona's council passed into nationalistic and republican hands, Ferrán was prosecuted for maladministration and finally driven out of the municipal institute in 1905.

From that time on, he devoted himself exclusively to his private 'Ferrán Institute', which moved from the city center to a luxurious garden house in the Barcelona suburbs in 1900. He continued to produce the same types of product and deliver exactly the same services as the public institution—a point that was used against him, with the charge that he could benefit from unclear accounting practices and the confusion of private and public costs. Because Ferrán sold vaccines and sera to the rest of Spain and to foreign countries, however, the range and volume of production was much larger than at the municipal institute, which basically served the public charities of the city and the Catalonian region.

A Last Challenge: To Defeat Tuberculosis

In 1897 Ferrán started working on tuberculosis. As usual, he began by developing a completely new morphology of the bacillus, which was completed by 1905. According to his proposal, the evolutionary cycle consisted of five different steps undergone by germs, with different pathological or immunological effects on the human body. These bacilli, which he named after the first five letters of the Greek alphabet, appeared as adaptations to changing environmental conditions and were designated 'mutations' in 1910, introducing a novel concept contrary to traditional Darwinian biology. Ferrán considered the first form, the Alpha bacillus, to be a universal saprophyte of the human species that could trigger an inflammatory response from the body. This substantial environmental change would lead to its metamorphosis into a Beta form, already endowed with the power to elicit an immunological response, which in turn would lead to the Koch bacillus form and to further degenerative forms. Therefore, he claimed that a vaccine made of Alpha bacilli would prevent tuberculosis in children, and he campaigned for the implementation of a broad program with this aim. With the agreement of the national authorities, he carried out massive tests of his vaccine in three Spanish towns (Alcira, Alberique, and Palma de Majorca), inoculating more than 19,000 people. In the 1920s, the vaccine was widely employed in Uruguay, Argentina, and Spain (with more than one million vaccines administered by 1927), while Ferrán claimed that its use in orphan homes had eradicated tuberculosis mortality. Opponents of the BCG vaccine were able to propose the antialpha vaccine as a practical alternative.

Bibliography

Primary: 1886. (with Gimeno, A., and I. Paulí) *La inoculación preventiva contra el cólera morbo asiático* (Valencia) [facs. edn. Valencia, 1985; edited by J. M. López Piñero et al.]; 1889. *Estudios acerca de la rabia y su profilaxis, 1887 a 1889* (Barcelona); 1910. *Errores doctrinales concernientes a la tuberculosis y a su bacilo . . . Nuevas orientaciones conducentes a la solución del problema de la profilaxis y de la terapéutica específicas de esta enfermedad* (Barcelona).

Secondary: Pinar, Susana, 2002. 'El bacteriólogo Jaume Ferrán y las mutaciones de Hugo de Vries' in Puig-Samper, Miguel A., Rosaura Ruiz, and Andrés Galera, eds., *Evolucionismo y cultura. Darwinismo en Europa e Iberoamérica* (Madrid) pp. 319–332; Báguena, María José, 1995. 'Jaume Ferran i Clua (Corbera d'Ebre, Terra Alta, 1852-Barcelona 1929). La primera vacuna bacteriana' in Camarasa, Josep M., and Antoni Roca, eds., *Ciència i tècnica als Països Catalans: una aproximació biogràfica als darrers 150 anys* (Barcelona) pp. 651–679; Fernández Sanz, Juan José, 1990. *1885: El año de la vacunación Ferrán. Transfondo político, médico, sociodemográfico y económico de una epidemia* (Madrid); Roca Rosell, Antoni, 1988. *Història del Laboratori Municipal de Barcelona de Ferran a Turró* (Barcelona); Bornside, George H., 1982. 'Waldemar Haffkine's Cholera Vaccines and the Ferran-Haffkine Priority Dispute.' *Journal of the History of Medicine and Allied Sciences* 37: 399–422; Bornside, George H., 1981. 'Jaime Ferrán and Preventive Inoculation against Cholera.' *Bulletin of the History of Medicine* 55: 516–532.

Esteban Rodríguez-Ocaña

FERRIAR, JOHN (b. near Jedburgh, Roxburghshire, Scotland, 21 November 1761; d. Manchester, England, 4 February 1815), *medicine, public health, literature.*

Ferriar was the son of Alexander Ferriar, a Presbyterian minister, and his wife Mary Burn. Nothing is known of his early schooling, but he attended Edinburgh University from 1776 to 1781, studying with Alexander Monro *secundus* (1733–1817), William Cullen (1710–90), Joseph Black (1728–99), and James Gregory (1729–73). He graduated MD (1781), and married Barbara Gair (1782). The couple had five children.

After graduation, Ferriar first practiced medicine at Stockton-on-Tees. In 1785 he moved to Manchester, and he became physician to the Manchester Infirmary in 1789. The Industrial Revolution was well underway, and Manchester had grown from a village to a city of 50,000 inhabitants by 1786, dominated by factories and suffering from environmental degradation and serious public health problems. In the eighteenth century, pollution, overcrowding, and poor sanitation were just beginning to be recognized as health hazards, and Ferriar's experience with his infirmary patients convinced him that public action was necessary to improve the health of the factory workers and to preserve that of the owners. He began a campaign to educate the public in his paper, 'Epidemic Fever of 1789, and 1790', describing the outbreak in Manchester and nearby Salford. He pointed to the dangers of many unsanitary practices, including filth and overcrowding, and called on the police to impose sanitary regulations on lodging houses and streets to ensure that they were kept clean and well-ventilated. He paid particular attention to the practices that spread infection, noting that even a few sick workers in a cotton mill could spread disease throughout the mill. In 1796 his efforts bore fruit when Manchester set up a Board of Health, one of the first in Great Britain.

Ferriar believed that fever, once it arose under dirty and unsanitary conditions, acted as a kind of tangible contagion, which could spread to the rich as well as to the poor. 'A minute and constant attention' to the wants of the poor, he noted, 'is not less an act of self-preservation' on the part of the rich, 'than of virtue' (Ferriar, *Medical Histories* vol. 1, p. 246). The remedy, Ferriar believed, was cleanliness, light, and fresh air. For this reason he believed that the sick poor should be removed from their own environment and sent to fever hospitals, such as the House of Recovery established through Ferriar's efforts in Manchester in 1796. He was instrumental in the founding of fever wards at Stockport as well. His ideas on fever, published in the 1790s in his *Medical Histories and Reflections*, influenced the next generation of sanitary reformers, including William Pulteney Alison (1790–1859). The cholera epidemics of 1832 and beyond made his warnings on the importance of public health for rich and poor alike appear prophetic.

Ferriar's other medical advocacy was for humane, though strict, treatment of the insane. Influenced by contemporary ideas of moral management, he believed that a system of rewards and punishments would allow insane patients to develop self-restraint and thus the ability to manage their disorder, if it could not be completely cured. He felt that, like fever patients, the insane were best treated in special hospitals, away from their families, who would be inclined to indulge them too much. 'Among strangers', Ferriar noted, 'they find it necessary to exert their faculties, and the first tendency to regular thinking becomes the beginning of recovery' (Ferriar, *Medical Histories* vol. 2, p. 110).

Ferriar was one of the leading physicians in Manchester, and his friends included Thomas Percival (1740–1804), with whom he shared an interest in hospital reform and public health. He was a member of the Manchester Literary and Philosophical Society, and wrote essays on Laurence Sterne's (1712–68) works, as well as others in the eighteenth-century literary canon.

Bibliography

Primary: 1792–98. *Medical Histories and Reflections* 3 vols. (Manchester); 1798. *Illustrations of Sterne; with other essays and verses* (London) [reprinted 1971, New York].

Secondary: Pickstone, John V., 1985. *Medicine and Industrial Society: A History of Hospital Development in Manchester and its Region, 1752–1946* (Manchester); *Oxford DNB.*

Lisa Rosner

FERRIER, DAVID

FERRIER, DAVID   (b. Woodside, Aberdeenshire, Scotland, 18 January 1843; d. London, England, 19 March 1928), *physiology, neurology.*

The sixth child and second son of a businessman, Ferrier initially studied classics and philosophy at Aberdeen University. He switched to medicine at the University of Edinburgh in 1865, graduating three years later and becoming briefly an assistant in general practice at Bury St Edmunds, Suffolk. At Edinburgh he had met the neurologist John Hughlings Jackson (1835–1911), and in 1870 he moved to the Middlesex Hospital Medical School, London for a year as a lecturer in physiology. In 1871 he moved again to King's College London, beginning his long career there as demonstrator in physiology. In 1872 he replaced William Guy as professor of forensic medicine (they coauthored the fourth edition of Guy's *Principles of Forensic Medicine*). He served as assistant physician (1874) and then full physician (1890) to King's College Hospital. In 1889 the post of professor of neuropathology was specially created for him, a position he held until retirement in 1908, while he was a cofounder of the influential journal *Brain* (1881) with James Crichton-Browne (1840–1938), Jackson, and J. C. Bucknill (1817–97). Nevertheless, he believed it important to maintain a general interest in medicine, and in routine clinical teaching would choose a topic outside his own specialty, such as discussing a patient with myxedema.

Ferrier spent three years studying the physiology of the nervous system in a variety of animals, from guinea pigs to monkeys, and was bitterly attacked by the antivivisectionists. Nevertheless, in 1876 he published *The Functions of the Brain*, which was an immediate success all over Europe and translated into several major languages and went into an enlarged second edition within a few years. Centering on the electrical stimulation of the brain in animals, or the destruction of various parts of the brain, his studies established the localization of sensory and motor functions to different but precise areas of the cortex. Furthermore, Ferrier argued that

there were association areas, which integrated the functions of these specialized centers. At the International Medical Congress in London in 1881 he gave a brilliant demonstration of cerebral function and localization. His localization of the visual area to the angular gyrus, however, proved to be wrong, given that the suggestion was based on short-term survival studies in monkeys, but even after the correct site had been demonstrated Ferrier was reluctant to correct his error, because the hypothesis fitted into a coherent pattern with his other, correct, findings.

Drawing on the results of these extensive researches, Ferrier came to the important conclusion that conditions affecting the brain could be treated surgically. His suggestion was triumphantly vindicated in 1883 by two neurosurgical pioneers—Sir William McEwen (1848–1924) in Glasgow and Rickman Godlee (1849–1925) in London—when they successfully removed brain tumors, and hence Ferrier could be described as one of the originators of modern neurosurgery. He was elected FRS (1876) and knighted (1911).

Bibliography

Primary: 1875. (with Guy, William) *Principles of Forensic Medicine* (London) (4th edn.); 1876. *Functions of the Brain* (London) (2nd edn., 1886); 1890. *The Croonian Lectures on Cerebral Localisation* (London).

Secondary: Young, R. M., 1990. *Mind, Brain and Adaptation in the Nineteenth Century* (New York); Balance, C., 1928. 'The late Sir David Ferrier.' *British Medical Journal* i: 525–526, 574–575; *DSB; Oxford DNB.*

Stephen Lock

FIASCHI, THOMAS HENRY [TOMMASO ENRICO]

FIASCHI, THOMAS HENRY [TOMMASO ENRICO] (b. Florence, Italy, 31 May 1853; d. 17 April 1927, Darling Point, Australia), *surgery, viniculture.*

The son of University of Florence mathematics professor Lodovico Fiaschi and his English-born wife, Clarissa Fisher, Thomas Fiaschi studied medicine in Florence before moving to Australia. There he spent a brief period practicing medicine in the Queensland goldfields before becoming a house surgeon at St. Vincent's Hospital, Sydney. There he married an Irish nun from the hospital and the couple returned to northern Italy, where he graduated MD and ChD (Pisa and Florence) in 1877.

Fiaschi returned to Australia with his family in February 1879, setting up practice in Windsor, a small town on the outskirts of Sydney, where he joined the honorary medical staff at the local hospital. He was one of the pioneers of Listerian antiseptic surgery in Australia, employing liberal use of carbolic acid in treating septic wounds. His reputation quickly spread due to the unusually low mortality rates. Four years later he moved to Sydney, where he became president of the local branch of the British Medical Association (1889–90). Following another visit to Italy, Fiaschi went to the United States to study advances in aseptic and abdominal surgery, adding these skills to his repertoire.

He became honorary surgeon to Sydney Hospital in 1894, chairman of the board of medical studies in 1909, and consulting surgeon in 1911. A sound rather than brilliant operator, Fiaschi was noted for his orthopedic surgery, as well as his treatment of goiter and hydatid disease. Keenly interested in the progress of medical students at the hospital, he is said to have been the first person in Australia to deliver systematic lectures on the history of medicine.

His cultural versatility became manifest in his distinguished military career, during which he served with both the Italian and Australian forces. He joined the Italian army in Abyssinia in 1896, was decorated for bravery, and afterwards wrote about the mistreatment of Italian prisoners of war. During the South African War (1899–1902) he commanded the 1st Field Hospital of the New South Wales Lancers. While searching for wounded troops, he accepted the surrender of some Boer forces, a feat for which he was again decorated. In World War I, Fiaschi commanded the 3rd Australian General Hospital on Lemnos, supporting the Gallipoli campaign. After being sent back to England because of illness, he temporarily resigned from the Australian army to work as a surgeon in an Italian military hospital. When he retired from the Australian Army Medical Corps Reserve in 1921, Fiaschi held the rank of brigadier-general. Doubtless his battlefield experience enhanced his surgical skills, particularly in orthopedics, where he excelled.

Fiaschi was prominent among the Italian community in Australia, being a founder and president of the Dante Alighieri Literary Society. Widely read, he was equally adept at writing or translating articles for Italian, French, or British journals. Like many Italians he was convinced of the value of wine as a medicament. Fiaschi introduced the chardonnay grape variety to Australia, first grown on his Tizzana vineyard near Windsor. He acquired another winery at Mudgee and had cellars in the city where his wines were sold. He found a new outlet for his surgical knowledge by introducing aseptic conditions to winemaking. Tizzana wines won many prizes, with Fiaschi acting as president of the Australian Wine Producers' Association for twenty-five years (1902–27).

Fiaschi's son Piero (1879–1948) was a genito-urinary specialist who, like his father, practiced at Sydney Hospital. A bronze replica of the Florentine *Il Porcellino* monument in front of the hospital commemorates both father and son. The day surgery unit at Hawkesbury Hospital in modern Windsor is named after Thomas Fiaschi.

Bibliography

Primary: 1896. *Da Cheren a Cassala. Note di viaggio* (Florence).

Secondary: 1927. 'Obituary.' *Medical Journal of Australia* i: 732–735; *DAuB.*

Peter J. Tyler

FIBIGER, JOHANNES ANDREAS GRIB   (b. Silkeborg, Denmark, 23 April 1867; d. Copenhagen, Denmark, 30 January 1928), *bacteriology, pathology, clinical trials.*

Fibiger was born in the provincial town of Silkeborg. He lost his father, district physician Christian Emanuel August Fibiger, as a young boy and grew up in Copenhagen with his older sister and his mother, Elfride (née Müller). He studied medicine at the University of Copenhagen, graduating in 1890. He worked as an assistant to Carl Julius Salomonsen at the bacteriological laboratory of the university (1891–94), as a resident at Blegdamshospitalet (1894–97), and as prosector at the Institute of Pathology at the university (1897–1900). During the 1890s, Fibiger was primarily concerned with diphtheria, perhaps inspired by his visit in 1891 to Emil von Behring in Berlin. In 1895 he defended his thesis on the bacteriology of diphtheria. He then went on to perform a study, with Thorvald Madsen, on the therapeutic effects of diphtheria serum on patients at Blegdamshospitalet (1896–97). Fibiger allocated the patients to a treatment group or a control group according to day of admission, a very early example of a randomized clinical trial. In the published paper, he also discussed the principles of controlled, therapeutic research.

In 1900 Fibiger assumed the professorship of pathological anatomy at the University of Copenhagen, a position he held for the rest of his life. He prepared for the job by visiting important pathological anatomists in Europe, and upon his return he began work on tuberculosis with the veterinarian Carl Oluf Jensen. In 1902 they were able to show that bovine tuberculosis could be transmitted to humans through unheated milk, thus rejecting the claim made by Robert Koch the previous year that the bovine bacteria posed no threat to humans.

In 1907 Fibiger joined the Cancer Committee set up by the Danish Medical Association and increasingly turned his research interest to this field. That same year, when examining rats as part of his research on tuberculosis, he observed what appeared to be cancerous growths in the mucous membranes of the animals' stomachs. Fibiger also found that the animals were infected by a roundworm, which he named *Spiroptera neoplastica*. He embarked on a lengthy research project to establish the connection between the worms and the cancer in rats. In 1913 Fibiger published his results, arguing that a toxin produced by the worms caused the cancer, and claiming that he had discovered a way to experimentally induce malignant tumors in rats. These findings brought him international fame, and he was immediately recognized as having performed a breakthrough in the field of cancer research, which had come to a standstill mainly as a result of a lack of experimental models. Fibiger was awarded the 1926 Nobel Prize in Physiology or Medicine in October 1927. He died of stomach cancer three months later.

Fibiger was acknowledged as a meticulous and persistent researcher, but his reputation was blemished when the theory that brought him the Nobel Prize was disproved.

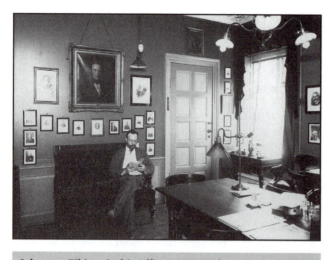

Johannes Fibiger in his office, *c.* 1910. Photograph, Medical Museion, University of Copenhagen.

During the 1930s, it was agreed that the tumors in the rats were not cancer, but benign growths caused by vitamin A deficiency. This has overshadowed his achievements as a source of inspiration to the cancer research field. Also, his pioneering contributions to the development of clinical trials have only recently been recognized.

Bibliography

Primary: 1898. 'Om Serumbehandling af Difteri.' *Hospitalstidende* 6: 309–325, 337–350; 1913. 'Über eine durch Nematode (Spiroptera sp. n.) hervorgerufene papillomatöse und carcinomatöse Geschwultzbildung im Magen der Ratte.' *Berliner klinische Wochenschrift* 50: 289–298.

Secondary: Nielsen, Anita Kildebæk, and Eivind B. Thorling, 2001. 'Backing the Wrong Horse?' in Nielsen, Henry, and Keld Nielsen, eds., *Neighbouring Nobel: The History of Thirteen Danish Nobel Prizes* (Århus) pp. 461–493; Hróbjartsson, Asbjørn, Peter C. Gøtzsche, and Christian Gluud, 1998. 'The Controlled Clinical Trial Turns 100 Years: Fibiger's Trial of Serum Treatment of Diphtheria.' *British Medical Journal* 317: 1243–1245; Secher, Knud, 1947. *The Danish Cancer Researcher Johannes Fibiger* (Copenhagen); Jensen, Carl Oluf, 1928. 'Johannes Fibiger.' *Oversigt over det kongelige danske Videnskabernes Selskabs Forhandlinger* pp. 101–117.

Søren Bak-Jensen

FICINO, MARSILIO   (b. Figline, Italy, 19 October 1433; d. Careggi, Italy, 1 October 1499), *philosophy, medicine.*

Ficino, son of the physician Dietifeci and Alessandra da Montevarchi, studied philosophy in Florence with Niccolò Tignosi. In the 1450s, after reading Platonic and Hermetic works, Ficino started to associate Hermes Trismegistus with Plato. Cosimo the Elder and Cristoforo Landino encouraged Ficino to study Greek texts and discover the sources of Platonism. It is believed that Ficino then attended the University of Bologna, studying philosophy and medicine. (Although scholars disagree on the exact nature of this training, a medical education is undeniable.) In the 1450s and 1460s Ficino worked on many treatises and in 1457 read and commented on Lucretius' *De rerum natura*, but he then burned his Lucretian works, fruit of 'levitas iuvenilis' [youthful vanity] (Vasoli, 1997, p. 381b).

The study of Platonic sources led Ficino to translate such texts as *Oracula Chaldaica*, Orphic hymns, and pseudo-pythagorean works. In the 1460s Ficino obtained the *Academia* of Careggi from Cosimo and started to work on a translation of the Platonic dialogues, thus becoming the restorer of Platonic philosophy. In 1463 he finished the Latin translation of the first fourteen treatises of the *Corpus Hermeticum*, first published in 1471. By 1464 Ficino had also translated ten Platonic dialogues, in addition to other Platonic works.

During the *signoria* of Cosimo's son, Piero (1464–69), Ficino lectured on Plato's *Philebus*, probably after having commented on Plato's *Symposium*, the most famous of Ficino's commentaries. Ficino then started to work on Christianizing Platonism with his *Theologia Platonica* and *De christiana religione*; he later became a deacon and priest. His *Disputatio contra iudicium astrologorum*, never published, was written against judiciary astrology, to defend providence and freewill.

After the difficult period of the *congiura de' Pazzi* (1478) and the plague (1478–80), Ficino wrote the *Consilio contro la pestilenzia* (1481). Ficino described plague as a poisonous steam, enemy of the heart spirit, and originating in the conjunction of Mars with Saturn. After a short section on symptoms, the majority of the treatise was dedicated to preservation from plague, giving suggestions on diet and on improving and disinfecting the environment. There follows a section on therapeutics, with description of drugs, such as *tiriaca*, *mitridato*, and *bezoar*, phlebotomy, and many recipes. Final chapters were devoted to the protection of doctors and those caring for the sick. According to Ficino, contagion functioned between individuals who were similar in complexion, qualities, and horoscope (Katinis, 2003).

In the 1480s Ficino strengthened his friendship with Lorenzo (d. 1492) and continued to work on the translation and commentary of Plato's dialogues. He dedicated the *Theologia Platonica* (1482) to Lorenzo and published Plato's dialogues in 1484. In the same period he started work on the translation and commentary of Plotinus's *Enneads*, first published in 1492. To grasp Plotinus's philosophy, Ficino needed to translate many other neoplatonic and neopythagorean works. He also continued to work on medicine, but refused to translate Hippocrates' works into Latin, arguing it was better to practice medicine than to write on medical theory.

In 1489 Ficino published *De vita triplici*, a series of three books. The first, *De vita sana*, dealt with the preservation of health, especially that of geniuses and literary men, who were often troubled by melancholy. The book ends with a series of recipes. The second book, *De vita longa*, was about the rules for lengthening life, with a series of suggestions on complexion and diet, especially relevant for old men. The third book, *De vita coelitus comparanda*, which began as a commentary on Plotinus's *Ennead* IV 3, 11, is the most famous and complex of the three books. Starting with a theory of the sympathy between astral and sublunar bodies, by the mediation of the *mundi spiritus*, the book deals with the means of grasping celestial gifts by knowledge of the cosmos. Ficino followed the neoplatonic theory of chains of being, developing the doctrine of a complex series of manifest and occult qualities communicating from the heavens to the earth. Ficino then showed how to use celestial bodies in medicines and exploit occult powers from the stars. His heavenly medicine culminated in a well-structured musical healing, where the *musica humana* found her therapeutic tools in the harmony of the spheres. The correspondence between human sounds and astral sounds was of use in taking care of human souls and bodies, because of the physical power of harmony.

In the last years of his life, Ficino faced a charge of practicing magic in *De vita coelitus comparanda* and was caught up in the difficulties surrounding Girolamo Savonarola's (1452–98) preaching and execution. Ficino continued to work on many translations and books, including *De sole*. In 1496 he published the first volume of *Commentaria in Platonem*, his life's work.

Bibliography

Primary: 1975–81. (Kristeller, Paul Oskar, preface) *The Letters of Marsilo Ficino* 5 vols. (London);1983. (Musacchio, Enrico, ed.) *Consilio contro la pestilenzia* (Bologna); 1989. (Kaske, Carol V., and John R. Clark, eds.) *Three Books on Life* (Binghamton, NY).

Secondary: Katinis, Teodoro, 2003. 'Sulle fonti aristoteliche e platoniche del *Consilio contro la pestilentia* di Ficino.' *Bruniana & Campanelliana* 9: 445–451; Vasoli, Cesare, 1997. 'Ficino, Marsilio' *DBI*, 47: 378a–395b.

Concetta Pennuto

FINLAY Y BARRES, CARLOS JUAN (b. Puerto Principe [now Camaguey], Cuba, 3 December 1833; d. Havana, Cuba, 21 August 1915), *yellow fever, epidemiology.*

An important member of Havana's scientific community in the late nineteenth and early twentieth centuries, Carlos Finlay was best known for his theory that yellow fever was transmitted through an independent agent, the mosquito. Born in Cuba to a Scottish father and a French mother, Finlay was educated in France and the United States, where he graduated from the Jefferson Medical College in Philadelphia in 1855. For the next several years he traveled and continued his education. After a yearlong sojourn in Peru, he returned to Havana in 1857 and began

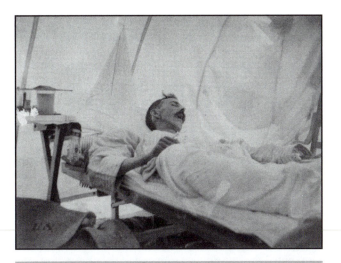

A man with yellow fever in hospital at Siboney, Cuba, July 1898. Photoprint courtesy of the National Library of Medicine.

his practice in ophthalmology and general medicine. Three years later he traveled to Paris for one year and then returned to Havana. Except for brief periods in the United States, Finlay lived for the rest of his life in Havana, where he died in 1915.

Finlay duplicated his cosmopolitan background with his own marriage. In 1865 he married Adele Shine, the daughter of an Irishman who had migrated to Trinidad, British West Indies. Born in Trinidad, Adele had lived in Canada and the Island of Guernsey as a teenager before coming to Cuba, where she met Finlay. Their children were born in 1868, 1870, and 1876. One son, also named Carlos, became a physician and authored a book about his father, *Carlos Finlay and Yellow Fever* (1940).

Finlay's involvement with yellow fever began in 1879 with his appointment to the United States Commission to study yellow fever. This commission was created as a result of an epidemic in New Orleans in 1878, which prompted the National Board of Health, under the auspices of the American Public Health Association, to create a commission to study yellow fever in Havana. During the course of this investigation Finlay developed the theory that yellow fever was transmitted through the *Culex* mosquito (also known as *Stegomyia fasciata* and later as the *Aedes aegypti*). Although the theory of mosquito transmission was not new, it was not particularly popular, as most physicians at the time held to a miasmic theory of contagion. An additional contribution of Finlay was his identification of the specific mosquito species, which he deduced by noting that this mosquito could be found at the same altitudes and temperatures in which yellow fever was prevalent.

Finlay began publicizing his theory in 1881, first at the International Sanitary Conference in Washington, DC, where he represented Cuba and Puerto Rico, and later that year in Havana, at the Academy of Sciences. He initially published his ideas in Spanish in the paper 'El Mosquito Hipoteticamente Considerado como Agente de Transmission de la Fiebre Amarilla' (1881) and later in English in a paper titled 'Yellow Fever: Its Transmission by the Means of the Culex Mosquito' in the *American Journal of the Medical Sciences* (1886).

Finlay's theories met with a measure of skepticism from the medical community. Although he conducted a number of experiments in Cuba between 1881 and 1900, it was not until 1901 that the theory was accepted as definitive. The lack of acceptance of his theory was in part due to a perceived lack of rigor in his experiments. In the early experiments, which he conducted between 1881 and 1900, Finlay allowed mosquitoes to first bite infected patients, then healthy volunteers. Enough of the volunteers contracted a mild case of yellow fever for him to conclude that he had pinpointed the cause of transmission of the disease. But critics pointed out that the volunteers were also exposed to other species of mosquitoes as well as to yellow fever patients themselves, arguing that there were too many uncontrolled factors for the experiment to be conclusive.

But the additional, and some historians argue more definitive, reason for this prolonged period of skepticism about Finlay's theory was the United States' inattention to the problem of yellow fever. Although the United States had supported yellow fever research in the past, the matter became much more urgent when it occupied Cuba in the aftermath of Cuba's final war of independence, (1895–98). Disease ravaged U.S. troops in Cuba, where for every one soldier dying in combat another twenty-five became ill and died. Moreover, in Havana yellow fever afflicted both U.S. troops and civilians. Once the United States became the occupying power, the matter of disease eradication took on a new urgency.

In 1899 the U.S. provisional government in Cuba named a Yellow Fever Board, which Finlay was to chair. Its members included Cuban doctors Diego Tamayo and Juan Guiteras, U.S. Army Surgeon General William Gorgas, Chief Sanitary Officer of Havana John G. Davies, and H. R. Carter of the Marine Hospital Service. Their mandate was to demonstrate the cause of yellow fever and eradicate the disease. They would also work closely with John Ross, director of Las Animas Hospital. Finlay was finally able to persuade Ross and Gorgas to take his theory seriously enough to test it. This was due in part to the failure of Gorgas's own attempts to eradicate yellow fever in Havana the previous year, in which extensive sanitation measures had done nothing to attenuate outbreaks of the disease. Through a series of experiments for which Finlay provided not just the hypothesis but also the mosquito eggs themselves, the U.S. Army's board finally demonstrated to its satisfaction the role of the mosquito in the transmission of yellow fever.

The experiments are remembered by both Cubans and Americans as dramatic acts of heroism. The only other theory about the transmission of yellow fever claimed that contamination and infection resulted from soiled clothing and bedding, so researchers divided volunteers into two groups. One group spent a night in a mosquito-free room filled with soiled clothing and bedding, while the other group allowed itself to be bitten by mosquitoes that had bitten infected patients. This proved that the soiled clothing was not the source of infection. Further experiments proved definitively that the mosquito, after a period of incubation, was the only agent of transmission of yellow fever. But several volunteers died in the course of this experiment, including Dr Jesse Lazear.

Once the source of yellow fever was proved, William Gorgas embarked on a mosquito eradication campaign that included destroying larvae as well as ensuring that mosquitoes did not come into contact with yellow fever patients. These efforts proved successful, and Havana saw its final death from yellow fever in September 1901. In 1902 Finlay was appointed Chairman of Commission for Hygiene and became a member of Cuba's National Board of Health. Cuba's first president, Tomás Estrada Palma, named him Chief Sanitary Officer of Cuba. In this capacity he formed the National Sanitary Board, with support from Juan Guiteras and Diego Tamayo, who was Secretary of Government at the time. He initiated a number of campaigns against other diseases, including tuberculosis, tetanus, glanders, infantile paralysis, malaria, typhoid, and smallpox. He retired from this post in 1909, at the age of seventy-six. He died six years later in Havana.

Although his published selected papers primarily contain publications on yellow fever, Finlay published extensively on a number of medical subjects. These publications include the first Cuban reports on diseases such as trichinosis (1885) and beriberi (1885), numerous reports on cholera, articles on public health and sanitation, and a number of publications in his original field of specialization, ophthalmology. Finlay was nominated for the Nobel Prize in Physiology or Medicine seven times, in 1905, 1906, 1907, 1912, 1913, 1914, and 1915, but he never won the prize.

Bibliography

Primary: 1965–81. *Obras Completas.* Havana: Academia de Ciencias de Cuba, Museo Histórico de las Ciencias Médicas 'Carlos J. Finlay' 6 vols. (Havana); 1881. 'El Mosquito hipotéticamente considerado como agente de transmisión de la Fiebre Amarilla.' *Anales de la Academia de Ciencias* 18: 147–169; 1886. 'Yellow Fever: Its transmission by means of the *culex* mosquito.' *American Journal of the Medical Sciences* (n.s.) 92: 395–409;

Secondary: López Sánchez, José, 1999. *Carlos J. Finlay: His Life and His Work.* (Havana); Stepan, Nancy, 1978. 'The Interplay between Socio-Economic Factors and Medical Science: Yellow Fever Research, Cuba and the United States.' *Social Studies of Science* 8(4): 397–423; Roig de Leuchsenring, Emilio, 1965. *Médicos y medicina en Cuba: Historia, Biografía, Costumbrismo.* (Havana); Finlay, Carlos E, 1940. *Carlos Finlay and Yellow Fever* (New York); DSB.

Alejandra Bronfman

FINSEN, NIELS RYBERG   (b. Tórshavn, Faroe Islands, 15 December 1860; d. Copenhagen, Denmark, 24 September 1904), *physiology.*

Finsen was a son of Hannes Christian Steingrim Finsen, Danish prefect in the Faroe Islands, and Johanne Sophie Caroline Christine Formann, who died when Finsen was four years old. Finsen grew up in the Faroe Islands, and he attended Herlufsholm Boarding School in Denmark (1874–76), Reykjavik Grammar School in Iceland (1876–82), and University of Copenhagen (1882–90), where he received his MD.

His years in school were difficult. His grades were modest and he suffered from a chronic heart disease, which had a major impact on his life and caused his death at the age of forty-three. A postmortem diagnosed the condition as constrictive pericarditis.

Johan Henrik Chievitz, professor of anatomy at the University of Copenhagen, recognized Finsen's significant talent for dissection and engaged him as prosector (1890–93), together with another young physician, Sophus Bang (1866–1950), who became an inspiring partner and a close colleague and friend to Finsen, until their estrangement in 1902. In 1892 Finsen married Ingeborg Dorthea Balslev. They had four children.

From 1892 Finsen investigated the positive and negative effects of light. His research focused on the use of light in the treatment of skin diseases and on the examination of the biological effect of light. Finsen believed that protection from ultraviolet light ('the red room') could have a curative effect on smallpox patients, which successful use during the Scandinavian smallpox epidemics in 1893–94 confirmed.

Early experiments by Finsen and Bang in 1893 separated the heating effect of infrared light from the 'chemical' effect of ultraviolet light and thus confirmed Downes and Blunt's observations (1877–78) that ultraviolet light impedes the growth of, or even kills, bacteria. Finsen was the first to examine and use radiotherapy. In 1896 he published his most important paper on the use of concentrated ultraviolet light in medicine, proposing its use in the treatment of skin diseases.

Finsen's unusual and simple methods and approach to scientific work were described as 'his greatest weakness and his greatest strength' (Hessenbruch and Petersen, 2001, p. 399). It distanced him from Danish academia, but quickly led him to an effective treatment of skin tuberculosis (lupus vulgaris), and in 1896 he founded the Finsen Medical Light Institute in Copenhagen where hundreds of patients were successfully treated. Finsen and his team developed arc lamps and special devices with lenses in order to obtain sufficient intensity of ultraviolet light. As a result of Finsen's ingenuity an effective device was soon launched (around 1900), which for more than twenty-five years was used in this therapy. The spectacular treatment of lupus made Finsen a public hero in Denmark, and at the Paris World Fair in 1900 his phototherapy was internationally acknowledged.

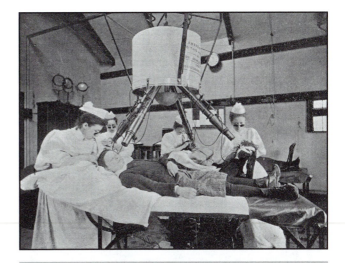

Finsen lamp with four tubes enabling four patients to be treated simultaneously. This lamp was presented to the London Hospital in 1900 by Princess Alexandra of Wales, who was Danish by birth. Wellcome Library, London.

Finsen's major contribution was his demonstration of the beneficial effects of concentrated ultraviolet light in the treatment of lupus vulgaris. In 1903 he was awarded the Nobel Prize for the foundation of phototherapy. It has been emphasized that Finsen's Nobel Prize should have been shared with his colleague, Sophus Bang.

Finsen also conducted early research on salt and water metabolism (1894 and 1904), on the seasonal variation of hemoglobin in blood (1894), and on the reaction of animals to light (1895), for which he has been considered a pioneer of ethology, which much later was attributed to Wolfgang Köhler (1887–1967) and Konrad Lorenz (1903–89).

Bibliography

Primary: 1899. *Ueber die Anwendung von concentrirten chemischen Lichtstrahlen in der Medicin* (Copenhagen) [First published in 1896 in Danish]; 1901. *Phototheraphy: (1) The Chemical Rays of Light and Small-pox, (2) Light as Stimulant, (3) The Treatment of Lupus Vulgaris by Concentrated Chemical Rays* (London); 1903. *Die Bekämpfung des Lupus Vulgaris. Mit 24 Tafeln und einer Statistik über 800 behandelte Fälle* (Jena).

Secondary: Lyngbye, Jørgen, 2003. *Lyssagen. Niels Finsen og hans team på Finseninstituttet* (Copenhagen); Hessenbruch, Arne, and Flemming Petersen, 2001. 'Niels Finsen (Physiology or Medicine 1903). Banishing Darkness and Disease' in Nielsen, Henry, and Keld Nielsen, eds., *Neighbouring Nobel* (Aarhus) pp. 393–429; *DSB.*

Signe Lindskov Hansen

FISCHER, EUGEN   (Karslruhe, Germany, 5 June 1874; Freiburg im Breisgau, Germany, 9 July 1967), *anthropology.*

Fischer is known for having introduced anthropology based on genetics, preparing the rise of human genetics in

Germany. Son of businessman Eugen Fischer Sr. and Josephine Salinger, Fischer studied medicine at the University of Freiburg im Breisgau (1893–98). He attended the lectures of anatomist Robert Wiedersheim and zoologist August Weismann, who was known for his theory on the continuity of germ plasma. After receiving a degree in anatomy, Fischer worked as an assistant at the Institute of Anatomy and gave lectures on anthropology, which at that point was still coupled with anatomy.

In 1908 he traveled to the German colonial area of South-West Africa to study a population of half-caste descendants of Dutch Buren and black Hottentots. He intended to show that racial characteristics, such as skin color, texture of hair, and color of the eyes followed Mendelian laws. The results of the research carried out in what is now Rehoboth, Namibia, were published in 1913, and brought Fischer much recognition in the anthropological circles of the time.

After returning to Freiburg, Fischer carried out local heritage studies and became interested in racial hygiene. He also met Alfred Ploetz, the founder of the eugenics movement in Germany, and Fischer founded a local branch of the German Racial Hygiene Society in Freiburg (1910). In 1918 he succeeded Wiedersheim as head of anatomy in Freiburg. In 1920 he coauthored the book known as Baur-Fischer-Lenz, which covered all knowledge of genetics up to that point.

Fischer cofounded the German Society for Physical Anthropology in 1925 and two years later accepted the post of director at the new Kaiser-Wilhelm-Institute for Anthropology, Human Heredity, and Eugenics. At the same time, he became head of anthropology at the University of Berlin and developed this institute into a leading research institution, with a focus on examining how environment and heredity shaped races. Muckermann headed the eugenics department, and Helmut Freiherr von Verschuer led the department for human heredity.

Not long after Hitler came to power, Fischer became vice-chancellor of the University of Berlin (May 1933). Despite his strong commitment to racial hygiene, Fischer was at first in a precarious position as a result of his heterosis theory, which said that half-castes are not inferior to individuals from allegedly pure races. Moreover, he distanced himself from race classifications based on skull measurements and did not support Nazi racial theory as it idealized the Nordic race. Nevertheless, Fischer's position was reinforced by 1935 and his institute, in the end, played a large part in the implementation of Nazi racial hygiene. As head of the Upper Hereditary Health Court in Berlin, Fischer supervised the enforcement of the compulsory sterilization law in his district.

After the beginning of World War II, Fischer succeeded in restructuring and reorienting his institute around new research goals. A department for comparative genetic pathology, led by Hans Nachtsheim, was founded at the beginning of 1941 and carried out experimental research on gene expression up to the end of the war.

In 1942 Fischer retired from his post as director of the Kaiser-Wilhelm-Institute and supported the appointment of Helmut Freiherr von Verschuer as his successor. He returned to Freiburg, but later went to live with his daughter in Sontra, near Berlin, after Freiburg was heavily bombed in December 1944. There he penned his autobiography and continued to publish scientific works. In 1950 he finally returned to Freiburg and helped Verschuer, who had been prosecuted by the Allies for his involvement in Nazi racial hygiene, obtain a chair for human genetics at the University of Münster. There Fischer had a major influence on postwar human genetics in Germany.

Bibliography

Primary: 1913. *Die Rehobother Bastards und das Bastardierungsproblem beim Menschen. Anthropologische und ethnologische Studien am Rehobother Bastardvolk in Deutsch-Südwestafrika* (Jena); 1921. (with Baur, Erwin, and Fritz Lenz), *Grundriß der menschlichen Erblichkeitslehre und Rassenhygiene* (Munich).

Secondary: Gessler, Bernhard, 2000. *Eugen Fischer (1874–1967). Leben und Werk des Freiburger Anatomen, Anthropologen und Rassenhygienikers bis 1927* (Frankfurt am Main); Lösch, Niels C., 1996. *Rasse als Konstrukt. Leben und Werk Eugen Fischers* (Frankfurt am Main).

Anne Cottebrune

FISHBEIN, MORRIS (b. St Louis, Missouri, USA, 22 July 1889; d. Chicago, Illinois, USA, 27 September 1976), *medical journalism, medical history, medical reform.*

Born to a father who imported porcelain and glass, Fishbein entered the University of Chicago in 1906 and then studied at Rush Medical College, qualifying in 1913. After a short internship at Durand Hospital, Chicago, in 1913, he obtained a temporary post at the *Journal of the American Medical Association*, subsequently serving as assistant editor until 1924. He became editor in the latter year, remaining in this post until 1949, when the American Medical Association forced him to retire.

Fishbein achieved a high profile to both the profession and the public. Transforming the AMA's publishing activities, he widened the scope of its journal, writing many signed and unsigned articles himself and also starting journals devoted to the newly burgeoning medical specialties. His books included histories of the AMA, of quackery, and of doctors in World War II. For many years secretary of the American Association for the History of Medicine, he was to present a large number of rare books to the University of Chicago.

Besides writing a stream of syndicated news columns, magazine features, and pamphlets on health subjects, Fishbein was also a popular speaker, both in public and on the radio. Such attainments led to his featuring in the prestigious cover photograph in *Time* magazine in 1937, though his prolonged and strident campaigns against quackery and state medicine also earned him the epithets of 'medical Mussolini' and the 'best known and least liked doctor in the United States'. And inevitably such forceful views disseminated from such a prominent platform brought him into conflict with the powerful AMA, which forced his resignation. Retirement, however, did little to sap his energies, and Fishbein continued his involvement with both lay and professional publications, maintaining a host of friendships at home and abroad and writing an extended autobiography.

Although subsequent generations would hardly recognize his name, Fishbein had an immense and lasting influence on medical journalism, both for the profession and for the public. For the former he showed that journals need not be dry repositories of unintelligible and irrelevant scientific articles, but could be attractive and readable, including discussions of topical political and ethical issues as well as humor (for many years he wrote the popular anonymous 'Dr Pepys' series in *JAMA* himself). His wide international friendships were important in the immediate postwar period in establishing such influential organizations as the World Medical Association. His enthusiasm for and wide knowledge of medical history were enshrined in the establishment of the Morris Fishbein Center for the History of Science and Medicine opened at the University of Chicago in 1970.

For the public his numerous articles and radio features showed that doctors need no longer hide behind a cloak of anonymity or refrain from discussing conditions that had traditionally been surrounded by embarrassment. Welcomed today by both the profession and the public, such characteristics are now taken for granted, but without Fishbein's pioneering energy they would have taken much longer to be introduced and to be accepted.

Bibliography

Primary: 1929. *An Hour on Health* (Philadelphia); 1969. *An Autobiography* (New York).

Secondary: Bealle, Morris Allison, 1938. *Medical Mussolini* (Washington, DC); *DAMB*.

Stephen Lock

FLEMING, ALEXANDER (b. Lochfield farm, near Darvel, Scotland, 6 August 1881; d. London, England, 11 March 1955), *pathology, therapeutics.*

Born to Hugh Fleming, farmer, and Grace Sterling Morton, Alexander was the third child of his father's second marriage. He received a good education to age thirteen at local schools and in 1895 moved to Marylebone to live with siblings, one of whom had studied medicine. After six years spent studying and working in commerce, Fleming inherited a small legacy and in 1901 he enrolled in St Mary's Hospital Medical School, a small school with a reputation for sports.

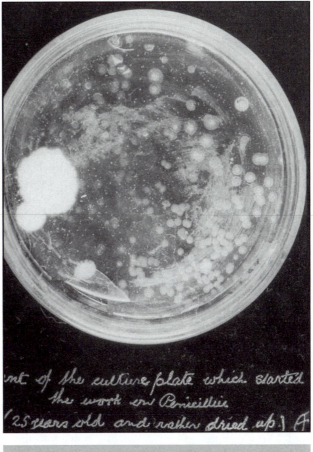

Alexander Fleming's original culture plate containing *Pencillium notatum*. Photograph, Wellcome Photo Library, London.

Gifted with both academic and athletic abilities, Fleming did well, winning many prizes. He took the conjoint exam in 1906, the MBBS (London) in 1908, and the FRCS in 1909, but already he had effectively become a pathologist.

In 1906 Fleming was hired as an assistant to Sir Almroth Wright (1861–1947), the chief pathologist at St Mary's and one of the leading scientific researchers of the day. From 1907, Fleming's name began to appear on papers from the St Mary's laboratory in favor of therapeutic vaccination. Fleming became Wright's right-hand man: he solved technical problems, built tricky apparatus, organized bacteriological tests and treatments, and wielded a deft syringe. In 1909 alone, he developed a therapeutic vaccine for acne, began the earliest English injections with salvarsan, and developed a simplification of the Wassermann test. Fleming followed Wright to France in 1914, where they produced vaccines and wrestled with the problem of wound infection, which they treated with irrigation, thereby enraging surgeons who preferred antisepsis.

The work on vaccines continued into the 1920s, but Fleming also developed two new lines of work: lysozyme and penicillin. In 1922 he noticed that his nasal mucous, and other bodily fluids, contained an antimicrobial substance: it lysed or killed some forms of bacteria. Fleming, a taciturn man at the best of times, was a poor public speaker and failed to generate interest in the work. However, his observations with lysozyme prepared him well for the events of September 1928. On returning from a holiday, he noticed that a colony of bacteria had been lysed by *Penicillium notatum,* a contaminating mold. Subsequent experiments confirmed that penicillin was a powerful antimicrobial, effective against many common bacteria, but also revealed obstacles to its use. Student assistants couldn't purify the extract and it was unstable and quickly depleted. Fleming continued to experiment with the substance, sent strains to other research labs, and published papers expounding the substance's uses as a laboratory technique for killing unwanted organisms in culture media; he also successfully treated patients. But once again he failed to arouse interest in his antibiotic and by 1936 he was concentrating on sulfonamides. Howard Florey (1898–1968) and Ernst Chain (1906–79) took up penicillin as one of several substances worthy of further investigation in 1940 and when he read of their early success in *Lancet* in August 1940 Fleming introduced himself and was given some role in developing the purified antibiotic. While the Oxford scientists rebuffed journalists, Fleming—coming from a small and entrepreneurial school—did nothing to discourage them and so received the lion's share of the publicity and became a popular hero. Professor of bacteriology at St Mary's in 1928, he succeeded Wright as principal of the Wright-Fleming Institute of Microbiology from 1946 to 1948, when he retired. FRS in 1943, FRCP and knighted in 1944, and Nobel laureate in 1945, Fleming spent the last decade of his life traveling and receiving honors.

Fleming married Sarah Marion McElroy in 1915; they had a son, Robert, who became a doctor. She died in 1949, and he married Amalia Koutsouri-Voureka in 1953.

Bibliography

Primary: 1929. 'On the antibacterial action of cultures of a *Penicillium.*' *British Journal of Experimental Pathology* 10: 229.

Secondary: Macfarlane, Gwyn, 1984. *Alexander Fleming: The Man and the Myth* (London); Hare, Ronald, 1970. *The Birth of Penicillin and the Disarming of Microbes* (London); Maurois, André, 1959. *The Life of Sir Alexander Fleming* (London); *DSB*; *Oxford DNB*.

E. A. Heaman

FLEXNER, ABRAHAM (b. Louisville, Kentucky, USA, 13 November 1866; d. Falls Church, Virginia, USA, 21 September 1959), *medical education, philanthropy.*

Flexner was born in Louisville, Kentucky, the sixth of nine children of Morris Flexner and Esther Abraham, Orthodox Jewish immigrants. Morris started as an itinerant peddler and later built a successful wholesale hat business. However, he lost the business during the panic of 1873, and the family grew up in poverty. Though Flexner

MEDICAL EDUCATION
IN THE
UNITED STATES AND CANADA

A REPORT TO
THE CARNEGIE FOUNDATION
FOR THE ADVANCEMENT OF TEACHING

BY
ABRAHAM FLEXNER

WITH AN INTRODUCTION BY
HENRY S. PRITCHETT
PRESIDENT OF THE FOUNDATION

BULLETIN NUMBER FOUR

576 FIFTH AVENUE
NEW YORK CITY

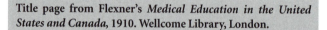

Title page from Flexner's *Medical Education in the United States and Canada,* **1910. Wellcome Library, London.**

always professed the highest respect for his parents' religious views, he and his siblings ultimately became indifferent to the ancient beliefs and customs of Judaism. Flexner did absorb his parents' love of education, learning, and liberal culture, and he benefited from the warm and caring home environment they provided as well.

An intellectually precocious child, Flexner spent six years at the Louisville Male High School, two years in the preparatory division and four years in high school. Despite his later claim that his public school education was inferior, he undertook a demanding course of study—Latin, Greek, German, French, mathematics, natural science, psychology, English literature, physics, and chemistry. He excelled in every subject except mathematics, receiving several academic prizes. He was chosen salutatorian of the graduating class of 1884 and gave an oration on reform of the civil service system, a reflection of his keen interest in politics.

In 1884, with financial aid from his oldest brother Jacob, who had become a pharmacist, Flexner entered the newly created Johns Hopkins University. Flexner was the first member of his family to attend a university, and Johns Hopkins was on its way to becoming one of the most influential American universities of the nineteenth century. At Hopkins, he undertook a heavy course load, which allowed him to graduate with an AB degree in classics in 1886. He was highly impressed with the Hopkins system of education, particularly its emphasis on research and scholarly inquiry, which was patterned on the German university system. Flexner was particularly influenced by Daniel Coit Gilman, the first president of the university, who imparted to him an appreciation of the importance of original research in all scholarly fields. This value Flexner carried with him throughout his career. 'Those who know something of my work,' he later recalled, '. . . will recognize Gilman's influence in all I have done or tried to do' (Flexner, 1940, p. 52).

After returning to Louisville in 1886, Flexner taught in a local high school for four years, then organized a private high school of his own. 'Mr. Flexner's School', as it came to be known, provided intensive tutoring to wealthy, often unruly, boys, to prepare them for Eastern colleges. So well did graduates of the school perform that Flexner came to the attention of Charles W. Eliot, the president of Harvard University.

In 1905 Flexner closed his school to pursue graduate work at Harvard. There he studied philosophy and psychology for their possible bearings on educational problems. In 1907 he traveled in Europe, where he closely observed the various educational systems. In 1908 he published his first book, *The American College*, a critique of higher education in the United States. The book criticized the lecture and elective system and called for universities to pay more attention to intellectual matters, and less to extracurricular affairs.

The Flexner Report

In the early 1900s, medical education in the United States was in ferment. A consensus had emerged among medical educators regarding how medicine should be taught and learned. In their view, rigorous entrance requirements should be established; the scientific subjects must be added to the curriculum; and students should be active learners through laboratory work and clinical clerkships, and not just passive learners relying solely on the memorization of lectures, as before. In addition, a new view had emerged as to what the medical school should look like as an institution—namely, that it should become part of the university, with full-time faculty committed to research as well as to teaching. Many, though certainly not all, medical educators of the time thought that there was no longer room for 'teaching schools' that provided good instruction but undertook no research.

However, such a system of medical education had not yet been created. Ever since the Civil War, medical schools had progressed enormously, but further improvements were needed to elevate the average school to a minimum standard of excellence as well as to institute additional improvements at the stronger schools. In addition, many notorious 'proprietary schools'—commercial ventures, operated for profit, that had extremely low standards and typically advertised scientific and clinical opportunities that did not exist—continued to operate.

This situation concerned the Council on Medical Education of the American Medical Association, which in 1906 conducted a private survey documenting these conditions. Believing that it was politically imprudent for a medical organization to be publicly critical of medical schools, the Council invited the Carnegie Foundation for the Advancement of Teaching to conduct a similar study, and Henry Pritchett, the president of the Carnegie Foundation, readily accepted the invitation. The person selected by Pritchett to conduct the inspection of medical schools was Flexner.

How Flexner came to Pritchett's attention is not known. Perhaps Pritchett had learned of him through his first book, *The American College*. It is possible that Flexner's younger brother, Simon, a distinguished virologist who had attended the Johns Hopkins Medical School and then directed the Rockefeller Institute for Medical Research, played a role. In any event, the choice proved to be fortunate. Aggressive, articulate, and outspoken, Flexner became a forceful spokesman for modern methods of medical teaching and the most loyal friend that academic medicine in America had ever had.

Flexner began his work at the Carnegie Foundation in December 1908. He knew little about medicine or medical education as he began the project. He read voraciously on the subject, conferred regularly with the Council on Medical Education, and made many trips to Johns Hopkins, whose medical school stood above all others and to Flexner represented the ideal. Indeed, he later spoke frequently of the great intellectual debt he had to the medical school's dean, William Welch, and other members of the pioneering medical faculty at Johns Hopkins.

Though Flexner learned much from his visits to Johns Hopkins, he was not a mere tool of Welch and the Hopkins faculty. A sophisticated educator, Flexner had already developed a coherent philosophy of education prior to embarking on the study of medical education. Flexner maintained that students at all levels should 'learn by doing' and be 'active learners'. He believed that John Dewey's ideas of the experiential nature of learning were generally applicable in education. And, influenced as he was by Gilman, Flexner needed no convincing about the importance of original research at institutions of higher learning. Flexner's conceptual framework, in short, had already been developed. Welch and the others merely provided the details as they pertained to medicine.

Following his crash course on medical education, Flexner began a busy year of travel to each of the 155 medical schools in the United States and Canada. His visits were quick but thorough. He knew what he was looking for, and in a remarkably short time he could understand the salient features of a school. The resultant report, *Medical Education in the United States and Canada*, issued in June 1910 as Bulletin Number Four of the Carnegie Foundation for the Advancement of Teaching (Flexner, 1910), made newspaper headlines and created an immediate sensation.

The Flexner report emphasized the work remaining to be done in medical education rather than the progress that had already been made. It pointed out the need for entrance requirements. It also pointed out the importance of providing students with laboratory work in the scientific subjects and clerkships in the clinical fields so they could be active learners. It further discussed the great need for money and hospital facilities so that the desired educational reforms could be implemented. With devastating candor, the report, a classic of muckraking journalism, directed its fiercest attack at the proprietary schools, exposing the scandalous conditions and outright fraud that existed at these wretched schools. Although the report was not original—everything in it had been said by academically-inclined medical educators since the 1870s—it had a galvanizing effect on public sentiment, making the achievement of the ideal much more attainable. In the next fifteen years, catalyzed by the report, the proprietary schools were forced to close, many weak schools merged, and all surviving schools acquired the money and hospital facilities to place medical education on a firm educational footing.

The Flexner report was notable for another reason. It made possible a choice among the competing models of what medical schools should look like as institutions. Flexner had argued that only one type of medical school was acceptable: university schools, with large full-time faculties and a vigorous commitment to research. He held the new school at Johns Hopkins as the model of excellence to be emulated by all. Thus, the report not only influenced the speed at which medical education in the United States developed thereafter, but the form it ultimately assumed.

Philanthropist and Educational Statesman

Medical Education in the United States and Canada established Flexner as the arbiter of the reconstruction of medical education. For two more years he remained at the Carnegie Foundation, where schools would routinely consult him when making important faculty appointments or launching major developmental programs. While there, he also published a second study, *Medical Education in Europe* (Flexner, 1912), which further enhanced his reputation as an authority in the field.

In 1913 Flexner received the opportunity to wield even greater influence when he became assistant secretary, and later secretary, of the General Education Board, a huge private foundation established by oil magnate John D. Rockefeller. There, Flexner not only continued his activities as an advisor to medical schools, but he also created and directed philanthropic programs that financed the reorganization of many private and public medical schools. During his fifteen years at the foundation, Flexner guided $61 million of Rockefeller money into medical education. Because of matching stipulations, Flexner estimated that the original grants eventually led to $600 million in new resources for U.S. medical schools. At Flexner's insistence, this money was used to construct new facilities, hire full-time faculty, and support medical research. Flexner's extraordinary opportunity to support medical schools willing to follow the Hopkins model accounts for his most lasting impact on medical education.

At the General Education Board, Flexner also continued to write on educational matters. He focused not only on medical education but also on all aspects of education. Notable works included *Public Education in Maryland* (1916), *Public Education in Delaware* (1919), and *Medical Education: A Comparative Study* (1925). The unifying theme in all his writings was his conviction that John Dewey's ideas of progressive education, embodied by the term 'learning by doing', applied to every level of education. Indeed, Flexner's celebrated essay of 1916, 'A Modern School', inspired the creation the following year of the Lincoln School, the outstanding private progressive school of the period.

In 1928 Flexner left the General Education Board. He continued writing, most notably *Universities: American, English, German* (1930). More significantly, in 1930 he persuaded Louis Bamberger and his sister, Mrs Felix Fuld, to donate $5,000,000 to create the Institute for Advanced Study at Princeton. Flexner organized the Institute, served as its first director, and, in that capacity, brought Albert Einstein to the United States.

Flexner retired from the Institute in 1939. He died of old age in 1959. More than any other single individual, he had helped to create the American system of medical education. His work epitomized the view that medical education was not medicine but education.

Bibliography

Primary: 1910. *Medical Education in the United States and Canada* (New York); 1912. *Medical Education in Europe* (New York); 1925. *Medical Education: A Comparative Study* (New York); 1940. *I Remember: The Autobiography of Abraham Flexner* (New York).

Secondary: Bonner, Thomas Neville, 2002. *Iconoclast: Abraham Flexner and a Life in Learning* (Baltimore); Ludmerer, Kenneth M., 1985. *Learning to Heal: The Development of American Medical Education* (New York); Fox, Daniel, 1980. 'Abraham Flexner's Unpublished Report: Foundations and Medical Education, 1909–1928.' *Bulletin of the History of Medicine* 54: 475–496; Hudson, Robert P., 1972. 'Abraham Flexner in Perspective: American Medical Education, 1865–1910.' *Bulletin of the History of Medicine* 46: 545–561; *DAMB*.

Kenneth M. Ludmerer

FLICK, LAWRENCE FRANCIS

FLICK, LAWRENCE FRANCIS (b. Carrolltown, Pennsylvania, USA, 10 August 1856; d. Philadelphia, Pennsylvania, USA, 7 July 1938), *medicine, tuberculosis.*

Flick was born on a farm, the son of John Flick and Elizabeth (Sharbaugh) Flick. He married Ella Josephine Stone in 1885, with whom he had seven children. Flick attended St Vincent College in Philadelphia. When he found that he suffered from tuberculosis, in order to heal himself he decided to enroll at Jefferson Medical College, also in Philadelphia, from which he received his MD in 1880. He then did an internship at Philadelphia General Hospital. Flick had intended to become a lawyer after healing himself, but his health deteriorated from tuberculosis while working in a law office and he moved to California, where he made orange crates at two cents each. There his health improved. He gained sixty pounds and concluded that eating free oranges and finding other inexpensive, nutritious food had helped cure his disease. Flick returned to Philadelphia, where he spent the rest of his life becoming a leader in the fight against tuberculosis.

Although Koch described the organism we now believe defines tuberculosis in 1882, the debate over what causes tuberculosis continued for many years thereafter. Flick was an early and prominent proponent of the idea that tuberculosis was not hereditary, but could be spread from person to person, and he was one of the first to argue for registration of people with tuberculosis. The dual goals of both treating the disease in individuals and controlling (and perhaps eradicating) the disease in the community could be accomplished by segregating people with tuberculosis in special institutions called 'sanatoria'. Flick established several such institutions in and around Philadelphia. In 1903 he persuaded the steel manufacturer Henry Phipps to endow an institute for the study and treatment of tuberculosis, an institute for which Flick served as director.

Flick's most long-lasting accomplishment came through his role in creating organizations that served as the basis for the voluntary health movement. In 1892 Flick founded the first organization to control tuberculosis, the Pennsylvania Society for the Prevention of Tuberculosis. The use of the term 'prevention' in this and similar organizations signaled a role not only for scientific study of the disease but also for public health action designed to improve community health. Indeed, organization members saw their role as encompassing everything from hospital and medical care to working with boards of health, to lobbying for the passage of appropriate legislation. Another important characteristic of Flick's early group was the emphasis on belief in the contagious nature of the disease. Other local organizations followed. In 1904 Flick played an instrumental role in creating the National Association for the Study and Prevention of Tuberculosis, which became the National Tuberculosis Association in 1918 and eventually the present-day American Lung Association in 1937. This group served as the model for several other disease-specific public health organizations, such as the American Cancer Society (1913), the American Heart Association (1922), and the National Foundation for Infantile Paralysis (1938).

In addition to his work on tuberculosis, Flick had a long-standing interest in the history of the Catholic Church in the United States, publishing in the area as well as serving as president of the American Catholic Historical Society.

Bibliography

Primary: 1904. *Consumption, A Curable and Preventable Disease: What a Layman Should Know about It* (Philadelphia); 1925. *Development of Our Knowledge of Tuberculosis* (Philadelphia); 1937. *Tuberculosis—A Book of Practical Knowledge to Guide the General Practitioner of Medicine* (Philadelphia).

Secondary: Bates, Barbara, 1992. *Bargaining for Life: A Social History of Tuberculosis 1876–1938* (Philadelphia); [Obituary], 1938. *New York Times* 8 July, p.17; *DAMB*.

Joel D. Howell

FLINT, AUSTIN, SR

FLINT, AUSTIN, SR (b. Petersham, Massachusetts, USA, 20 October 1812; d. New York, New York, USA, 13 March 1886), *medicine.*

The son, grandson, and great-grandson of physicians dating back to the American Revolutionary War, Flint attended Amherst College for two years and Harvard Medical School (1830–33), graduating at the age of twenty-one. His marriage to Anne Skillings in 1835 produced a son, Austin Flint, Jr., who became an important physiologist and professor. He practiced first in Northampton and Boston, Massachusetts (1833–36), and then in Buffalo, New York (1836–44, 1845–52), in Chicago, Illinois (1844–45), in Louisville, Kentucky (1852–56), in New Orleans, Louisiana (winters of 1858–61), and in Long Island College Hospital and New York City (1859–68). Flint was a founder of the Buffalo School of Medicine (1847) and the Bellevue Medical College (1861) and the professor of the principles and practice of medicine at Rush Medical College in Chicago, the University of Louisville, the New Orleans Medical School, and Long Island College. His honors included prizes from the American Medical Association for his essays on physical diagnosis of the chest (1852, 1859), a Doctor of Laws degree from Yale University (1881), and honorary membership in the Medical Society of London. He was a strong defender of the medical profession and its standards, serving as the president of the New York Academy of Medicine (1872–75) and the American Medical Association (1884). In addition, he was a delegate and principal speaker at the International Medical Congress (1876, 1881, and 1884) and its president-elect (1887). Flint continued to be a reforming educator and strong visionary leader in the medical profession until 1886, when he died from a stroke at the age of seventy-four.

The young Flint was greatly influenced by James Jackson, his teacher at Harvard Medical School, who was an early advocate of the stethoscope and physical diagnosis. Although Laennec's classic 1819 monograph describing the stethoscope and its great value had been published in Philadelphia in 1823, stethoscopy was not rapidly accepted in America. American physicians, mostly schooled by a proprietary system of lectures and postgraduate apprenticeship, and practicing in small villages, did not have the broad exposure to the clinical and autopsy findings of heart and lung diseases that was readily available in the large Paris teaching hospitals. Nor were there experienced teachers like Laennec and his disciples to explain the complicated technique and point out the abnormal auscultatory findings. This would become the self-appointed role of Flint, a peripatetic teacher, who would come to be described as 'the American Laennec' (Gross, 1887, p. 161). Flint was a careful observer and a prolific writer who compiled extensive notes—he left almost 17,000 handwritten pages of observations about his patients, which were the basis of his books. His publications, beginning in 1840 with an account of twenty-four cases of rubeola, eventually numbered over 240. He founded the *Buffalo Medical Journal* in 1845, which he edited for ten years and to which he contributed many articles, and he authored several of the most influential textbooks of medicine in nineteenth-century America. These texts included *A Practical Treatise on the Diagnosis, Pathology and Treatment of Diseases of the Heart* (1859), *A Treatise on the Principles and Practice of Medicine* (1866), *Manual of Auscultation and Percussion* (1876), *Clinical Medicine, a Systematic Treatise on the Diagnosis and Treatment of Diseases* (1879), and *Physical Exploration of the Lungs by Means of Auscultation and Percussion* (1882). His publications, many of which were reprinted in Great Britain, brought him national and international attention. His book *A Treatise on the Principles and Practice of Medicine* went through six editions, sold 40,000 copies, and was heralded as the best medical text written by an American. *Lancet*, in a posthumous review of the book, published 12 March 1887, stated, 'America may well be proud of having produced a man whose indefatigable industry and gifts of genius have done so much to advance medicine and all English reading students must be grateful for the work he has left behind.'

His earliest writings were on fever. He studied epidemics of typhoid fever and typhus showing that the two diseases were separate entities, and he was among the first to accept the germ theory of Koch in 1882. He was conservative in his use of mercury and phlebotomy, popular remedies of the time, and advocated exercise and a low-fat diet to avoid weakness and 'fatty degeneration' of the heart. Flint disapproved of the common practice of polypharmacy, commenting that 'Nothing is easier than to prescribe drugs . . . to refrain from their use may require not a little firmness and independence. An ignorant or weak practitioner therefore may be tempted to pursue a medical treatment in opposition to his judgment or to cover up his lack of knowledge' (Evans, 1958, p. 239). The natural history of untreated diseases was an area of special interest through which he could show that many patients spontaneously recover without popular treatment. To support his conviction, he studied and published large series of untreated cases of tuberculosis, pleurisy, dysentery, pneumonia, and Bright's disease.

In his teachings on auscultation, Flint sought to simplify Laennec's unwieldy classification, in which each abnormal cardiac and pulmonary sound was thought to signify a separate disease. Like his counterpart Josef Skoda in Vienna, he analyzed and correlated the pitch of the sounds with the disease, thus providing a more understandable and therefore less discouraging clinical approach prior to the electrocardiogram and chest x-ray. Flint's Law stated that 'An elevation of pitch always accompanies a diminution of resonance in consequence of pulmonary consolidation.' He introduced his concepts in an 1856 monograph on the practical use of the stethoscope, and his *Manual of Percussion and Auscultation* was popular from 1876 until 1922. William Osler commented to his students at the University of Pennsylvania that 'Not one of you who takes a stethoscope into his hand but is a debtor to Dr. Flint for simplifying much that was complicated in the auscultation of the heart and lung' and praised him as 'the Nestor of clinical medicine in this country'.

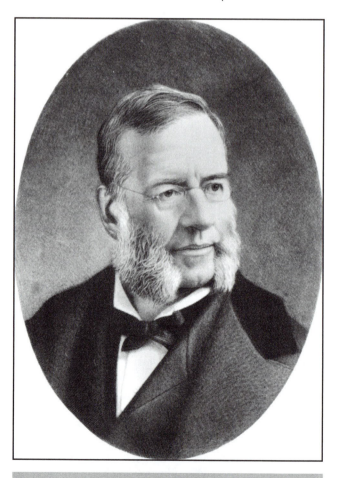

Austin Flint. **Halftone reproduction from William B. Atkinson,** *The Physicians and Surgeons of the United States*, **Philadelphia, 1878. Wellcome Library, London.**

A tall, handsome man with an excellent voice, Flint was greatly admired for his progressive thoughts, diagnostic acumen, and inspiring teaching. A professor at six medical schools, he fought for improved standards of medical education and basic science. He became a leader in the growing communities where he practiced and organized clinics where a large following of students and practitioners fell under his influence. He insisted that his students thoroughly study and follow up their patients with carefully kept records, not just attend the lectures. He stated, 'The ability to observe is not a natural gift nor does it accompany as a matter of course the acquisition of knowledge that one acquires from reading or didactic lectures. It is an art to be acquired.' His emphasis on the examination of the patient, centered on the use of the stethoscope to arrive at a carefully reasoned differential diagnosis, set an example that his students would learn and follow. At Bellevue Hospital in New York City, a large audience of students from three medical schools attended his hour-and-a-half, twice daily instructions. It was said that '. . . he is a lecturer at once clear, distinct, and inspiring. During his hour in the classroom, no student ever falls asleep' (Gross, p. 160).

In 1862 Flint reported a presystolic murmur at the apex associated with severe aortic regurgitation, which he had first noted at the Charity Hospital in New Orleans: 'In some cases in which free aortic regurgitation exists, the left ventricle becoming filled before the auricles contract, the mitral curtains are floated out and the valve closed when the mitral current takes place, and, under the circumstance, this murmur may be produced by the current just named, although no mitral lesion exists.' Although Flint well deserves to be remembered as one of the most important physician leaders, clinicians, and teachers in nineteenth-century America, his name is now recalled primarily as an eponym—'the Austin Flint murmur'.

Bibliography

Primary: 1852. 'On the variations of pitch in percussion and respiratory sounds, and their application to physical diagnosis.' *American Medical Association Transactions* 5: 75–123; 1859. *A Practical Treatise on the Diagnosis, Pathology and Treatment of Diseases of the Heart* (Philadelphia); 1862. 'On cardiac murmurs.' *American Journal of Medical Sciences* 44: 29–54; 1866. *A Treatise on the Principles and Practice of Medicine* (Philadelphia); 1876. *Manual of Auscultation and Percussion* (Philadelphia).

Secondary: Berman, Paul, 1988. 'Austin Flint—America's Laennec Revisited.' *Archives of Internal Medicine* 148: 2053–2056; Smith, Dale C., 1978. 'Austin Flint and Auscultation in America.' *Journal of the History of Medicine* 33(2): 129–149; Shaftel, Norman, 1960. 'Austin Flint, Sr. (1812–1886): Educator of Physicians.' *Journal of Medical Education* 35: 1122–1134; Thorn, George W., 1959. 'Austin Flint—A Biographical Study of a Founding Member.' *Transactions of the American Clinical and Climatologic Association* 71: li–lxvi; Evans, Alfred S., 1958. 'Austin Flint and His Contributions to Medicine.' *Bulletin of the History of Medicine* 32: 224–241; Gross, Samuel W., 1887. *Autobiography of Samuel D. Gross, MD* (Philadelphia); Osler, William, 1886. 'Remarks to the class in clinical medicine, University of Pennsylvania.' *Canada Medical Surgical Journal* 1886: 572; *DAMB*.

Mark E. Silverman

FLOREY, HOWARD WALTER   (b. Adelaide, South Australia, 24 September 1898; d. Oxford, England, 21 February 1968), *experimental pathology, penicillin research.*

Florey was the youngest child of a bootmaker, Joseph Florey (1857–1918), from the village of Standlake in Oxfordshire. Joseph's wife, Charlotte, suffered from tuberculosis and in 1885 the family, including two young daughters, moved to Australia to benefit her health. Joseph set up business in Adelaide, but the following year Charlotte died and in 1889 Joseph married Bertha Wadham, daughter of an Australian widow who had nursed his wife. They had two more daughters before their last child, Howard, was born in 1898.

At the age of ten Florey was enrolled at Kyre College, transferring in 1911 to St Peter's Collegiate School in Adelaide. He excelled academically and athletically, and he resolved to follow his sister Hilda by applying to study medicine at Adelaide University. Florey entered the Medical School in March 1916 and passed the preclinical examinations with honors in 1918. His father died in September of that year, leaving the family heavily in debt, but scholarships enabled him to continue his studies and he graduated MB BS in 1921. At the university Florey was attracted to clinical laboratory medicine, intensifying an early conviction that his future lay in research. Florey applied for a Rhodes Scholarship at Oxford University in August 1920 and it was awarded in December that year, with a proposed start date of October 1921. However, Florey was not due to graduate in Adelaide until December 1921 and he sought leave to defer the start until January 1922. Surprisingly, after much argument, the Oxford authorities agreed.

Oxford and Cambridge

Oxford was a culture shock for the brash colonial, but Florey soon fell under the spell of its intellectual vigor and the close proximity of fine scientific minds. In July 1923 he took a first in physiology, and Sir Charles Sherrington offered him a post as demonstrator in his department. Florey took up his duties in October and started research involving microscopic observations on the circulation of blood in the cerebral capillaries of cats, a study that required considerable patience and technical ingenuity. Sherrington was sufficiently impressed to encourage Florey to apply for the John Lucas Walker studentship in experimental pathology at the University of Cambridge under Professor Henry Dean. He took up the studentship in 1924 after spending the long vacation as medical officer to the Oxford University Arctic Expedition.

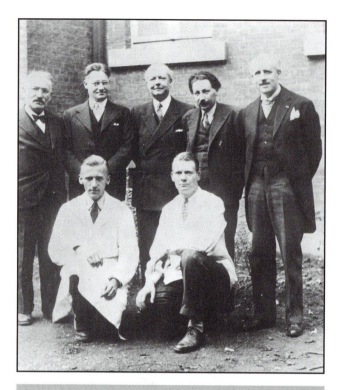

Group portrait (back row, L–R), Selman Waksman, Howard Florey, J. Trefouel, Ernst Chain, Andre Gratia; (front row, L–R), P. Fredericq, Maurice Welsch. Oxford. Photograph, Wellcome Library, London.

At Cambridge Florey immersed himself in a continuation of the work on the response of brain capillaries to inflammation and various external stimuli. During 1925 he obtained a Rockefeller Foundation Fellowship for study in the United States. He set sail for New York on 19 September 1925 with the intention of working at Cornell University with Robert Chambers, an international expert on micro-dissection of tissues. When this offer fell through, Florey arranged at short notice to go instead to the laboratory of the pharmacologist Alfred Newton Richards in Philadelphia. It was a providential move.

Prelude to Penicillin

While in America, Florey received the offer of the Freedom Research Fellowship, newly endowed by an unknown benefactor at the London Hospital in East London. The conditions of the appointment (freedom to choose his own line of research, a fully equipped laboratory, no clinical work or teaching, and a salary of £850 per annum) were too tempting to refuse; Florey curtailed his stay in America by two months and returned to England in May 1926. In London Florey was joined by Mary Ethel Hayter Reed (1900–66), daughter of a prominent Adelaide family and a fellow medical student with whom he had maintained an intense correspondence since leaving Australia. She arrived in England in late September 1926, and they were married at Holy Trinity Church Padding-

ton on 19 October. A courtship conducted by long-distance correspondence was not the best preparation for marriage and the relationship was not an easy one. Nevertheless, the marriage survived until Ethel's death in 1966, and she was very supportive professionally, not least by carrying out many of the early clinical trials of penicillin in Oxford during World War II. They had two children, Paquita and Charles.

In London Florey started work on mucus secretion, an interest that he had developed in America, partly stimulated by personal problems with recurrent dyspepsia. London was not to his taste and he felt drawn back to Cambridge. A successful thesis for a fellowship at Gonville and Caius College, and the support of Sherrington and Dean, enabled Florey to become an Unofficial Fellow of Caius in 1926 and to return to the university the following year as the Huddersfield Lecturer in Pathology. Another thesis gave him a Cambridge PhD in 1927. It was also during this year that he acquired the services of a fourteen-year-old boy, James Kent, as a laboratory technician. He was to remain Florey's skilled assistant for forty years.

Florey stayed in Cambridge until 1932, consolidating his reputation as an experimental pathologist with a keen intellect and a reputation for bluntness. His research interests expanded to include the role in the body's natural defenses of lysozyme—a substance discovered in 1921 by Alexander Fleming in nasal mucus and other bodily secretions. Although life at Cambridge was stimulating and conducive to the development of his talents, the prospects of a professorship, on which he had set his sights, were remote, and Florey began looking elsewhere. In 1931 he applied for the Joseph Hunter Professorship in Pathology at Sheffield University Medical School, which boasted two influential Fellows of the Royal Society: the physiologist John Beresford Leathes, and Edward Mellanby. Although Florey had little of the teaching and clinical experience required of a conventional Professor of Pathology, he was duly appointed and took up his duties in March 1932.

Leathes and Mellanby both left Sheffield in 1933 and, when Georges Dreyer, the Professor of Pathology at Oxford, died suddenly in 1934, it was no surprise when Florey leaped at the opportunity. With powerful backers, the outcome was scarcely in doubt, and Florey returned to Oxford in 1935 to head Dreyer's former department at the Sir William Dunn School of Pathology.

Florey set about organizing his new department and strengthening his team. He had long felt the need for a dedicated biochemist to help carry his research forward and when he learned of the availability of a talented young Jewish refugee from Nazi Germany, Ernst Boris Chain (1906–79), he was happy to offer him a job. Chain was a volatile character and sparks often flew in the Dunn School, but Florey's team was soon to be responsible for one of the most remarkable developments in twentieth-century medicine: turning penicillin from a laboratory curiosity into a 'miracle drug'.

Florey had ironically missed several opportunities to learn about penicillin. He was almost certainly aware of Fleming's work, since he was an editor of the *British Journal of Experimental Pathology*, where Fleming's famous paper first appeared. He was also in contact with Fleming, who performed some lysozyme assays for him. Among Florey's staff at Sheffield was a young pathologist, Cecil George Paine, who had studied at St Mary's Hospital. While working at Sheffield Royal Infirmary in 1930, Paine had experimented with Fleming's 'mould juice' and used it to successfully treat gonococcal eye infections of newborn infants. Florey was aware of this work, but took little interest at the time.

Penicillin and After

Among the tasks Florey gave to Chain was the investigation of the mode of action of lysozyme. In reviewing the literature on natural antibacterial compounds, Chain happened upon penicillin, which also became included in the study. Though the Oxford work was conceived simply as a biochemical research exercise, talk of antibacterial chemotherapy was then in the air: Gerhard Domagk published details of Prontosil (the first sulfonamide) in 1935 and in 1939 René Dubos's tyrothricin work was causing a stir in America. In September 1939, three days after the outbreak of war, Florey applied to his former colleague, Edward Mellanby, now Secretary of the Medical Research Council, for a grant to explore the therapeutic potential of penicillin. He was awarded £25, with the possibility of a further £100. An application to the Rockefeller Foundation yielded a more generous response: $5,000 per year for five years.

Chain's flair and the technical ingenuity of Norman Heatley soon produced enough crude penicillin for proper microbiological investigations and, in May 1940, a scientifically derisory but convincing experiment on eight infected mice. After further tests the landmark penicillin paper appeared in *Lancet* in late August. The department was now turned into a factory for the production of enough penicillin for clinical trials. By early February 1941, the scene was set for the first clinical use of penicillin; by June it was clear that they had uncovered something very special.

It was impossible to purify and produce penicillin on a large scale in wartime Britain so Florey turned to America for help. Accompanied by Norman Heatley (and to the fury of Chain, who had not been consulted) Florey set off in great secrecy for the United States on 27 June 1941. He got little response from American drug companies, but there was support from his old friend Newton Richards, who had an influential position on the National Defense Research Committee. With Richards's help (and government money) the cooperation of the pharmaceutical industry was secured. By the end of World War II problems of the mass production of penicillin had virtually been solved. In the meantime, Ethel Florey was continuing clinical trials in

England, and in May 1943 Howard traveled with his fellow-Australian Hugh Cairns (another Rhodes Scholar) to North Africa to oversee trials of penicillin in battle wounds. Later that year, he went on a secret mission to Russia with his bacteriological colleague Gordon Sanders to share their expertise with the wartime ally.

Florey shunned the media spotlight, and public adulation for penicillin fell on Fleming, much to the derision of those who knew the true facts. Though popular recognition was lacking, official accolades came thick and fast. Florey was knighted in 1944, and in 1945 he received the Nobel Prize, together with Fleming and Chain. He had been elected to the Royal Society in 1942 and in 1960 became one of its most effective presidents. In 1962 he was elected Provost of The Queen's College, Oxford. A baronetcy (Baron Florey of Adelaide and Marston) and the Order of Merit followed in 1965. In Australia Florey refused a State Governorship but became very involved with the foundation of the Australian National University and with the John Curtin School of Medical Research in Canberra. He became Chancellor of the University in 1965. Florey received innumerable medals, honorary degrees, and international prizes, including the Légion d'honneur (1946), and the United States Medal for Merit (1948).

Lady Florey died suddenly in October 1966. In June 1967 Florey married his longtime laboratory colleague and confidante, Margaret Jennings. It was to be a short but happy union. Florey died of a heart attack at The Queen's College, Oxford on 21 February 1968.

Bibliography

Primary: 1940. (with Chain, E., A. D. Gardner, N. G. Heatley, M. A. Jennings, J. Orr-Ewing, and A. G. Sanders) 'Penicillin as a Chemotherapeutic Agent.' *Lancet* ii: 226–228); 1941. (with Abraham, E. P., E. Chain, C. M. Fletcher, A. D. Gardner, N. G. Heatley, and M. A. Jennings) 'Further Observations on Penicillin.' *Lancet* ii: 177–189; 1949. (with Chain, E. B., N. G. Heatley, M. A. Jennings, A. G. Sanders, E. P. Abraham, and M. E. Florey) *Antibiotics. A Survey of Penicillin, Streptomycin and Other Antimicrobial Substances from Fungi, Actinomycetes, Bacteria and Plants* (Oxford).

Secondary: Lax, Eric, 2004. *The Mold in Dr Florey's Coat. The Remarkable True Story of the Penicillin Miracle* (New York); Williams, Trevor I., 1984. *Howard Florey. Penicillin and After* (Oxford); Macfarlane, Gwyn, 1979. *Howard Florey: The Making of a Great Scientist* (Oxford); Bickel, Lennard, 1972. *Rise Up to Life. A Biography of Howard Walter Florey Who Gave Penicillin to the World* (London); *DSB*; *Oxford DNB*.

David Greenwood

FLOYER, JOHN   (b. Hints, Staffordshire, England, 3 March 1649; d. Lichfield, England, 31 January 1734), *medicine.*

Floyer was the third child and second son of Richard Floyer, a barrister, and Elizabeth Babington. At the age of fifteen, he entered Queen's College, Oxford, to read medicine.

After graduating BA (1668), MB (1674), and MD (1680), Floyer returned to practice as a physician in Lichfield, near his place of birth. In 1680 he married Mary Fleetwood (née Archbold), with whom he had two sons. Floyer remained in Lichfield until his death in 1734, contributing extensively to the development of medical theory and practice through his many publications and also becoming a leading figure in the local community. Knighted by Charles II in 1684, he also served as a justice of the peace, a bailiff, a regular member of the grand jury, and a trustee of the Lichfield turnpike trust.

Floyer based his approach to health and disease particularly on Galenic formulations of humoral medicine and published medical treatises in a wide variety of areas. In 1687 his first book, *The Touchstone of Medicines*, attempted to classify plant remedies according to taste and smell and in line with the previous work of John Ray (1627–1707), with which Floyer was acquainted.

In 1698 Floyer published what is probably the first English monograph on asthma, *A Treatise of the Asthma*, which went through several English editions and was translated into French (1761). Himself a sufferer from the condition, Floyer strove to separate different types of shortness of breath, to identify the immediate causes of asthma attacks, and to determine the efficacy of certain treatments. In particular, his close observation of the onset and natural history of the symptoms of asthma enabled him to identify the lungs as the organic seat of the condition and to stress the importance of contraction of the 'muscular fibres of the Bronchia' in the pathogenesis of asthma. In addition, Floyer speculated on the significance of a family history of asthma and focused clinical attention on the role of environmental triggers, such as dust, feathers, atmospheric pollution, tobacco smoke, climate change, certain foods, exercise, and emotions.

Inspired both by Galen's studies of the pulse in health and disease and by Chinese approaches to pulse diagnosis, and using his studies of elderly almsmen in the hospital of St John the Baptist in Lichfield, Floyer devised a 'pulse watch' with a second hand in order to provide an exact measurement of the speed of the pulse. Floyer's meticulous approach to pulse diagnosis was published in 1707 as *The Physician's Pulse-Watch*.

Floyer also made substantial contributions to other areas of medical practice. For example, having visited many springs and wells around the country, he promoted the use of hydrotherapy, advocating in particular the value of cold bathing for infants and children. In addition, in 1724 he published an important medical study on care of the elderly, *Medicina Gerocomica: or, the Galenic Art of Preserving Old Men's Healths*. As in many of his other works, Floyer stressed the importance of fresh air, exercise, a regular diet, and moderation in alcohol and tobacco consumption. Floyer also wrote *Advice to a Young Student of Physic*, intended to provide a program of medical education for his grandson, who unfortunately died in childhood.

Floyer's publications exemplify the ambiguities inherent in early Enlightenment medical thought. Although skeptical of the impact of the natural sciences and clearly committed to traditional Hippocratic and Galenic medicine, Floyer was also pioneering in his emphasis on careful observation and experiment and in his use of novel technologies to enhance diagnosis and prognosis. Like many of his contemporaries, he was extremely well-read; his library, which contained medical treatises by leading European physicians and scholars, was donated to Queen's College, Oxford, where he had begun his lifelong commitment to medicine.

Bibliography

Primary: 1687. *The Touchstone of Medicines* (London); 1698. *A Treatise of the Asthma* (London); 1707. *The Physician's Pulse-Watch* (London).

Secondary: Jenner, Mark, 1998. 'Bathing and Baptism: Sir John Floyer and the Politics of Cold Bathing' in Sharpe, Kevin, and Steven N. Zwicker, eds., *Refiguring Revolutions: Aesthetics and Politics from the English Revolution to the Romantic Revolution* (Berkeley) pp. 197–216; Gibbs, D. D., 1969. 'Sir John Floyer, M.D. (1649–1734)' *British Medical Journal* i: 242–245; Townsend, Gary L., 1967. 'Sir John Floyer (1649–1734) and His Study of Pulse and Respiration.' *Journal of the History of Medicine and Allied Sciences* 22: 286–316; *Oxford DNB*.

Mark Jackson

FOLEY, HENRY L. H. (b. Vignory, Haute Marne, France, 11 April 1871; d. Vignory, France, 2 August 1956), *military medicine, oriental studies.*

The son of a civil servant, Foley started his education in his native village of Vignory, where he constantly won prizes. In 1890–1891 he graduated from the secondary school with a BA in philosophy and mathematics. In 1892 he joined the L'Ecole du Service de Santé Militaire in Lyon as one of fifty-six students, and graduated in 1895, sixth in his class. On completion of his doctoral thesis, he was promoted to the post of senior medical assistant, second-class. Unsuccessful in his desire to serve in China, Foley held a number of posts in France (in the rank of Médecin Major de 2me Classe) before becoming attached to the hospital in El Aricha and Oran, Algeria. This country became his destiny. Following the orders of General Lyautey, Foley was given charge of the hospital Beni-Ounif de Figuig, south of Oran near Algeria's border with Morocco. In 1914 Foley became the chief medical officer of the Maillot hospital in Algeria. His work was rewarded in January 1917 when Emile Roux, Director of the l'Institut Pasteur, nominated Foley for the Prix Monthyon of the Academy of Sciences for his work on recurrent fever and typhus.

At the end of World War I Foley was put in charge of the Saharan laboratory of the l'Institut Pasteur in Algeria. He was particularly concerned with training French medical servicemen, who were specialists in tropical diseases, his students obtaining unique information on these conditions. During a number of his appointments in Algeria, he modified the rules of the local public health administration and often introduced strict hygiene for the native medical personnel. He organized the public health services in the Algerian Sahara from 1918 to 1955. He was equally active in vaccination programs for the indigenous population. In 1908 he discovered the role played by the louse in the transmission of relapsing fever. This discovery led to the incrimination of the louse in the transmission of exanthematic typhus, of which the epidemiology is similar.

Foley also authored various works concerning aspects of pathology affecting the Saharan people.

Bibliography

Primary: 1930. *Moeurs et médecine des Touareg de l'Ahaggar* (Algiers); http://www.pasteur.fr/infosci/archives/fly1.html

Secondary: Doury, Paul, 1998. *Henry Foley. Apôtre du Sahara et de la medicine* (Hélette).

Nikolaj Serikoff

FØLLING, (IVAR) ASBJØRN

(b. Kvam, Norway, 23 August 1888; d. Oslo, Norway, 24 January 1973), *clinical biochemistry.*

Følling, the son of farmer Iver Følling and Mathilde Kaldal, grew up in a rural area in the middle part of Norway. His ancestors had been farmers for generations. At age fourteen he broke with this tradition, left the farm, and attended a secondary school in Trondheim. He continued his education at the Norwegian Institute of Technology in Trondheim and graduated in 1916 as a civil engineer in organic chemistry. He then moved to Oslo as an assistant at the Institute of Physiology, Faculty of Medicine, University of Oslo. Three years later he became assistant professor in the medical department, National Hospital (Rikshospitalet), where he was responsible for the management of the Clinical laboratory.

In addition to his full-time duties, first at the Institute of Physiology and later at Rikshospitalet, Følling also studied medicine, graduating as a medical doctor in 1922. From 1926 to 1930 he was a university fellow in clinical physiology, and with additional support from the Rockefeller Foundation he visited several of the leading medical centers in the United States. In 1929 he finished a PhD thesis on the renal reactions to the metabolic acidosis induced by ingestion of ammonium chloride (NH_4Cl). Three years later he was appointed professor in nutritional physiology, still working at Rikshospitalet. In the period from 1935 to 1953 he was professor of physiology and biochemistry at the Norwegian College of Veterinary Science. In 1953 he returned to Rikshospitalet as professor and head of the new Department of Clinical Chemistry. He resigned in 1958, at the age of seventy.

One day in January 1934 a young mother of two mentally retarded children knocked on Følling's door at the clinical laboratory at Rikshospitalet. She begged him to help find out why her children had become retarded. Being a kind and friendly person, he agreed to try, although his expectations were very small. After a clinical examination, which apart from the severe mental retardation did not yield any clues, he began to apply the different analytical methods of the laboratory on blood and urine from the siblings.

At that time Gerhardt's reaction in urine was a test that was used in the treatment of patients with diabetes mellitus. If the addition of ferric chloride ($FeCl_3$) to the urine resulted in a mahogany-like color, the urine contained abnormal quantities of some degradation products from fat ('ketone bodies'), indicating improper control of the disease. When applied to the urine of the two children, Gerhardt's reaction revealed an olive-green color, which then rapidly disappeared. Følling had never before seen this rapidly disappearing color. He set out to find the structure of the compound responsible for the phenomenon. After several weeks of intensive chemical detective work, he showed that the compound was phenylpyruvic acid. This acid was already known to the biochemical world, but it had never before been found in humans. Følling correctly suggested that it stemmed from the amino acid phenylalanine and that the accumulation in the two children was due to a metabolic defect in the degradation of phenylalanine. The first patients with 'oligophrenia phenylpyrouvica', or Følling's disease, had been discovered. Later the disease was named phenylketonuria, or PKU. For the rest of his professional life, Følling worked on different aspects of the disease and on the metabolism of phenylalanine.

The association between a genetically based disturbance in the intermediary metabolism and a profound mental defect had never been shown before. This discovery led to considerable optimism in the medical world regarding the possibilities for understanding and treating mental illness. Følling became highly decorated, receiving several national and international awards for his contributions.

Bibliography

Primary: 1934. 'Über Ausscheidung von Phenylbrenztraubensäure in der Harn als Stoffwechselanomalie in Verbindung mit Imbezilität.' *Hoppe-Seylers Zeitschrift für physiologische Chemie* 227: 169–176 [English trans. in Boyer, Samuel, ed., *Papers on Human Genetics* 1963 (Englewood Cliffs, NJ)].

Secondary: Scriver, Charles R., and Seymour Kaufman, 2001. 'Hyperphenylalaninemia: Phenylalanine Hydroxylase Deficiency' in Scriver, C. R., A. L. Beadet, W. S. Sly, and D. Valle, eds., *The Metabolic & Molecular Bases of Inherited Disease* (New York) pp. 1667–1724.

Oddvar Stokke

FOREEST (FORESTUS), PIETER VAN

(b. Alkmaar, the Netherlands, 15 November 1521; d. Alkmaar, 10 March 1597), *medicine.*

Van Foreest descended from a notable family, being the son of Jordaen van Foreest, bailiff of Bergen, and Margriet Nanning Beyersdochter. He attended the celebrated Latin school of Alkmaar, where Laurens Jacobsz. Zas, a Reformation leader in Holland, was among his teachers. In 1539 he enrolled at Louvain University. Unhappy with the theoretical character of the medical curriculum, he returned to his birth town the same year, to study with the Alkmaar town physician Melis Cornelisz, who was teaching from Arnald of Vilanova (1240–1311). Arnald, a follower of Avicenna (Ibn Sīnā), attached great importance to sensory observation. In 1540 van Foreest went to Italy to study at the universities of Padua (where he met Andreas Vesalius), Venice, and Ferarra. He graduated on 29 November 1543 in Bologna, where he studied with Benedictus Faventinus Hippocrates. After that, he worked in Rome, Paris, and Pithiviers (near Orleans). In May 1546 he set up practice in Alkmaar, where he married Eva van Teylingen, the daughter of a mayor. Although his tasks were those of a town physician, he was not appointed or paid accordingly.

In Alkmaar, van Foreest put his astronomical knowledge to use by compiling prognostications on a yearly basis: almanacs explaining the correlations between astronomical movements and morbidity patterns. In 1558 van Foreest was called to give medical assistance to the town of Delft, which was suffering heavily from a plague epidemic. He was to stay there for thirty-seven years. In 1575 he gave an inaugural address on the occasion of the opening of Leiden University. He did not, however, become professor. Preferring practice to teaching, he returned to Delft, where Prince William of Orange (whose corpse he embalmed in 1584) was among his patients. After the death of his wife, van Foreest returned to Alkmaar, where he practiced during the final two years of his life. His native town decided to honor him by appointing him as town physician with a princely salary.

Van Foreest is known for his criticism of quacks, uroscopists, and Paracelsians. Most of all, however, he is known as a keen observer, whose observations earned him the epithet 'the Dutch Hippocrates'. His Hippocratism 'seems to reflect the increasing flexibility of approach of traditionalist physicians in general from the 1560s onward, as they abandoned some of the more textbased approaches to medicine' (Nutton, 1989). Forestus' Observationes set a standard by supplying the 'observationes' and the 'scholia' of approximately 1,350 case histories. During the seventeenth century, his Opera omnia went through many reprints.

Bibliography

Primary: 1609–14. Observationum et curationum medicinalium ac chirurgicarum Opera Omnia (Frankfurt).

Secondary: Vis, Jurjen, 1998. 'Alkmaarse stadsdoctoren in de zestiende eeuw.' Gewina 21: 65–80; Bosman-Jelgersma, Henriëtte A., ed., 1996. Pieter van Foreest. De Hollandse Hippocrates (Krommenie); Nutton, Vivian, 1989. 'Pieter van Foreest and the Plagues of Europe: Some Observations on the Observationes' in Houtzager, H. L., ed., Pieter van Foreest. Een Hollands medicus in de zestiende eeuw (Amsterdam).

Jurjen Vis

FOREL, AUGUST (b. La Gracieuse, Switzerland, 1 September 1848; d. Yvorne, Switzerland, 27 July 1931), *entomology, psychiatry, hypnosis, neurology.*

In his youth Forel was fascinated by insects. He later recalled that his reading of Darwin's *Origin of Species* convinced him of the inseparability of psychology and brain physiology. Between 1866 and 1871 he studied medicine in Zurich, but did not pass his examinations. He went on to study brain anatomy with Theodor Meynert in Vienna, and graduated in 1872 with a thesis on the thalamus opticus of mammals. He then went to Munich, where he became an assistant physician under B. A. Von Gudden, with whom he had studied in Zurich. In 1875 Forel completed the first microscopic section of the whole brain, having contributed to making a useable brain microtome. He studied the topography of the trigeminal, pneumogastric, and hypoglossal nerves, and discovered the origin of the acoustic nerve. His depictions of the hypothalamus led to part of it being called the 'Campus Foreli'. In 1874 his *The Insects of Switzerland* appeared, which won several prizes. Forel sent a copy to Darwin and corresponded with him about ants. Thereafter, he continued to publish numerous significant works in entomology and went on study trips to collect specimens.

In 1879 he was appointed professor of psychiatry at the University of Zurich and Director of Burghölzli Asylum. There he established a laboratory for brain anatomy. In 1886, against the prevailing view that ganglion cells connected through anastomoses, he argued that they were directly connected by intertwining, similar to trees in a dense forest. His views were published the following year in a paper titled 'Einige hirnanatomische Betrachtungen und Ergebnisse' [Some brain anatomical considerations and results]. At the same time, Wilhelm His was coming to similar conclusions from a different basis, and they are jointly credited for formulating what was later called the neuron theory.

In 1883 Forel married Emma Steinheil, with whom he had six children. On reading Hippolyte Bernheim's *De la suggestion et de ses applications à la thérapeutique*, [Of suggestion and its applications to therapeutics] he became fascinated with hypnosis. In 1887, after a brief study with Bernheim in Nancy, he returned to Zurich and played a prominent role in promoting the practice of hypnotism and psychotherapy. Forel utilized hypnosis not only on the patients at the Burghölzli, but also on other doctors, attendants, and nurses. His 1889 work, *Der Hypnotismus und seine strafrechtliche Bedeutung* [Hypnotism and its criminal significance], went through many editions. In 1892 he founded the *Zeitschrift für Hypnotismus* with Jonas Grossmann. In 1902 this was renamed the *Jahrbuch für Psychologie und Neurologie*. In 1909 he founded the international society for medical psychology and psychotherapy. The aim of the society was to foster the development of a general science of psychotherapy through holding annual conferences, and Forel campaigned against the sectarianism of psychoanalysis.

Rejecting any form of dualism, Forel was a convinced monist. Thus he saw his wide-ranging interests—from brain anatomy and entomology to psychiatry and social reform—as essentially related. It was from ants, he claimed, that he learned the value of industry and community. Forel developed the conviction that a principal cause of insanity was alcoholism, and he became an active proponent of the temperance movement. It was for this reason that in 1898 he took early retirement from the Burghölzli, where he was succeeded by his former student Eugen Bleuler, and dedicated himself to the cause of social hygiene.

In 1905 he published *Die sexuelle Frage: Eine naturwissenschaftliche, psychologische, hygienische und soziologische Studie für Gebildete* [The sexual question: a natural scientific, psychological, hygienic, and social study for the educated]. The work was an encyclopedic study of sexuality in its evolutionary, biological, ethnological, pathological, and social aspects. In it Forel promoted social reform and the emancipation of women, militated against pornography and alcoholism, and controversially, was in favor of eugenics. The first edition sold out in two weeks, and it became a bestseller and was widely translated. In 1938 the work was banned in Germany by the National Socialists. In 1911 Forel suffered a stroke, which left him hemiplegic, but he learned to write with his left hand. During the war, he was active in the pacifist movement. In 1921 he joined the Bahá'i faith, which represented the religious expression of his monism. Forel maintained that it formed the basis through which all religions could be united.

Bibliography

Primary: 1874. *Les Fourmis de la Suisse* (Basel); 1906. *Hypnotism, or Suggestion and Psychotherapy* (London); 1908. *The Sexual Question* (New York); 1937. *Out of My Life and Work* (London).

Secondary: Meier, R., 1988. *August Forel 1848–1931: Arzt, Naturforscher, Sozialreformer* (Bern); Walser, H. H., 1968. *August Forel. Briefe Correspondance 1864–1927* (Bern).

Sonu Shamdasani

FOURCROY, ANTOINE FRANÇOIS DE   (b. Paris, France, 15 June 1755; d. Paris, 16 December 1809), *chemistry, medical education, politics, administration.*

Fourcroy's father, the scion of a noble family that had fallen on hard times, was a pharmacist employed in the household of the Duke of Orléans. One of his lodgers, the physician Félix Vicq d'Azyr, took an interest in the son and encouraged him to study medicine. They remained close as Vicq d'Azyr worked to build the new Royal Society of Med-

icine, chartered in 1778. Fourcroy received his doctorate from the Paris Medical Faculty in 1780, after his supporters in the Society paid the fee, which he could not afford. However, the Faculty, which was engaged in a bitter turf battle with the Society, refused him admission as a doctor regent, which would have allowed him to become a professor. As a result, the Society formally made him an associate. He actively contributed to its work, particularly the examination of mineral waters and proprietary medicines. Fourcroy had a very limited medical practice; instead he devoted himself to a career as chemist, teacher, and public official. He received appointments in chemistry at the Royal Veterinary School in Alfort (1783) and the Jardin du Roi (1784), the royal center for natural history in Paris. In 1785 the Academy of Sciences elected him as an associate member in chemistry.

Fourcroy welcomed the outbreak of the French Revolution in 1789. After the monarchy was overthrown in August 1792, he was elected as an alternate for the new National Convention; in July 1793 he filled the vacancy created by the assassination of Jean-Paul Marat. Fourcroy joined the radical Jacobin Club and played an active role in the Convention's Committee on Public Instruction. Following the fall of the Jacobin leadership in July 1794, he served on the Convention's Committee of Public Safety. As a member of a special commission he was charged with developing a plan for training medical practitioners, which the army desperately needed. The final legislation (4 December 1795) provided for a School of Health in Paris, with smaller ones at Strasbourg and Montpellier, to teach both medicine and surgery. Fourcroy became professor of chemistry at the Paris school. After Napoleon seized power in November 1799, Fourcroy joined the new Council of State; in 1802 he assumed additional responsibilities as Director General of Public Instruction. He played a key role in drafting major new laws regulating medical and pharmaceutical education and practice (1803) and other plans for the reform of French education. In 1808 Napoleon made him a count.

Fourcroy was an early exponent of the new quantitative chemistry. He conducted research linking chemistry, pharmacy, natural history, and medicine, often with collaborators, especially his former student Louis-Nicolas Vauquelin. Much of his work dealt with animal substances, including brain, bone, muscle fiber, mucus, bile, urine, bladder, and gallstones. He and Vauquelin isolated and named urea. In pharmacy he opposed the traditional practice of combining many different drugs and insisted that the clinician needed to know the precise properties of each ingredient.

Fourcroy's analysis of drugs and his work on the chemistry of living things contributed to a major reform of the materia medica and to the development of what we now call organic chemistry. The reorganization of medical and pharmaceutical education and practice, which he led, helped shape the modern health professions in France.

Bibliography

Primary: 1785. *L'Art de connaître et d'employer les médicaments dans les maladies qui attaquent le corps humain* 2 vols. (Paris); 1791–92. *La Médecine éclairée par les sciences physiques; ou, Journal des découvertes relatives aux différentes parties de l'art de guérir* 4 vols. (Paris).

Secondary: Viel, Claude, 2002. 'Antoine-François de Fourcroy (1755–1809), promoteur de la loi de Germinal an XI.' *Revue d'Histoire de la Pharmacie* 51: 377–394; Kersaint, Georges, 1966. *Antoine François de Fourcroy (1755-1809): sa vie et son œuvre* (Paris); Smeaton, William Arthur, 1962. *Fourcroy: Chemist and Revolutionary, 1755–1809* (Cambridge).

Matthew Ramsey

FOURNIER, JEAN-ALFRED (b. Paris, France, 12 May 1832; d. Paris, 23 December 1914), *venereal disease.*

Fournier was the child of Vincent Fournier, who worked in a customs office, and Anaïs Élisa Dumas. Raised in modest circumstances, Fournier first attended the Institution Jauffret before entering Lycée Charlemagne as a scholarship student. Fournier studied at the Paris Faculté de Médecine (graduated in 1860) before holding a series of internships under Edouard Chassaignac (1855), Germain Sée (1857), Bergeron (1858), Boucher de la Ville-Jossy (1859), and, most importantly, Philippe Ricord (1856). Fournier always recognized Ricord as 'his master' and he was widely regarded as Ricord's most important scientific legatee.

Fournier's early works, his studies of the nature of syphilitic contagion (1857), the syphilitic chancre (1860), and the incubation period of syphilis (1865), remained within the Ricordian mold. But while Fournier remained wedded to the methods of clinical observation championed by Ricord, Fournier tended to rely less on his hospital experience and more on his vast private practice for his most important research materials. Over the course of his career, Fournier maintained a detailed set of files on all his patients, a collection that by the end of his life was said to contain in excess of 30,000 case records, some of which tracked his patients for as long as twenty-five years after their initial infection. It was these records that provided Fournier with the material for his best-known contributions to medical science: his demonstration of the syphilitic origins of tabes dorsalis (1876) and general paresis (1893). These findings were challenged by many of the leading neurologists of the day. But if certain of Fournier's claims regarding 'parasyphilitic hysteria', 'hereditary hystero-syphilis', and the syphilitic origins of Little's disease (spastic diplegia) were exaggerated, the most important elements of his description of advanced syphilis were subsequently confirmed by modern bacteriology.

A prolific writer, Fournier authored more than a dozen books and innumerable articles, pamphlets, and reports, nearly all of which were devoted to the study of venereal disease. Named 'doctor of hospitals' in 1863, Fournier was appointed head physician at the Hôpital de Lourcine in 1868 before succeeding Alfred Hardy at the Hôpital Saint-Louis in 1876, where he remained until his retirement in 1902 (and where one can still visit the collection of pathological specimens Fournier helped to create). Beginning in the 1860s Fournier offered a regular course on venereal disease, first at Lourcine, subsequently at Saint-Louis. In 1879 he was named to the Paris Faculté de Médecine's newly created chair for Cutaneous and Syphilitic Diseases. In the same year he was elected to the Académie de Médecine.

Beginning in the 1870s Fournier increasingly turned his attention to questions of public health and 'antivenereal prophylaxis'. A founding member of the Société Française de Prophylaxie Sanitaire et Morale (1901), Fournier played a major role in delineating the precise outlines of the 'syphilitic peril' that was said to threaten the French nation and race. These concerns do much to explain Fournier's advocacy of mercurial cures lasting up to six years and more, a recommendation that appears to have had some effect on therapeutic trends. But most of Fournier's other recommendations (the passage of legislation regulating prostitution, the creation of special dispensaries for the treatment of venereal disease, the mandatory study of venereal disease for medical students, and public education of the dangers of venereal disease) remained a dead letter in his own day.

Bibliography

Primary: 1860. *De la contagion syphilitique* (Paris); 1882. *De l'ataxie locomotrice d'origine syphilitique (tabes spécifique)* (Paris); 1903. *Prophylaxie de la syphilis* (Paris).

Secondary: Tilles, Gérard, and Daniel Wallach, 2002. *La Dermatologie en France* (Paris); Corbin, Alain, 1990. *Women for Hire: Prostitution and Sexuality in France after 1850* (Cambridge); Crissey, John Thorne, and Lawrence Charles Parish, 1981. *The Dermatology and Syphilology of the Nineteenth Century* (New York).

Alex Dracobly

FRACASTORO, GIROLAMO (b. Verona, Italy, 1476–78; d. Incaffi, Italy, 6 August 1553), *medicine, contagion.*

Fracastoro, son of Paolo Filippo and Camilla Mascarelli, studied at the University of Padua, graduating *in artibus* in 1502 (*promotores:* Giovanni dell'Aquila, Girolamo della Torre, Gabriele Zerbi, Pietro Trapolino, and Marcantonio della Torre; *testes:* Tiberio da Bologna, Francesco Burana, and Marco Faella). At Padua Fracastoro studied philosophy with Pietro Pomponazzi and Nicolò Leonico Tomeo, and medicine with Marcantonio, Girolamo della Torre, and Alessandro Benedetti. In 1501 Fracastoro began lecturing in logic and in 1502 became *conciliarius anatomicus.* He maintained these engagements until 1509, when he left Padua because of the invasion by the Cambrai league. In 1508 Fracastoro was invited to enter the Academia Forojuliensis in Pordenone, under the patronage of Bartolomeo of Alviano. Here Fracastoro met with many men of letters, including Giulio Camillo Delminio, Giovanni Cotta, and Andrea Navagero. After Alviano's defeat at Agnadello in 1509, Fracastoro went back to Verona. He married Elena Clavi, with whom he had four sons and a daughter. In 1505 Fracastoro entered the Collegium of Physicians at Verona, becoming councilor and prior. In Verona Fracastoro also entered the Academia Gibertina of Gian Matteo Giberti (Bishop of Verona), becoming his personal physician. Here Fracastoro met scholars such as Ludovico Nogarola, Reginald Pole, and Marcantonio Flaminio. When in 1510 plague broke out, Fracastoro left Verona and retreated to Incaffi, on the slope of Monte Baldo, near the Lake of Garda. Here he created 'a private paradise' (Fracastoro, 1984, p. 3), where he worked on his treatises. However, he continued to practice medicine and alternated his stay at Incaffi with Verona. In 1545 he was appointed first physician of the Council of Trent and was the guest of cardinal Cristoforo Madruzzo. In 1547, with the physician Balduino de' Balduini, Fracastoro drew up the medical report of petechial typhus, which was used by Pope Paulus III to move the Council from Trento, which happened to be under the imperial jurisdiction of Charles V, to Bologna, a Church town. Fracastoro was then accused of having satisfied the pope's wishes of removing the Council from imperial control. This was another good reason for Fracastoro to return to Incaffi.

Among the people Fracastoro knew were men of letters such as Ludovico Ariosto, Mattia Bandello, and Aretino. Fracastoro quite certainly met Nicolaus Copernicus (1473–1543) at the University of Padua. It is possible he also met Albrecht Dürer (1471–1543) and Desiderius Erasmus (*c.* 1466–1536) during their visits to Padua. Fracastoro was tied to the world of the visual arts, and scholars have discussed his likely links with Raphael, Titian, Giorgione, and Mantegna. One of his close friends was the famous geographer Giambattista Ramusio, author of *Navigazioni e viaggi* (1550), dedicated to Fracastoro. The friendship between Ramusio and Fracastoro was demonstrated not only by the dedication, but also by Fracastoro's active contribution to Ramusio's work (for instance, Fracastoro was interested in purifying sugar) and the suggestions Ramusio wrote for Fracastoro's *De sympathia* (on sugar, on the functioning of the compass, and on the subject of antiperistasis). There is a collection of letters written by Fracastoro to Ramusio concerning botany, geography, astronomy, and medicine. This link was sealed by Fracastoro's friendship with Ramusio's son, Paolo, who was the editor of the first edition of Fracastoro's *Opera omnia* (Venice, 1555) and who is considered the likely author of Fracastoro's biography, first published in this edition. There are letters by Fracastoro to Paolo Ramusio, too, and a critical study of the Venetian edition of 1555 shows that Paolo worked on Fracastoro's texts many times. This editorial process was greatly praised by humanists, such as Ludovico Nogarola, who wrote an epigram on Paolo's work.

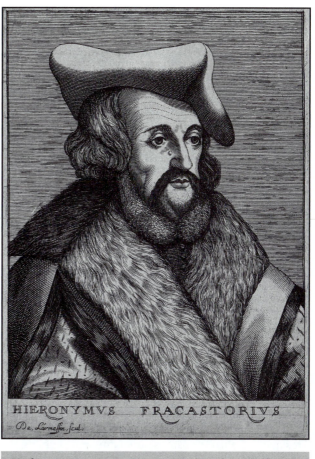

HIERONYMVS FRACASTORIVS
De. Larmessin. scul.

Girolamo Fracastoro. Line engraving by Nicolas de Larmessin, 1682. Iconographic Collection, Wellcome Library, London.

In addition Conrad Gesner visited Fracastoro in 1544 at Verona. The Zurich physician inserted Fracastoro's works in his *Bibliotheca Universalis*. And in 1541 Charles V, traveling from Germany to North Italy, stopped at Peschiera. When riding in the city, Cardinal Madruzzo pointed out Fracastoro, whom the emperor rewarded with a gesture of recognition.

Syphilis

Fracastoro started the poem *Syphilis sive morbus Gallicus* in the 1510s, and it was published in 1530 in Verona. The poem was dedicated to Pietro Bembo. The editors are not named in the first edition, but it is likely they were the Da Sabbio brothers, whom Bishop Giberti brought to Verona from Venice especially to print Greek texts. This edition was preceded by a Venetian pirated edition, published with many errors and without the author's *imprimatur*. In 1525 Fracastoro presented the poem in two books to Bembo, who especially praised the second book, full of Virgilian figures. He commended the description of the Holy Tree (*Guaiacum*), but invited Fracastoro to eliminate the mercury myth. He was worried because of Fracastoro's intention to write a third book, including the myth of Syphilus, and to let the mercury myth remain in the second book. But Fracastoro went on in his own way and published his work in 1530.

From the end of the fifteenth century, there was a great debate about the spread of syphilis, its American origin, and ways of propagation. Fracastoro was among those scholars who refuted the disease's American origin, as claimed in Book I of *Syphilis*, even if he recognized that it was an unfamiliar disease in Europe. This did not mean, however, that it was a very new disease; instead, he viewed it as an example of the way nature acted, spreading her *genitalia semina* [seeds] through the earth, water, and air. These seeds could become active after different periods of gestation, that is, a short time or a long period, with syphilis belonging to the last category. Fracastoro underlined the role of air and sky in the spread and origin of syphilis, comparing it to the Black Death. He then dwelt on the description of symptoms. Book II was dedicated to prophylaxis, describing the role of *atra bilis*, of environment, of exercise and diet; and then to therapy, where readers found the myth of Ilceus to justify treatment by mercury. Book III dealt with the discovery of the New World, especially *Hispana*. Here the *Guaiacum* tree presented the only hope for those for whom syphilis was an eternal plague. The Spaniards violated the paradise of the New World by their guns, attracting the wrath of Apollo, who sent syphilis to them. This myth recalled the natives on Atlantis and Syphilus, the shepherd, who aroused Apollo's wrath by his impiety. The disease was God's punishment; *Guaiacum* was the therapy for this disease. But Fracastoro concluded his poem by confirming that syphilis spread in Europe independently from America. The name given to the disease comes from Fracastoro's poem title and his myth of Syphilus.

Fracastoro worked on syphilis on two other occasions. First, he wrote an unpublished prose treatise on syphilis, always addressed to Bembo (Fracastoro, 1939). Here Fracastoro dealt more carefully with the medical issues, free from the constraints of poetical rules. Confirming the native origin of syphilis over notions of an American origin, nevertheless he rejected its identification with elephantine disease and leprosy, and claimed a humoral—phlegmatic—origin. Fracastoro showed the same attitude in the chapters on syphilis in *De contagione*, in which he claimed that the disease was new not because of its foreign origin, but because its signs rested unknown for a long time. Fracastoro again maintained the phlegmatic nature of syphilis and the efficacy of mercury and Holy Tree therapy.

Critical Days

In 1538 Fracastoro published *Homocentricorum sive de stellis liber unus* with a short treatise on the doctrine of critical days, *De causis criticorum dierum libellus*. In the vast field of astrological medicine, a critical day was the day during a disease, especially fever, when the patient experienced a crisis. Galen elaborated a complex astrological and astronomical doctrine in his *De diebus decretoriis*, linking the crisis with lunar phases. This doctrine gave rise to a huge tradition, ranging from Jewish and Arabic medicine to the medieval and Renaissance medicine of Europe. Fracastoro wrote against this tradition, attacking the physicians who followed the astrologers. In his opinion, the critical days of fevers should not to be related to lunar phases, but to overlapping cycles of humoral paroxysms, particularly of yellow and black bile. The complex calculation of critical days was based on the sliding of the humoral paroxysms.

Fracastoro fought against astrology and astrological medicine according to Giovanni Pico's *Disputationes adversus astrologiam divinatricem* and raised a violent reaction. In the second half of the sixteenth century, physicians and astronomers such as Andrea Turini, Michelangelo Biondo, and Luca Gaurico wrote against Fracastoro's treatise. Only in the seventeenth century was Fracastoro defended by Jacques Fontaine and his text translated into Italian by Troilo Lancetta.

Contagion

In 1546 Fracastoro published in Venice, with the help of the heirs of Lucantonio Giunti, *De sympathia et antipathia rerum liber unus* and *De contagione et contagiosis morbis et eorum curatione*. *De sympathia*, conceived as a commentary on *De contagione*, gave it a theoretical framework devoted to refuting astrological doctrines traditionally tied to the argument of contagion. Contagion was considered but one of the *mirabilia* [marvels] of nature. To demonstrate that all marvelous natural phenomena can be explained without recourse to astrological arguments, Fracastoro grasped the concept of sympathy from the neoplatonic tradition and inserted it into an Aristotelian physics. He dealt with physical, alchemical, physiological, and psychological phenomena, expounding the principles of natural philosophy necessary to the interpretation of contagion. The first book of *De contagione* dealt with the theory of contagion, its nature, the many kinds of contagion, the causality, the difference between contagious disease, noncontagious disease, and poisons, and the signs of contagion. The second book analyzed the different kinds of contagious disease, such as contagious fevers, poxes and measles, pestilential fevers, exanthematous typhus (namely *lenticulae vel puncticulae*), plague, contagious phthisis, rabies, syphilis, elephantiasis, leprosy, scabies, and cutaneous infections. The third book was concerned with therapy, discussing treatment of each of the contagious diseases mentioned.

Fracastoro has frequently been considered the forerunner of modern bacteriology and the notion of *contagium vivum*, because of his theory of contagious disease's seeds (*seminaria*) and the doctrine of affinity between the seed and its recipient.

It has also been claimed that Fracastoro revived the atomistic tradition of Lucretian *semina* and built his idea of contagion on it. But when reading *De contagione* accompanied by its commentary, *De sympathia*, Fracastoro's epistemological strategy becomes clearer. For instance, even if a Lucretian influence is undeniable (especially on the poetry), the Aristotelian corpuscular doctrine expounded in *De sympathia* to explain the structure of bodies, but not matter, where atomism was suggested, was used to reject atomism itself. Bodies were composed of particles and not atoms. *Seminaria* were the product of the putrefaction and dissolution of such structured bodies and *seminaria* therefore became compatible with Aristotelian physics and the Neoplatonic sympathy. In fact, their way of acting was ruled by their affinity (*analogia*) with the body that they entered. This *analogia* is one of the major subjects of *De sympathia*.

Bibliography

Primary: 1538. *Homocentricorum sive de stellis liber unus. Eiusdem De causis criticorum dierum per ea quae sunt in nobis* (Venice); 1546. *De sympathia et antipathia rerum liber unus, De contagione et contagiosis morbis et curatione libri tres* (Venice); 1930. *De contagione et contagiosis morbis et eorum curatione, libri III.* Translation and notes by Wilmer Cave Wright (New York and London); 1939. (Pellegrini, Francesco, ed.) *Trattato inedito in prosa di Gerolamo Fracastoro sulla sifilide* (Verona); 1984. *Fracastoro's Syphilis.* Introduction, text, translation and notes with a computer-generated word index by Geoffrey Eatough (Liverpool).

Secondary: Peruzzi, Enrico, 1997. 'Fracastoro, Girolamo.' *DBI* 49: 543b–548a; Nutton, Vivian, 1983. 'The Seeds of Contagion: An Explanation of Contagion and Infection from the Greeks to the Renaissance.' *Medical History* 27: 1–34; Martellozzo Forin, Elda, 1969. *Acta graduum academicorum ab anno 1501 ad annum 1525* (Padua): schedule no. 174; *DSB*

Concetta Pennuto

FRAGA, CLEMENTINO   (b. Muritiba, Brazil, 15 September 1880; d. Rio de Janeiro, Brazil, 8 January 1971), *clinical medicine, medical education, public health.*

Fraga graduated in 1903 from the School of Medicine of Bahia, city of Salvador, and became assistant professor at the school the following year. In 1906 he moved to Rio de Janeiro, then the capital of Brazil, where he worked as sanitary inspector in the campaign against yellow fever led by Oswaldo Cruz. Fraga also practiced medicine at Santa Casa de Misericórdia Hospital, the main medical establishment of its kind in the city.

In 1910 Fraga returned to Salvador, resuming his position at the School of Medicine. In 1914 he received the title of full professor, continuing to teach the course of Medical Practice. In 1917 he was appointed chief of the National Sanitary Commission in charge of yellow fever in Bahia; between September and December 1918 he helped organize emergency services for Spanish influenza victims in Rio. Through his work he established a strong reputation among official and medical agencies. From 1921 to 1926 he was elected to represent Bahia in the Chamber of Deputies and participated in the debates concerning health and educational reforms. Because of his parliamentary activities, in 1926 he moved to Rio de Janeiro and became professor at the School of Medicine of Rio de Janeiro.

In 1926 Fraga replaced Carlos Chagas in the direction of the National Department of Public Health. From the highest position in the emergent Brazilian public health system, he led the fight against the return of yellow fever to Rio between 1928 and 1929. It is important to mention that the fever had been controlled by Oswaldo Cruz some twenty years before in the city, and its reemergence in the late 1920s implied a rethinking of the earlier concepts and methods used to control the fever. Public health under Fraga's administration strengthened the cooperation between Brazil and the International Health Division of the Rockefeller Foundation in the fight against yellow fever. After the so-called 1930s Revolution, a populist and authoritarian movement that overthrew the elected government, Fraga resigned.

The new regime kept Fraga out of public office. He instead devoted his time to teaching, medical practice, and the study of tuberculosis. Seeking to innovate the study of tuberculosis in Rio's Medical School, in 1930 he created a special training course. For twelve years, until his retirement in 1942, Fraga taught the course, which attracted hundreds of young doctors and a number of renowned foreign professors such as Émile Sergent, Robert Debré, and Edouard Rist. In the late 1930s Fraga was appointed Professor Emeritus at the Schools of Medicine of Bahia and Rio and a member of the Brazilian Academy of Medicine. From 1937 to 1940 he was the Director of Health and Assistance in the country's capital. In 1954 he briefly returned to politics, representing Rio de Janeiro in the House of Deputies. Fraga remained active as a physician, lecturer, and educator, participating in many congresses and scientific societies. Following a literary tradition of Brazilian physicians, Fraga published several works of biographies and memoirs. In 1938 he was elected member of the prestigious Brazilian Academy of Literature.

Fraga died at age ninety. His was one of the longest and most important medical careers in Brazil during the twentieth century. His career was exemplary in combining so many aspects, namely medical education, public health, clinical research, politics, and literature.

Bibliography

Primary: 1929. *A Febre Amarela no Brasil—Notas e documentos de uma grande campanha sanitária* (Rio de Janeiro).

Secondary: 2001. 'Clementino Fraga' in Beloch, Israel, and Alzira Abreu, eds., *Dicionário histórico-biográfico Brasileiro: 1930–1983* (Rio de Janeiro) pp. 1340–1341; Coutinho, Afrânio, et al., eds., 1980. *Clementino Fraga: itinerário de uma vida* (Rio de Janeiro).

Gilberto Hochman

FRANCO, ROBERTO (b. Chimbe, Colombia, 1 June 1874; d. New York, New York, USA, 4 July 1958), *tropical medicine.*

Franco was born in a small country town in Colombia and attended the Universidad Nacional de Colombia (UNC) (1891–97), graduating MD. He continued his medical studies at the Paris School of Medicine and at the Paris Institute of Colonial Medicine (1903). In the same year, he also worked briefly with Charles Nicolle in Tunisia and spent four months at the London School of Tropical Medicine. In short, he received a remarkable education studying tropical medicine in Europe.

After returning to Bogotá, in 1904 Franco founded the Chair of Tropical Medicine at UNC, with a laboratory attached to the chair. He was the holder of the chair from 1905 to 1940. In 1907 Franco and two students investigated an epidemic in Muzo's emerald mines, located in a valley near the Colombian Andes. They concluded that it was yellow fever, acquired by laborers during the day in the nearby jungle, not in the urban zones. However, they did not identify the vector that transmitted the disease. This was the first formulation of the concept of 'jungle yellow fever', which went against the common idea that the fever was an urban disease transmitted only by the *Aedes aegypti* mosquito (inspired by the sanitation of Havana in 1901 and Rockefeller Foundation campaigns in the early 1920s). Franco's reports, published only in local medical journals (1907 and 1911), explain why the discovery was internationally unknown. Eventually the epidemic subsided, and the group shifted its interest to hookworm, which was widespread in Colombia. Franco organized the first campaign against this disease (1911) among coffee growers, who produced the main export product of the country. Some years later this work was supported by the Rockefeller Foundation hookworm campaign (1920–35), with Franco serving as an advisor.

Franco's early work on yellow fever became a matter of debate with the Rockefeller Foundation. Members of the Foundation visited Muzo frequently between 1916 and 1930 and rejected Franco's conclusions because they could not find *Aedes aegypti*. In 1932 Kerr and Patiño-Camargo from Rockefeller used mice protection tests to demonstrate that people from Muzo had been exposed to jungle yellow fever some time ago. They argued that Franco's 1907 diagnosis was correct, but they did so in Rockefeller terms. In 1934 Fred L. Soper from Rockefeller 'rediscovered' jungle yellow fever in Brazil and recognized the priority of Franco's discovery. Soper's discovery established the disease's natural reservoir in the Amazon and suspected it could be transmitted by several kinds of mosquitoes. Thanks to this recognition, Franco was considered a national celebrity (his 1911 report was republished in 1936).

Franco was appointed Dean of the Faculty of Medicine of UNC (1924–26), and President of the prestigious National Academy of Medicine. He was also on the editorial board of the Academy's journal, *Revista Médica de Bogotá.* He helped to organize a number of major national medical events and gave a scientific status to the study and practice of tropical medicine in his home country. In 1937 he was appointed President of the UNC. Some years later he became the head of the new University of Los Andes in Bogotá (1948–51), a school created by a group that followed the North American models of higher education.

Bibliography

Primary: 1907. 'Informe presentado al sindicato de Muzo por la misión encargada de estudiar la epidemia de fiebre observada en la mina en los meses de marzo y abril de 1907.' *Revista Médica de Bogotá* 28(331): 93–105; 1910. 'Anemia tropical, uncinariasis o anquilostomasia.' *Revista Nacional de Agricultura* 8/9: 229–281; 1911. 'Fiebre amarilla y fiebre espiroquetal; endemias y epidemias en Muzo, de 1907 a 1910.' *Sesiones Científicas del Centenario.* vol. 1 (Bogotá).

Secondary: Quevedo, Emilio, et al., 2005. *Café y gusanos, mosquitos y petróleo. El tránsito de la higiene hacia la salud pública en Colombia, 1873–1953* (Bogotá).

Emilio Quevedo

FRANK, JOHANN PETER (b. Rodalben near Pirmasens, Germany, 19 March 1745; d. Vienna, Austria, 24 April 1821), *medicine, social medicine.*

Frank was born in the Palatinate, the eleventh of fourteen children. His father was a merchant, his mother the daughter of a bailiff. He entered the university in Metz at the age fifteen, studied philosophy, and earned a doctoral degree. In 1763 he registered as a medical student at the University of Heidelberg. After graduating in medicine, he practiced as a physician in the vicinity of Pirmasens. There he became the deputy of the district doctor and the court physician to the margrave. But his actual career did not begin until 1774, when he became the personal physician of the Prince-Bishop of Speyer. In this function, he found an opportunity to combine the wealth of personal experience he had gathered during his practice as a doctor with his ideas for reform in the health care system. In 1783 he published the first three volumes of his *System einer vollständigen medicinischen Polizey* (*A System of Complete Medical Police*). In part in response to this work and its reception, he was appointed to the chair for Practical Medicine at the University of Göttingen. A year later he accepted an appointment as successor to S. A. Tissot at the University of Pavia. In 1786 he was entrusted with the task of reforming the health care system in Lombardy. In 1795 he entered the Austrian state medical system when he was appointed director of the Vienna Hospital. In 1804 he was called to fill the chair of Professor of the Medical Clinic at the University of Vilna. Three years later he was appointed to the staff of the Medical-Surgical Clinic in St Petersburg; at the same time he became the personal physician of the Russian tsar. For reasons of health he returned to Freiburg in 1809, and after the death of his daughter who resided there, he relocated once again to Vienna. After he had turned down Napoleon's offer to

FRANK, JOHANN PETER 515

become inspector general of his health care system, Frank remained as a personal physician in Vienna until his death.

The State, Health Care, and Medicine

Frank became known not only for his medical writings but also for his program to reform the state health care system in the second half of the eighteenth century. This reform program was in keeping with the political aims of the territories in the German Empire. In order to strengthen the economy, there was interest in increasing industrial production. Necessary for this was not only a large force of workers but a strong and healthy population. Population policy became a centerpiece of measures in economic policy. The guiding concept was that the wealth of a state could be measured by the size of its healthy population. Care for the health of the individual thus became a political obligation for the benefit of the state. This was the point of departure for Frank and several other academically trained physicians. On the basis of their competence, they considered themselves able to present programs to the authorities to achieve these goals. The medical profession and the government regarded themselves here as partners, sharing a joint responsibility for the care of the general population.

Frank's working assumption was that disease is a social phenomenon. His interest was centered not on the individual but rather on the factors in social life that might cause disease. He viewed human society in analogy to the human body. Both were subject to similar laws. In keeping with this concept, the physician was able to investigate and treat both the human being and society, utilizing medical and biological means for this purpose.

Frank viewed eighteenth-century society as a sick patient. In order to heal this patient, it was first necessary to analyze the causes of the malady in order to recommend appropriate therapeutic measures. In his eyes, this was the task of medicine. It was the job of the authorities to implement the proposals. Their task was to regulate and control the social life of the subjects by laws and corresponding police directives.

Frank and his associates relied on two main pillars in order to achieve the goal of a healthy population and thus a healthy state: a reform of the health care system and prophylaxis by means of public enlightenment. In reforming the system, Frank drew on his wealth of experience as a practical physician. Already at that time, he had been busy engaged in working out regulations for midwives and the establishment of a school for midwifery, as well as a code of regulations for restructuring the system of military surgery. Along with the training of medical practitioners, government programs were to be developed dealing with protection from infectious diseases and care for the poor, the sick, and orphaned.

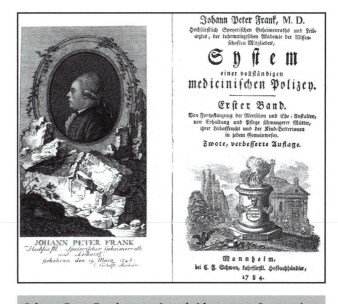

Johann Peter Frank, portrait and title page to *System einer vollständigen medicinischen Polizey.* Mannheim, 1784. Rare Books, Wellcome Library, London.

But each individual was expected to care for his own health as well in order to promote the well-being of the state as a whole. Using pamphlets and other written material on good health practices, attempts were made to reach and instruct the general population.

Medical Police

Against the backdrop of this relationship between the state, health, and medicine, Frank developed his concrete measures for the 'medical police', as they were termed in the discourse of the era. In his six-volume treatise *System einer vollstaendigen medizinischen Polizey,* he spelled out his conceptions. The concept 'medical police' pointed to the obligation of the authorities to deal with the life and health of the subjects and to monitor their behavior. Frank worked on this fundamental study for much of his life. The first three volumes appeared between 1779 and 1783, and volume four in 1788. He completed the two final volumes in 1813 and 1817–19, after he had withdrawn from his official functions.

In this work Frank was guided by two main tasks. He wished to investigate social living conditions with respect to the possible threat they posed for health, while at the same time making recommendations to the authorities about how the government could deal with this danger by means of state laws and regulations. Such an extensive undertaking demanded a *system,* as indicated in the work's title. Its systematic qualities were anchored in the normal biography of the human being. It began with conception, then went on to birth and upbringing, dealt with dietary measures such as movement and proper food, and included other factors such as clothing, housing and cleanliness, and public hygiene in the towns; it concluded with the burial of the citizen.

Operating under the premise that the state should intervene at the earliest possible point in time, Frank looked at the reproductive behavior of the subjects of the state. This thematic complex was of greatest importance in respect to the quantitative and qualitative improvement of the condition of the population. Frank analyzed it in two ways: in regard to the society and to the individual. For society it was important to take steps to ensure that as many children as possible were conceived who could survive in good health, and thus be useful to the state. For the individual, it was important that the sexuality of the state's subjects, which they could not control and supervise themselves, was regulated in such a way by government measures so as to achieve the overarching aim.

Frank pinpointed several conditioning factors that led to a bad physical constitution in offspring. Thus, he considered the age of the parents—either too young, too old, or unequal in age—as a factor influencing a weak constitution in their descendants; poor health of the parents was also a factor. In Frank's view, the only institution that could guarantee any improvement in this condition was matrimony. That was why it should be subject to very strict government supervision.

For example, Frank called for legal limits to be set for the age for marriage. In order to heighten prospects for healthy progeny and to prevent unhealthy offspring, documents should be obtained attesting to the state of health of the prospective marriage partners. Unhealthy couples should be prevented from procreating, while healthy individuals should be encouraged by means of financial incentives to have children. This program should be bolstered by educational measures, because it was important to better not only the physical condition of the human being but also his moral constitution.

Frank's work contained similar restrictive proposals for all spheres of life. Frank took into account everything that could endanger the person from the moment of conception to death, and thus ultimately could restrict him in his primary task as a 'useful' citizen of the state. With the aid of laws, reforms in medical policy, and educational measures, Frank hoped to eliminate illnesses and other negative influences for society over the long term.

Impact

Even during his lifetime, Frank's work attracted great attention and respect, but it also sparked criticism. The extensive powers that Frank accorded the authorities over the lives of their subjects led to the criticism that his reform proposals were excessively oriented to favor laws and regulations of the state. Thus, those reforms were never implemented. However, they would have also been very difficult to put into practice due to economic reasons and technical problems of administration.

But precisely as an idealistic program, Frank's conception subsequently provided rich soil for differing patterns of interpretation. With his focus on the state as the arbiter of the health of society, Frank raised basic questions dealing with the relationship between society, illness, and health. This problematic area was the core focus in the fields of social medicine and public hygiene that established themselves at the end of the nineteenth century. Therefore it is only natural to attempt to identify lines of continuity between Frank and these disciplines. His ideas were also compatible with the later eugenic and race-political concepts of National Socialism. So it is not surprising that in the Nazi era, Frank was widely read and cited. Aside from these linear influences, in more recent research Frank is interpreted against the backdrop of the concepts of social disciplining and the medicalization of society. The intent to regulate and supervise society emerges in great clarity in Johann Peter Frank's work and ideas. It was indeed a hallmark of the territorial states and principalities of the German Empire in the eighteenth century.

Bibliography

Primary: 1779–1819. *System einer vollständigen medicinischen Polizey* . . . 6 vols. (Mannheim, Tübingen, Vienna); 1976. (Lesky, Erna, ed. and intro) *A System of Complete Medical Police* (Baltimore).

Secondary: Pieper, Markus, 1998. 'Der Körper des Volkes und der gesunde Volkskörper. Johann Peter Franks "System einer vollstaendigen medicinischen Polizey".' *Zeitschrift für Geschichtswissenschaft* 46: 97–119; Seidler, Eduard, 1996. 'Anfänge einer sozialen Medizin. Johann Peter Frank und sein "System einer vollständigen medicinischen Polizey"' in Schott, Heinz, ed., *Meilensteine der Medizin* (Dortmund) pp. 258–264; Seidler, Eduard, 1991. 'Johann Peter Frank (1745–1821)' in Engelhardt, Dietrich von, and Fritz Hartmann, eds., *Klassiker der Medizin. Von Hippokrates bis Christoph Wilhelm Hufeland*, vol. 1 (Munich) pp. 291–308; Barthel, Christian, 1989. *Medizinische Polizey und medizinische Aufklärung. Aspekte des öffentlichen Gesundheitsdiskurses im 18. Jahrhundert* (Frankfurt and New York).

Jürgen Helm and
Karin Stukenbrock

FREEMAN, JOHN (b. Leeds, England, 18 July 1876; d. ?, 18 January 1962), *allergy, clinical immunology.*

Freeman, the son of J. J. Freeman, CBE, a solicitor, was educated at Charterhouse School before beginning his medical degree at Oxford. After serving with the Oxfordshire Light Infantry in South Africa, Freeman resumed his medical studies at St Mary's Hospital in London. After graduating in 1905 and then studying at the Pasteur Institute in Paris, he joined the Bacteriology Department at St Mary's run by Sir Almroth Wright (1861–1947). In 1907, after his marriage to Violet Alice Leslie Hadden, Freeman spent a year in Vienna on a Radcliffe Travelling Fellowship before returning to St Mary's to take up a research position in Wright's department, contributing initially to Wright's influential studies of vaccine therapy.

In 1907 Freeman persuaded an old school friend, Leonard Noon (1877–1913) to join him at St Mary's. Together, Freeman and Noon began to expand their clinical interest in immunization to the development of vaccines against hay fever. The study of hay fever was to occupy Noon until his premature death from tuberculosis in 1913 and, together with research on other allergic conditions, came to dominate the whole of Freeman's professional life, both in the laboratory and the clinic, until his own death in 1962.

The central features of Freeman and Noon's approach to hay fever first appeared in *Lancet* in 1911. Convinced that active immunization was preferable to the passive immunization that had been developed by William P. Dunbar (1863–1922) at the State Hygienic Institute in Hamburg, Freeman and Noon attempted to vaccinate hay fever sufferers against the effects of pollen by injecting them subcutaneously with increasing doses of pollen extract. Encouraged by the results, Freeman subsequently not only expanded this approach to other allergic diseases (such as asthma, food allergies, and reactions to bee stings) but also devised novel treatment protocols to suit the demands of his many private patients. The central features of Freeman's rather idiosyncratic approach to allergy were clearly set out in his major monograph, *Hay-Fever: A Key to the Allergic Disorders* (1950).

Adopted by allergists across Europe and North America, desensitization or immunotherapy rapidly became the cornerstone of clinical allergy practice, constituting the treatment of choice even after the introduction of new pharmaceutical agents, such as antihistamines and inhaled steroids, during the post–World War II decades. In the 1980s, however, as doubts about the safety and efficacy of the procedure escalated, intervention from the Committee on Safety of Medicines sparked controversies about the role of immunotherapy, and the practice was effectively curtailed in Britain.

In spite of ongoing disputes about his major therapeutic innovation, Freeman's unique brand of clinical holism, his commitment to fostering a close relationship between laboratory research and clinical practice, and his contributions to professional societies for pathologists and allergists clearly shaped the development of allergy and clinical immunology in Britain, Europe, and North America. Under Freeman's directorship, St Mary's Allergy Department housed the largest allergy clinic in the world, not only attracting eminent visiting researchers from many countries and generating media interest, but also training subsequent generations of allergists through programs of postgraduate lectures and research fellowships. In 1976 a feature article in *The Times* paid expansive tribute to Freeman's legacy by referring to the extent to which St Mary's had become 'to allergies what the Pasteur Institute is to viruses'.

Bibliography

Primary: 1911. 'Further observations on the treatment of hay fever by the hypodermic inoculations of pollen vaccine.' *Lancet* ii: 814–817; 1914. 'Vaccination against hay fever.' *Lancet* i: 1178–1180; 1950. *Hay-Fever: A Key to the Allergic Disorders* (London).

Secondary: Jackson, Mark, 2003. 'John Freeman, Hay Fever and the Origins of Clinical Allergy in Britain, 1900–1950.' *Studies in History and Philosophy of Biological and Biomedical Sciences* 34: 473–490; [Anon.], 1963. 'Obituary: John Freeman.' *Journal of Pathology and Bacteriology* 85: 243–247.

Mark Jackson

FRERICHS, FRIEDRICH THEODOR (b. Aurich, Fresia [now Germany], 24 March 1819; d. Berlin, Germany, 14 March 1885), *medicine.*

The son of a landowner, Frerichs studied medicine in Göttingen from 1838 to 1841, and then practiced as an ophthalmologist in Aurich. He returned to Göttingen in 1846 in order to prepare his habilitation, and was then appointed extraordinary Professor of Special Pathology and Therapy. Frerichs started to conduct chemical investigations during this period of study (*Investigations into the physiological and pathological role of bile*, Thesis 1845). Following his appointment, he continued this work, leading Rudolf Wagner to entrust him with a number of contributions to his *Companion to Physiology* (1842–53), including the chapter on digestion. Frerichs would remain faithful to the study of this topic throughout his whole scientific career. In 1850 he was recruited at Kiel, and in 1852 he was appointed both Professor of Special Pathology and Therapy and Director of the Medical Clinic in Breslau. Frerichs was able to transfer from this small teaching clinic to the City Hospital, where he had access to all patients. He set up a chemical and microscopy laboratory in two rooms of the hospital, which enabled him to combine bedside observations with chemico-physiological investigations. This allowed him to be the first to identify the elimination of tyrosine and leucine in the urine of patients suffering from kidney disease, as well as identifying other metabolic products. Thus, Frerichs's research contributed significantly to knowledge about kidney disease and diabetes, confirming his place as a pioneering figure in both clinical chemistry and experimental patho-physiology.

In 1859, at the height of his fame as a clinician, Frerichs succeeded Lukas Schönlein as the director of the University Medical Clinic in Berlin; in addition he became a Medical Advisor to the Minister of Culture. Overworked, he no longer had any time to conduct experiments in the small laboratory that had been built for him under a staircase of the 'Old Charité'. At Frerichs's request, the new anatomy building constructed in 1865 included a three-room laboratory in which numerous pupils, including Bernhardt Naunyn, Marcel Nencki, and Carl Anton Ewald, were able to further Frerichs's research interests by conducting experiments into the composition of bodily fluids and the analysis of metabolic processes. Frerichs himself increasingly focused his attention on clinical teaching, and his lectures based on clinical cases became famous because of their clarity and his use of everyday language. Frerichs especially impressed his audience with his extremely precise clinical information, his nuanced descriptions of pathological changes, and his reliable diagnoses, even though Rudolf Virchow refuted many of them, albeit in a friendly spirit.

Frerichs was also active in the sphere of the organization of science. In collaboration with Ernst von Leyden, he founded the *Zeitschrift für klinische Medizin* in 1879, as well as the Verein für Innere Medicin zu Berlin in 1881, the forerunner of the Society for Internal Medicine founded in 1882 of which Frerichs was the first president. Although never proven, Frerichs's death in 1885 was tinged with the suspicion of suicide. As he suffered from colic, the thesis of an opium overdose cannot, however, be ruled out.

Bibliography

Primary: 1851. *Die Bright'sche Nierenkrankheit und deren Behandlung* (Braunschweig); 1858–61. *Klinik der Leberkrankheiten* 2 vols. (Braunschweig) [English trans., 1861 (London)]; 1884. *Ueber den Diabetes* (Berlin).

Secondary: Franken, Franz Hermann, 1994. *Friedrich Theodor Frerichs (1819–1885). Leben und hepatologisches Werk.* Thesis, Freiburg.

Volker Hess

FREUD, ANNA   (b. Vienna, Austria, 3 December 1895; d. London, England, 9 October 1982), *psychoanalysis, child analysis, child care.*

Freud was the youngest of six children of Martha and Sigmund Freud. She studied to be a teacher, but from an early age her interests were drawn toward psychoanalysis. Commencing in 1918, Freud analyzed her himself. Highly questionable, perhaps even constituting malpractice from the standpoint of psychoanalytic theory, this fact was kept as a tightly maintained secret. Anna Freud quickly became a central figure in the institutional world of psychoanalysis. In 1922 she became a member of the Vienna Psychoanalytic Society and began practicing in the following year. In 1924 after the departure of Otto Rank (1884–1939), she took his place in Freud's 'secret committee', which controlled the psychoanalytic movement behind the scenes. In 1925 she became involved with the Internationale Psychoanalytische Verlag (publishing house), and became the secretary of the newly founded Vienna Psychoanalytic Institute. From 1927 to 1934, she was general secretary of the International Psychoanalytic Association.

Child analysis was the field in which she found her métier. In 1927 she published her first book, *Einführung in der Technik der Kinderanalyse* [Introduction to the Technique of Child Analysis]. In the 1930s, she established the Jackson nursery with Dorothy Burlingham (1891–1979) in Vienna, who became a lifelong companion. In 1936 she published what has been considered her main contribution to psychoanalytic theory, *Das Ich und das Abwerrmechanismen* [The Ego and the Mechanisms of Defense], in which she classified a series of defense mechanisms. This work is credited with playing an important role in the development of 'ego psychology' in psychoanalysis.

During this period, Anna Freud played a central role in her father's life, managing his affairs. In 1938 she came to England with him, where she was to remain for the rest of her life (she would be awarded a CBE in 1967). During the war, together with Dorothy Burlingham, she established the Hampstead war nurseries, which provided foster care for children of single parents. They coauthored two books based on this work: *War and Children* (1943) and *Infants without Families* (1944).

In 1952 she founded the Hampstead Child Therapy Clinic, which established a training in child analysis. Her views on child analysis brought her into conflict with Melanie Klein (1882–1960), who had emigrated to London in the 1920s and established a considerable following in the British Psycho-analytical Society. As a consequence, a series of 'controversial discussions' took place in the society between 1941 and 1945. There is no better example, one without parallel in the history of medicine, of how psychoanalysis came to furnish the basis for a new scholasticism.

After Sigmund Freud's death, she held the central position of authority and power in the psychoanalytic movement and was the guardian of orthodoxy. Her collected works span eight volumes, but it is arguable that her most lasting effects do not lie here, but in the manner in which she cultivated and perpetuated the Freud legend. The main pillars of this effort were James Strachey's Standard Edition of Freud's psychological writings, edited 'in collaboration with Anna Freud', Ernest Jones's three-volume biography of Freud, Kurt Eissler's Sigmund Freud archives at the Library of Congress in Washington, and the censored editions of Freud's correspondence. Anna Freud was closely involved with all these enterprises, and all concerned deferred to her wishes. Jones's biography, dedicated to Anna Freud, utilizing documents some of which have not yet been made generally available, transformed Freud's self-fashioned heroic legend into what was long taken as the definitive portrait of Freud and the rise of psychoanalysis. Strachey presented an internalist edition of Freud, dissociating his work from its medical, psychiatric, scientific, philosophical, and cultural contexts. Eissler sequestered documents, some of which were not scheduled to become available until 2113, to withhold potentially damaging information and to impede independent historical investigation into the origins of psychoanalysis. Commencing with the edition of Freud's correspondence with Wilhelm Fliess, Anna Freud was principally responsible for the censorship of Freud's correspondence. Thus she was centrally responsible for shaping the image of Freud, and what could and could not be generally known about him, which played a great part in the impact on society at large that psychoanalysis came to have.

Bibliography

Primary: 1968–83. *The Writings of Anna Freud* (New York); 1954. (with Bonaparte, Marie, and Ernst Kris, eds.) *Origins of Psychoanalysis: Letters to Wilhelm Fliess, Drafts and Notes, 1887–1902 by Sigmund Freud* (London).

Secondary: Borch-Jacobsen, Mikkel, and Sonu Shamdasani, 2006. *Le Dossier Freud. Enquête sur l'histoire de la psychanalyse* (Paris); King, Pearl, and Ricardo Steiner, eds., 1992. *The Freud/Klein Controversies 1941–45* (London); Young-Bruehl, Elisabeth, 1988. *Anna Freud: A Biography* (New York); *Oxford DNB.*

Sonu Shamdasani

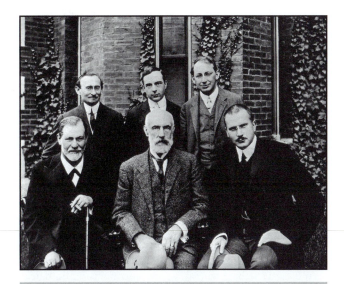

Sigmund Freud (left front) with Stanley Hall and Carl Gustav Jung (see biographical entry); back row (L–R) Abraham Arden Brill, Ernest Jones, and Sándor Ferenczi, Worcester, Massachusetts, 1909. Photograph, Iconographic Collection, Wellcome Library, London.

FREUD, SIGMUND (b. Freiberg, Austrian Empire (now Píbor, Czech Republic), 6 May 1856; d. London, England, 23 September 1939), *neuropathology, psychology.*

The son of Kallamon Jacob Freud (1815–96) and Amalie, née Nathanson (1835–1930), Sigismud, later Sigmund, Freud was born the eldest of eight children into a Jewish lower-middle-class family. Jacob Freud, a wool merchant, had married for the third time in 1855; his young wife Amalie was then as old as the eldest sons from Jacob's first marriage.

Due to economic difficulties in Freiberg, Jacob Freud and his family moved first to Leipzig and shortly thereafter to Vienna, the commercial and financial center of the Austrian Empire, which was likely to offer better market opportunities than the provincial town in Moravia. From childhood on, Sigmund Freud could thus witness almost on a daily basis what the struggle for decent incomes in families of modest social status meant. In addition, he was exposed, as his autobiographical writings reveal, to latent or manifest, yet increasing anti-Semitism until he left Vienna for British exile in 1938.

Freud, age eleven, was admitted to the Viennese Leopoldstädter Communal-Realgymnasium, where he received the baccalaureate with distinction in 1873. The topic of the examination in classical Greek was, by mere chance, Sophocles's *Oedipus*, a tragedy the linguistically gifted young man had read in its original version some weeks earlier.

Freud was driven in later youth by passionate curiosity for themes relating to the humanities, and especially for historical, anthropological, and political topics. This may explain why he first was unsure which faculty to choose: law, medicine, or the humanities. After having read *Die Natur*, a text whose authorship was (wrongly) attributed to Goethe, he finally decided to study medicine. Yet, after registration as a regular student at the University of Vienna in 1873, he still attended lectures offered in the Faculty of Medicine as well as in the humanities; he even intended to obtain a doctorate in both faculties. Forced by the university's statutes to choose, he finally opted for medicine alone.

During the first semesters, Freud particularly enjoyed studying zoology. He did some research of his own, for which he was twice granted a stay at the Zoological Station at Trieste; the results of this research were published in 1877 in two articles, one of which dealt with the posterior nerve roots in the spine of European brook lamprey (*Petromyzon planeri*), the other with the microstructure of the testicles in eels (both in 1877). Freud then shifted to yet another biomedical subdiscipline and joined the physiological laboratory of the University of Vienna. This research institution was headed by Ernst Brücke, a highly regarded experimentalist who shared the scientific-materialist approach with Hermann von Helmholtz, Emil du Bois-Reymond, Carl Ludwig, and some younger physiologists. Freud's focus of attention now was the nervous system. He analyzed the structure of nerve cells and nerve fibers in the crawfish, and elaborated new histological techniques; one of these new methods was published in 1884 in the British journal *Brain* under the title *A New Histological Method for the Study of Nerve-Tracts in the Brain and Spinal Cord.*

Freud received his MD in 1881. At that time, his plan was to seek a permanent research and teaching position within academia. Brücke, however, convinced him that this plan was likely to fail due to economic conditions. Without private financial resources, the outlook of a professional career as researcher in physiology was too much overcast with risks of all sorts. The only realistic option for Freud was that of a medical practitioner. He therefore decided to prepare himself for the opening of a private practice. He entered the General Hospital at Vienna, worked first in the ward of internal medicine headed by Hermann Nothnagel and, subsequently, in that of neurology and psychiatry headed by Theodor Meynert. During this period he acquired the clinical knowledge that permitted him to become a specialist for paralytic disorders, particularly in children. Indeed, in 1891, 1893, and 1897 he published texts of considerable length on Little's disease, diplegia, atonic-diplegic cerebral palsy, and kindred ailments. Another clinical field in which Freud undertook research in 1884–85 was that of the application of cocaine. Not only did he write a substantial report on Parke's cocaine, but also collaborated with his friend Carl Koller on the exploration of the local anesthetic effects of this substance. These investigations eventually led to the discovery of the usefulness of cocaine in surgical inventions on the eye (Freud came close to this discovery, but granted, in full fairness, priority to his friend).

In 1885 Freud received the habilitation in neuropathology and was named *Privatdozent* by the Minister of Education. He also applied successfully for a research grant, with the purpose of studying various clinical aspects of hysteria, then a hotly debated neurological and neuropathological topic. He had previously dealt with hysteria, as several brief articles, mostly review articles, amply document.

Freud's medical grand tour led him to the neurological department of the La Salpêtrière hospital in Paris. This department was run by Jean-Martin Charcot, the leading authority in neuroanatomy and neuropathology in Parisian medicine.

Charcot's epistemological creed was that of positivist medicine, which may be summarized in one sentence: no disease, no disturbance, and no symptom without a cause, the latter being understood as a recognizable temporal or permanent modification within or on the surface of the human organism. This creed entailed that pathogenic causes be systematically sought either in congenital deteriorations of specific tissues, in damages brought about immediately or mediately by infectious or poisonous agents, or in traumatic modifications of specific parts of the body due to mechanical or other physical injuries. Diseases without causes *in materia* were judged to be impossible on metaphysically plausible grounds.

But it was also part and parcel of the positivist approach to the whole array of biomedical problems to take seemingly unusual or non-normal occurrences of symptoms into consideration if, and only if, these symptoms were not ascribable to errors of expert observers or to patients' faking.

Within the context of these epistemologically constraining criteria, hysterics turned out to provide a set of exceptional cases. On the one hand, their symptoms constituted more or less stable clusters. On the other hand, their symptoms were observed by many physicians over several years according to the same rules. Judging from the semiological perspective, the signs of hysteria were real. But no concomitant pathological modification in living matter could be traced. This was a sufficient reason for a major nosological revision within the traditional positivistic frame. It was not that Charcot could easily be convinced of the absence of *material* (i.e., physiologically or post mortem) anatomically

traceable causes. But his department—which included a laboratory and a museum and relied on experts in the fine arts, in physiological measurement by means of the newest available equipments, on anatomists, on neurologists with long experience, etc.—produced so much evidence of palsy, ataxia, hemianopia, and other sensory and motor impairments *without* any recognizable material cause that Charcot recognized the theoretical and practical interest of further studying the multifarious phenomena of hysteria.

When visiting La Salpêtrière, Freud thus not only acquainted himself as a participant observer with the practices of experimental and therapeutic hypnosis, but he also became familiar with the performances of the fine-grained registration techniques of the sphygmograph, the myograph, and other such measuring devices applied to hysterics proper or to sane, but experimentally hypnotized, subjects.

The setting at Charcot's neuropathological department also showed that the boundaries between the (physiological) laboratory and the (clinical) ward had become permeable in both directions—contrary to the dogma of experimental medicine as purported, e.g., by Claude Bernard, who thought that both settings should remain strictly apart.

The accumulation of clinical data and of experimentally reproduced symptoms relating to hysteria suggested a far-reaching revision of nosology. Hysteria came to be conceived as a paradigmatic nervous trouble belonging to an entire family of similar disturbances, such as neurasthenia or phobias, all characterized as fully fledged pathological conditions without recognizable causes *in materia*. Since persons who did *not* suffer from *physiologically* conspicuous conditions would still display, without faking anything or without otherwise behaving in a theatrically made-up way, the symptoms resembling those of organic illnesses, the latter's causes were *psychical*. The new challenge to neuropathology thus was nosologically relevant syndromes *sine materia*.

Though Charcot did not entirely give up hope of still finding some physical cause(s) of hysteria, phobias, and similar conditions, he admitted, at least provisionally, mental or psychological events in a person's life (such as terrorizing fright, shaking experiences, shocks, but also enduring frustrations and the like) as pathogenic causes. In other words, Charcot and his collaborators did not reject the necessity of identifying pathogenic causes, but rather allowed for a broader definition of such causes so that it could apply to the mental realm as well.

During his stay at La Salpêtrière, Freud had many opportunities to familiarize himself with the diagnostic techniques and spirit of the Charcot group. He could also gather extensive firsthand information on the use of hypnosis. Though he was led to give up hypnotism even before the publication of *The Interpretation of Dreams*, his founding monograph of psychoanalysis, in the fall of 1899, the nosological (and ontological) revision motivated by the study of hysterics had a decisive impact on Freud's later development. Indeed, he seems to have been most impressed by partial paralyses in hysterics, a phenomenon that was amenable to replication under experimental conditions that pointed to the breakdown of willful motor activity due to *psychical* pathogenic causes without modifications in the nervous matter. As he emphasized in his 1893 essay in tribute to Charcot, hysterical palsies were the outcome of phantasies, which had occurred in traumatic moments in the brain of patients. The paralyzed parts of the body did not concord topologically with the knowledge of scientific anatomy, but rather invaded in anarchic ways the patients' bodies according to their phantasmagoric anatomy.

In the controversies regarding Freudian psychoanalysis, the continuity-discontinuity issue has attracted a great deal of attention since the early 1920s. In one respect—namely that of the cure itself—Freud certainly departed from the methods of hypnotism. In another respect, Freud's theory of psychical pathogenic causes of neuroses and other troubles was elaborated in continuity with the medical school of Charcot. Speaking in unqualified terms of either continuity or discontinuity does thus not make much sense from the point of view of the history of medicine.

Back in Vienna, Freud opened his private practice on Easter Sunday of 1886. In September of that year, he married Matha Bernays, to whom he had been engaged since 1882.

His therapeutic methods were then either common electrotherapy or hypnosis. At that time, Freud was perceived as a somehow rebellious promoter of hypnosis, who did not hesitate to pay a visit to Hippolyte Bernheim's ward in Nancy with the purpose of receiving information on further methods for the treatment of neurotic patients. His social status was quite ambiguous: on the one hand, doctors sought his help on problems of organic paralyses, but on the other, his views on hysteria, especially on male hysterics, evoked outrage and hostility on the part of traditional practitioners. Freud, however, continued to treat neuroses as before and published a monograph on aphasia in 1891, a critique of strict localizationism, in which he drew from John Hughlings Jackson and where he coined the technical term 'Agnosie' (agnosia). He extended his collaboration with Josef Breuer with whom he published a monograph on hysteria in 1895, wrote dozens of reviews of neurological and neuropathological publications, and began analyzing dreams, mainly his own.

Within the next four years, he worked on interrelating topics that were intended to be presented in a monograph that could be read as an introduction to psychoanalysis and at the same time as a kind of user manual for practicing neuropathologists. Paradoxically, these topics were all centered on dreaming, a very common phenomenon occurring in nearly every person of nearly every age. But rather than taking dreams to be either hardly credible premonitions or short-lived, chaotic expressions of bodily sensations during sleep mixed with remembered visual or acoustic impressions,

Freud redefined them as a window open to the processes of the unconscious in man that manifested itself in fanciful nocturnal scenes. This inaugural monograph thus made the boundaries between pathological and sane conditions permeable. Indeed, he argued that the 'language' of dreams and its lawful 'grammar' were translatable into the vocabulary of scientific psychology, or, rather, into the vocabulary of a new science of psychology. The result of this theoretical innovation was twofold: on the one hand, one could study the unconscious in man by way of systematic analyses of a common phenomenon and could thus apply the theoretical insights to the cure of neuroses of all sorts; on the other hand, one could dispense with hypnosis, since a rational, analytic reconstruction of one's mental condition could reveal the pathogenic cause of neurotic malfunctioning, which could be remedied by the 'talking cure', the verbal reenactment of the 'forgotten', that is, repressed, traumatic event.

In 1902 Freud was promoted to the rank of an 'ausserordentlicher Titular-Professor' (extraordinary professor) at the Faculty of Medicine in Vienna. In the same year, he published a monograph on *The Psychopathology of Everyday Life*, in which he analyzed various types of parapraxis, defined, similar to dreaming, as symptomatic manifestations of unconscious processes (such as repressed wishes).

From 1903 to 1904 on, the circle of like-minded physicians, psychologists, and interested laypersons who would regularly gather at Freud's apartment on Wednesdays grew. The first congress of psychoanalysis took place in Salzburg in 1908; in the following year, Freud was invited to deliver lectures at Clark University in the United States. In 1910 the International Psychoanalytic Association was founded at Nuremberg; Freud was elected as its first president.

The period of time between 1903–04 and the outbreak of World War I was marked by both collaborative work on psychoanalytic issues and by quarrels between the 'founding father'—as Freud came to be denoted later by partisan historians of psychoanalysis—and some of his followers. The study of symbols in dreams, which was nearly absent in the first edition of *The Interpretation of Dreams* but received prominent visibility in the second edition of the monograph in 1909, was in fact the outcome of intense collaborative work and, on Freud's own view, the result of a subtle compromise between divergent psychoanalytic approaches.

The period following World War I, during which the psychoanalytic movement endured a setback while the number of Freud's patients in Vienna significantly decreased, brought at once an unexpected international recognition of the new approach. Indeed, the thousands of soldiers suffering from 'war neurosis', without physical trauma, confirmed the cogency of psychoanalysis. In addition, Freud's works were read far more frequently outside the medical discipline than within medicine. Psychoanalysis thus received attention from novelists, journalists, historians, filmmakers, artists, etc., and became a subject of public, though often controversial, attention.

From 1915 to 1918 Freud wrote a number of important theoretical articles that not only addressed metapsychological themes, that is, themes relating to the theory construction of the psychoanalytic approach, but also themes of public interest, including the issue of war and peace, artistic creation, mass political movements, religion, and the role of sexual emancipation.

In 1930 Freud was awarded the Goethe Prize of the City of Frankfurt. On that occasion, he admitted in a letter to Alfons Paquet that he welcomed this honor as a compensation for the public recognition that had been denied to him until then.

From 1923 on, Freud suffered from cancer. His illness and the political situation brought about after 30 January 1933 by National-Socialist politics in Germany seems to have enforced his pessimistic worldview. Jewish members of the German branch of the International Psychoanalytic Association were removed from office and were banned from practicing; in 1936 the Psychoanalytic Publishing Company at Leipzig was closed. In March 1938, after the 'Anschluss' of Austria, Freud's daughter Anna, herself a practicing psychoanalyst, was interrogated by the secret police. On the initiative of Marie Bonaparte, the Freud family left Austria in June 1938 for British exile. In the last months of his life, Freud completed his last book, *Moses and Monotheism.* Three weeks after the outbreak of World War II, Freud died after having been administered heavy doses of morphine—it seems, upon his own request.

Bibliography

Primary: 1891. *Zur Auffassung der Aphasien* (Vienna); 1895 (with Breuer, Josef). *Studien über Hysterie* (Vienna); 1974. (with Jung, Carl Gustav). *Briefwechsel* (Frankfurt am Main); 1985. *Briefe an Wilhelm Fließ* (Frankfurt am Main) [English translation: *The Complete Letters of Sigmund Freud to Wilhelm Fliess* (Cambridge, MA, and London)]; 1989. *Jugendbriefe an Eduard Silberstein* (Frankfurt am Main); 1993–2005. (with Ferenszi, Sándor) *Briefwechsel* (Vienna); 1995. *The Standard Edition of the Complete Psychological Works* (London, reprint); 1996. *Schriften über Coca* (Frankfurt am Main); 2002. *Unser Herz zeigt nach dem Süden. Reisebriefe 1895–1923* (Berlin).

Secondary: Marinelli, Lydia, and Andreas Mayer, 2003. *Dreaming by the Book: Freud's "The Interpretation of Dreams" and the History of the Psychoanalytic Movement* (New York); Ginsburg, Nancy, and Roy Ginsburg, 1999. *Psychoanalysis and Culture at the Millennium* (New Haven); Lohmann, Hans-Martin, 1998. *Sigmund Freud* (Reinbek bei Hamburg); Appignanesi, Lisa, and John Forrester, 1992. *Freud's Women* (London); Gay, Peter, 1988. *Freud: A Life for Our Time* (London and New York); Laplanche, Jean, and J. B. Pontalis, 1974. *The Language of Psycho-Analysis* (New York); Schur, Max, 1972. *Freud: Living and Dying* (New York); Jones, Ernest, 1953–57. *The Life and Work of Sigmund Freud* 3 vols. (New York).

Alexandre Métraux

FRIDERICHSEN, CARL (b. Copenhagen, Denmark, 5 June 1886; d. Copenhagen, 14 April 1982), *pediatrics.*

Friderichsen, the son of army doctor Carl Friderichsen and his wife Ady Henriette, grew up in Copenhagen. He studied medicine at the University of Copenhagen, receiving the medical degree in 1912. After brief visits to London and Paris, he worked in several hospital departments in Copenhagen (1912–15). Eventually pediatrics became his main focus, and he held positions as house physician in children's departments in various Copenhagen hospitals (1915–19), in addition to posts as assistant in the departments of pathological anatomy and pharmacology at the University of Copenhagen. After serving as a resident at the Queen Louise Children's Hospital (1919–24) and as head of the pediatric department of the Frederiksberg Polyclinic (1924–31), he became chief physician at the pediatric ward of Sundby Hospital, a post he held until his retirement in 1956.

In January 1917, while working in the pediatric ward of Rigshospitalet, Friderichsen observed the case of a six-month-old boy who died from acute degeneration of the suprarenal glands due to hemorrhages, only a few hours after the first symptoms (notably small areas of bleeding under the skin) had been observed. Friderichsen examined records from other Copenhagen hospitals and found two other cases similar to the one he had observed. Literature studies led him to twenty-five similar cases, including the case reported by Rupert Waterhouse in 1911, and since Friderichsen found these to differ from suprarenal bleeding in infants and adults, he suspected a new type of adrenal apoplexy. He first published his findings in Danish in 1917, speculating that infection or intoxication might be the cause. In 1918 he published his results in German, generating international attention. In 1933 this serious and well-known disease was named the Waterhouse-Friderichsen syndrome.

Friderichsen continued to monitor developments regarding the etiology and therapy of the syndrome, but he also did research on other subjects. His thesis from 1923 explored the clinical aspects of acidosis in infants due to nutritional disturbances, and in 1934 he presented a case of tetany in an infant caused by a latent osteitis fibrosa in the mother. Later works addressed the treatment of pneumonia and of febrile convulsions and vitamin A deficiency.

Throughout his career and up until shortly before his death, Friderichsen maintained a large private practice and acted as physician to the children of the royal family. He actively promoted cooperation among pediatrics in the Nordic countries and served as chairman of the Danish Pediatric Society (1928–34). He divorced his first wife, Kate Riise, in 1942, and married Ruth Skøde Billund the following year, surviving her by only a few months.

Bibliography

Primary: 1918. 'Nebennierenapoplexie bei kleinen Kindern.' *Jahrbuch für Kinderheilkunde und physische Erziehung* 87: 109–125.

Secondary: Varon, Joseph, Karen Chen, and George L. Sternbach, 1998. 'Rupert Waterhouse and Carl Friderichsen: Adrenal Apoplexy.' *Journal of Emergency Medicine* 16: 643–647; Melchior, J. C., 1982. 'Carl Friderichsen.' *Ugeskrift for Læger* 144: 1733–1734; Plum, Preben, 1956. 'Carl Friderichsen.' *Acta Pædiatrica* 45: 329–333.

Søren Bak-Jensen

FROST, WADE HAMPTON   (b. Marshall, Virginia, USA, 3 March 1880; d. Baltimore, Maryland, USA, 1 May 1938), *epidemiology, poliomyelitis, influenza, tuberculosis.*

Frost was the seventh child of a country doctor, Henry Frost, and a schoolteacher, Sabra Walker Frost. Both parents were well educated and provided higher education for their children. Two sons became physicians, two daughters, nurses, and another son, an accountant. In 1898 Frost entered the University of Virginia, at the time among the most prestigious academic institutions in the United States. He received a BSc (1901) and an MD (1903). Possibly motivated by a strong tradition of public service among the graduates of the University of Virginia, Frost joined the Public Health and Marine Hospital Service (1905) and was assigned to clinical duties at the Baltimore Marine Hospital. However, he was soon assigned to investigative activities in a yellow fever outbreak in New Orleans. The effective control of the epidemic, and Frost's role, did not escape notice by his superiors and in 1908 he was transferred to the Hygienic Laboratory, forerunner of the National Institutes of Health. There he sharpened his epidemiological skills and carried out classic studies of waterborne diseases, poliomyelitis, and influenza. In 1919, on assignment at the newly established Johns Hopkins School of Hygiene and Public Health, Frost became the first professor of epidemiology in the United States. He remained on the faculty until his death.

In 1941 Kenneth Maxcy, Frost's successor at Johns Hopkins, edited a selection of Frost's publications. He classified them into five categories, namely, epidemic investigations, stream pollution, acute infectious diseases, public health principles and practice, and chronic endemic infectious diseases. In the first category, Maxcy included one of three publications from *Hygienic Laboratory Bulletin No. 90* (1913). In this publication, Frost laid out the complete descriptive epidemiology of poliomyelitis, including the recognition of the roles of healthy carriers and nonparalytic cases in the transmission of infection and the extremely low infectivity of the causal agent. Three papers in the second category contained Frost's observations on the problem of stream pollution generated by the increasing urbanization of the United States. The third category included seven papers, two on influenza, three on minor respiratory disease, and two on diphtheria. In 'Statistics of Influenza Morbidity, with Special Reference to Certain Factors in Case Incidence and Case Fatality' (1920), Frost introduced the morbidity sample survey as a methodology to provide a more comprehensive understanding of epidemics than could be obtained from mortality or morbidity registration. The fourth category, containing four papers, included Frost's only attempt to define the content, scope, and theory of epidemiology. Maxcy's fifth category contained three papers of great interest: the first, on the use of the secondary attack rate to study the familial aggregation of tuberculosis; the second, expounding the application of cohort analysis; and the third, discussing a strategy for the control of tuberculosis.

Frost's most far-reaching influence lay in the development of the teaching of epidemiology. There were no precedents when he came to the Hopkins in 1919. He drew heavily on his own experiences and developed a case-study strategy that galvanized his students, who, in turn, emulated his methods as they scattered about the country.

Frost's words describing epidemiology, in his introduction to the reprint of Snow's classic study of cholera, are often quoted: 'Epidemiology at any given time is something more than the total of its established facts. It includes their orderly arrangement into chains of inference which extend more or less beyond the bounds of direct observation. Such of those chains that are well and truly laid guide investigation of the facts of the future, those that are ill made fetter progress . . . .' (Richardson, 1936, p. ix).

Bibliography

Primary: 1936. Richardson, B. W., *Snow on Cholera*, introduction by Frost, W. H. (New York); 1941. (Maxcy, Kenneth F., ed.) *Papers of Wade Hampton Frost* (New York).

Secondary: Daniel, Thomas M., 2004. *Wade Hampton Frost, Pioneer Epidemiologist 1880–1938* (Rochester, NY); *DAMB*.

Warren Winkelstein, Jr.

FRUGARD, ROGER   (aka ROGER FRUGARD OF PARMA) (fl. Italy, twelfth century), *surgery.*

Roger's name first appears during the last half of the twelfth century, when he was recognized as the foremost surgeon in Italy. He has since been acknowledged as a primary figure in the rebirth of the art and science of surgery in Western Europe. But we know little about him and whence he came. The following is a consensus.

Roger was the son of an old Parmesan family, and today he is known as Roger Frugard of Parma. He lived at least until the end of the twelfth or early thirteenth century. The erudition exhibited in his works indicates that he knew the few Latin translations of the classic and Arabic masters, which were appearing in Italy at that time. Because he could read Latin, we assume that he was educated in the schools provided by Italian priests and monks at, or near, Parma. Some of the clerical physicians—a very few of them also practiced surgery—took priestly orders or became monks. The constraints that prevented the clerical physicians from acting as surgeons were not severe in Italy in Roger's epoch.

But where did he learn the rudiments of practical surgery? Early in the twelfth century, Salerno was the only place in Italy where some formal medical education was obtainable and where some standards of excellence were exhibited. By mid-century Bologna had accepted some of the translations and personnel and began to grow as a center that in the thirteenth century came to rival Salerno, along with Padua, Parma, and Naples. But Roger had Salerno and he became its star. Salerno had offered some schooling in medicine for at least a century and its status allowed it to grant a sort of license, or permit, to practice medicine and surgery. It was a certificate of competence, which by 1220 was accepted everywhere in Italy, and later on, in all of northern Europe, by decree of Emperor Frederick ll. For more than seven centuries the surgical treatise attributed to Roger, his *Chirurgia*, was credited as the first European surgical text, a product of a Salernitan.

We know that Roger did not put his pen to his own book; *Chirurgia* was compiled by a group of his pupils and issued sometime between 1170 and 1180, probably in Parma. The editor and leader of the compilers was Guido II of Arezzo. Some believe that Roger was alive at the time and participated and approved the work. We know that the book had immediate success in Salerno and elsewhere in Italy, where it was reproduced by copyists. Many of those manuscripts are now in medical libraries through the world, in Latin and in other languages.

Even before the dawn of the thirteenth century, Roger's *Chirurgia* was the accepted standard text in medical schools. The practical experience of the surgeons who had been enlightened by it led them to emend Roger and to provide glosses that supplemented what they felt was deficient, and they rearranged the presentation of the materials, which at first had been randomly ordered by Roger's amanuenses. The orderly arrangement of the pioneer surgical text and the list of its contents were proposed by Roger and modified by Roland Capelutti. They were copied with few changes for more than three centuries.

Bibliography

Primary: 1170. (Ruggiero da Parma) *Chirurgia* (Italian edn. by Stroppiana, Luigi, and Dario Spallone); 1853. (De Renzi, Salvatore) *Collectio Salernitana* 5 vols. (Bologna) [V 01.11 contains the Venetian edn. (1546) of a thirteenth-century Ms of Roger, pp. 425–496]; 1957. *Istituto Di Storia Della Medicina Della Universita Di Roma* (Rome) [English translation Rosenman, L. D., 2002 (Philadelphia)].

Secondary: Hunt, Tony, 1994. *Anglo-Norman Medicine* vol. I. (Cambridge); Tabanelli, Mario, 1965. *La Chirurgia ltaliana Nell'Alto Medioevo* (Florence).

Leonard D. Rosenman

FUCHS, LEONHART

FUCHS, LEONHART (b. Wemding, Germany, 17 January 1501, d. Tübingen, Germany, 10 May 1566), *medicine.*

Fuchs was born into an old patrician family in Wemding, near Nördlingen. His grandfather had been the local mayor and his mother, Anna, was the daughter of another patrician family. His brother, Hans, later became a priest; two sisters, Barbara and Anna, married in Wemding. Although his father died young, Fuchs enjoyed an excellent education. At age ten he started attending a Latin school in Heilbronn. A year later he moved on to Erfurt, and at age twelve his name already figured in the matriculation records of Erfurt University. Having obtained his baccalaureate, he returned home and established a private school in Wemding. He did not stay long, however. In 1519 he went to Ingolstadt, where he studied Latin and Greek with Reuchlin and Ceporinus and received a master's degree. Still in Ingolstadt, he then began to study medicine while he continued his Greek studies, reading the original Greek medical texts. With a doctoral degree in medicine he left Ingolstadt in 1524 and settled in Munich, probably to work in free medical practice. In Munich he married Anna Fridberger, with whom he had six daughters and four sons.

In May 1526 he returned to Ingolstadt as a professor of medicine but quit in 1528 to work as personal physician to the Margrave of Brandenburg in Ansbach. His departure seems to have been motivated by the growing animosities that he faced as a result of his sympathies with the Protestant reformation. At the same time, Georg von Brandenburg developed plans to establish a Protestant university in Ansbach, but that plan was never achieved. Nevertheless, when Fuchs accepted another professorial appointment in Ingolstadt, in 1533, he stayed for only a few months, presumably because of the massive resistance that he encountered in Ingolstadt. He returned to Ansbach and soon afterward, when an epidemic broke out, accompanied the court to nearby Kulmbach.

Finally, in 1535 his life as an itinerant academic came to an end. Fuchs accepted a professorship in Tübingen. He soon played a major—and sometimes quite controversial—role in the university. Seven times he served as its rector and pushed successfully for a thorough reform of the medical curriculum along the principles of medical humanism. Confessional strife continued to overshadow his work and life in Tübingen as well, though now as a result of the growing animosities between Lutherans and Zwinglians. Fuchs was on the verge of going to Copenhagen as a personal physician to King Christian but decided against it in the end. He also turned down an offer from Cosmas de' Medici to come to Pisa. Fuchs remained in Tübingen until his death.

Fuchs entered the stage of European science and medicine as one of the first major Northern representatives of medical humanism and anti-Arabism. His first major publication, the *Errata recentiorum medicorum*, did not meet with unequivocal enthusiasm but it immediately gained him a prominent place among contemporary medical writers. Drawing very generously from, if not plagiarizing, a similar work by the leading Italian medical humanist Leoniceno, Fuchs vehemently attacked the academic medicine of his time for relying largely on the works of Avicenna

(Ibn Sīnā), Averroes (Ibn Rushd), and other 'Arabic' writers. Fuchs called them butchers and murderers who had strayed from the path of truth of the ancient physicians. In accordance with humanist principles he wanted to see their teachings replaced by those of Galen, Hippocrates, and the other ancient authorities. Since he himself had little access to original Greek manuscripts, Fuchs focused on revising extant editions and translations of the Galenic and Hippocratic works. In 1532 he published a new translation with commentary of the sixth book of the Hippocratic 'Epidemics'. In the 1540s he followed suit with various Galenic treatises. In 1538 he accepted a commission from several publishers in Basel to undertake, together with Joachim Camerarius and Hieronymus Gemusaeus, a new complete Greek edition of the works of Galen. His ambition to establish himself as the leading humanist physician in the German lands also provided the background for a vehement public dispute with another leading German medical humanist, Janus Cornarius, who had accused Fuchs of plagiarism.

As Fuchs realized, the original Hippocratic and Galenic works provided no easy access for the aspiring physician. They lacked the systematic and comprehensive structure that was a major reason for the outstanding success that Avicenna's *Canon of medicine* still enjoyed in Fuchs's time. Fuchs understood that medical humanism would be able to assert itself on a large scale only if painstaking philological analysis and reconstruction went hand in hand with the publication of new propaedeutic texts that taught the principles of Hippocratic and Galenic medicine to beginners without resorting to the 'Arabic' authorities. In 1531 he published his *Compendiaria ac succincta admodum in medendi artem eisagoge* and continued to revise and expand it over the following years. By 1541 he had turned it into a voluminous medical handbook titled *Methodus seu ratio compendiaria perveniendi ad veram solidamque medicinam*. In 1555 the work appeared under the title *Institutionum medicinae . . . libri quinque*, now without the sections on pharmaceutics, which were published independently as *De usitata huius temporis componendorum miscendorumque medicamentorum ratione libri quatuor*.

Fuchs's 'Institutions' continued to rank among the most popular medical textbooks long after his death. Today, however, Fuchs's name has come to be associated above all with his botanical work (the 'Fuchsia' still commemorates his botanical achievements). Together with Otto Brunfels and Hieronymus Bock he was one of the German founding fathers of modern scientific botany. His *De historia stirpium commentarii insignes* of 1542 are generally acknowledged as a highlight of sixteenth-century botany. In this work, Fuchs presented more than five hundred plants to his readers, with brief descriptions of their outward appearance, preferred habitat, and time of flowering and seeding as well as, in most cases, philological remarks about the different terms and synonyms by which the ancient authorities

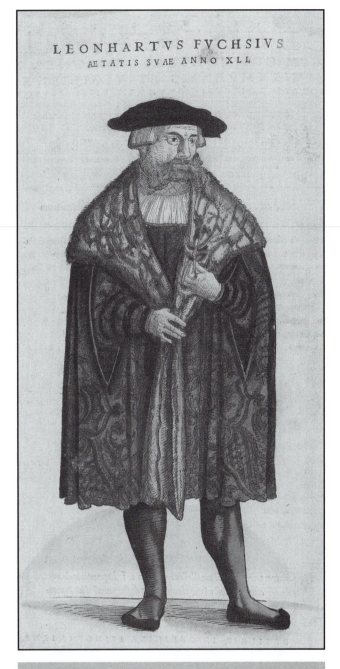

Leonhart Fuchs, aged 41. Engraving from *De historia stirpivm commentarii insignes . . .* Basel, 1542. Rare Books, Wellcome Library, London.

referred to the plant in question. His detailed comments on the temperament and powers of the individual plants consisted largely of a juxtaposition of the relevant passages from the ancient works. Like his predecessor Brunfels, Fuchs aimed first at clearly identifying the medicinal plants that ancient and more recent authors had mentioned and recommended, often under various names. The task was of eminent practical importance: when contemporary physicians erroneously mistook a plant for the one that Galen,

Dioscorides, and other pharmaceutical authorities had recommended for a certain condition or desired effect, their treatment was bound to be wrong, useless, or even dangerous. Fuchs differed from Brunfels to the degree that he accepted very little that the 'Arabic' physicians had written. But like Brunfels, Fuchs realized that an unequivocal identification of the plants that the ancient authorities referred to could not be achieved by painstaking philological analysis alone. Botanical fieldwork involving a careful empirical study of northern European medicinal plants was also indispensable. The book's lasting fame is owed above all to the excellent large-scale woodcuts drawn 'from nature' by Heinrich Füllmaurer and Albert Mayer and sculpted by Rudolph Speckle under Fuchs's guidance. With very few exceptions, they each covered a whole folio page. Even in black and white they offered a highly detailed and realistic illustration that, much more than the rather vague verbal description, could serve as a fairly reliable basis for a correct identification of the plants found in nature or in a pharmacist's shop.

In spite of its undisputed scientific merits, Fuchs's *De historia stirpium commentarii* were not quite the commercial success Fuchs and his publisher Isingrin had hoped for. Even though Fuchs resented vernacular editions of medical books for fear of encouraging self-treatment, he agreed to a heavily revised German edition that appeared under the title *New Kreüterbuch* in 1543. It maintained the folio-size woodcuts and the original order according to the Greek names of the plants, which in the German translation appeared entirely arbitrary. The book became easier to use and addressed a much wider readership. The extensive quotes from the works of ancient authorities were replaced by a single, more concise characterization of the individual plants. A new index of diseases was added, which permitted the reader to look for different plants that were recommended for the disease in question.

Revised editions followed, some of them much cheaper, in octavo and with correspondingly smaller illustrations. A fair number of mostly unauthorized editions in German followed as well. Among others, Walther Ryff, author of a number of highly successful medical works, made generous use of Fuchs's illustrations for his own herbal, provoking a vitriolic polemical exchange between Fuchs and Ryff's publisher Egenolph. There were also Dutch, French, and Spanish translations. Fuchs himself continued to work on expanding and completing his *De historia stirpium commentarii* in the years after 1542. In the end, the work was to present some 1,500 plants. But Fuchs could not find a publisher who was prepared to take the financial risk involved in producing such a voluminous and costly book. It was never published, and after Fuchs's death the manuscripts and most of the printing blocks were lost and never found again.

Bibliography

Primary: 1566–67. *Leonhardi Fuchsii opera omnia in tribus tomis digesta* (Frankfurt); 1530. *Errata recentiorum medicorum, LX. numero, adiectis eorundem confutationibus* (Hagenau); 1531. *Compendiaria ac succincta admodum in medendi artem eisagoge, seu introduction* (Hagenau); 1542. *De historia stirpium commentarii insignes* (Basel); 1555. *Institutionum medicinae, ad Hippocratis, Galeni, aliorumque veterum scripta recte intelligenda mire utiles libri quinque* (Lyons); Hizler, Georg, 1566. *Oratio de vita et morte clarissimi viri, medici et philosophi praestantissimi, D. Leonharti Fuchsi, artis medendi in Academia Tubingensi Professoris doctissimi* (Tübingen).

Secondary: Brinkhus, Gerd, and Claudine Pachnicke, eds., 2001. *Leonhart Fuchs (1501–1566). Mediziner und Botaniker* (Tübingen); Fichtner, Gerhard, 1968. 'Neues zu Leben und Werk von Leonhart Fuchs aus seinen Briefen an Joachim Camerarius I. und II. in der Trew-Sammlung.' *Gesnerus* 25: 65–82; Stübler, Eberhard, 1928. *Leonhart Fuchs. Leben und Werk* (Munich); *DSB*.

Michael Stolberg

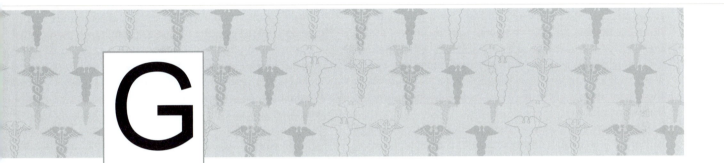

G

GAAZ, FEDOR PETROVICH (FRIEDRICH JOSEPH HAAS) (b. Munstereifel, Germany, 8 August 1780; d. Moscow, Russia, 16 August 1853), *medical philanthropy, public health.*

Born into an old Cologne family with medical traditions, Gaaz was educated at the Academic School in Cologne and received his medical education at the universities of Jena and Göttingen, completing a doctorate of medicine at Göttingen University in 1805. He specialized as an ophthalmologist at Vienna under A. Schmidt.

He arrived in Russia in 1806 in the capacity of personal doctor to Princess V. Repina. Gaaz completed two trips to the Northern Caucasus, about which he published a book in Moscow in French, *Ma visite aux eaux de Alexandre en 1809 et 1810* (1811). This was the first scientific description and appraisal of medical treatment from the springs at Zheleznovodsk and Essentuksk. Gaaz was the founder of treatment by Trans-Caucasus mineral waters and one of the founders of resort treatment, climate therapy, medical meteorology, and balneology in Russia. He suggested a system of measures with the aim of creating a general Russian resort in the district of the Caucasian Mineral Waters.

In 1817, after an epidemic of diphtheria in Moscow, Gaaz published 'Découverte sur la croup, ou L'astma synanchicum acutum' ['The discovery of croup or acute asthma'] under the pseudonym Sutamilli. This led to his book on the same theme, *Beitrage zu den Zeichen des Croups* [Report about the symptoms of croup], put out by Moscow University in 1818, in which he generalized on the evidence about croup reported by more than sixty authors. In this first fundamental work on pediatrics in Russia, he created a new interpretative apparatus and clarified the terminology, which established a differential diagnostics of croup due to diphtheria. This research helped develop a nosological orientation in Russian medicine and played a positive role in studies on diphtheria.

Extending the work of his teacher from Göttingen, J. F. Blumenbach, Gaaz formulated the speculative (without experimental proof) 'physiological theory of assimilation', in which he explained basic principles taking their course in the vital processes in the organism. He argued that when an organism is healthy, the constancy of its internal characteristics is preserved.

From 1807 to 1812 he was head doctor of the Pavlovskii hospital in Moscow, and from 1825 to 1826 he was state-physician for Moscow, responsible for the medical well-being of the city. He advised on improving the organization of medical services for the population, put together regulations for the examination of psychiatric patients, and envisaged measures for vaccination. He first formulated the need for a service for emergency medical stations in Moscow (1811) and on-site emergency care (1848).

At the time of the cholera epidemic in Moscow in 1830–31, Gaaz was appointed a member of the provisional medical council for the struggle with cholera and head doctor of the Iauzskaia temporary cholera hospital. He spoke out against the application of bloodletting as an irrational medical measure when treating cholera patients.

In 1829 he became the chief doctor for Moscow prisons. He significantly improved the maintenance of prisoners, abolishing the shaving of half the head of women and exiles, the iron bars that held eight to twelve prisoners when they walked to penal exile, and the iron shackles that lacerated the skin. Gaaz took the sensitive position that punishment was first of all a form of penitence that excluded elements of civic vengeance.

By his initiative Moscow prisons were reconstructed, a prison hospital was built (1832), a school for the children of the arrested was established, and a police hospital for the homeless opened; he lived in a small apartment next to the hospital for the homeless. The Moscow police hospital for the homeless became the first special hospital for emergency medical care in Russia. From 1840 to 1843, Gaaz was the head doctor of the Staro-Ekaterina hospital for unskilled laborers.

The name 'Gaaz' even during his lifetime acquired significance as a symbol of impartiality, of medical selflessness, and of the struggle with the difficult conditions of prison life in Russia. In 1848 in Moscow, he founded jointly with Baroness S. Shcherbatova the Nicholas society of nurses, which was later renamed the society 'in memory of Baroness S. S. Shcherbatova and Doctor F. P. Gaaz'.

In 1909 a monument to his work was installed in the courtyard of the hospital where Gaaz had lived. On the pedestal was the motto of Gaaz: 'hurry to do good'. These words were also left on the gravestone of Gaaz at the German cemetery in Moscow.

His humanitarian principles of the professional service of the doctor inspired many Russian doctors.

Bibliography

Primary: Rossiiskaia gosudarstvennaia biblioteka. [Russian state library]. Nauchno-issledovatel'skii otdel rukopisei. [Scientific research department for manuscripts]. 'Documents relating to the period of residence of Gaaz in Moscow (1809–12).' f. 153, op. 6–9 (Moscow); Rossiskii gosudarstvennyi istoricheskii arkhiv. [Russian state historical archive]. 'Documents connected to the visit of Gaaz to the district of the Caucasian Mineral Waters and others.' f. 759, op. 1, d. 329, l. 40; d. 330, l. 21; d. 332, l. 13; f. 1297, op. 56, d. 107, l. 42–72. (St Petersburg); Gosudarstvennyi arkhiv Rossiskoi Federatsii. [The State Archive of the Russian Federation]. f. 564, op. 1, ed. khr. 279, 281, 288–289, 292. (Moscow); Tsentral'nyi istoricheskii arkhiv g. Moskvy. [Central historical archive of the city of Moscow]. f. 1, op. 1, d. 3488–3489, 3504, 3514–3515, 3522, 3532. (Moscow).

Secondary: Bliukhina, N., 2004. 'Vklad vracha-gumanista F. P. Gaaz v Meditsinskuiu nauku i praktiku' ['The Contribution of Doctor-Humanist F. P. Gaaz to Medical Science and Practice'] (Dissertation for the degree of MSc) (Moscow); Kopelev, L. Z., 1993. *Sviatoi doctor Fedor Petrovich* [*The saintly doctor Fedor Petrovich*] (St Petersburg); Muller-Dietz, H., 1980. *Friedrich Joseph Haas als Arzt in Moskau* (Berlin); Hamm, A., 1979. *Doctor medizin Friedrich Joseph Haas . . .* (Bonn); Koni, A. F., 1904. *Fedor Petrovich Gaaz* (St Petersburg).

Mikhail Poddubnyi

GABALDÓN, ARNOLDO (b. Trujillo, Venezuela, 1 March 1909; d. Caracas, Venezuela, 1 September 1990), *malaria eradication, epidemiology.*

Born to Joaquín Gabaldón and Virginia Carrillo Márquez in an upper-middle–class family, Gabaldón attended high school in his hometown and entered the Central University of Venezuela, Caracas, to study medicine. In 1931, a year after his graduation, he was sent by the government to pursue specialized studies at the Institute of Tropical Diseases in Hamburg. He also visited Rome's antimalaria Experimental Station sponsored by the Rockefeller Foundation. Also thanks to the Foundation, he received a fellowship to study at the Johns Hopkins School of Hygiene and Public Health (1933–35). In Baltimore, he became familiar with bacteria, helminthes, protozoa, and disease-carrying viruses as well as their vectors. He crowned his studies at Johns Hopkins with a doctoral degree and a thesis on protozoology. Before returning to his home country, he visited the laboratories of the Rockefeller Foundation in New York City, beginning a long and fruitful collaboration with this institution.

Shortly after his return, Venezuelan political authorities declared malaria the country's main health problem because of its vast incidence in rural areas, where the majority of the population lived. In the recently created Ministry of Health and Social Assistance (1936), a Division of Malariology was envisioned. The young Gabaldón was entrusted with its organization and asked to carry out malaria investigations and campaigns with a national scope.

The Organizer

Gabaldón was head of the Division during the years 1936–50. He began his work with comprehensive studies of the disease and mosquito-specimen gathering, including their identification and classification. He also mapped the distribution of the *Anopheles* species, their behavior in endemic regions, the malaria endemicity and epidemicity of towns, the seasonal distributions of malaria, and malaria's annual cycles. On the basis of his own collected data, Gabaldón argued for a new climatic zone, the 'paraequatorial', not considered by geographers before. Eventually, his finding proved to be correct and useful for antimalaria work.

Thanks to these sound studies on the country's different vectors and their respective potential in malaria transmission, it was possible to organize an effective campaign aimed at controlling mosquito populations, especially—

but not exclusively—*Anopheles albimanus* and *Anopheles darlingi*, the latter being the most important malaria vector in the country. The campaign consisted of the use of larvicide fish; environmental sanitation to diminish the number of larva reservoirs; the education of physicians, schoolteachers, and leaders of rural communities on malaria; and the distribution of quinine and other drugs in vulnerable groups.

Gabaldón's staff was initially badly prepared. He progressively transformed the Division of Malariology's personnel into an efficient, specialized, and full-time staff. Gabaldón's care and charisma enforced a remarkable discipline, self-confidence, and a strong motivation that induced all the Division's members, regardless of their position, to perceive their work as part of a vital mission for their motherland. Hierarchies were based on merit rather than political influence. A link and educational instrument for field officers was the *Tijeratazos* newsletter (literally 'snippings'), published in Spanish between 1938 and 1946. Each issue carried relevant information from newspapers, news on administrative issues, and summaries of academic works from Venezuela and other parts of the world (sometimes translated into Spanish). Because of its valuable content in Spanish, the newsletter also circulated in several Latin American countries.

The increased efficiency of antimalaria activities in Venezuela facilitated the governmental provision of funds to Gabaldón's Division. Thanks to this support (and to Rockefeller Foundation grants), an infrastructure for malaria control developed in the country. In 1941 Gabaldón acquired more experience with the clinical dimension of malaria. In that year he was in charge of the malaria ward at the Civil Hospital of Maracay, evaluating diverse therapeutic schemes and using new drugs such as atebrine and chloroquine. He also used this location to train antimalaria health experts in Venezuela. As a result, in 1943 Gabaldón inaugurated a School of Malariology in Maracay. Its students were physicians and technicians willing to become malariologists: respected health experts at the time. In a few years, the school's high quality made it a regional center for malaria training.

At the same time, Gabaldón promoted health engineering in Venezuela, a relatively new profession in the country. He considered these professionals as essential for malaria control. Venezuelan engineers, as well as physicians working under Gabaldón, were sent to U.S. universities for further training, with fellowships from the Venezuelan government and the Rockefeller Foundation. He also artfully promoted the link between the reduction of malaria and improvements in national health indicators, such as health expectancy, and the improvement of living conditions in the rural areas.

The Antimalaria Campaign

Gabaldón became acquainted with the residual power of DDT against *Anopheles* toward the end of World War II during a lecture tour on malaria for U.S. military personnel assigned to serve in the Pacific. Aware of its potential use in Venezuela, he obtained and used the insecticide rapidly. He also trained personnel in the proper handling of the dangerous chemical. House registers in rural Venezuelan areas were compiled, and educational procedures were carefully elaborated to gain the collaboration of rural inhabitants for spraying activities. A nationwide DDT-based campaign was launched in 1945, the first of its kind attempted in a developing country. The campaign managed to temporarily interrupt transmission and reduced the numbers of individuals infected. Gabaldón was confident that isolation and vigilance of residual cases would contribute to eradication. After three years, around 115,000 houses had been sprayed. The mortality rate from malaria—which during the five-year period 1941–45 was 109 deaths per 100,000—was reduced to 3.5 in 1949, 0.5 in 1955, and 0.0 in 1962 (Otero et al., 1988). Thus, in 1961 Venezuela became the first country to register a significant malaria-free zone with the World Health Organization: a total of 407,945 square kilometers of its territory.

Paradoxically, the more successful the campaign became (in spite of refractory foci and the existence of insecticide-resistant species of *Anopheles*), the sooner malaria research efforts were abandoned. As a result, the local examination and proper response to unanticipated biological, administrative, and political situations was feeble. Starting in the late 1950s and early 1960s, antimalaria work in Venezuela began concentrating instead on routine DDT spraying and supervision visits. The Venezuelan political authorities considered it unnecessary to maintain an energetic and comprehensive campaign because the disease was apparently disappearing. It was difficult for Gabaldón himself to change this trend. During the final years of dictatorship of General Marcos Pérez Jiménez (who ruled the country from 1948 to 1958), Gabaldón was just an adviser to the malaria Division (during the years 1950–58), and his role mainly reinforced its international support. During that period he was also director of the School of Malariology, which since the 1950s, and with the support of the Pan American Sanitary Bureau, had become an international center for the training of malaria eradicators.

The Expert and His Return to Research

With a new democratic government of President Rómulo Betancourt, Gabaldón was appointed Minister of Health and Social Assistance in 1959, a position that he held until 1964. One of his achievements as minister was his rural-housing program aimed at providing peasants with decent and hygienic accommodation at low cost. He also became involved in a great number of Venezuelan health administrative duties and in international advisory activities that took away time from his direct intervention in the Venezuela malaria program. As minister, Gabaldón tried to maintain the malaria-eradication campaign by transforming the old Division into the new Division of Rural Endemics and Environmental Health. The new Division also dealt with diarrheal diseases and Chagas disease, among other tasks. However, it was difficult to preserve sufficient funds and high status for malaria eradication. Despite the fact that the research unit of the Division of Rural Endemics became part of the School of Malariology, Gabaldón's efforts to reactivate malaria research were unsuccessful. Also, Maracay's international malaria course began to dilute, including other diseases such as gastroenteritis, colitis, typhoid, yellow fever, dengue, filariasis, recurrent fevers, leishmaniasis, Chagas disease, and bilharzias.

In a parallel development, during the 1960s, Gabaldón's international reputation as an expert increased. His active participation in advisory boards can be traced to his membership in the Malaria Commission of the Pan American Sanitary Bureau that met from the 1940s. Gabaldón's initial success in controlling malaria in a large area of Venezuela raised high hopes that eradication was possible in the Western hemisphere. With Fred L. Soper, director of the Pan American Sanitary Bureau, he supported at the bureau's fourteenth conference, which took place in Santiago in 1954, the malaria-eradication decision based on indoor spraying of DDT. From 1946 to 1970 Gabaldón was also a prominent member of the World Health Organization's Malaria Committee, another multilateral agency that supported eradication between the mid-1950s and the late 1960s. As member of this commission, he played an active role in the writing of a number of reports that became blueprints for malaria control and eradication all over the world. Among his many foreign invitations and distinctions was his appointment as Simon Bolivar Chair and Fellow of Trinity College, Cambridge University (1968).

During the early 1970s Gabaldón remained loyal to the idea that malaria eradication was possible, even though malaria was furiously coming back in Venezuela and other countries of Latin America (however, never at the level of incidence of the 1940s). He became more interested in the analysis and diffusion of Venezuela's early success with malaria. He disagreed with the return to malaria control and with the idea, promoted by WHO, that the development of basic health services should precede any disease-oriented campaign in rural and medically underserved areas.

In 1972, a year before his retirement from a distinguished career in public service and international health, Gabaldón founded a laboratory in the National Institute of Health to carry out research on avian malaria in Venezuelan birds. He established a malaria parasite model for turkeys, ducks, and pigeons, creatively linking mosquitoes with plasmodiums. In 1985 he was elected a member of the Venezuelan Academy of Physical, Mathematical, and Natural Sciences, delivering a paper on avian malaria in the neotropical region of Venezuela.

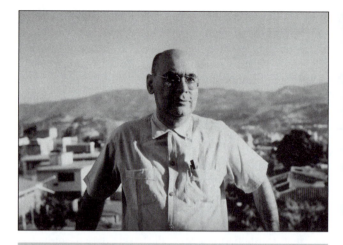

Arnoldo Gabaldón. Photograph by Leonard-Jan Bruce-Chwatt, Iconographic Collection, Wellcome Library, London.

Gabaldón's remarkable studies and leadership allowed Venezuela to overcome an obstacle in its economic and social development. For many writers, Venezuela's progress during the second half of the twentieth century (based in the productivity of oil camps located in rural areas and the raising of living standards of peasants) was partly explained by the control of malaria. Gabaldón also set an example of how a medical scientist from a developing country could do original research and improve the health of its population.

Bibliography

Primary: 1948. 'The Malaria Problem in the Neotropical.' *Proceedings of Fourth International Congress of Tropical Medicine and Malaria* 1: 913–927; 1954. (with Berti, Arturo Luis) 'The First Large Area in the Tropical Zone to Report Malaria Eradication: North Central Venezuela.' *American Journal Tropical Medicine and Hygiene* 5: 793–807; 1965. *Una política sanitaria* (Caracas); 1983. 'Malaria Eradication in Venezuela: Doctrine, Practice, and Achievements after Twenty Years.' *American Journal Tropical Medicine and Hygiene* 32: 203–211; 1998. *Malaria Aviaria en un país de la región neotropical: Venezuela* (Caracas).

Secondary: Gutiérrez, Ana T, 1998. *Tiempos de Guerra y Paz. Arnoldo Gabaldón y la investigación sobre Malaria en Venezuela (1936–1990)* (Caracas); Berti, Arturo Luis, 1997. *Arnoldo Gabaldón: Testimonio sobre una vida al servicio de la gente* (Caracas); Litsios, Socrates, 1988. 'Arnoldo Gabaldón's Independent Path for Malaria Control and Public Health in the Tropics: A Lost "Paradigm" for WHO.' *Parassitologia* 40(1–2): 231–238; Otero, Miguel, Rolando Sifontes, and Andrés Sucre, 1988. 'Evolución y estado actual del Programa antimalárico en Venezuela. Informe sobre la situación malárica en Venezuela. Año 1986.' *Gaceta Médica de Caracas* 4–6: 341–361; Gotteberg, Carlos, 1987. *Imagen y Huella de Arnoldo Gabaldón* (Caracas).

Yajaira Freites
Translation: Claudio Mendoza

GALE, GEORGE WILLIAM (b. Durban, South Africa, 21 May 1900; d. London, England, 24 March 1976), *social medicine, public health.*

The third child and only son of missionaries, Gale grew up in northern Zululand, spoke fluent Zulu, and was precociously bright. As a youngster he decided to train as a doctor and work among the Zulu. This ambition was made possible by a string of scholarships, which took him to school in Durban, at the Universities of Natal and South Africa (BSc, 1919, and MSc, 1921), and Edinburgh (MB, ChB, 1927, and Diplomas in Tropical Medicine, 1928, and Public Health, 1935).

Throughout his life Gale saw medicine as his Christian mission, and on qualification he returned to Natal to practice among rural Zulu communities (1928–1936). Hoping to address the dearth of rural health personnel, he joined a scheme at Fort Hare College (Eastern Cape) to train African medical aids (1936), but resigned within a year, convinced the program produced insufficient numbers and frustrated the trainees, who underwent lengthy training without achieving the status or rewards of a medical degree.

Seeking a position in the Union's Department of Public Health, he took appointments as Assistant Medical Officer of Health in Pietermaritzburg (Natal) and Benoni (Transvaal), to familiarize himself with urban health conditions. A pamphlet he published at his own expense discussing the health needs of rural Africans (Gale, 1938) led to his appointment in the Department of Public Health, where the rising tide of African ill-health was causing official alarm.

Within the department (1938–52), Gale was a powerful advocate of social medicine. His 'brilliant public health medicine' (Kark and Kark, 1999, p. 83) and knowledge of the Pholela health center informed the National Health Services Report (1944), much of which he probably wrote. Appointed the Secretary of Health and Chief Medical Officer of Health (1946–52), his reasoned defense of the health centers and the Clairwood Institute of Family and Community Health (IFCH) ensured their survival through the 1950s.

Thwarted by government health policy, Gale left the civil service to become dean of the new black medical school in Durban (1952). As dean, Gale incurred much official displeasure. Defeated in his desire to create a non-racial medical school for Africa, he nonetheless insisted it accept non–South African (black) students and be on par with other medical schools in the country—and regularly overspent his budget to achieve this. He also ensured that work at the IFCH was integrated into the students' clinical training. Despite his best efforts, however, the segregated medical school was deeply embedded in the racist norms of apartheid South Africa and provoked much student disaffection.

Constant problems with state and students led Gale to an appointment as professor of preventive medicine at Makerere, Uganda (1955–60), where he established the teaching of preventive medicine in students' clinical years and introduced health centers. On his retirement, he was appointed WHO Visiting Professor of Social and Preventive Medicine to the medical schools of Thailand (1960–64) and Kuala Lumpur, Malaysia (1965–69), integrating ideas of social medicine in the university curricula he drafted.

In fostering social medicine and a new form of medical education, Gale was in advance of most of his medical contemporaries in South Africa. His ideas were, however, recognized by the WHO at the time and still have relevance to the health needs of the developing world.

Bibliography

Primary: 1938. *A Suggested Approach to the Health Needs of the Native Rural Areas of South Africa* (Benoni, South Africa); 1944. U.G. 30-44. *Report of The National Health Services Commission* (Pretoria); 1970. 'The Aftermath—an Abiding Value' in Gluckman, Henry, *Abiding Values. Speeches and Addresses* (Johannesburg) pp. 495–518; 1999. Kark, Sidney, and Emily Kark. *Promoting Community Health. From Pholela to Jerusalem* (Johannesburg).

Secondary: Marks, Shula, 2000. 'George Gale, Social Medicine and the State in South Africa' in Dubow, Saul, ed., *Science and Society in South Africa* (Manchester) pp. 188–211; Marks, Shula, and Neil Andersson, 1992. 'Industrialization, Rural Health and the 1944 Health Services Commission in South Africa' in Feierman, Steven, and John M. Janzen, eds., *The Social Basis of Health and Healing in Africa* (Berkeley) pp. 131–161.

Shula Marks

GALEN OF PERGAMUM (b. Pergamum, Mysia, Asia Minor [now Bergama, Turkey], 129; d. Rome, Italy, *c.* 210), *medicine.*

Galen was the most influential and prolific medical author of antiquity. His extant works run to thousands of pages in Greek, and some additional works survive only in Arabic, Latin, or other translations, covering topics from logic and scientific method through anatomy, physiology, disease classification, element theory, hygienic (including diet and exercise), theory of the soul (or mind), and pharmacology.

Introduction

The sheer volume of Galen's output makes it difficult to summarize his work and the progress of his thought, and there are further problems for analysis. First is the lack of historical evidence for his career outside his own writings. There is almost no mention of him by any even near-contemporary author, so we are reliant on Galen himself for the facts of his career, with no independent yardstick to judge his significance or influence within his own lifetime. Other problems arise from certain peculiar features of his literary output, which result from important characteristics of his intellectual and cultural environment. These are the overwhelmingly polemical nature of his work and its 'mimetic', or classicizing, quality. Galen came from both an intensely competitive intellectual world and an educational formation in which rhetoric and philosophy (and more generally the 'classics' of Greek literature) took center stage. Galen's procedure of expressing his theories (a) by means of lengthy attacks on other individuals and schools, (b) by 'blinding with science' in the elaboration of his philosophical or technical distinctions, and (c) by assembling a rank of 'ancient' authorities (usually Plato and Hippocrates, but a shifting range of others according to specific contexts) who, he claimed, supported his views in any given area, leads to difficulty at times both in pinning down with precision Galen's own scientific theories and in determining the nature of consistency or connection between different areas of his thought.

Galen was, or appears to have been, a great systematizer: he spent pages outlining the fundamental definitions and distinctions in a topic, and his work was also full of cross-reference, suggesting a series of links between different works in different subject areas and an overall body of knowledge that was somehow spanned by the full range of his own writing. This suggestion was made even more explicitly by the two books of self-summary *My Own Books* and *The Order of My Own Books*. Yet the differences in technical language, use of authority, and intellectual approach—one may even say, genre—between treatises in the different areas mean that relationships between different styles of explanation are problematic. The text *Mixtures*, for example, and, relatedly, *The Soul's Dependence on the Body* give a far-reaching account of the determining effect of 'low-level' physical entities (the hot, cold, wet, and dry) on the individual's characteristics. Yet when we turn to other works—for example, works on organ-based physiology (*Natural Faculties*, *Doctrines of Hippocrates and Plato*) or disease classification—we encounter different sets of theoretical concepts, or jargons, in play in each 'genre'. It is not so much that the different types of account are physically inconsistent with each other, but rather that Galen left the precise nature of the connections unclear, as he moved between the different medical or philosophical languages given by the tradition in the particular field in which he was writing.

Biography and Intellectual Influences

Born in the city of Pergamum (Pergamon, Pergamos) on the western seaboard of Asia Minor in the Roman Empire, the son of an architect, Galen received the elite Greek-speaking education of the second century, specializing in philosophy until, supposedly in response to a god-sent dream, his father turned him to the study of medicine. His early exposure to philosophy, however, was crucial; for Galen throughout his career was to put philosophical modes of argument (and the specifics of Platonic and Aristotelian doctrine) at the heart of his peculiar medical-philosophical synthesis. More specifically, it seems that an early exposure to Skepticism (then a prominent strand in Platonist philosophy) left him not just with an abiding intellectual hatred of Skepticism, but with a powerful sense of the need to combat it by founding scientific propositions on as secure a logical basis as possible. From his early twenties he spent several years completing his education by travel and study, including in Alexandria, coming into contact with anatomists and experts in the Hippocratic texts; and it was from this early period that some of his first major anatomical and logical works date. He then spent some time as a doctor to the gladiators, and in his first Roman period (162–66), he took part in public displays of (animal) anatomy as well as writing on physiology/anatomy. In 168, he went as military doctor on campaign with the army of Marcus Aurelius in Germany, returning the following year. Galen gained the patronage of several elite members of Roman society (including the emperor himself) and over the next forty or so years wrote the rest of his vast output on physiology, diagnosis and therapy, hygienic, pharmacology, Hippocratic commentary, and soul theory.

Logic and Epistemology

Galen's interest in philosophy, and his abhorrence of Skepticism and of what he considered sophistical modes of argument, led him to a serious engagement with logic. On the one hand, this brought about certain technical developments of interest to the specialist logician; of more significance for Galen's scientific work was the way in which he attempted to bring Platonic concepts of truth and certainty and Aristotelian ways of presenting a proof (syllogistic) to bear on arguments about biological and therapeutic matters. At one level this insistence on rigor can be seen as a rhetorical tool: Galen used superior knowledge of philosophy to impress and trump rival practitioners who may in some cases have been less well-educated or of artisan background. But Galen's devotion to rationality, as well as the ruthless rigor of his logical arguments (though it is a rigor that cannot always be consistently pursued), won him admirers, including in the modern age. Within the medical context of his own time, Galen engaged with (and provided us with the major evidence for) the divergent medical 'sects'—Rationalists (or Dogmatists), Empiricists, and Methodists (a kind of theoretical minimalists). While asserting the importance of observation and claiming his own personal superiority in this field, Galen always put to the fore the need for a strong theoretical framework, in the sense of a clear understanding of physiological causation and the ability to reason logically.

Anatomy and Physiology

Galen's extensive work here put him in the tradition of Alexandria, in particular of Herophilus and Erasistratus. Whereas in Hellenistic Alexandria, dissection of human cadavers seems to have taken place, it is unclear whether or to what extent Galen was experienced in human anatomy. Most of his dissections were apparently performed on Barbary apes, although presumably at least his work as a doctor for the gladiators and his stint as a military doctor on campaign gave him some first-hand exposure to human anatomy. He wrote extensively on anatomical procedures, and his vast work—*The Usefulness of the Parts of the Body*—showed a high degree of accuracy in anatomical description. For Galen, though, anatomy was more than just anatomy: *The Usefulness of the Parts* is better described as a work of Aristotelian anatomy-physiology, the main aim throughout being to show that 'nature does nothing in vain' and to demonstrate the way each part of the body has been perfectly created for its function. Anatomy thus becomes a 'hymn to the creator'. This belief in purpose or function in nature, and in particular in physiology, was a constant philosophical theme; alongside the Skeptics, as the target of Galen's philosophical ire, were those (following the Epicurean school in philosophy, or doctors like Erasistratus) who attributed physiological events to purely mechanistic causes. Here Galen was heavily influenced by the biological works of Aristotle.

Physiological System

Galen's physiological theories were not always clear in all their details: the exact processes of sense perception, for example, or exactly what a *dynamis* (power or faculty)—a commonly used explanans of organ-function—was. In its overall scheme, though, his physiological system can be seen as a fascinatingly ambitious synthesis of Platonic-Aristotelian philosophy (in particular, the theory of the 'three-part soul') with developments from the Alexandrian anatomical-physiological tradition already mentioned. Central to this system was the role of brain as the 'source of perception and voluntary motion' and as the seat of rational thought—a view that Galen supported with an impressive (from a modern standpoint) array of experimentally backed arguments (especially in *The Doctrines of Hippocrates and Plato*, a text that clearly bears some relation to a public demonstration before a crowd). He showed, for example, that ligation of the spinal cord of a pig led to loss of function (e.g., voice, limb movements) at any level below that of the ligation. This clarity regarding brain function, however, could be said to contrast with two much cloudier areas: first, the precise content of his theories regarding vital heat, respiration, the vascular system, and the heart; and second, quite how Galen's *physiological* account of the functions divided between his major organs—brain, heart, and liver—could be mapped onto a theory of the soul deriving from Plato. (Plato's three-part theory was essentially concerned with accounting for moral conflict within the soul and the need for the supremacy of reason over the passions).

In Galen's version, at any rate, brain, heart, and liver were the chief *archai* (sources or principles) in the body: the brain as already described; the heart, the source of 'the blood that courses vigorously' and of involuntary motion (in the sense that the heart continued to govern the functions that maintained life without conscious input from the brain); and the liver of nutrition, related to vegetative function and to desires for food and sex. It should be added that *The Art of Medicine*, now doubted as an authentic work of Galen but of great influence on medieval Galenism, includes the genitals as a fourth *archê*. Each source then had its own network of distribution and instrument (*organon*) by which it performed its function: the liver (seen as the producer of blood) was the source of the veins; the heart was the source of the arteries, with the instrument being blood mixed with a particular kind of air, the *pneuma zôtikon* or life-supporting breath; the brain was the source of the nerves, and the instrument was another *pneuma*, the *pneuma psychikon* (mental), this latter being 'elaborated' from the former. Note here that in his physiology of the vascular system, Galen took issue with his most noted forebear Erasistratus, who believed there was *only* pneuma in the arteries. Galen thus arrived at a distinction between arteries and veins, which bears some resemblance to our understanding, while in no way approaching a theory of circulation or indeed a fully worked-out conception of the function of the heart. For Galen, breathing had a role in both fuelling and moderating the vital heat (closely connected with the heart), and respiration also took place through pores in the skin, enabling pneuma to enter the arteries at their fine ends. It was essentially the state of knowledge as left by Galen that Harvey took as his starting point (with specific reference to the Galenic works) in his *De motu cordis*. With regard to perception and the motion of the muscles, Galen was clear about the role of the nerves as channel of transmission (or 'flow'), but less clear as to whether or in what way the pneuma was involved in this transmission.

Fundamental Qualities

Galen's 'element theory', perhaps more properly described as a theory of qualities (the fundamental entities, he believed, were 'the hot', 'the cold', 'the wet', and 'the dry'), was one derived from a long tradition. In line with his preferred affiliations, he was at pains to ascribe it to 'Hippocrates' (drawing mostly on the Hippocratic *Airs, Waters, Places*); but in its specifics, it owed as much to Aristotle. The theory, most fully laid out in *Mixtures*, was one that gave an account both of the balance or 'mixture' most conducive to health in the individual and of the congenital differences *between* individuals (and races), as well as of the ways in which environment (winds, ambient heat, and so on) and diet affected health. Particular substances (e.g., poppy, mandragora, and hemlock) could be described as cold, in the sense that they had a cooling effect on the body; Galen's element or 'quality' theory was thus of close relevance to his theory of health (hygienic), to his pharmacology, and also to aspects of his soul theory (because the balance or mixture of the brain was a key determinant in mental matters).

Hygienic

As stated, the theory of elements was of central importance to the conception of health, as it determined both the analysis of the individual's state (e.g., too hot, too wet) and the analysis of which foods, physical environments, and forms of exercise or rest could be prescribed for that state. At the same time, in his *Hygienics* (the actual Greek title of his major work in the area, usually translated as *De Sanitate Tuenda*, or *On the Preservation of Health*, and incidentally a work widely read and translated—by Thomas Linacre for Henry VIII, for example—in early modern times), Galen doubtless took on much that was traditional in terms of perceptions of the properties of individual foods and other prescriptions. Hygienic was the study of what the healthy or near-healthy individual should do to remain healthy or return to perfect health, as opposed to the study of disease proper and its cure. It thus resembled the modern study of diet or of exercise more than anything in modern orthodox medicine. Particular foods, as well as types of bath, massage, and exercise, were prescribed for particular conditions, but this procedure was distinguished from the prescription of *pharmaka*, which only applied in the case of actual illness. It is noteworthy not just that 'health' in this conception seemed only available to the person with sufficient resources of wealth and leisure, but also that the pursuit of health was potentially an all-day, lifelong pursuit, which could sit alongside the other pursuits of an educated gentleman: one might have included a doctor in one's entourage in the same way that one surrounded oneself with poets, artists, or philosophers. It is also worth noting that in this area, too, Galen (and doctors generally) worked in a highly competitive environment. There were—as today—a host of athletic or gymnasium trainers who believed that their prescriptions on diet and exercise were the path to health, and these trainers were the object of Galen's particular virulent polemical attack (see his *Exhortation to Study the Arts*), partly for training the body in a dangerously unbalanced way, partly because they—unphilosophically—concentrated on the body at the expense of the soul.

Disease Classification, Diagnosis, and Cure

In a range of works on the classification of diseases and symptoms and on the nature of diagnosis and healing, Galen offered definitions and systems of categorization of considerable complexity, often preferring to remain at the abstract level for long stretches of text. Disease was understood in terms of impairment of the function of an organ, and at the same time there was a causal relation with imbalances of qualities as outlined previously. There were also, however, distinct 'disease entities' (e.g., phrenitis, mania, dropsy, and fever), all of them already extant in the Greek medical tradition, which seemed to exist to some extent in isolation from the overarching theoretical system. Where fever was concerned, the disease category admitted a bewildering system of categorization in its own right. Both here and in the realm of diagnostic tools (especially the urine and the pulse, both of them subjects of extensive texts, again laying out systems of bewildering divisions and subdivisions), Galen the philosopher-doctor seemed brilliantly to have had his cake and eaten it too, demonstrating his unsurpassed ability to endlessly refine *definitions* while simultaneously at pains to stress that it was only through lifelong practical *experience* that one would be able to identify any of these distinctions in an actual patient. A few of his texts, most notably *Prognosis*, used anecdote to give a vivid flavor (one tainted by extravagant self-publicism) of the day-to-day practice of Galen as a doctor in elite Roman circles and of the range of observational techniques he used. The actual therapeutic tools included dietary prescriptions/restrictions, *pharmaka*, and the much-favored phlebotomy.

Pharmacology

Although again linked to his broader theories of the human body, in particular his theories of the fundamental qualities, Galen's pharmacology stands as perhaps a more independent body (and a very large one) than any other branch of his work. As in other areas, but in a different way, Galen looked back over a vast tradition of previous work and incorporated it within his own. The analysis of *pharmaka* (which were mainly of plant origin but included some of an animal or mineral nature) fell within the framework of the hot, the cold, and so on—and incidentally involved an unusual element, within Greek medicine, of *quantification*, as drugs were categorized in terms such as 'one degree hot'. Yet we may suspect that the actual use of a drug in a particular context essentially relied above all on the long tradition of received wisdom on drug use, which stretched back, at all sorts of literate and nonliterate levels, to the times of the Hippocratics and beyond. In any case, Galen recorded the pharmacological use of a great range of substances, and his work—while making interesting claims with regard to empirical methodology—stood alongside that of such authors as Dioscorides as a main source of evidence for herbal pharmacology in the ancient world.

Psychology/Soul Theory

To talk of Galen's theory of the soul or mind (*psychê*—the Greek word is used in discussions in both the philosophical and the medical context) is problematic because what we

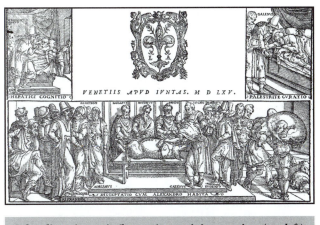

Galen dissecting a pig (bottom), examining a patient (top left), and bleeding a patient (top right). Woodcut, title page from *Opera omnia . . .* **1565. Rare Books, Wellcome Library, London.**

actually have is a series of discussions of the soul in quite different contexts, which in some ways seem to belong within different theoretical frameworks. We have seen how the soul in one sense belonged within Galen's theory of the *physiology* of the major organs. In another context, *The Soul's Dependence on the Body*, which considered the soul not from a physiological point of view but from that of its moral characteristics, Galen came close to a physicalist-determinist account in terms of the mixture of qualities in the brain. In yet another text he considered *The Affections and Errors of the Soul*—again in the moral sense—in terms that relied purely on cognitive and relational approaches. In each of these contexts the language used to discuss the 'soul' was Platonic, but in each case with different propositions and aims in view. There was, furthermore, a medical vocabulary of the soul, involving such traditional disease concepts as melancholy and mania. Discussion of the latter were found more in Galen's generalist works on health and disease than in his specific works on the soul; and it is perhaps striking that the 'disturbances' of the soul in this medicalized sense were discussed less, and less interestingly, by Galen than the soul's 'affections' (the Greek word *pathos* is used in both contexts), as understood in the moral-philosophical sense. Galen also wrestled with the larger 'philosophy-of-mind' question as to the definition or 'substance' of the soul—a question that he explicitly raised on a number of occasions and to which he always refused a final answer. Drawn (perhaps increasingly) to a physicalist answer in terms of the mixture in the brain, he seemed reluctant to commit himself to it definitively, while at the same time expressing doubt as to why a nonphysical soul would leave the body the result of physical causes.

Galen the Scholar

We have seen how Galen was keen to father his own theories on the great 'ancients', in particular Plato and Hippo-

crates; in the process, he engaged in scholarly analysis of the texts. Such scholarly analysis was in evidence *passim* in his important works (*The Doctrines of Hippocrates and Plato* and *The Soul's Dependence on the Body* being prominent examples); on some texts (Plato's *Timaeus* and a range of Hippocratic works), he went so far as to write detailed commentaries. Though the enterprise was a partial one and entailed specific beliefs about texts that a modern scholar would find incredible (the notion that Hippocratic authors had anatomical knowledge but did not bother to write it down, for example, or more specifically, the attempt to bring into line with Galen's own physiological theory a Hippocratic text that does not even have the distinction between veins and arteries), what is interesting is the level of scholarly sophistication at which Galen operated. Aware both of the apparent difficulties of reconciling the ancient texts with his views and of a 'Hippocratic question' as to authorship of the texts, he addressed points of detail about the shift in meanings of terms over time, the way in which a text was determined by the intended audience, and questions of authorship and consistency of view over a range of texts, in a way that made him in a sense a forerunner of modern Hippocratic scholarship.

Bibliography

Primary: (English translations of those works that either are the most important or are accompanied by particularly helpful introduction/commentary, or both.) 1968. (May, M. T., trans.). *Galen on the Usefulness of the Parts of the Body* (Ithaca, NY); 1978–84. (De Lacy, P., trans., ed., and comm.). *Galen on the Doctrines of Hippocrates and Plato* 3 vols. (Corpus Medicorum Graecorum, v. 4.1.2, Berlin); 1979. (Nutton, V., trans., ed., and comm.) *Galen on Prognosis* (Corpus Medicorum Graecorum v. 8.1, Berlin); 1984. (Furley, D. J., and J. S. Wilkie, trans., eds., and comms.) *Galen on Respiration and the Arteries* (Princeton); 1985. (Frede, M., and R. Walzer, trans. and eds.) *Galen: Three Treatises on the Nature of Science* (Indianapolis); 1997. (Singer, P. N., trans., introd., and notes) *Galen: Selected Works* (Oxford).

Secondary: Rocca, J., 2003. *Galen on the Brain: Anatomical Knowledge and Physiological Speculation in the Second Century AD* (Leiden and Boston); Garcia-Ballester, L., 2002. *Galen and Galenism: Theory and Practice from Antiquity to the Early Renaissance,* Arrizabalaga, J., M. Cabré, L. Cifuentes, and F. Salmón, eds. (Aldershot); Debru, A., ed., 1997. *Galen on Pharmacology: Philosophy, History and Medicine.* Proceedings of the 5th International Galen Colloquium, Lille, 16–18 March 1995 (Leiden, New York, Köln); Haase, W., and H. Temporini, eds., 1994. *Aufstieg und Niedergang der römischen Welt* [Rise and Decline of the Roman World], part 2, vol. 37.2 (Berlin); Barton, T. S., 1994. *Power and Knowledge: Astrology, Physiognomics and Medicine under the Roman Empire* (Ann Arbor); Nutton, V., 1988. *From Democedes to Harvey: Studies in the History of Medicine* (London), *DSB*.

P. N. Singer

GALL, FRANZ JOSEPH (b. Tiefenbronn, near Pforzheim, Germany, 9 March 1758; d. Paris, France, 22 August 1828), *neuroanatomy, psychology, craniology.*

Gall was the son of a modest wool merchant and sometime mayor of Tiefenbronn. Both his parents were devout Roman Catholics who intended their son for the church. Gall duly received his early education from an uncle who was a priest, before attending schools in Baden and Bruchsal. But although he remained nominally religious and was even to include a cerebral faculty for religion in his theory of brain structure, he was neither devout nor seen to be. Castigated for propagating materialism, atheism, fatalism, and immorality, he saw his books placed on the Index, and he was denied a religious burial. He is also alleged to have had many mistresses and to have sired an illegitimate son. In 1777, the same year that he married a young Alsatian girl, he began medical studies at Strasbourg, and in 1781 he moved to Vienna, where he received his MD in 1785. Until his death, he ran a conventional, if highly successful, medical practice, first in Vienna and then in Paris, where he took up permanent residence in 1807 and became a French citizen in 1819. Among his patients were the novelist Stendhal, the social theorist Comte de Saint-Simon, and the politician Prince Metternich, as well as the staff of twelve embassies. In 1825, after the death of his wife in Vienna, Gall married his mistress of many years, Marie Anne Barbe. The following year, he showed signs of cerebral and coronary sclerosis, and two years later, he died of an apoplectic stroke.

Gall's first publication, *Philosophisch-Medicinische Untersuchungen über Natur und Kunst im kranken und gesunden Zustande des Menschen* (1791), was largely a diatribe against metaphysics, and idealist and romantic speculations. Gall regarded himself as an empiricist revealing 'Nature's truths' and took as his particular mission the integration of scientific problems of mind and brain with those of life and society. From the mid-1790s he began collecting and studying human and animal skulls, as well as conducting extensive anatomical dissections of the brain. He developed his ideas (and showmanship) in public lectures and demonstrations in Vienna from 1796 until 1801, when the Emperor of Austria forbade them for being socially subversive in tending to materialism and atheism. In 1805, with his assistant, the medical student Johann Gaspar Spurzheim (1776–1832), he undertook a lecture tour of Germany, Denmark, the Netherlands, Switzerland, and France, which lasted until October 1807, when he settled in Paris. The tour was a resounding success, earning him considerable fame and fortune. The illustrious and fashionable flocked to his lectures, which were lavishly illustrated by a large assortment of casts and skulls as well as, initially at least, a performing monkey (rather in the manner of popular outdoor entertainments). Within scientific and medical circles, however, Gall's ideas were a source of intense and often acrimonious debate. Some contemporaries rightly detected that his cerebral theory did not in fact depend on his neuroanatomical and neurophysiological researches (which were generally admired), but simply drew credibility from association with them. Partly for this reason and partly because Napoleon took steps to restrict his influence in Paris, Gall's doctrines were rejected by the Institut de France in 1808, and in 1821 he failed to gain admission to the French Academy.

Gall's 'skull doctrine' (*Schädellehre*), or 'Organologie', as he preferred to call what others were to denominate 'craniology' and (after 1815) 'phrenology', was based on six propositions, none of which was strictly original. The first was that humans and animals were born with innate faculties or aptitudes. This was a commonsensical notion, which was partly born out of Gall's schoolboy observation that students who were better than he at memorizing had large, protruding eyes. Nevertheless, when forwarded as scientific doctrine, the notion flew in the face of Gall's contemporaries, the French *idéologues* who emphasized the importance of environment and learning over innate endowment.

Gall's second proposition—that the brain was the organ of the mind—was equally familiar, having been reiterated since the beginning of anatomy and physiology. But it, too, was also hugely controversial in that it radically challenged both the notion of the indivisibility of mind and the mind-body dualism posited by René Descartes. According to Gall, the mind (as brain) was a part of the organization of the body as a whole, not something separate from it. In thus treating the problem of brain and mind as analogous to that of any other organ and its function, Gall was original in bringing the mind–body problem into the domain of dynamic physiology and biology. The experimental physiologist Marie-Jean-Pierre Flourens (1794–1867), who opposed Gall's theory of cerebralization, nevertheless granted that it was wholly as a result of Gall that the proposition that the brain was the exclusive organ of the mind came to reign in nineteenth-century science.

Third, Gall proposed that the brain was not a homogeneous unity, but an aggregate of cerebral organs ('faculties') with discrete functions. Hitherto, within philosophies of mind, 'mental faculties' indicated nonspecific functional parameters; in Gall's system, however, they were physical operational vectors in unitary self-contained compartments of brain-matter. Cerebral ganglia, Gall believed, served as centers for determinate talents or propensities. Ultimately, after correlating many observations made of inmates of insane asylums, prisons, schools, and persons in public life, Gall concluded that there were twenty-seven such fundamental faculties in humans, nineteen of them shared by men and animals. From the point of view of the history of psychology, this assigning of specific mental functions to specific anatomical organs was the most revolutionary aspect of Gall's system. For the historian of philosophy, George Henry Lewes, who was no partisan of phrenology, it merited Gall 'the Kepler of Psychology' (Lewes, 1857, p. 640). As with his concept of cerebral localization, so with his psychophysiology a functional approach predominated—and endured. The term 'function', as applied to psychological and social phenomena, can in fact be traced back from its late-nineteenth-century and twentieth-century uses to the writings of Gall and his followers.

Gall further maintained that the cerebral organs were topographically localized and that, other factors being equal, the relative size of any one of them could be taken as an index to its power of manifestation. The 'organ of the sense for collecting and retaining facts', for instance, which Gall located just above the nose, would be larger in persons with that propensity.

Finally, and no less controversially, Gall proposed that because the skull ossified over the brain during infant development, external craniological means could be used to detect the internal state of these mental organs or faculties. Striking talents and propensities were correlated with the prominences on the skulls of men and animals. (So, too, in this correlation, were particular 'passions', phenomena hitherto associated not with the brain but with particular glands, such as the thyroid.) Here Gall's theory intersected with, and profited from, contemporary interest in physiognomy, especially as rekindled in the late eighteenth century by the Reverend Johann Caspar Lavater (1741–1801). Significantly, the first full account of Gall's doctrine (which was written by Spurzheim) was not entitled a 'craniological system' or 'brain organology', but rather, *The Physiognomical System of Drs. Gall and Spurzheim* (1815). Gall's physiognomy was profoundly different from that delineated by Lavater, however. Not only did it give no scope to immaterial and occult forces, but crucially, it related external signs of character to internal neurophysiological functions. Although Gall saw himself simply as recasting psychology from a branch of philosophy to one of biology, his physiognomy also fitted with a broader and more fundamental contemporary European project: the perception of the self in terms of psychological interiority.

Gall's organology and craniology as a basis for divining character and directing personality change were widely taken up in the early nineteenth century, especially in Britain and the United States. After lecture tours by Spurzheim and popularizations by Spurzheim's Scottish disciple, George Combe (1788–1858), there emerged a social reformist phrenology movement that was crucially important in the popular dissemination of scientific naturalism. Phrenology also had a profound impact in education, penal reform, and improvements in the care of the insane, as well as on such scientific writings as those of G. H. Lewes, Robert Chambers, and Charles Darwin's cotheorist, A. R. Wallace. Other luminaries who took phrenology seriously included G. W. F. Hegel, Otto von Bismarck, Karl Marx, Balzac, the Brontës, George Eliot, Walt Whitman, and Queen Victoria.

Although it is only the craniological aspect of Gall's doctrine that is recalled at the mention of phrenology today, for most of the nineteenth century, Gall's basic ideas were perceived as pivotal to reconceptualizing psychology, neu-

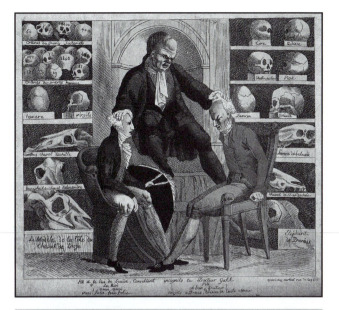

In a room filled with skulls of the famous, Franz Joseph Gall examines Pitt the Younger and Gustavus IV of Sweden, 1806. Etching with watercolor, Iconographic Collection, Wellcome Library, London.

roanatomy, and philosophy. Although neither his detailed classification nor his faculty psychology were to stand the test of time, contemporary opponents and advocates alike appreciated that his reduction of questions of mind and brain to the single domain of dynamic physiology constituted a historically significant means to sweeping away centuries of metaphysical speculations and reflections. According to his most astute modern biographer, his neuroanatomical work 'helped to alter the context of the study of brain from the prevailing mechanical and humoral theories to an organic, biological perspective' (Young, 1972, *DSB* vol. 5, p. 251). Indeed, the dust had hardly settled on the phrenology movement of the first half of the nineteenth century when the neurological fundamentals of Gall's ideas were significantly reinforced. Beginning in the 1860s, clinical support for cerebral localization emerged in France with the work of Jean-Baptiste Bouillaud and Pierre-Paul Broca; in Germany, epochally in 1870, through the physiological evidence of G. T. Fritsch and E. Hitzig; and in Britain, through the research of John Hughlings Jackson and David Ferrier, among others. Although these pioneers in brain function set aside Gall's specific concepts, they adopted his general principles, rendering the concept of the localization of brain function central to neurology and neurosurgery. So, too, as in psychology, where Gall's ideas shifted the context of study from metaphysical speculation on the nature of mind and thought to general biology, in sociology—not least through the work of its modern founders, Herbert Spencer and Auguste Comte—Gall's biological approach paved the way for fundamental and enduring reconceptualizations of man's place in nature.

Bibliography

Primary: 1808. *Recherches sur le système nerveux en general, et sur celui du cerveau en particulier; mémoire présenté à l'Institut de France, le 14 mars 1808* (Paris); 1810–19. *Anatomie et Physiologie du Système Nerveux en général, et du Cerveau en particular* 4 vols. and atlas of 1,000 plates (vols. 1 and 2 coauthored by Spurzheim, J. G.) (Paris); 1822–1825. *Sur les functions du cerveau et sur celles de chacune de ses parties* 6 vols. (Paris) [1835. Lewis, W. Jr., English trans. 6 vols. (Boston)].

Secondary: Wyhe, John van, 2002. 'The Authority of Human Nature: The *Schädellehre* of Franz Joseph Gall.' *British Journal for the History of Science* 35: 17–42; Heintel, Helmut, 1986. *Leben und Werk von Franz Joseph Gall: Eine Chronik* (Würzburg); Young, Robert M., 1970. *Mind, Brain and Adaptation in the Nineteenth Century* (Oxford); Lewes, George Henry, 1857. 'Phrenology' in his *Biographical History of Philosophy* (2nd revised edn., London) pp. 629–645; *DSB*.

Roger Cooter

GARCÍA SOLÁ, EDUARDO (b. Malaga, Spain, 17 February 1845; d. Granada, Spain, 13 January 1922), *histopathology, microbiology.*

García Solá studied at the School of Medicine of Granada University, where he graduated in 1867. He was taught by Mariano López Mateos (1802–63), who introduced Spain to the cell theory of Theodor Schwann. He was also taught by Aureliano Maestre de San Juan (1828–90), professor of anatomy, whose main interest was microscopic research and who later moved to Madrid to occupy the first professorship created in this field. García Solá spent his entire scientific life at the School of Medicine in Granada, where he was professor of pathology (1872–87) and then professor of normal histology and histochemistry (1887–1917). He also served as Rector of the university from 1891 to 1909.

García Solá was an early follower of laboratory medicine in Spain, supporting the application of basic science to attain a better clinical understanding of diseases. He was possibly the most important Spanish histologist and pathologist before the arrival on the scene of Santiago Ramón y Cajal. Two stages can be distinguished in his scientific production. In the first, from 1872 to 1880, he focused on pathology (histopathology) in active collaboration with Benito Hernando Espinosa (1846–1916), a fellow professor at Granada and director of San Lázaro Hospital. Visitors to this hospital, which specialized in leprosy, included Rudolf Virchow in the 1880s. During this period, García Solá published numerous papers that demonstrated his excellent knowledge of the main theories of his time, especially Virchow's version of cell theory.

From 1880 onward García Solá concentrated on microbiology, first parasitic diseases and then medical microbiology, producing more than thirty publications in this field. Of particular note were his studies on the specific action of germs (1884) and on natural immunity (1888) and especially those on cholera and leprosy. García Solá was one of the experts called to Valencia during a cholera epidemic in 1885 to assess the effectiveness of the vaccine against this disease discovered by Jaime Ferrán Clúa (1851–1929). In a report of great scientific rigor, he experimentally demonstrated that the disease was indeed cholera. He was highly critical of Ferrán for his reticence in permitting experimental studies to demonstrate the efficacy of his vaccine. In relation to leprosy, he developed a laboratory technique to distinguish the tuberculoid and lepromatous forms of the disease (1891).

As rector of Granada University, García Solá contributed to improving the facilities at the university. He was also a convinced defender of university autonomy and decentralization and of the teaching model applied in Germany, where laboratory medicine began. Finally, he championed the inclusion of new subjects in medical studies, such as ophthalmology, neurology, and microbiology.

Bibliography

Primary: 1874. *Tratado de patología general y anatomía patológica* (Madrid); 1885. 'El cólera de Valencia y la vacunación anticolérica.' *Gaceta médica de granada* 3: 417–436; 449–467; 481–489; 1888. *Tratado elemental de histología e histoquimia normales* (Madrid).

Secondary: Olagüe de Ros, Guillermo, 2001. *Sobre sólida roca fundada. Ciento veinte años de labor docente, asistencial e investigadora en la Facultad de Medicina de Granada (1857–1972)* (Granada) especially pp. 64–68; López Piñero, José María, 1983. 'García Solá, Eduardo' in López Piñero, José María, et al., eds., *Diccionario histórico de la ciencia moderna en España.* (Barcelona) vol. 1, pp. 383–384; Torres López, Antonio Jesús, 1959. 'Eduardo García Solá.' *Actualidad Médica* 35: 811–820.

Guillermo Olagüe de Ros

GARCÍA-MEDINA, PABLO (b. Tunja, Colombia, 12 August 1858; d. Bogotá, Colombia, 11 July 1935), *hygiene, public health.*

García-Medina, nephew of the physician-pharmacist Bernardino Medina (a university professor of materia medica and pharmacy), attended the Universidad Nacional in Bogotá, graduating MD in 1880. He worked and later shared his uncle's office and drugstore and joined Bogotá's Society of Medicine and Natural Sciences in 1889. Influenced by the 1890 medical congress held in Cuba, García-Medina organized similar medical events, meetings that started in 1893 in Colombia under his guidance.

In 1886 the Colombian government created the Central Board of Hygiene (CBH) to control the spread of diseases and epidemics, to inspect the quality of food and water, to provide adequate waste disposal, and to establish quarantines in city ports. This was the first attempt to establish a national state-supported organization of public health. García-Medina became the secretary of the CBH in 1891, and from that date until 1932 he was its main leader and took the task of establishing a national public health administration for Colombia. He was convinced that the state had the main responsibility for the population's health. García-Medina found that the structure of a board made decision making difficult and in 1918 managed to convince the political authorities of this, so the Congress enacted a law replacing the CBH with the centralized National Direction of Hygiene (it is interesting to note that the term used was 'hygiene', because of French medical influences). García-Medina was its director until 1932. At the same time he taught hygiene and physiology at the Universidad Nacional and held prestigious positions, such as secretary of the National Academy of Medicine (1891–1903). He was also the president of this institution (1910–12). He used these positions to help gain prestige for hygienic activities. Before then, the status of Colombian physicians was tied mainly to clinical and private practice.

Around the turn of the twentieth century, an institutionalized poor-relief system, in which private charity and state beneficence worked together, was organized in Colombia. A number of hospitals, medical-care services for the poor, asylums for mentally ill individuals, and leprosy-control activities were part of the charitable endeavor. A key achievement of García-Medina was the incorporation of these matters into a public health policy changing the system. Poor relief was considered no longer a charitable option but a state obligation. In 1925 the National Direction of Hygiene became the National Direction of Hygiene and Public Assistance, and García-Medina kept its directorship until 1932, when a new liberal government removed him from his post. The reason for his removal was that he had worked with the previous conservative regime.

Over forty years, García-Medina's leadership established a centralized direction of public health for the country and fulfilled all of Colombia's international sanitary regulations. García-Medina was committed to progress and civilization, which was understood as synonymous with participation in the world market. Sanitation of seaports was considered essential to Colombia's development of an export economy in agriculture and to the opening of markets with Europe and the United States. García-Medina participated in the Sixth International Sanitary Conference held in Montevideo (1921), where he was named vice-president, and in the first conference of national directors of health, carried on in Washington (1926), where he was appointed honorary president of the Pan American Sanitary Bureau. Throughout his career he worked with international health organizations such as the Rockefeller Foundation, which helped organize campaigns in Colombia against hookworm and yellow fever.

Bibliography

Primary: 1910. *Tratado elemental de higiene y nociones de fisiología para la enseñanza de estas materias en las escuelas y colegios de Colombia* (Bogotá); 1932. *Compilación de leyes, decretos, acuerdos y resoluciones vigentes sobre higiene y sanidad en Colombia* 2 vols. (Bogotá).

Secondary: Hernández Álvarez, Mario, 2002. *La salud fragmentada en Colombia, 1910–1946* (Bogotá); Aparicio, Julio, 1951. 'Elogio del doctor Pablo García Medina.' *Revista de la Facultad de Medicina* 20: 9–20.

Diana Obregón

GARIOPONTUS (aka GUARIMPOTUS) (fl. *c.* 1035–1050, Salerno, Italy), *medicine.*

Gariopontus of Salerno was the author of a large medical treatise, the *Passionarius* or *Book of Diseases*. The text, a practical manual arranged in head-to-foot order and treating both particular and universal conditions, was widely popular with learned physicians throughout the Middle Ages and was published in its entirety three times in the Renaissance.

Relatively little is known about Gariopontus's personal life. Peter Damian, a monk at the Abbey of Monte Cassino and a cardinal under Pope Leo IX, referred to Gariopontus at mid-century as 'an old man to me, a most upright gentleman, and a scholarly physician outstandingly learned in medicine' (Glaze, 2005, pp. 71–72). Similarly, Lawrence of Amalfi, former monk of Monte Cassino, addressed a letter to Gariopontus at about the same time; he discussed allegorical interpretations of biblical topics in such a reverential tone as to suggest that Gariopontus's own scriptural interpretations were vastly superior to Lawrence's and others'. The signature or subscription of Gariopontus appears in several Salernitan documents and charts the progression of his clerical career: he is 'clericus', 'subdiaconus', 'yppodiaconus', and 'presbiter'.

Gariopontus's considerable efforts at compiling a synthetic manual for medical practice were motivated by the sorry state of medical literature in his day. His *Passionarius* interweaves chapters from several distinct treatises of the Early Middle Ages that circulated often as a loose unit of treatises. These represent excerpts, translations, and adaptations of ancient, largely Greek medical literature, as rendered into Latin by the sixth and seventh centuries. These include the early medieval Galenic *Ad Glauconem de medendi methodo, Liber tertius, Aurelius, Esculapius,* and some excerpts from Theodorus Priscianus. To these were added, probably in the eleventh century, a series of chapters 'On Gout' taken from Alexander of Tralles's *Therapeutics.* In addition to presenting a more logical order useful to practical utility, Gariopontus's version clarifies through editorial intervention both the Latinity of his source texts and the considerable Greek technical terminology that saturated them—for example, the names of diseases, symptoms, and materia medica. The order of treatment begins with diseases of the head and progresses downward with successive books treating thorax, abdomen, and pelvic viscera; muscles and articulations; and skin and eruptive conditions with spasms and paralysis; and the book concludes with two books on fevers. In the Renaissance printings of the text, one printer divided it into eight books, and modern scholars have suggested in error that the books on fevers represent a separate text. Neither of these proposals is justified by the more than fifty surviving manuscripts, in which the text is always arranged in seven books, with books six and seven on fevers counted as integral components of Gariopontus's work.

The *Passionarius* was composed just prior to the new wave of translations of Greco-Arabic material produced in the region by Constantine the African and others. In spite of this, Gariopontus's text enjoyed ready popularity with the twelfth-century and early thirteenth-century Salernitan scholars, among whom it was cited widely as an authority and was often coupled in Salernitan *practicae* with the very useful *Viaticum* of Constantine. The absence of the full text of the *Pantegni, Practica* may account in part for this situation. Because of Gariopontus's Salernitan associations, in the later Middle Ages, university-trained physicians often found his text both desirable and useful for their own collections. In the end, the logical arrangement and practical utility of Gariopontus's treatise guaranteed its popularity well into the sixteenth century.

Bibliography

Primary: 1526. *Passionarius Galeni* (Lyons); 1531. *Garioponti vetusti admodum medici ad totius corporis aegritudines remediorum* (Basel); 1536. *Habes sincerioris medicinae amator . . . Garioponti medici* (Basel).

Secondary: Glaze, Florence Eliza, 2005. 'Galen Refashioned: Gariopontus in the Later Middle Ages and Renaissance' in Furdell, Elizabeth Lane, ed., *Textual Healing: Essays in Medieval and Early Modern Medicine* (Leiden).

Florence Eliza Glaze

GARROD, ARCHIBALD EDWARD (b. London, England, 25 November 1857; d. Cambridge, England, 28 March 1936), *medicine, biochemistry, genetics, pediatrics.*

Garrod was the fourth son of Alfred Baring Garrod (1819–1907), who was a physician at University College Hospital, London, and an authority on diseases of the joints. After attending Marlborough College, Wiltshire, the younger Garrod went to Christ Church, Oxford (1877–80), graduating with a first in the natural sciences. He followed his father into medicine rather than pursuing a purely scientific career, training at St Bartholomew's Hospital, London (1880–84), under Samuel Gee (1839–1911) and William Russell (1830–1909). He rejected the empiricism of Gee and was inspired by Russell to take an interest in chemistry. Further study in Vienna (1884–85) at the Allgemeines Krankenhaus confirmed Garrod's enthusiasm for clinical science. Shortly after returning to England, he was appointed to the staff at St Bartholomew's as a house physician (1885) and took his MD from Oxford in 1891. He also worked as physician to the Marylebone General Dispensary, served as assistant physician at the West London Hospital, joined the visiting staff of the Alexander Hospital for Children with Hip Disease, and was assistant physician (1892–99) and then physician (1899–1920) at the Hospital for Sick Children, Great Ormond Street. During World War I, he served on the staff of the 1st London General Hospital at Camberwell. In 1915 he was promoted to temporary colonel in the Army Medical Service, serving in Malta, where he was consulting physician (1915–19) to the Mediterranean forces. For his services he was appointed CMG (1916) and KCMG (1918).

However, until the 1920s Garrod's reputation was closely connected to St Bartholomew's. He was elected casualty physician (1888–1903) to the hospital, followed by medical registrar (1895–1902), assistant physician (1903–12), and physician to children's department (1904–10), which he helped establish. At the age of fifty-five he was elected consulting physician (1912–20), and he went on to direct the newly established medical unit (1919–20) before leaving London to take up the Regius chair of medicine at Oxford University (1920–27). In the interwar period he also served on the Medical Research Council (1923–28). However, his clinical work never entirely satisfied him. His bedside manner was said to be limited to his interest in the color of his patients' urine samples. It was this enthusiasm for the biochemistry of urine that came to dominate his work and ideas.

Physiological Chemistry

Although much of Garrod's early focus was clinical, his research concentrated on the chemical and metabolic changes in disease, and as his career progressed, he increasingly moved into biochemistry. He worked with his father in a study of rheumatoid arthritis while assistant physician at the West London Hospital. Whereas Garrod senior had devoted himself to chemical pathology and had previously differentiated rheumatoid arthritis from gout, Archibald adopted a different approach shaped by his interest in chemical and metabolic changes. He wanted to confine the term 'rheumatism' to a definite set of phenomena, which he believed depended on specific morbid processes, seeing rheumatism as a systemic disease. As a result of his work with his father, he published *A Treatise on Rheumatism and Rheumatoid Arthritis* (1890). Later, he drew a distinction by classifying osteoarthritis separately in an article he contributed to Thomas Clifford Allbutt's *System of Medicine* (1907). Garrod also co-edited the first edition of *Diseases of Children* (1913) with F. E. Batten and Hugh Thursfield.

After collaborating with his father, he started researching the chemical aspects of urine with Frederick Gowland Hopkins (1861–1947), who won the Nobel Prize in 1929 for his biochemical research. Garrod sought to examine the nature of chemical substances that colored urine, energetically employing the spectroscopic methods he had acquired during his undergraduate studies at Oxford. Work with Hopkins encouraged a passion for the rigorous application of physiological chemistry to clinical problems at a time when many were trying to find specific causes of disease.

Inborn Errors

Work on urinary chemistry led Garrod to investigate alkaptonuria after coming across a number of patients at St Bartholomew's with this rare disease. At the time, alkaptonuria—a disorder that turns the urine black and that often led to arthritis—was attributed to a bacillus. Garrod adopted a different interpretation, his curiosity being aroused by the familial pattern in his patients, which he believed 'can hardly be ascribed to chance' (Garrod, 1901). For him there was an apparent pattern of inheritance: although the affliction was most often not passed on from parent to child, it did reappear later in their descendents. On the basis of discussions with his friend, the naturalist and Mendel advocate William Bateson (1861–1926), he considered the possibility that alkaptonuria was a recessive disorder. Mendelism offered a theoretical explanation for the effects of consanguinity that Garrod saw in his patients. This thesis encouraged him to investigate the metabolism behind urinary abnormalities. As a result, Garrod incorporated biochemistry and Mendelian laws into the study of disease. Later, he would play down his contribution, arguing that it was Bateson who had seen the 'daylight'.

Garrod argued that the buildup of homogentisic acid, which caused the urine's characteristic pigmentation, was the result of a failure of a 'ferment' or enzyme. He speculated that the lack of enzyme function resulted from a defect inherited at birth. This led him to think about metabolic pathways and to recognize that variation in Mendelian heredity could explain an 'inborn error of metabolism'. Garrod had no idea about the nature of a gene, but he asserted the idea of metabolic variation, or what he called 'chemical individuality', arguing that the information for producing specific enzymes in humans was inherited. Such inherited variations could lead either to a simple 'metabolic sport', such as alkaptonuria, or to congenital abnormalities, such as Down syndrome. Through his work on alkaptonuria, he introduced a paradigm that biochemistry was dynamic and different from the static nature of organic chemistry.

After ten years of research, Garrod outlined his ideas in the RCP's 1908 Croonian Lectures: 'Inborn Errors of Metabolism'. He summarized a large body of evidence and suggested that four metabolic disorders—albinism, alkaptonuria, cystinuria, and pentosuria—had certain features in common and should be regarded as recessively inherited. He explained that only occasionally would the heredi-

tary 'chemical individuality' result in overt disease. A revised edition was subsequently published in 1909.

Inborn Errors of Metabolism (1909) was Garrod's most important work and has been seen as providing a foundation for later genetic research. However, although the book was positively reviewed, contemporaries overlooked its significance. Despite the simplicity of Garrod's interpretation of 'inborn errors of metabolism' as gene defects, his work had relatively little influence on the thinking of early geneticists or on eugenics. Garrod was not active in the Genetical Society, and he was not involved in the Eugenics Society. His ideas were only briefly discussed in a few works, such as in Bateson's *Mendel's Principles of Heredity*, which discussed the early science of genetics and Mendelism. Contemporary clinicians and reviewers assumed that his research focused on rare diseases rather than fundamental questions about living systems. Hence, his findings were interpreted as providing clinical recognition of alkaptonuria and other glycogen-related diseases. Garrod later admitted that such work 'lay on the very fringe of knowledge' (*Lancet*, 1936, i, p. 807).

Academic Medicine

Garrod's enthusiasm for research and chemical pathology shaped by clinical experience influenced his views on how medical education should be organized. Though he had, like many of his contemporaries, received an empirical education that stressed the importance of anatomy and the bedside, the 'lack of scientific spirit and atmosphere' he perceived in England alarmed him (*St Bartholomew's Hospital Journal*, November 1908, p. 21). Influenced by William Osler and the style of academic training he had established at Johns Hopkins, Garrod argued that England's apparent scientific lethargy could be reversed only by merging a culture of research and scientific study with the bedside: the clinical laboratory had to be closely associated with the wards for medicine to progress. His ideas fit into a growing strand of opinion that English medicine was falling behind Germany, reflecting wider cultural and imperial fears about England's position. Through the organization of English medical schools into German-style clinics, the perceived defects of the English system could be overcome. His support for research and the development of academic clinics was a reaction to shifts in medical practice that were encouraging a sense of optimism about the value of science to medicine. For Garrod, a system of academic medicine under the guidance of full-time professors would allow science and research to flourish by bringing together bench and bedside and would also reverse the perceived decline of English medicine.

To promote these ideas, he worked with Osler to found the Association of Physicians of Great Britain and Ireland for the academically minded. Its purpose was to facilitate discussion and publication of fundamental research that had no immediate clinical application. This was to be achieved through the *Quarterly Journal of Medicine*, and Garrod was appointed to the editorial board. He also actively supported the need to establish academic clinical units in teaching hospitals. He propounded their benefits for medicine to the press and to the Royal Commission on university education in London, and at St Bartholomew's he helped facilitate the creation of two academic units at the hospital in 1919. Garrod was appointed professor of medicine to head the new medical unit. Mourning the loss of two of his three sons in World War I, he threw himself into organizing the new unit, which gave him a new lease of life. However, he resigned in the following year to succeed Osler as Regius professor of medicine at Oxford.

Oxford

At Oxford Garrod hoped to develop his ambitions for the medical unit at St Bartholomew's. He believed that the type of academic clinic he envisaged would be better furthered in a university environment that was not so dominated by a culture where considerations of establishing a medical career dominated. Garrod found that the Oxford medical faculty and the atmosphere promoted by Osler provided him with greater opportunities for developing his plans. In the university he encouraged the improvement of research and laboratory facilities, though most of his efforts were directed at furthering biochemistry. Garrod had become an enthusiastic supporter of biochemistry since his early work with Gowland Hopkins, and at Oxford he worked with the Rockefeller Foundation and private donors to establish a new biochemistry laboratory in 1926 under Rudolf Peters.

At Oxford he also continued his own work on 'inborn errors of metabolism', presenting his ideas in the 1927 Huxley Lecture on 'Diathesis' at the Charing Cross Hospital, published in a fuller form as *The Inborn Factors in Disease* (1931). Garrod never considered the work a book; he saw it as an 'essay' emphasizing the role of individual genetic susceptibility in human disease. This placed the nature-nurture controversy on a scientific basis. *The Inborn Factors in Disease* demonstrated Garrod's medical outlook that sought to fuse clinical practice with biochemical and laboratory study.

Garrod's work initially had a limited impact. Although his understanding of alkaptonuria was included in a number of biochemistry textbooks, it was not until the 1950s that his concept of 'chemical individuality' was developed following the rediscovery of his work by the Nobel Prize–winning (1958) microbial geneticists George W. Beadle (1903–89) and Edward Tatum (1909–75). His 'inborn errors of metabolism' had an important influence on their 'one-gene–one-enzyme' hypothesis and the role that genes played in determining protean structure. Bea-

INBORN ERRORS OF METABOLISM

The Croonian Lectures delivered before the Royal College of Physicians of London, in June, 1908

By

ARCHIBALD E. GARROD

D.M., M.A. OXON.

Fellow of the Royal College of Physicians.
Assistant Physician to, and Lecturer on Chemical Pathology at St. Bartholomew's Hospital.
Physician to the Hospital for Sick Children, Great Ormond Street

" ἐν πᾶσι τοῖς φυσικοῖς ἔνεστί τι θαυμαστόν."
Aristotle, Περὶ ζῴων μορίων, I. 5.

LONDON

HENRY FROWDE   HODDER & STOUGHTON

OXFORD UNIVERSITY PRESS   20, WARWICK SQUARE, E.C.

1909

Title page of *Inborn Errors of Metabolism*, 1909. Wellcome Library, London.

dle expressed regret that he had been slow to recognize the importance of Garrod's work and acknowledged how close Garrod had come to the 'one-gene–one-enzyme' hypothesis. However, whereas Beadle's work helped shape the development of human genetics in the 1950s and 1960s, Garrod never regarded himself as a geneticist, and it was only in retrospect that his contribution to genetics was recognized.

Bibliography

Primary: 1890. *A Treatise on Rheumatism and Rheumatoid Arthritis* (London); 1901. 'About alkaptonuria.' *Lancet* ii: 1484–1486; 1909. *Inborn Errors of Metabolism* (London); 1913. *Diseases of Children* (London); 1931. *The Inborn Factors in Disease* (Oxford).

Secondary: Bearn, Alexander G., 1993. *Archibald Garrod and the Individuality of Man* (Oxford); Bearn, Alexander G., and Elizabeth D. Miller, 1979. 'Archibald Garrod and the Development of the Concept of Inborn Errors of Metabolism.' *Bulletin of the History of Medicine* 53: 315–328; *Oxford DNB*.

Keir Waddington

GAUBIUS, HIERONYMUS DAVID   (b.   Heidelberg,

Germany, 24 January 1705; d. Leiden, the Netherlands, 29 November 1780), *medicine, chemistry.*

Gaubius, son of cloth-merchant Johann Christoffel Gaub, received his primary education at a Jesuit college in his native town, even though he was of protestant origin. He continued his studies at the school of the pietist A. H. Francke in Halle, where the severely repressive discipline caused him to fail completely. His uncle Johan Gaub, a well-known medical doctor in Amsterdam, took him under his care and sent him to the University of Harderwijk in 1722. At the time, the entire medical curriculum was entrusted to Bartholomaeus de Moor, who died in 1724. Gaub then went to the University of Leiden where Herman Boerhaave, Bernard Siegfried Albinus, and Herman Oosterdijk Schacht were the leading men. In 1725 he graduated with a thesis entitled *Specimen inaugurale medicum exhibens ideam generalem solidarum corporis humani partium.* In this description of the solid human body parts, he followed Boerhaave's views: the fibers are the elementary body structures, consisting of water, volatile salts, spirits, and—as fundamental ingredient—earth.

After a study tour to Paris and Strasbourg, he practiced medicine in Deventer for a short while and then, from 1727, in Amsterdam. In 1731 he was appointed lector of chemistry in Leiden, taking over that part of Boerhaave's commission. His inaugural address emphasized the importance of chemistry for the physician. Yet, when he was appointed full professor in chemistry in 1734, his oration forcefully rejected the chemists' claim that they could prolong human life.

Shortly afterward, in June 1735, he married Constantia Gaub, his cousin from Amsterdam. In 1738 Boerhaave's chair in theoretical medicine was given to Gaubius, and in 1744 he took over the teaching of medical practice from Oosterdijk Schacht. He did not, however, continue Boerhaave's famous bedside teaching in the Caecilia Hospital. Gaubius's theoretical lessons, the sole instruction for prospective physicians, were highly rated by the students. In addition to his professorship, Gaubius became a consulting physician to stadtholder William V and his family in 1760. He retired from his academic positions in 1775 and died five years later after a short illness.

His most important publications include a textbook of general pathology entitled *Institutiones pathologiae medicinales* and two of his rectorial addresses, both entitled *De regimine mentis.* The textbook was translated into French, German, English, and Dutch and widely used until the 1830s. It had an eclectic character and provided different views on human physiology and on the relationship between body and soul. Influenced by the irritability principle of Haller (propagated in Leiden by Gaubius's colleague Winter), Gaubius emphasized the *vis vitalis* as a force in all living creatures, which was activated by stimuli from without and within the body. Therefore, it consisted of a sensitive and a moving component. In addition, he conceived of a *vis animalis*, the force in charge of the senses, communicating between the *vis vitalis* and the soul. Body and soul form a *mixis*, a kind of interpenetration. He used this construction to elucidate 'psychosomatic' phenomena.

In his 1747 address, he dealt with the influence that the (condition of) the body has on the soul, sometimes causing psychic symptoms. In this regard he named the *vis animalis* and the *vis vitalis* the mental and the corporeal *enormoon*. In his 1763 address, he discussed the influence of the soul on the body, which sometimes gave rise to corporeal illnesses. Thus, Gaubius's significance may be said to lie in his efforts to incorporate new findings in the field of anatomy and microscopy in a meaningful new synthesis.

Bibliography

Primary: 1747. *Sermo academicus de regimine mentis* (Leiden); 1758. *Institutiones pathologiae medicinalis* (Leiden); 1763. *Sermo academicus alter de regimine mentis quod medicorum est* (Leiden).

Secondary: Pogány-Wnendt, Peter, 1991. *Das mechanistische Denken in der modernen Medizin im Spiegel ihrer geschichtlichen Entwicklung: Hieronimus David Gaub (1705–1780)* (Frankfurt am Main); Hamers van Duynen, S. W., 1978. *Hieronymus David Gaubius* (Assen); Rather, L. J., 1965. *Mind and Body in Eighteenth-Century Medicine. A Study Based on Jerome Gaub's* De Regimine Mentis (London).

G. van der Waa

GE, HONG 葛洪   (b. Danyang, Jiangsu province, China, *c.* 283; d. Mount Loufu, Guangzhou, China, 343/363), *self-cultivation, formulary literature, Chinese medicine.*

Ge Hong was born into a prominent aristocratic clan in southern China with deep roots in the practice of supernatural powers, physical and spiritual cultivation, and longevity. His great-uncle, Ge Xuan 葛玄 (164–244), is known as a famous magician and revered as the founding patriarch of the Lingbao School of Daoism. Ge Hong's official biography, however, suggests that he grew up in such poverty that he was forced to cut firewood in the mountains to support his studies. Despite poverty, he apparently stood out in his youth for intelligence and studiousness. Throughout his adult life, he filled several eminent government positions, but also declined many appointments in order to remain in seclusion and pursue his goals of physical and spiritual self-cultivation. Toward the end of his life, he took a post as county magistrate in China's extreme south, purportedly because of the availability of local cinnabar, a major ingredient in his alchemical experiments. He was engaged in writing and the pursuit of immortality when he died.

Ge Hong is most famous for having composed a text named *Baopuzi* 抱朴子 [The Master Who Holds on to Simplicity], which is a key source for reconstructing the religious history of early medieval China. Consisting of two parts, the 'exoteric writings' contain fifty scrolls on 'Confucian' subjects such as the ordering of society, morality, and the governing of the country. The 'esoteric writings', also in fifty scrolls, cover what he calls 'Daoist' material on the individual cultivation of supernatural powers with the final goal of sublimating the body physically and spiritually to the point of immortality. Though not synthesized into a systematic whole, these essays offer insights into the religious and medical practices that were current in southern China in the early medieval period. They describe techniques of immortality aimed at the ultimate metamorphosis of the physical body, either by way of 'release from the corpse' or by 'ascending to Heaven in broad daylight'. Ge Hong believed in the need for faith and initiation by a supreme master in possession of sacred texts and techniques to complete this difficult undertaking. But beyond that, he stressed the importance of perseverance, a reclusive life, and the continuous practice of specialized techniques, such as purification, alchemy, sexual cultivation, dietary restrictions, breathing and other exercises, rituals, and visualization meditation. Although he is perhaps most famous as an alchemist, this was only one of many techniques he employed in his lifelong quest for immortality. As such, he is representative of early Chinese medical and religious authors who emphasized the need for living in harmony with the natural world and familiarizing themselves with the extensive materia medica of early Chinese medicine (plants, animals, and minerals), as well as with the formulas used to combine them for purposes ranging from treatment of disease to preservation of health and reversing the process of natural aging.

In addition to the *Baopuzi*, Ge compiled a formulary called *Bei ji zhou hou fang* 備急肘後方 [Emergency Formulary to Keep Up One's Sleeves] and the *Shen xian zhuan* 神仙傳 [Biographies of Spirit Immortals], a collection of Daoist hagiographies in ten scrolls. Last, he is credited with two collections, one on anomaly accounts and one on biographies of recluses, both of which are lost. From autobiographical statements and the content of his writings, Ge Hong emerges as a Daoist proselytizer who valued arcane wisdom over worldly knowledge and aimed at substantiating claims of transcendence and immortality that were questioned or ignored by more secular writers.

Bibliography

Primary: 317. *Baopuzi* 抱朴子 [The Master Who Holds on to Simplicity] 70 scrolls; (n.d.) *Bei ji zhou hou fang* 備急肘後方 [Emergency Formulary to Keep Up One's Sleeves] 6 scrolls; (n.d.) *Shen xian zhuan* 神仙傳 [Biographies of Spirit Immortals] 10 scrolls.

Secondary: Campany, Robert, 2001. *To Live as Long as Heaven and Earth: A Translation and Study of Ge Hong's Traditions of Divine Transcendents* (Berkeley); Robinet, Isabelle, 1997. 'Ge Hong and His Tradition' in *Taoism. Growth of a Religion*, trans. Phyllis Brooks (Stanford) pp. 78–113; Sailey, Jay, 1978. *The Master Who Embraces Simplicity: A Study of the Philosophy of Ko Hung (A.D. 283–343)* (Hong Kong); Ware, James R., trans., 1981. *Alchemy, Medicine and Religion in the China of A.D. 320: The Nei P'ien of Ko Hung* (Cambridge, MA) [reprinted 1981 (New York)].

Sabine Wilms

GEAR, JAMES HENDERSON SUTHERLAND

(b. Germiston, South Africa, 8 April 1905; d. Johannesburg, South Africa, 19 July 1994), *virology, poliomyelitis, tropical diseases.*

The second of three brothers, all of whom had illustrious medical careers, James Gear was educated at St John's College, Johannesburg, and entered the Medical School at the University of Witwatersrand (Wits) after completing a BSc there (1926). He completed his residency at the Johannesburg Hospital before taking up a position in the South African Institute of Medical Research, where he remained throughout his distinguished career, becoming its deputy director in 1950 and then serving as director from 1960 to 1973. He returned to Wits as honorary professor of tropical diseases in 1960.

During World War II, Gear joined the South African Medical Corps, eventually becoming the officer commanding the Medical Laboratory Services, with the rank of major. A severe outbreak of yellow fever in the Sudan took him in 1942 to the Rockefeller Foundation in New York, which at that time supplied all the vaccine for the African continent, to study the manufacture of yellow fever vaccine so that a plant could be started in South Africa. He played an important role in developing the vaccines for yellow fever and typhus, which saved the lives of Allied soldiers in North Africa and Eastern Europe.

The 1940s and 1950s saw Gear at the height of his powers, often making discoveries whose true significance was not realized until later. This was true of the antigen he found in jaundiced U.S. servicemen vaccinated against yellow fever, which seems to have been the Australia antigen rediscovered twenty years later. Similarly, he noted at this time the pathological responses of the body's immune system, which were later to be rediscovered as the autoimmune diseases. His discovery of the role of the Coxsackie B virus in the etiology of neonatal myocarditis, a subject on which he became a world authority, first brought him international attention, although it was his contribution to the discovery and systematic mass application of the polio vaccine that ultimately brought him the greatest recognition.

The establishment of a South African Polio Research Foundation (1953) was largely his inspiration: Gear was the Foundation's director until it was taken over by the government and transformed into the South African Institute of Virology in 1976. During the major 1955 polio outbreak in

South Africa, he organized the immunization of thousands of children with the newly discovered Salk vaccine, and he introduced the routine national use of the oral polio vaccine in 1960.

As a virologist, Gear contributed to the understanding of enteroviruses (work he began in the 1930s) and did some of the earliest work on the viral hemorrhagic fevers and the arboviruses, as well as researching bilharzia, river blindness, malaria, trypanosomiasis, rickettsial and chlamydial diseases, relapsing fever, and fungal diseases. He published between two and three hundred articles, and before South Africa left the WHO (1964), he served on four of its expert committees and four of its working parties. He also served on most important national health bodies including the first Board of the South African Medical Research Council (1969).

Gear was one of the most formidable of South Africa's twentieth-century medical scientists. His receipt of the Medical Association of South Africa's Bronze Medal as the most outstanding graduate of his final year was the first of his many highly prestigious national and international honors. He has rightly been described as 'one of the last of the world's great generalists who attained specialist status across a vast spectrum of tropical disorders' (Gear, 1995, pp. 20–21).

Bibliography

Primary: 1988. *Handbook of Viral and Rickettsial Hemorrhagic Fevers* (Boca Raton, FL); 1996. *History of the Polio Research Foundation* (Johannesburg).

Secondary: Schoub, Barry D., 2003. *National Institute of Contagious Diseases, Annual Report* (Johannesburg); Gear, John, 1995. 'On the 1st Anniversary of the Death of James Gear (1905–94).' *Adler Museum Bulletin* 21: 20–21; Schoub, Barry D., and J. van den Ende, 1994. 'Professor J.H.S. Gear 1905–1994.' *Adler Museum Bulletin* 20: 3–13; 1986. 'Festschrift for James Gear.' *South African Medical Journal* 71 (Supplement): 1–84.

Shula Marks

GEE, SAMUEL JONES (b. London, England, 13 September 1839; d. Keswick, Lake District, England, 3 August 1911), *medicine, pediatrics.*

Gee was the only surviving child of William Gee, a dealer in china and glass, and his wife Lydia Sutton. He was educated by his mother before attending school at Enfield, Middlesex (1847–49), and then at home under his father's tutelage. He was sent to University College School, London (1852–54) before entering University College London (1857–61) to study medicine. He graduated MB (1861) from the University of London, and then MD (1865). He initially worked as house surgeon at University College Hospital (1865–66) and at the Hospital for Sick Children (1865–66), Great Ormond Street, where he was made assistant physician (1866–75) and then physician (1875–94). He

was elected assistant physician (1868–78) to St Bartholomew's Hospital, London, where he served as physician (1878–1904) and consulting physician (1904–11). In the hospital's medical school he lectured in pathological anatomy (1872–78), in the principles and practice of medicine (1878–93), and in clinical medicine (1880–1904). Gee also had a considerable private practice and was physician to the Prince of Wales (1901–11).

His position at the Hospital for Sick Children saw him become an expert on childhood diseases. His early papers on chicken pox, scarlet fever, and tubercular meningitis appeared in John Russell Reynolds's *System of Medicine* (volumes 1 and 2, 1866, 1868). Gee was the first to identify celiac disease: in 1888 he laid the foundation for describing symptoms of the condition as a loss of appetite, diarrhea, and marked failure to thrive, and he established the criteria for treating the disease with a dietary approach. He also worked on splenic cachexia in children and in 1882 was the first to write about cyclic vomiting syndrome, and his description of the child's head in hydrocephalus demonstrated that it was distinct from the enlarged skull of rickets.

Gee was a highly respected clinician and teacher. It is said that his observation was acute and systematic and that the treatment he prescribed was judicious. His work bore evidence of a deep knowledge of the history of medicine, philosophy, and literature. Gee was convinced of the merits of classical learning and resisted any dilution of traditional clinical training. He remained a self-confessed empiric and taught students accordingly. As a traditionalist, he celebrated the bedside and learned his dogmatic method from William Jenner (1815–98). In his book *Auscultation and Percussion, Together with Other Methods of Physical Examination of the Chest* (1870), Gee justified his clinical principles with an appeal to classical traditions in medicine and in particular to Hippocrates. *Auscultation and Percussion* became a standard text for students, and his *Medical Lectures and Aphorisms* confirmed his Hippocratic approach and faith in the value of bedside clinical teaching. For Gee, experience was to be gained on the ward and then supplemented by hours in the postmortem room. He therefore stressed the importance of painstaking analysis of physical signs and asserted that morbid anatomy gave meaning to the bedside. In students he instilled the value of postmortems and contempt for physiology. House officers therefore liked working with him because they knew exactly what was expected of them. As an intellectual chauvinist who was well read in German ideas on bacteriology and pathology yet dismissive of those ideas, Gee told students to forget their physiology when entering the wards because physiology was an experimental science that in his view had contributed little to practical therapeutics, and medicine was an empirical art. Gee went so far as to doubt the value of experiment in the natural sciences. By the end of the nineteenth century, he had become alarmed about the changes that were occurring in medical practice. He remained adamant that the naked eye was better than the laboratory analysis and until his death continued to extol a style of bedside medicine that was becoming increasingly anachronistic.

Bibliography

Primary: 1870. *Auscultation and Percussion, Together with Other Methods of Physical Examination of the Chest* (London); 1888. 'On the coeliac infection.' *Saint Bartholomew's Hospital Reports* 24: 17–20; 1915. *Medical Lectures and Aphorisms* (London).

Secondary: Lawrence, Christopher, 2000. 'Edward Jenner's Jockey Boots and the Great Tradition in English Medicine 1918–1939' in Lawrence, Christopher, and Anna-K. Mayer, eds., *Regenerating England: Science, Medicine and Culture in Inter-War Britain* (Amsterdam) pp. 45–66; *Munk's Roll*; *Oxford DNB*.

Keir Waddington

GENTILE DA FOLIGNO (b. ?, *c.* 1280; d. Perugia, Italy, 18 June 1348), *scholastic medicine.*

Little is known about Gentile da Foligno's youth. He was most likely born in the last quarter of the thirteenth century in Foligno, and his father was a renowned physician who probably passed on some of his knowledge to his son. There is some speculation as to what university he attended and who his teachers were. Taddeo Alderotti and Peter of Abano were once thought to be among them, although there is no evidence to support this claim. However, Dino del Garbo, who was his colleague at Sienna at the beginning of the 1320s, was very likely one of his masters. Gentile was surely associated with this group of academic physicians from Bologna, considering that many references to the group's work appear in his own writings.

In 1322 Gentile da Foligno was teaching at the University of Sienna. He remained there until October 1324 and then left for the University of Perugia, where he taught at least until 1327. The paucity of documentation provides little information about his life from this date up to 1338. However, it has been well attested that he taught at Perugia from 1338 until his death. Gentile was not only a famous scholar, but also a successful practitioner. For instance, he was summoned to the bed of sickly Ubertino da Carrara, the ruler of Padua from 1338 to 1345. His skills were held in such high regard that numerous prominent figures from Umbria employed his services during this period. Gentile's medical practice is well documented in his *Consilia*, a compilation of medical consultations and prescriptions written for specific individuals that was widely distributed after his death.

Most of what we know about Gentile comes from his writings, which include almost every genre of medical literature of his time. He authored commentaries on such works as Hippocrates' *Aphorisms* and Galen's *Tegni*. His *questiones* or *dubia* mirror the academic practice of the *disputatio* (disputation), which was a sort of public debate between scholars about controversial issues. He also wrote a number of treatises on several subjects, including pharmacology and hygiene, but his most famous work is his commentary on Avicenna's (Ibn Sīnā) *Canon*. By the end of the thirteenth century, the *Canon* had become the foundation of the teaching of medicine in Italian universities. Gentile da Foligno was the first author to produce an almost comprehensive commentary on that medical encyclopedia, an endeavor to which he consecrated the last thirty years of his life. This commentary displays his particular interest in pedagogical matters and the epistemological foundations of medical science. It was widely circulated; eleven editions of at least part of it were printed, and forty-nine manuscripts remain today.

The end of Gentile da Foligno's life was marked by the outbreak of the Black Death in Europe. From the beginning of the epidemic, he treated the sick and attempted to discover a remedy, according to his *Consilium de pestilentia*, which was one of the first treatises on the subject. Shortly thereafter, on 12 June, he fell sick, and he died six days later, most likely of the plague.

Despite the fact that he did not revolutionize the medical science of his time, Gentile da Foligno can be considered one of the most brilliant representatives of scholastic medicine in fourteenth-century Italy. He insisted on the importance of reason in medical practice as well as the use of anatomy. Furthermore, the logical complexity and the formal perfection of his writings earned him the nickname of 'Speculator'.

Bibliography

Primary: 1520. *Questiones et Tractatus extravagantes* (Venice); 1520–1522. *Expositiones super Canones Avicennae* 4 vols. (Venice).

Secondary: Chandelier, Joël, 2002. 'Gentile da Foligno. Médecin et universitaire du XIVe siècle' in *École nationale des chartes. Positions des thèses* pp. 21–28; French, Roger K., 2001. *Gentile da Foligno and Scholasticism* (Leiden, Boston, and Cologne); Ceccarelli, Lino. 'Gentile da Foligno.' *DBI* 52: 162–167.

Joël Chandelier

GERHARD, WILLIAM WOOD (b. Philadelphia, Pennsylvania, USA, 23 April 1809; d. Philadelphia, 28 April 1872), *medicine.*

Gerhard was the son of William Gerhard and Sarah Wood, both Moravian. He married the daughter of a British officer named Dobbyn in 1850; they had three children. Gerhard graduated from Dickinson College in 1826. He then went to study with one of the most distinguished Philadelphia physicians of the day, Joseph Parrish, also becoming a resident at the Philadelphia Almshouse. Thus—like many other people of that time who wanted to become physicians—he did his apprenticeship before attending the University of Pennsylvania Medical School, from which he received an MD in 1830.

Gerhard then went to study in Paris, which was a hotbed of intellectual fervor, the place to which students traveled from all over the world to learn about the latest and most important changes in medical science. Gerhard studied with many great figures of the day, but spent much of his time learning from Pierre Louis, who introduced into medicine the idea of the 'numerical method', a way of carefully counting the evidence that one used to draw conclusions. Gerhard and a few other American students studied privately with Louis. While in France, Gerhard wrote several important papers, including one on Asiatic cholera and one that may have been the first description of tuberculosis as a cause of meningitis in children. He also took the opportunity to visit Great Britain before returning to the United States.

In 1833 Gerhard returned to Philadelphia and in 1834 became a resident physician at the Pennsylvania Hospital. The next year he was elected to the staff of the Philadelphia Almshouse, and he helped to create a hospital within, known as 'Blockley'. When an epidemic struck Philadelphia in 1836, Gerhard studied the disease and reported the next year on the epidemic in a paper that was the first to clearly differentiate typhoid fever from typhus fever. This paper attracted considerable attention in Europe, at that time an unusual event for original research from the United States. In 1838 he became an editor of the *Medical Examiner*, where he published many of his clinical lectures. In 1842 he wrote a highly regarded book on diseases of the chest.

Bibliography

Primary: 1837. 'On the Typhus Fever, Which Occurred at Philadelphia in the Spring and Summer of 1836.' *American Journal of the Medical Sciences* 19: 289–322; 1842. 'Typhoid and Typhus Fever' in Tweedie, Alexander, *A System of Practical Medicine* vol.1 (Philadelphia) pp. 199–204; 1850. *The Diagnosis, Pathology, and Treatment of Diseases of the Chest*, 3rd edn. (Philadelphia).

Secondary: Smith, Dale C., 1980. 'Gerhard's Distinction between Typhoid and Typhus and Its Reception in America, 1833—1860.' *Bulletin of the History of Medicine* 54: 368–385; 1937. 'Editorials: Centenary of Gerhard's Publication on Typhus Fever.' *Annals of Medical History* 9: 280; Middleton, William S., 1935. 'William Wood Gerhard.' *Annals of Medical History* 7: 1–18; Osler, William, 1909. *An Alabama Student and Other Biographical Essays* (New York); *DAMB*.

Joel D. Howell

GEROULANOS, MARINOS (b. Patras, Greece, 21 February 1867; d. Athens, Greece, 1960), *surgery.*

Following his high school studies in Lixouri and Argostoli on Kefalonia island, Geroulanos moved to Munich, where he enrolled in medical school and completed his university studies during the years 1887–1892, while working for a living at the same time. He obtained his doctoral degree from the Medical School of Munich University in 1892. In order to study further, he went to Berlin, but he later returned to Munich to be appointed initially as external assistant to Professor Ziemmsen and then as a permanent assistant in St Hedwig Hospital in Berlin. Later, he became permanent assistant in the surgical clinic of Greifswald University, alongside Professor Helferich, whom he followed to Kiel, where he obtained a fellowship and became a temporary professor.

Invited to Athens by Queen Olga in 1902, Geroulanos returned to undertake management of the surgical department in Evangelismos Hospital. Established in 1881 by Queen Olga and the Ladies Association for the Education of Women, the hospital was intended to educate female nurses, a novel institution in that era. Geroulanos worked in the surgical department of Evangelismos Hospital for twelve years. Together with pathologist Antonios Christomanos, he contributed significantly to the scientific organization of the institution.

In 1911 Geroulanos became a permanent professor of the Medical School of Athens University, lecturing and operating in the state hospital Elpis, which had become a university-standard clinic of the School of Medicine in 1841. He served as Dean from 1916 to 1917. In 1917, for political reasons, he was prevented from performing his duties at the university, but he regained his position in 1921. In the meantime, he was elected as a member of parliament for Kefalonia Island in 1920, and he continued to lecture at the university until 1939.

Geroulanos offered his services as a doctor-in-chief during Greece's military conflicts of that era (the Balkan wars and the Asia Minor expedition). Being a member of the Red Cross Committee, he worked diligently for hospitals established by the Red Cross during the war period. In 1909 he was in charge of the Red Cross mission in Sicily, set up to assist earthquake-stricken Messina.

In 1933 Geroulanos became a permanent member of the Athens Academy and, in 1938, its chairman. He was one of the founders, and the first chairman, of the Hellenic Surgical Society (1929) and was chairman of the Athens Medical Society between 1906 and 1914. In 1907 he founded a private clinic, known today as the Geroulanos Foundation. Because of his excellent education, surgical abilities, and gentle character, Geroulanos became the chosen surgeon in Greece. He participated decisively in the improvement and configuration of medical, hospital, and training procedures in the field of medicine in Greece between 1900 and 1950.

Geroulanos wrote more that one hundred essays in Greek and in German.

Bibliography

Primary: 1892. *Über Metastasenbildung maligner Geschwulste im Gehirn* (Thesis, Munich); 1894. *Über die Wirkung des Ferattins* (Munich); 1896. *Tuberkulose der Gelenke und der Wilbelsaule* (Berlin); 1897. 'Über Radiallislahmung.' *Deutsche Zeitschrift für Chirurgie*

47: 17; 1898. 'Studie über den operativen Pneumothorax.' *Deutsche Zeitschrift für Chirurgie* 49: 497; 1900. 'Lungenkomplikationen nach operativen Eingriffen.' *Deutsche Zeitschrift für Chirurgie* 57: 361; 1901. 'Chirurgische Belandlung der Lungennkrankheiten.' *Deutsche Arztezeitung* vol. 9; 1996. *Memories 1867–1957. Pages from the History of the Modern Hellenic Medicine* (Athens).

Secondary: 1929. *The Great Hellenic Encyclopedia* vol. 8; 1985, 1996. *The Papyros Larousse Britannica* vol. 16.

Maria Korasidou

GERSDORFF, HANS VON (b. ?, *c.* 1455; d. Strassburg, Alsace [now Strasbourg, France], *c.* 1529), *medicine, surgery.*

Little is known about Gersdorff's background and life. There are doubts that he was related to the line of nobility von Gersdorff in the Upper Lusatia. Rather, it is likely that he was the son of Heinrich von Gersdorff, a shearer and burgher in the city of Strassburg. According to his own statements, Gersdorff trained as a surgeon around 1475 and was active as a field doctor with the Strassburg troops in Granson, Murten, and Nancy during the Burgundian wars. He mentioned a 'master Nicklaus' as his teacher; recent research indicates that this very probably was Klaus von Matrei. When Gersdorff published his *Feldtbuch der Wundartzney* in 1517, he could look back on many years of activity as a surgeon in Strassburg, where he had performed more than 100 amputations in the Antoniter Hospital.

Gersdorff gained fame as a result of his *Feldtbuch der Wundartzney*, a folio volume with ninety-nine sheets and numerous illustrations. The woodcuts are probably the work of Strassburg painter Hans Wächtlin and are still reprinted today in works on the history of medicine and surgery. They show instruments, operations in progress, and, in two large figures, a skeleton and a scene from anatomy. The numerous reprints and editions of the work reflect its great popularity, especially among barbers and surgeons. Just in Strassburg alone, the book was reprinted at least seven times by 1542. A new edition prepared by Walter Ryff and published in 1551 in Frankfurt am Main was printed there for the last time in 1606. There were also translations into Dutch and Latin.

Often compared with Hieronymus Brunschwig's *Buch der Chirurgia* (1497), the *Feldtbuch* is considered a late work of the medieval surgical tradition. Organized in tractates of varying length, the *Feldtbuch* presents human anatomy and the treatment of wounds, injuries, and fractures and also covers how to deal with patients suffering from leprosy. The fourth and last section consists of three Latin–German glossaries on anatomy and medicine as well as various medicines. In the main the *Feldtbuch* is a very clever compilation of older writings and traditions. About a third of the text is based on Guy de Chauliac's *Chirurgia magna* and *Chirurgia parva*. It also contains sections the author created himself and based on his experience. In them, Gersdorff described the St Anthony's fire as well as techniques for performing amputations and orthopedic procedures. For treating gunshot wounds, he recommended washing out the wound with warm hemp oil, probably to prevent poisoning.

Bibliography

Primary: 1517. *Feldtbuch der Wundartzney* (Strassburg).

Secondary: Vollmuth, Ralf, 1996. 'War Klaus von Matrei der Lehrer Hans von Gersdorffs?' *Sudhoffs Archiv* 80: 109–117; Frederiksen, Jan, 1983. 'Johannes (Hans) von Gersdorff (Schielhans)' in Ruh, Kurt, et al., eds., *Die deutsche Literatur des Mittelalters. Verfasserlexikon* vol. 4 (Berlin and New York) pp. 626–630; Stannard, Jerry, 1972. 'Botanical Nomenclature in Gersdorff's Feldtbüch der Wundartzney' in Debus, Allen G., ed., *Science, Medicine and Society in the Renaissance* (New York) pp. 87–103; *NDB* 6, 322–323.

Jürgen Helm and Karin Stukenbrock

GESELL, ARNOLD LUCIUS (b. Alma, Wisconsin, USA, 21 June 1880; d. New Haven, Connecticut, USA, 29 May 1961), *child psychology, pediatrics.*

Gesell was born in Alma, Wisconsin, in 1880. He studied at the University of Wisconsin, and his initial interests were in the field of education. He went on to do doctoral work in psychology at Clark University, where he came into contact with Stanley Hall. Hall had played a pivotal role in establishing the child study movement, which set out to study childhood from a broad interdisciplinary basis. Under the impact of Darwinism, Hall attempted to establish a 'genetic psychology', which situated the study of human development within a broad evolutionary (and ultimately Haeckelian) framework. Hall maintained that the study of childhood would transform schools and institutions—and ultimately society as a whole. Gesell viewed Hall as the 'Darwin of psychology' and adopted his agenda. At the same time, Gesell embraced the experimental ethos that was prevailing in American psychology, an ethos from which Hall distanced himself. Gesell obtained his PhD in 1910, after which he moved to New York City to teach in an elementary school. In 1911 he became an assistant professor at Yale University. There, he established the Yale Psycho-Clinic (later to be the Clinic of Child Development). While at Yale, he also studied for a medical degree, which he obtained in 1915. His first book, coauthored with his wife, was published in 1912.

Gesell was initially concerned with the issue of retarded development. This led his research increasingly to focus on the question, what is a normal child? In his clinic, he placed children in a laboratory that he called the observation dome, where he could carefully control the environment and stimuli to which a child was subjected. He presented children with a variety of challenges and documented their behavior and responses at four weekly intervals. Gesell was interested in not just the field of intelligence, but the total developmental status of the child. As he put it, his aim was to study 'normality as a clinical entity'. Through his work, Gesell constructed an 'age atlas' of the child. He codified three thousand items of behavior in relation to ten major areas of the child's development and correlated this to seventeen age levels up to ten years. Gesell developed a scale of developmental norms (which ultimately had a hereditary basis) that he held was biologically and sociologically typical. His scale permitted a 'developmental diagnosis', which indicated how far ahead of or behind the norm any particular child was. The scale was widely used in medicine and education in the interwar period, and Gesell held out great hopes that his scale would enable haphazard practices such as adoption to take place on a more scientific basis. Gesell was primarily responsible for the widespread belief that normal development shows typical regularities against which deviations can be measured and established.

The evolving technologies of photography and film played a pivotal role in Gesell's work. From 1924, Gesell utilized 'cinemanalysis' to attempt to capture and codify the developmental process in children, who were filmed through a one-way mirror. From 1928, he established a vast photographic and film library at the Yale clinic, having filmed around 12,000 children. From 1922 to 1936, Gesell was president of the American Psychological Association. In 1950 the Gesell Institute of Child Development was founded in New Haven, where he was a consultant until his death in 1961.

Bibliography

Primary: 1912. (with Gesell, Beatrice) *The Normal Child and Primary Education* (Boston); 1934. *An Atlas of Infant Behavior* (New York); 1949. (with Ilg, Frances L.) *Child Development: An Introduction to the Study of Human Growth* (New York).

Secondary: Herman, Ellen, 2001. 'Families Made by Science: Arnold Gesell and the Technologies of Modern Child Adoption.' *Isis* 92(4): 684–715; Lindley, Pamela, 1991. 'Dr. Arnold Lucius Gesell: Philosopher, Child Psychologist, Pediatrician, Clinical Researcher.' PhD thesis, Texas Woman's University; *DAMB*.

Sonu Shamdasani

GIBBON, JOHN HEYSHAM (b. Philadelphia, Pennsylvania, USA, 29 September 1903; d. Philadelphia, 5 February 1973), *surgery.*

Gibbon, whose father was a surgeon, came from a long line of doctors. He graduated from Jefferson Medical College (1927) and later became professor of surgery there, following his father. More than half of his life was devoted to mechanizing support of the heart and lungs. But his later life was devoted to general thoracic surgery, not cardiac surgery.

His name is associated with the development of the heart lung machine, which from the mid-1950s allowed surgery within the heart under direct vision, while the work of the heart and lungs was done mechanically. It is less well-known that he played a part in promoting the use of mechanical ventilators. In 1942 curare was introduced into anesthesia, allowing positive-pressure mechanical ventilation to become routine. This was an important component of thoracic surgery, in which, with the chest open, spontaneous breathing is impossible. The practice had been taken up in Europe, but hand ventilation with a rubber bag filled with the gas mixture remained usual in the United States. The 1952 polio epidemic in Scandinavia resulted in many cases in which life was saved by ventilation, delivered by hand, day after day, by about 1,400 medical students. This led to the mass production of ventilators in Europe. The Jefferson ventilator was developed for Gibbon's thoracic service and introduced in 1957 as the first American ventilator for controlled ventilation.

Gibbon's interest in supporting the heart as well as the lungs began in 1931 at the bedside of a woman deteriorating with a massive pulmonary embolism. Operation to remove the clot was to be tried only in extremis because fewer than one in ten had survived the operation. Gibbon wished for a way to support the heart and lungs: a way to take the deoxygenated blood dammed back by the clot and oxygenate it and deliver it into the oxygen starved arterial system. When the patient's circulation eventually petered out, an operation was performed by Edward Churchill (1895–1972), but as had happened on most occasions, she did not survive. Twenty years later, Gibbon was successful in supporting a child through open-heart surgery to survival with a machine.

Gibbon's is a well-documented story of tenacity. He worked in Philadelphia for three years but applied to Churchill to return to Boston and in 1934 was given laboratory space. With very few funds, the help of his wife (who was a laboratory technician), and stray cats lured with tinned tuna fish, he continued his research. In 1935 he had his first success in the animal laboratory when he kept a cat alive on a pump. However, only a few animals recovered their circulation, and most of these died soon after.

World War II intervened, and afterward he returned to Jefferson Medical College. He was given practical and moral support by his institution, colleagues, and IBM engineers and continued experimenting. Eventually, he had a machine that he thought might be adequate. Between February 1952 and July 1953, he operated on four patients. The second survived, but when the third and fourth patients died, both five-year-old girls, he would do no more. He was encouraged to report the survivor. John Kirklin (1917–2004) took on the project at Mayo Clinic in 1953 and, using a modified version called the Mayo Gibbon pump, began to have success—four of the first eight survived.

At that time there were clearly competing approaches to the problem of operating on the heart and yet having the patient survive. The problem had been clearly stated by Henry Sessions Souttar (1875–1964) when he reported his first and only mitral valvotomy in the *British Medical Journal*

(1925). Opening a valve within the beating heart was being done regularly, and more complicated means were being explored. Charles Drew and Russell Brock were experimenting with hypothermia in London to achieve 'suspended animation'. William Thornton Mustard (1914–1987) in Toronto was experimenting with animals' lungs as the oxygenators. Clarence Walton Lillehei (1918–1999) in Minneapolis was poised to start human mother-to-child cross-circulation. In the view of many who were banking on a biological solution to the problem, a mechanical pump oxygenator was the least likely to succeed. It turned out that machines based on Gibbon's concept enabled cardiac surgery to be offered to tens of thousands of individuals, in growing numbers from the 1960s. But by then, Gibbon had ceased to operate on the heart.

Bibliography

Primary: 1954. 'Application of Mechanical Heart and Lung Apparatus to Cardiac Surgery.' *Minnesota Medicine* March: 171–185.

Secondary: Johnson, Stephen L., 1970. *The History of Cardiac Surgery, 1896–1955* (Baltimore); *DAMB*.

Tom Treasure

GILBERT THE ENGLISHMAN (aka GILBERTUS ANGLICUS, GILBERTUS DE AQUILA, GILBERT DE L'EGLE) (b. ?; d. ?; fl. *c.* 1250), *medicine, surgery.*

Biographical information on Gilbertus Anglicus is limited. It is uncertain whether the multiple names refer to the same person. A manuscript of his *Compendium medicinae* dated 1271 refers to him as Gilbertus de Aquila Anglicus. He was a descendant of a prominent Essex family. Gilbert may have cared for the archbishop of Canterbury, Hubert Walter, and may have been the royal physician to King John. There is no record of his education. The place and year of his death are unknown.

Gilbert's *Compendium medicinae* was one of the most important medical and surgical works of the English Middle Ages. Excerpts of the text were translated from the original Latin into New High German, Hebrew, Catalan, and Middle English. The English translation was one of the most popular medical texts in England and was also highly regarded throughout parts of central Europe up to the 1700s.

Gilbert's *Compendium* offered a summary of all learned medicine and surgery. Gilbert cited Arabic medical authorities such as Avicenna (Ibn Sīnā) and Averroes (Ibn Rushd). The text was organized first by diseases that affected the entire body and then by parts of the body, which made it an accessible and useful text for a wide range of readers. He based his observations and suggestions on humoral medicine. For example, he wrote about red eye and observed that the condition presented itself because of the redness of blood. He believed that the blood showed through the eyes when infection or imbalance of the humors caused the spleen to fail or the liver to overheat. He recommended telling the patient not to touch the eye, bloodletting, and finally described a remedy giving precise mixing instructions and ingredients. Gilbert was renowned for his medical recipes. Throughout his writing, he emphasized that medicine should be directed toward stimulating the power of the body to heal itself. Like many physicians of his day, Gilbert cared not only for the body but also for the soul of his patients.

Bibliography

Primary: 1991. (Getz, Faye Marie, ed.) *Healing and Society in Medieval England: A Middle English Translation of the Pharmaceutical Writings of Gilbertus Anglicus* (Madison, WI).

Secondary: Getz, Faye Marie, 1998. *Medicine in the English Middle Ages* (Princeton); Riha, Ortrun von, 1994. 'Gilbertus Anglicus und sein "Compendium medicinae".' *Sudhoffs Archiv.* 78(1): 59–79; Getz, Faye Marie, 1992. 'The Pharmaceutical Writings of Gilbertus Anglicus.' *Pharmaceutical History* 34(1): 17–25.

Amy Eisen Cislo

GILLBEE, WILLIAM (b. Hackney, London, England, 10 July 1824?; d. Melbourne, Australia, 4 January 1885), *surgery.*

Gillbee was the eldest of four children born to William and Sarah Gillbee ('Gilbee' in some early records). His father, an army captain, died shortly after the birth of the last child, and his mother remarried. The younger William remained behind while the rest of his family migrated to Tasmania in 1836. In 1844 Gillbee became a student at Edinburgh University Medical School, where he studied under John Goodsir, Robert Christison, and James Young Simpson. Moving to London in 1847 to take up the post of clinical clerk at Guy's Hospital, where Bransby Cooper was senior surgeon and William Gull was professor of physiology, Gillbee conducted himself well enough to attract excellent professional references and personal testimonials, facilitating his membership of the Royal College of Surgeons of England in 1848.

After a somewhat unsuccessful sojourn with his family, by now in Melbourne, and a working sea voyage to California, a bout of fever sent Gillbee back to London for medical treatment and thence to further study in Edinburgh. During this time, he renewed his association with James Simpson, by then one of the leaders of the profession, who was to become a friend and, in later years, a correspondent. In 1852 Gillbee yet again set sail for the Australian colonies, and by 1854 he had set up a medical practice in Collins Street, Melbourne, joined the Volunteer force as assistant surgeon (later principal medical officer), and been appointed honorary surgeon to the Melbourne Hospital.

During the next thirty years, Gillbee rose to be one of the leading lights in medical practice and society in the colony of Victoria: he was a 'committee man' in both his professional and private capacity; a promoter of and examiner in surgery at the new Medical School; a member of the founding committee of the *Australian Medical Journal*, to which he was a frequent contributor; a member, and later president, of the medical board and first president of the British Medical Association (Victorian Branch). He remained a bachelor all his life.

Following the 1867 publication of Lister's papers on antisepsis in *Lancet*, Gillbee read a paper of his own, entitled 'On the Treatment of Abscess and Compound Fracture by Mr Lister's New Method', to the Medical Society of Victoria on 4 December 1867. This paper was published in the *Australian Medical Journal* of January 1868 and is mentioned by Lister's biographer, Godlee, as having been sent by Gillbee to Lister himself. With Gillbee's use of carbolic acid (as a 'mopping out' agent), lint, tin foil, and putty, the treatment of this case followed closely the early Listerism of the period and was also certainly the first reported case in the colony, and probably in the Australian colonies as a whole. What is less evident in the paper is Gillbee's grasp of early germ theory. A subsequent outbreak of erysipelas at the Melbourne Hospital was to confirm this only too clearly, showing his confusion as to the causes of contagion and putrefaction and as to whether disease was an invading entity or a bodily process. However, in this mid-century period, Gillbee was simply reflecting a general etiological confusion and ambivalence in the profession that was not to be resolved until the bacteriological research of the 1880s.

In spite of his eminence, Gillbee's final years saw disputes at the Melbourne Hospital, causing him to lose his positions there, and he retired depressed and ill in 1883. Travel brought no recovery, and he died of a 'lung complaint' in 1885.

Bibliography

Primary: Gillbee Archive Files 657, 1507, 1524, 1995 (Brownless Biomedical Library, University of Melbourne).

Secondary: Dyason, Diana, 1984. 'William Gillbee and Erysipelas at the Melbourne Hospital.' *Journal of Australian Studies* 14: 3–28; Godlee, R., 1918. *Lord Lister* (London).

Susan Hardy

GILLES DE CORBEIL (aka AEGIDIUS CORBOLIENSIS) (b. Corbeil?, France, *c.* 1140; d. ?, *c.* 1224), *medicine, pharmacology, theology.*

One of a series of bridge-figures between medical cultures, like Lanfranc of Milan, Gilles carried medical texts and didactics from Salerno to Montpellier to Paris at the turn of the thirteenth century.

Gilles probably was born or associated with Corbeil outside of Paris and of humble origins. From Gilles' writings, we know he studied with or through Romualdo, Musandinus, Platearius, Maurus, and Urso in Salerno, possibly

around 1160. He then migrated to Montpellier, where he ran afoul of the medical faculty, returning thence to Paris, variously suggested in 1174, 1181, or 1194, with good evidence favoring the latter year. It appears that soon after his return, he took up teaching on the Petit Pont off the Île-de-la-Cité, then well known for instruction in the arts, philosophy, and medicine. By 1198, he had attracted sufficient fame to be praised by the poet Gilles of Paris and to be slandered by several enemies.

The historiographic tradition of his court role under King Philip Augustus is highly uncertain, although such patronage would have dramatically simplified his reacceptance into Parisian culture. Philip's modern biographer is dubious of Gilles's status. Similarly, he has been identified as a canon of Notre Dame, but with little support.

Gilles certainly wrote four medical texts, a possible fifth, and one theological work with medical imagery. All six were written in Latin verse (including more than 16,000 hexametric lines). Following his training in Salerno, Gilles was probably exposed to the early *Articella*, with its emphasis on Theophilus's *On Urines* and Philaretus's *On Pulses*. Gilles in turn wrote texts on both subjects with the same names, essentially brief poetic distillates of the earlier works. Their greatest virtue for students no doubt lay in their ease of memorization. His texts were commented on by Gentile of Foligno, Gilbert the Englishman, Walter Agilon, a variety of anonymous figures, and Gilles himself; they survive in numerous manuscripts and were printed from the fifteenth century and cited into the eighteenth century. As a consequence, they represent the first authoritative expansion to the *Ars medicine*. In 1270–74 the Medical Faculty of the University of Paris established a textual curriculum. It included the optional reading of Gilles's two sets of verses.

On the Signs and Symptoms of Diseases is a poetic compendium of diagnostic findings for a wide variety of diseases. *On the Praise and Virtues of Compound Medicines* survives in a single manuscript and is a combination of Nicolaus Praepositus's *Antidotary* and the *Glosses* of Mattheus Platearius; Gilles dedicated his text to Romualdo, who may have been associated with the papal court. *On the Praise and Virtues* also indicates the incipient decline of the school of Salerno. Gilles may have written *On Aromatic Simples*, although some scholars assign it to Otto of Cremona or Gerard of Cremona. This poem discusses a narrower spectrum of drugs than is found in *Compound Medicines* and was associated with Gilles's name by 1272 at the latest.

Hierapigra for Purging Prelates also survives in a single manuscript. In it Gilles railed against the excesses of priests, involving all of the deadly sins. He referred to one priest by name, the papal legate to Philip Augustus, Cardinal Guala Bicchieri. Of particular note was a recent ecclesiastical ruling in favor of celibacy, which, according to the physician, was contrary to the exigencies of nature and medicine. Carnal desire, Gilles felt, was a cure for the clergy's arrogance and a release for human physiology. Although strictly a work of critical theology, *Hierapigra* takes its metaphoric power from a laxative common in elite medical texts.

Bibliography

Primary: Viellard, C., 1903. *L'Urologie et les médecins urologiques dans la médecine ancienne: Gilles de Corbeil, sa vie, ses oeuvres, son poème des urines* (Paris); Viellard, C., 1909. *Essai sur la société médicale et réligieuse au XIIe siècle: Gilles de Corbeil, médecin de Philippe-Auguste et chanoine de Notre-Dame, 1140–1224?* (Paris); Kliegel, P., 1972. *Die Harnverse des Gilles de Corbeil* (Bonn); Scheler, Dieter Josef, 1972. *Die ierapigra ad purgandos prelatos des Egidius von Corbeil* (Würzburg).

Secondary: Ausécache, Mireille, 1998. 'Gilles de Corbeil ou le medecin pedagogue au tournant des XIIe et XIIIe siécles.' *Early Science and Medicine* 3: 187–215; Riha, Ortrun, 1988. 'Harndiagnostik bei Isaak Judaeus, Gilles de Corbeil und Ortolf von Baierland.' *Sudhoffs Archiv für Geschichte der Medizin und der Naturwissenschaften* 72: 212–224; Schalick, Walton O., 1997. 'Add One Part Pharmacy to One Part Surgery and One Part Medicine: Jean de Saint-Amand and the Development of Medical Pharmacology in Paris, c. 1230–1303.' PhD dissertation, Johns Hopkins University (Baltimore).

Walton O. Schalick III

GILLES DE LA TOURETTE, GEORGES (b. Saint-Gervais-les-Trois-Clochers, France, 30 October 1857; d. Lausanne, Switzerland, 26 May 1904), *neurology.*

To a great extent, Gilles de la Tourette's professional interests were influenced by the history of his childhood home, Loudun, the site of the famous trial of Sister Anne des Anges, whose alleged possession led to the execution of Father Urbain Grandier. These events framed Gilles de la Tourette's lifelong fascination with the extent to which mental disturbances historically had been misconstrued as resulting from supernatural forces. They informed as well his later interests in involuntary movements and vocalizations as examples of how behaviors that formerly had been attributed to possession were the results of medical conditions. Loudun was also the birthplace of Dr Théophraste Renaudot, an important ally of Richelieu, who advocated medical treatment of the poor. Renaudot's example influenced the young Gilles de la Tourette's decision to become a physician. Later, Gilles de la Tourette would write biographies of both Renaudot and Sister Anne des Anges.

Gilles de la Tourette completed his medical studies at Poitiers and arrived in Paris in 1877. He impressed his contemporaries as driven, often over-exuberant, and extremely combative. In contrast, more senior physicians, especially Jean-Martin Charcot and Paul Brouardel, under whom he interned, thought Gilles de la Tourette brilliant and exceedingly reliable.

In 1885, at Charcot's behest, Gilles de la Tourette published a two-part article that identified a combination of multiple motor tics and 'involuntary' vocalizations as a distinct disorder that he called *maladie des tics convulsifs* (convulsive tic disease). Charcot had selected Gilles de la Tourette because of the younger man's clinical experience with patients with tics and other similar phenomena. In particular, Gilles de la Tourette had been fascinated by jumping and startle behaviors reported in Malaysia, Siberia, and Maine (USA), variously known as 'latah', 'myriachit', and 'jumping'. These bizarre behaviors often were accompanied by echopraxia (imitation), echolalia, coprolalia, and copropraxia (sexual touching). In a review of these behaviors, he drew a parallel with similar cases that had presented at Charcot's clinic. The next year, when Gilles de la Tourette published his two-part study on convulsive tic disease, he included jumping, myriachit, and latah as variations of his typology.

In 1887, after finishing his thesis on locomotor signs of nervous disease and the diagnostic use of footprints (1885), Gilles de la Tourette was appointed Charcot's *chef du clinique* at the Salpêtrière. That same year, he published a study on hypnosis; he also married his cousin, Marie Detrois, with whom he would later have four children. During his tenure at the Salpêtrière, he published sixteen papers on hysteria, embarked on research into the effectiveness of suspension therapy on locomotor ataxia, and invented a vibrating helmet designed to treat neurasthenia, facial neuralgia, and vertigo. He joined with neurologist Paul Richer and photographer Albert Londe to establish the *Nouvelle Iconographie de la Salpêtrière* in 1888, and between 1891 and 1895 he published three volumes on hysteria inspired by Charcot. In 1893 a former female patient, who claimed that Gilles de la Tourette had hypnotized her against her will, fired three bullets into his head and neck. He recovered and soon accepted appointments as professeur Agrégé at Hôpital St Antoine and Chief Medical Officer to the 1900 World's Fair Exhibition. In addition to his extensive psychological and physiological works, Gilles de la Tourette also published theatrical and social criticism. Writing for *La Revue Hebdomadaire*, he used the pseudonym Paracelsus. In 1901, soon after the publication of his book on bromide treatment of epilepsy, Gilles de la Tourette developed what appeared to be syphilitic dementia. He entered a Swiss psychiatric hospital, where he died in 1904.

Bibliography

Primary: 1885. 'Étude sur une affection nerveuse caractérisée par de l'incoordination motrice accompagnée d'écholalie et de coprolalie (jumping, latah, and myriachit).' *Archives de Neurologie* 9: 19–42, 158–200; 1887. *L'hypnotisme dans les états analogue au point de vue médico-légal* (Paris); 1891–95. *Traité clinique et thérapeutique de l'hystérie d'après l'enseignement de la Salpêtrière* 3 vols. (Paris).

Secondary: Kushner, H. I., 1999. *A Cursing Brain? The Histories of Gilles de la Tourette Syndrome* (Cambridge, MA); Kushner, H. I., 1995. 'Medical Fictions: The Case of the Cursing Marquise and the (Re)construction of Gilles de la Tourette's Syndrome.' *Bulletin of the History of Medicine* 69: 224–254; Guilly, Paul, 1982. 'Gilles de la Tourette' in Rose, F. C., and W. F. Bynum, eds., *Historical Aspects of the Neurosciences* (New York) pp. 397–413.

Howard I. Kushner

GILLIES, HAROLD DELF   (b. Dunedin, New Zealand, 17 June 1882; d. London, England, 10 September 1960), *plastic surgery.*

Gillies was the son of Emily Street and Robert Gillies, a Scottish-born Dunedin estate agent who died shortly before Harold's fourth birthday. His mother was left comfortably off, and Gillies spent four years at a preparatory school near Rugby in England before attending Wanganui Collegiate in New Zealand from 1896 to 1900. He then returned to England to study medicine at Cambridge and St Bartholomew's Hospital Medical School, qualifying MRCS LRCP in 1908.

After graduation, Gillies pursued a career in otolaryngology until the horrific facial injuries inflicted by World War I opened up a new avenue. In early 1916 he reported to Cambridge Military Hospital in Aldershot for 'special duty in connection with plastic surgery'. By late 1917, based at Queen Mary's Hospital, Sidcup, he had introduced new grafting techniques, using pedicle tubes of living skin. (The Russian doctor Vladimir Filatov simultaneously but quite independently adopted the same technique in Odessa.)

At the outset Gillies enlisted Henry Tonks, a trained surgeon but then employed at London's Slade School of Fine Art, to produce detailed drawings of his operative techniques. Many illustrations were incorporated into Gillies's seminal *Plastic Surgery of the Face* (1920). The rediscovery of the Gillies Archive in the mid-1990s supplemented the published work and offers a unique insight into the development of this discipline. Gillies's second major textbook, *The Principles and Art of Plastic Surgery* (1957), compiled jointly with D. R. Millard, further enhanced his reputation; a stickler for high standards and accuracy, Gillies met the spiraling costs by selling his beloved Bentley car.

Gillies, in partnership with T. P. Kilner, dominated British plastic surgery in the 1920s. In addition to reconstructive work, he undertook many cosmetic operations, justifying these on psychological grounds. In 1930 he was knighted for 'valuable services in the treatment of facial disfigurement'. The partnership with Kilner was dissolved that same year, and Sir Harold established a new team with two young New Zealanders, Archibald McIndoe and Arthur Mowlem. By the late 1930s, Gillies was leaving much of the routine work to his colleagues as he pursued sporting and other interests.

The outbreak of World War II brought another change of direction: Gillies became consultant adviser to the Ministry of Health, with responsibility for training maxillofacial teams. It was around this time that he met Peter Medawar, whose interest in immunology was fired by a discussion with Gillies about the rejection of skin grafts in burn patients, many of whom were Battle of Britain pilots.

By 1945 the specialty had expanded to such an extent that the British Association of Plastic Surgeons, with Gillies as first president, had forty founding members. A decade later, Gillies was honorary president of the inaugural International Congress of Plastic Surgeons in Stockholm. In 1956, however, he complained about being reduced to picking up the small jobs that the 'big boys' did not want.

Gillies excelled at sport, rowing for Cambridge in his student days and playing competitive golf until his mid-seventies. He was an accomplished painter, still exhibiting in 1959. He also maintained a lifelong interest in professional affairs; in July 1960, just weeks before his death, the *Times* reported that Gillies had devised a special aluminum splint that might enable the South African cricketer Griffin to bowl again.

In 1949 McIndoe described his former mentor as 'a dynamic if unorthodox teacher who impressed by paradox, invective, cajolery and raillery'. Gillies apparently bore no grudge regarding this rather unflattering description. When McIndoe, eighteen years Gillies's junior, died in early 1960, Gillies's tribute in the *Times* noted, 'The last enemy leaves his family and all of us desolate but his record will be framed in immortality.' It was an epitaph that could have been repeated on Gillies's own demise just six months later.

Bibliography

Primary: 1920. *The Plastic Surgery of the Face* (London).

Secondary: Pound, R., 1964. *Surgeon Extraordinary* (London); *Oxford DNB.*

Derek A. Dow

GILLMAN, JOSEPH   (b. Pretoria, South Africa, 3 December 1903; d. Nice, France, 5 September 1981), *histology, nutrition, pathology.*

Born in Pretoria and educated on a scholarship at Jeppe High School in Johannesburg, Joseph (Joe) Gillman completed a BSc degree and graduated in 1929 from medical school at the University of the Witwatersrand (Wits). An outstanding student who was appointed to head the histology subdepartment of the anatomy department at Wits even before graduation, Gillman had an illustrious academic career at that university for thirty years (1930–60). During this period, he radically revised the curriculum in histology and physiology, founded the *South African Journal of Medical Sciences* and was one of its first coeditors (1935–39), and received a D.Sc. (1939). An honorary reader in experimental biology and medicine (1945–50), he ended his career at Wits as professor and head of physiology

(1950–61). He also headed the unit on nutrition funded by Wits and the Council for Scientific and Industrial Research (CSIR), was a member of the World Health Organization (WHO) Expert Committee on the teaching of physiology and preventive medicine (1958), and served as a member of the WHO Committee on Diarrhoeal Diseases in Children (1962). Among his many honors was the gold medal from the SAAAS (1953), in recognition of his outstanding contribution to the advancement of science.

Gillman inspired many of South Africa's most outstanding medical scientists. These included Sydney Brenner, a Nobel prizewinner, and the internationally renowned paleontologist Philip Tobias, both of whom have publicly acknowledged their enormous debt to Gillman's intellectual stimulation; others of his students proceeded to distinguished academic posts across the world.

A Marxist, Gillman was a controversial figure in University politics and outspoken in his opposition to the South African government's racial policies. Many senior colleagues thought his curriculum changes too drastic, accused him of intellectual arrogance, and questioned the integrity of his work. Irked by disagreements within the University and increasingly uncomfortable with apartheid, he accepted Nkrumah's invitation to head Ghana's Institute of Health and Medical Research. With Nkrumah's fall (1966), he left Ghana, working thereafter in London and Malta, before retiring to Nice, France (1972).

Over the years Gillman's 'research output was prodigious and versatile' (Tobias, 1982, p. 1008): he wrote over 230 articles and reviews in cytology, histology, embryology, and primatology. It is, however, for his work in nutrition that he is mainly remembered. Together with his brother Theodore, his long-term partner Christine Gilbert, and others, he coauthored numerous papers dealing with aspects of malnutrition. The 584-page volume with Theodore, *Perspectives in Human Malnutrition*, was the summation of this work. Focusing largely on pellagra, and backed by extensive histological research, the authors examined 'the clinical and pathological manifestations of malnutrition' in Africans and argued that it is best understood by concentrating on 'disturbed physiological regulations' and 'developmental processes', rather than by using an 'organ concept of disease' or looking for a missing dietary element. They saw malnutrition as lying behind 'the unusual incidence of various diseases in the Africans', and echoing the Gluckman Report, they argued that rapid urbanization, low wages, and race prejudice, rather than 'racial difference', had created 'nutritional problems of the first magnitude' in South Africa. Pellagra, among South Africa's 'commonest nutritional syndromes', had, they believed, increased at 'an alarming rate' since the war—for 'essentially' economic reasons, its 'most vicious single causative factor' being man-made poverty (Gillman and Gillman, 1951, pp. 1–14, 41–43, 62–64)—words that still resonate powerfully with contemporary concerns.

Bibliography

Primary: 1951. (with Gillman, Theodore) *Perspectives in Human Malnutrition: A Contribution to the Biology of Disease from a Clinical and Pathological Study of Chronic Malnutrition and Pellagra in the African* (New York).

Secondary: Murray, Bruce K, 1997. *Wits. The 'Open' Years* (Johannesburg); Tobias, Phillip V., 1982. 'In Memoriam.' *South African Medical Journal* 62: 1007–1008; Van Zyl, A., 1982, 'Professor A Van Zyl writes.' *South African Medical Journal* 62: 1008.

Shula Marks

GIMBERNAT I ARBÓS, ANTONI DE (b. Cambrils, Tarragona, Spain, 15 February 1734; d. Madrid, Spain, 17 November 1816), *surgery, anatomy.*

Gimbernat studied arts and philosophy at the University of Cervera. In 1756 he began his training as a surgeon at the Royal College of Surgery in Cádiz, an institution created by Pere Virgili in 1748 under royal patronage to improve the standards of naval surgeons.

He returned to Catalonia in 1763 and was employed to teach anatomy at the Royal College of Surgery in Barcelona, which had been founded three years previously for the training of military and civil surgeons. While he was teaching and practicing dissection in the school's anatomical theater, he described the configuration of the inguinal ligament that took his name and the surgical technique of the treatment of the crural hernia. Those findings were published in 1793 and translated into English two years later and into German and French sometime later.

Pensioned by the crown, in 1774 he embarked upon a journey of research, which took him through France, England, Scotland, and Holland over a period of five years. In London he attended lectures of John Hunter and had the opportunity to demonstrate the surgical technique of the crural hernia. The motive of his journey was to accumulate experience in order to create a center of surgery in Madrid on his return. The project aroused opposition among the court physicians who feared the development and consolidation of a new state profession integrated by civil and military surgeons trained in the three royal colleges.

Nevertheless, in 1787 he founded the Royal College of Surgery of San Carlos, near the rebuilt Hospital General building, in Madrid and was appointed as a codirector with Mariano Rivas. The students had to reach a high level of training, in both theory and practice, in anatomy, chemistry, pathology, medical therapeutics, and surgical skills. Apart from the compulsory classes, students were expected to attend periodical *juntas literarias* (literary meetings) where the most interesting clinical cases were discussed.

Gimbernat's sojourn in Edinburgh proved decisive in affiliating him with those who defended the union of medicine and surgery, an ephemeral union officially established in Spain between 1799 and 1801.

Being a great admirer of French surgery, he collaborated with the government of José Bonaparte (1808–13) and later presided over the Superior Council of Public Health, with the result that on the return of Fernando VII to the Spanish throne, he was accused of being an 'afrancesado' (Francophile) and was discredited and dishonored. He spent the last years of his life almost blind and in abject poverty.

Gimbernat can be considered the Spanish paradigm of the reform of surgical studies at his times. He was involved in the three royal colleges of surgery (Cádiz, Barcelona, and Madrid) that revolutionized knowledge and medical-surgical practice in Enlightenment Spain.

Bibliography

Primary: 1926–27. (Salcedo, E., ed.) *Obras de don Antonio de Gimbernat.* 2 vols. (Madrid); 1768. *Oración inaugural* (Barcelona); 1793. *Nuevo método de operar en la hernia crural* (Madrid); 1802. *Disertación sobre las úlceras de los ojos que interesan la córnea transparente* (Madrid).

Secondary: Pérez Pérez, Núria, 2004. 'El Hospital General de Santa Creu frente al Real Colegio de Cirugía de Barcelona: la controversia surgida en torno al suministro de cadáveres para el anfiteatro anatómico de Gimbernat.' *Medicina e Historia,* 4ª época (1): 1–15; Guardiola, Elena, and Josep E. Baños, 2004. *Eponímia mèdica catalana* (Barcelona); Astrain, Mikel, 1996. *Barberos, cirujanos y gente de mar. La sanidad naval y la profesión quirúrgica en la España ilustrada* (Madrid); Bujosa, Francesc, 1983. 'Gimbernat y Arbós, Antonio' in López Piñero, José María et al., eds., *Diccionario histórico de la ciencia moderna en España* vol. 2 (Barcelona); Burke, Michael E., 1977. *The Royal College of San Carlos. Surgery and Spanish Reform in the Late Eighteenth Century* (Durham, NC); Gimbernat, Carlos de, 1828. *Sucinta historia del Dr. D. Antonio de Gimbernat* (Barcelona).

Àlvar Martínez-Vidal

GIOVANNINI, GIOVANNI BATTISTA (b. Gravedona, Milan, Italy, 12 January 1636; d. Madrid, Spain, 26 December 1691), *surgery, medicine, natural philosophy.*

Giovannini was born somewhere near Milan. When still very young, he enrolled as a surgeon in the Spanish army and participated in the campaigns in Lombardy until 1663, when his regiment was transferred to Extremadura because of the Spanish war with Portugal. In 1667, as a result of the intervention of the royal doctor Lucas Maestro Negrete, he entered the service of Juan José of Austria, stepbrother of the recently crowned King of Spain Carlos II and a decisive figure in the political and cultural ambience of the time.

Until the prince's death in 1679, Giovannini ('Juanini', as appearing in his books, all published in Spanish) was his chamber surgeon and accompanied him to his military and political destinations. Giovannini established a close relationship with Joan d'Alòs, professor at the University of Barcelona, and with José Lucas Casalete at the University of Saragossa, both supporters, as was Giovannini, of the acknowledgment of both the blood circulation doctrine and its consequences on the corporal economy. Likewise, he corresponded with Juan Mathias de Lucas, a doctor of German origin and a resident in the court of Lisbon.

In his youth Giovannini studied anatomy at the University of Pavia, probably with Antonio Calvi, and during his life, he performed numerous public demonstrations in anatomical theaters in Salamanca, Saragossa, and Madrid, as well as in various French and Italian cities, according to his accounts. During his years in Saragossa serving Juan José of Austria, he performed diverse dissection experiments, including microscopic observation, vivisection, and autopsies carried out with diagnostic purposes.

In 1676, established at Saragossa, he corresponded with François Bayle, professor at the University of Toulouse, who was instrumental in the translation of Giovannini's book *Discurso político y phísico* [Political and Physical Discourse] into French nine years later. Dedicated to Juan José of Austria, it questioned the traditional vision regarding the quality of Madrid's air with arguments of a chemical nature far removed from the supposed Galenic imperatives. In 1689 a considerably amplified version was published that merited the praise of the royal doctor Andrés de Gámez, a former protophysician at the court of Naples.

In 1679, after the death of his patron, Prince Juan José, he devoted himself to the practice of surgery in Madrid. This did not impede his continued pursuit of intellectual interests, as demonstrated in the publication of the first part of his *Nueva idea physica natural* [New natural physical idea], in which he ascertained the origin of matter that moves things from the compared principles of 'acid salt' and 'alcali salt'.

As a result of the intervention of Andrés de Gámez, he corresponded with Francesco Redi, who proposed a personal meeting between the two in Florence in 1686. During this same journey through Italy, Giovannini also met Marcello Malpighi and Pompeo Sacco. In 1691 he published the most significant part of his writing relating to the nervous system. Influenced by the work of Thomas Willis and Raymond Vieussens, Giovannini conceived the animal spirits of *succus nerveus* in terms of 'atoms of acid salt and volatile alcali' and explained its movement as a fermentative process in which the *aerial nitre* theorized by John Mayow intervened.

Bibliography

Primary: 1679. *Discurso político y phísico que muestra los movimientos y efectos que produce la fermentación y materias nitrosas en los cuerpos sublunares* (Madrid) (2nd edn., 1689); 1685. *Nueva idea physica natural demostrativa, origen de las materias que mueven las cosas* (Zaragoza); 1689. *Carta escrita al mui noble aretino doctor don Francisco Redi, médico de su Alteza* (Madrid) (2nd edn., 1691).

Secondary: Cobo, Jesús, 2005. *Juan Bautista Juanini (1636–1691): medicina, cirugía y neurociencias* (PhD thesis, Universitat Autònoma de Barcelona); López Piñero, José María, 1976. 'Juan Bautista Juanini

(1636–1691) y la introducción en España de la medicina moderna y de la iatroquímica' in *Medicina moderna y sociedad española. Siglos XVI–XIX* (Valencia) pp. 149–173.

Àlvar Martínez-Vidal

GIRARD, GEORGES DESIRÉ (b. Isigny-sur-mer, Calvados, France, 4 February 1888; d. Paris, France, 20 February 1985), *medicine, bacteriology.*

The son of French civil servants, Girard won admission to the Navy Medical School at Bordeaux in 1909, graduating as a Naval physician four years later. He served in the medical corps of the French Colonial Army during World War I (1914–17), receiving the Croix de Guerre in 1916.

Girard's medical life changed forever after he was posted as resident physician to the French colonial hospital in Diego-Suarez, Madagascar, where he also ran the bacteriological laboratory (1917–20). Learning on the spot, Girard in 1922 became director of the Pasteur Institute in the Malagasy capital of Tananarive, a position he would hold until 1940. Here, Girard worked on leprosy, typhoid, tuberculosis, and especially bubonic and pneumonic plague, a subject on which he would make his mark internationally and on which he published thirty-six articles.

The highly virulent pneumonic form of plague dominated in successive outbreaks in Madagascar, beginning in 1921. Girard's research demonstrated that the virulence of the rat flea persisted for at least a year in the absence of infected rats. He showed the risks of infection caused by the Malagasy custom of 'Famadinha', the handling of cadavers at tombs a year after initial burial. Rat fleas were able to hibernate in the clothing of the plague dead and still infect mammals. Girard's solution was to create a special cemetery for the plague dead.

Concerned to find a safe and effective preventive vaccine for plague, Girard took leave in 1926 to enroll in a bacteriology course at the Pasteur Institute in Paris. On his return to Madagascar, Girard and his collaborator, Jean Marie Léopold Robic, set to work to develop a new vaccine. After six years of trials, in 1932 their so-called E.V. strain of attenuated plague bacilli was found to protect laboratory animals. To show its safety for humans, Robic and Girard vaccinated themselves several times. Soon the Girard-Robic vaccine was being used successfully in Madagascar, Senegal, South Africa, the Belgian Congo, and the Soviet Union. It remained the only treatment against plague until the arrival of antibiotics after World War II.

Girard spent most of the war years in Paris, where he was in charge of plague research at the Pasteur Institute. An exception was his research trip to Senegal (1944–45), where he spent six weeks studying the way in which the 1944 plague-control campaign had been organized and making recommendations for future campaigns. Girard's report was a devastating critique of what he described as shoddy work on plague in Senegal over the preceding thirty years. Especially neglected had been research on the role of the flea population in Senegal. Although not free of bias against Africans, Girard blamed the health authorities rather than the victims of plague and argued that colonial public health would only improve significantly with a change of political will by the French government leading to new investment in structural changes such as modern housing.

In his later years Girard enjoyed the prestige of a leading French scientist, serving as president of the Société de Pathologie Exotique (1954–58) before retiring from the Pasteur Institute in 1959. A meticulous and courageous scientist, Girard is remembered as a strict and demanding research director.

Bibliography

Primary: 1946. 'L'état actuel de la question de la vaccination antipesteuse.' *Presse Médicale* 54: 468; 1955. 'Plague.' *Annual Review of Microbiology* 9: 253–276.

Secondary: Echenberg, Myron, 2002. *Black Death, White Medicine: Bubonic Plague and the Politics of Public Health in Colonial Senegal, 1914–1945* (Portsmouth, NH); Dodin, André, 1985. 'La vie et l'oeuvre du Docteur G. Girard.' *Bulletin de la Société de Pathologie Exotique* 78: 413–415; Coulanges, P., 1983. 'Cinquantenaire du vaccin antipesteux EV (Girard et Robic).' *Bulletin de la Société de Pathologie Exotique* 76: 114–120.

Myron Echenberg

GLISSON, FRANCIS (b. Bristol, England, 1599; d. London, England, 14 October 1677), *medicine, hepatology, anatomy.*

Glisson was the third child of William Glisson, a tailor, and William's wife, Mary. He was educated at Rampisham in Dorset and then at Gonville and Caius College, Cambridge, where he earned a BA (1621) and an MA (1624). For the next ten years, he was a fellow of the College. In 1634 he gained his MD from Cambridge, and two years later, he was appointed regius professor of medicine of that university, holding the position until his death. Despite this, he also spent a good deal of time in London, becoming a Fellow of the College of Physicians in September 1635, and reader in anatomy and Goulstonian lecturer for the College in 1639 and 1640, respectively. He served as President of the College from 1667 to 1669, during which time he had the particular responsibility of raising the funds necessary for the rebuilding of the College after the Great Fire of 1666. The anatomy lectures that he gave at the College and other surviving manuscripts of his extensive anatomical investigations reveal him to have been a keen adherent of William Harvey's (1578–1657) ideas. In 1654 this work led to the publication of *Anatomia Hepatis*, a detailed anatomy of the liver (an organ whose function required complete re-examination after the discovery of the circulation of the blood) and of the lymphatic vessels. The book reveals him to have been a particularly skilled anatomist, using injection techniques to illustrate and investigate the vessels within the liver, and it contains the first detailed account of the capsule of the liver now known as Glisson's capsule.

Glisson did not work alone. From the mid-1640s he met regularly with other physicians and also with philosophers, including George Ent, John Wallis, and John Wilkins, in order to discuss medical research and natural philosophy. There is a clear connection between some of these informal group meetings and the emergence of the Royal Society after the Restoration, a body of which Glisson was a founder member. A more immediate result was the publication (1650) of *De rachitide sive morbo puerili*, with an English translation (*A Treatise of the Rickets: Being a Disease Common to Children*) the following year. Substantially, but not entirely, written by Glisson, this work grew out of the discussions of a group of physicians about the new condition, rickets. It provided a detailed description of the disease, distinguished it from scurvy and other afflictions, and interpreted its origin with reference to the notion of irritability.

Glisson developed this last interest in the remainder of his work. Through anatomical and philosophical investigations he, like William Harvey, critiqued dualistic understandings of the body and the soul. In *De natura substantiae energetica, seu, De vita naturae* (1672) Glisson argued that matter has a 'life' with perceptive, appetitive, and motive faculties. In *De ventriculo et intestinis*, his study of the stomach and intestines published in 1677, he paid particular attention to the fibers of the body in a way that anticipated Albrecht von Haller's (1708–77) work on the irritability of muscles in the eighteenth century. Shortly after the publication of this work, he died in London and was buried in St Bride's, Fleet Street.

Bibliography

Primary: 1993. (Cunningham, Andrew, ed.) *From Anatomia Hepatis (The anatomy of the liver), 1654* (Cambridge); 1998. (Cunningham, Andrew, ed.) *Lectures and Other Papers* (Cambridge).

Secondary: Henry, J., 1987. 'Medicine and Pneumatology: Henry More, Richard Baxter, and Francis Glisson's *Treatise on the energetic nature of substance*.' *Medical History* 31: 15–40; Frank, R. G., 1980. *Harvey and the Oxford Physiologists* (Berkeley and Los Angeles); Pagel, W., 1967. 'Harvey and Glisson on Irritability, with a Note on Van Helmont.' *Bulletin of the History of Medicine* 41: 497–514; *DSB*; *Munk's Roll*; *Oxford DNB*.

Mark Jenner

GLUCKMAN, HENRY

GLUCKMAN, HENRY   (b. Zager, Lithuania, 12 July 1894; d. Johannesburg, South Africa, 5 June 1987), *public health, venerology.*

Born in Lithuania, Gluckman came to South Africa as a child. After attending school in Randfontein and Johannesburg, he studied medicine at the London Hospital (1912–17). On qualification, he was commissioned into the South African Medical Corps with the rank of captain. Awaiting transport to the front, he worked as a house-surgeon in Monmouthshire and Cardiff and served as a locum in a coal-mining district in south Wales. These experiences probably sensitized him to the social causes of ill health and led to his lifelong commitment to social medicine.

After the war, Gluckman went into private practice in Johannesburg, but was swiftly drawn into more public roles. Appointed lecturer in the University of Witwatersrand's medical school (1922–39), he showed an early interest in STDs, serving as director of the Johannesburg City Council Special Treatment Centre (1920–40), chairman of the South African Social Hygiene Council (1920–37), and consultant venerealogist to the Johannesburg Hospital (1928–38). One of the handful of South African medical professionals who recognized the social roots of much ill health, he entered national politics as an MP (1938–58) and became the natural spokesman of those calling for a 'new order' in medicine. After unsuccessfully attempting to introduce national health insurance, he persuaded the government to set up a commission 'to enquire into, report and advise upon ... the provision of an organized National Health Service' that would ensure 'adequate' health services 'for *all* sections of the people of the Union of South Africa' (UG 30-1944, p. 1). He both drafted the Commission's wide-ranging terms of reference and chaired it (1942–44).

The commissioners took evidence from roughly 1,000 witnesses across South Africa. Their evidence stressed the gravity of the health crisis in South Africa and recommended the establishment of a unified national health service open to all, regardless of race, color, or creed, and paid for out of state taxation. 'The cure of ill health' was impossible, they declared, without state intervention in nutrition, housing, and environmental services—mere 'doctoring' was not enough (UG 30-44, p. 102). Distinguishing between personal and nonpersonal health services, they envisaged a three-tiered mode of delivery, based on 'the most modern conception of health'—promotive and preventive services based on 400 health centers as pioneered at Pholela, with local and regional hospitals providing curative care. In the South African context, these recommendations were virtually revolutionary, and the report was a tribute to Gluckman's 'superb political and chairmanship skills' (Kark and Kark, 1999, p. 83). He became the first Jew to have a cabinet appointment when he became Minister of Health, charged with implementing the commission's recommendations (1945).

Before the fall of the government (1948), Gluckman had established forty health centers and a training institute for their health workers. The government failed, however, to support the commission's central recommendation, the creation of a unified national health service, or to fund its far-reaching recommendations. The electoral victory of the pro-apartheid National Party was the final blow to the commission's report. Gluckman became the opposition's parliamentary spokesman on health (1948–58) and supported public health by chairing South Africa's National War Memorial Health Foundation (1952–87) and presiding over the National Tuberculosis Association (1947–87). In his memory the University of the Witwatersrand endowed the Henry Gluckman medal, awarded to distinguished candidates in the fellowship examination of the College of Public Health Medicine (1993), a sign of renewed interest in his ideas in the run-up to South Africa's post-apartheid elections (1994).

Bibliography

Primary: 1944. *UG30-44 Report of the National Health Services Commission* (Pretoria); 1970. *Abiding Values. Speeches and Addresses* (Johannesburg); 1999. (with Kark, Emily) *Promoting Community Health. From Pholela to Jerusalem* (Johannesburg).

Secondary: Marks, Shula, and Neil Andersson, 1992. 'Industrialization, Rural Health and the 1944 Health Services Commission in South Africa' in Feierman, Steven, and John M. Janzen, eds., *The Social Basis of Health and Healing in Africa* (Manchester) pp. 131–161; Lean, Phyllis, 1970. 'Profile' in Gluckman, Henry, *Abiding Values. Speeches and Addresses* (Johannesburg) pp. 3–31.

Shula Marks

GODLEE, RICKMAN JOHN   (b. London, England, 15 April 1849; d. Whitchurch, near Reading, England, 20 April 1925), *surgery.*

Godlee, youngest son of Quakers Rickman Godlee, a barrister, and Mary Lister, sister of the surgeon Joseph Lister (1827–1912), entered University College, London, in 1866. After completing his BA in a year, he joined the college's medical faculty. Even as a student, his abilities as a surgical operator were admired, and when he took his MB and MS degrees in 1872–73, he received gold medals for surgery.

After working in Edinburgh at the Royal Infirmary, Godlee returned to University College Hospital under his cousin, the surgeon Marcus Beck (1843–93). Beck was a major proponent of Joseph Lister's antiseptic surgery, and Godlee became a firm supporter and frequent practitioner of 'Listerism'. He was elected FRCS in 1876 and in the same year moved to Charing Cross Hospital to take the post of assistant surgeon and lecturer in anatomy. When a similar post became vacant at University College Hospital in 1877, however, Godlee came back to his alma mater and remained there for the rest of his career. He showed great concern for the teaching of surgical anatomy and wrote and illustrated an *Atlas of Human Anatomy* (1880) to accompany his lectures.

In addition to his success as a teacher, Godlee's reputation as an innovative operator continued to increase. His public standing grew in November 1884 when he and the neurologists David Ferrier (1843–1928) and John Hughlings

Jackson (1835–1911) used new diagnostic techniques to locate and remove a large brain tumor. The death of the patient a few days after the operation, however, provoked a small scandal. In the mid-1880s Godlee developed an interest in thoracic surgery: he wrote on the subject with the surgeon James Kingston Fowler (1852–1934) and was in 1884 made surgeon to the Brompton Hospital for Consumption and Diseases of the Chest in London.

In 1891 Godlee married Juliet Seebohm, daughter of the financier Frederic Seebohm. The couple bought a house on Wimpole Street in London, the very center of the capital's fashionable 'doctoropolis'. Godlee's professional standing at University College continued to increase: he took the chair of clinical surgery in 1892, and in 1900 he was appointed Holme Professor of Clinical Surgery. He assisted his uncle (by now Lord Lister) with his practice and supervised the editing and publication of Lister's papers. Godlee's belief in the power of 'Listerism' persisted until the end of his life; in *Lord Lister* (1917), a popular biography, he attributed the rise of modern surgery almost entirely to the introduction of the antiseptic method.

In the last decade of his career, Godlee received many honors. He was Librarian (1907–16) and President (1916–18) of the Royal Society of Medicine and President (1911–13) and Hunterian Orator (1913) of the RCS. In 1912 he was created a baronet. He resigned his professional posts in 1914 and was appointed emeritus professor of clinical surgery. In 1920 he retired and moved to his farm in Whitchurch.

Godlee's career must be seen in the context of his uncle's life and work. Although not as versatile a technical innovator as Lister, Godlee worked throughout his life for improvements in the status and knowledge base of surgery. In 1850 surgery was a bloody craft; by 1900 it had become a clinical science. This transformation took place largely through the efforts of surgeons such as Godlee.

Bibliography

Primary: 1880. *Atlas of Human Anatomy* (London); 1898. (with Fowler, James Kingston) *Diseases of the Lungs* (London); 1917. *Lord Lister* (London).

Secondary: *Plarr's Lives*; *Oxford DNB*.

Richard Barnett

GOLDBERGER, JOSEPH   (b. Girált, Hungary, 16 July 1874; d. Washington, D.C., USA, 17 January 1929), *medicine, epidemiology, public health.*

Born in 1874 in eastern Hungary, Goldberger was one of six children born to sheepherder and tenant farmer Samuel and his wife, Sarah Goldberger. After an epizootic ravaged their sheep flock, impoverishing the family, they emigrated to America, settling in the Lower East Side of Manhattan in New York City. There Samuel Goldberger opened a small grocery store catering to the poverty-stricken immigrant Jews living in the neighborhood. Education was the way out of this debilitating environment, and at age sixteen Joseph enrolled in the College of the City of New York (CCNY). He remained at CCNY for two years before entering Bellevue Hospital Medical College, receiving the MD degree, with honors, in 1895. After a two-year internship at Bellevue Hospital and a brief unprofitable effort to set up practice in Manhattan, Goldberger moved to Wilkes-Barre, Pennsylvania, where, presumably, competition would be less. Although his practice in Wilkes-Barre flourished, he found clinical medicine unfulfilling. Thus, in June 1899 he took and passed the weeklong written and oral examination for entry into the prestigious United States Marine Hospital Service. He would remain in the service, subsequently renamed United States Public Health Service, until his death (Kraut, 2003).

During his early years with the Marine Hospital Service, Goldberger served in various quarantine stations at home and abroad and was assigned to several special epidemic investigations. He studied outbreaks of yellow fever in Mexico and Louisiana, typhoid fever in Washington, D.C., dengue fever in Texas, and diphtheria in Detroit. In the Hygienic Laboratory of the Public Health Service, he studied the mode of transmission of typhus fever and the period of infectivity of measles. In 1909 he investigated an outbreak of Schamberg's Disease, a benign progressive dermatosis. In this investigation Goldberger demonstrated his investigative style, namely a combination of observational and experimental study. After observing a strong association between use of new straw mattresses by patients and the isolation of a tiny mite, *Pediculoides vetricosus*, from mattress stuffing, he colonized the mites and applied them to the skin of a volunteer to produce the typical lesions of the disease. To complete the experiment, he applied killed mites to the skin of another volunteer without effect. In these activities, Goldberger developed his research skills and established himself among the most able investigators in the Public Health Service. Then, in March 1914, the Surgeon General assigned him to take charge of the pellagra studies of the service. Goldberger would spend the rest of his professional career in this endeavor.

Pellagra, a recurrent multiorgan disease with a case-fatality rate of 40 to 50 percent, was essentially unknown in the United States before 1900. However, during the first decade of the twentieth century, it assumed epidemic proportions, with an estimated annual incidence of more than 100,000 cases, most occurring in the rural South. Its etiology was unknown, the dominant theories being consumption of spoiled corn and infection by an unknown microbial agent. It took Goldberger only a few weeks to reject these theories and propose an alternative paradigm. In his first publication on pellagra, only a little over three pages in length, he concluded that the disease could not be communicable, was due to a dietary deficiency, and could be prevented by increasing the consumption of fresh animal food components such as meat, eggs, and milk (Goldberger, 1914). These conclusions were based on the following observations: in institutions where pellagra was endemic, no nurse or attendant ever acquired the disease; in these institutions the nurses and attendants received a much more varied diet than inmates and had the opportunity to supplement their diet on the outside; and pellagra was most prevalent among the rural poor whose diets had been shown to be less varied than that of the urban poor who were rarely affected by the disease. Finally, in this first communication, Goldberger recommended 'reduction in cereals, vegetables, and canned foods that enter to so large an extent into the dietary . . . of the people in the South and an increase in the fresh animal food component, such as fresh meats, eggs and milk'. These conclusions were bolstered by subsequent studies extending over many years.

To test the hypothesis that pellagra was due to an unbalanced dietary—i.e., an excess of cereals, vegetables, and canned goods and a deficiency of fresh meat, eggs, and milk—and could be prevented, Goldberger and colleagues carried out a feeding experiment in two Mississippi orphanages and a Georgia mental hospital where pellagra was highly endemic. The initial observations covered one full year. In each institution, the U.S. Public Health service supplemented the diet of inmates by providing for an increase in the proportion of fresh meat and leguminous protein foods and providing eggs and milk, not previously included in the institutional dietary. The carbohydrate component of the diet in these institutions was reduced by curtailing the use of molasses and cane syrup. The results were striking. Of 244 pellagrins (persons with active disease or a history of the disease) consuming the modified diet, only one suffered a relapse in the year of observation, whereas among thirty-two pellagrins not receiving the modified diet, fifteen developed recurrent disease. Among 168 non-pellagrins, none developed the disease (Goldberger et al., 1915).

Concurrent with the prevention demonstration, Goldberger conducted an experiment to more rigorously test the hypothesis that a high carbohydrate diet deficient in fresh fruits, vegetables, and animal products such as meat, eggs, and dairy products was the cause of pellagra. The experiment was conducted at the Rankin prison farm of the Mississippi State Penitentiary. Prisoners at the Rankin farm routinely received a diet that included frequent servings of milk, cheese, butter, eggs, and fresh beef. Pellagra was not known to occur in Rankin farm inmates. Eleven convict volunteers, informed of the details of the experiment and assured of proper care and treatment if that should be needed, were guaranteed pardons by the Governor in return for their participation. These convicts, housed separate from the rest of the prison population and under guard day and night to prevent them from augmenting their experimental diet, were fed a diet similar to that provided the inmates of the institutions included in the prevention demonstration prior to that trial. The remainder of the convict population of the prison farm served as controls. Within five months, six of the eleven volunteers developed symptoms justifying a diagnosis of pellagra. Diagnoses were confirmed by two outside 'experts' experienced in the clinical diagnosis and care of pellagrins. None of the controls developed symptoms or signs of even a suspicion of pellagra (Goldberger et al., 1915).

To complete an understanding of the epidemiology of pellagra, Goldberger and associates from the Hygienic Laboratory, most importantly economist and statistician Edgar Sydenstricker, conducted community-wide surveys of seven cotton-mill villages in northwestern South Carolina beginning in the spring of 1916 and continuing throughout the year. In each village, a house-to-house survey was conducted at two-week intervals. A total of 115 new or recurrent cases of pellagra were ascertained, and extensive data on behavioral, social, economic, environmental, and, of course, dietary factors were collected. These data revealed a complex pattern of interactions that led to the conditions in the post–Civil War South conducive to the emergence of the pellagra epidemic (Goldberger et al., 1920). The mill village studies were innovative in providing a model for the comprehensive investigation of a disease of unknown etiology.

After 1920 Goldberger and his associates at the Hygienic Laboratory concentrated their efforts on identifying the specific dietary component the lack of which was responsible for pellagra. An amino acid component of protein—tryptophan—and brewer's yeast were demonstrated to have a curative effect. However, before he could unravel the complex chemistry that linked tryptophan, as a precursor, to niacin (nicotinic acid fraction of vitamin B complex), the component of brewer's yeast that was eventually identified as the pellagra preventive factor, Goldberger returned to the search for a practical preventive diet. His premature death at age fifty-five cut short his brilliant career.

Goldberger was nominated for a Nobel Prize five times. In support of the fifth nomination, the Director of the Hygienic Laboratory, George McCoy, wrote, 'It is not an exaggeration to say that many competent observers believe that no more important piece of medical research has been accomplished in this generation than has been done by Doctor Goldberger. It has put in our hands knowledge which when applied may be expected to lead to the eradication of pellagra.' Nevertheless, Goldberger did not receive a Nobel Prize

Despite the overwhelming evidence of the dietary etiology of pellagra, economic and cultural factors delayed implementation of widespread control actions, and the disease continued endemically in many areas of the rural South throughout the 1920s.

Bibliography

Primary: 1914. 'The Etiology of Pellagra. The Significance of Certain Epidemiological Observations with Respect Thereto.' *Public*

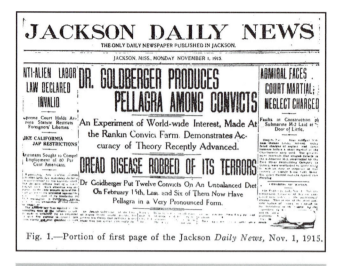

Fig. 1.—Portion of first page of the Jackson *Daily News*, Nov. 1, 1915.

Joseph Goldberger's pellagra experiment makes headline news. Halftone reproduction in 1916 from the *Journal of the American Medical Association* 66: 975–977. Wellcome Library, London.

Health Reports 26: 1683–1686; 1915. (with Waring, C. H., and D. G. Willets) 'The Prevention of Pellagra. A Test of Diet among Institutional Inmates.' *Public Health Reports* 30: 3117–3131; 1915. (with Wheeler, G. A.) 'Experimental Pellagra in the Human Subject Brought About by a Restricted Diet.' *Public Health Reports* 30: 3336–3339; 1920. (with Wheeler, G. A., and Edgar Sydenstricker) 'Pellagra Incidence in Relation to Sex, Age, Season, Occupation, and "Disabling Sickness" in Seven Cotton-Mill-Villages of South Carolina During 1916.' *Public Health Reports* 35: 1650–1664.

Secondary: Kraut, Alan M., 2003. *Goldberger's War: The Life and Work of a Public Health Crusader* (New York); Terris, Milton, ed. and introd., 1964. *Goldberger on Pellagra* (Baton Rouge, LA); *DAMB*.

Warren Winkelstein, Jr.

GOLDSTEIN, KURT (b. Kattowitz, German Upper Silesia (now Katowice, Poland), 6 November 1878; d. New York, New York, USA, 19 September 1965), *neurology, neuropsychology, psychotherapy.*

Goldstein, son of Abraham Goldstein (1836–1902) and Rosalie Cassirer (1845–1911), attended the universities of Breslau (now Wrocław, Poland) and Heidelberg; he received his medical degree at Breslau in 1903. His dissertation dealt with the structure of the posterior columns of the spinal cord. During a brief assistantship to Carl Wernicke, Goldstein became interested in aphasiology, a topic on which he was to write an innovative monograph paying special attention to the transcortical forms of this neuropathological condition (1915).

In 1906 Goldstein went to Königsberg, where he worked in psychiatry and neurology, and moved to Frankfurt am Main in 1914 as first assistant to Ludwig Edinger (1855–1918).

During World War I, he was involved in the treatment of brain-injured soldiers as head of the 'Institute for the Study of After-Effects of Brain Injuries' (Institut zur Erforschung der Folgeerscheinungen von Hirnverletzungen), founded in 1916 at Frankfurt. The rich clinical material obtained during and after the war was subsequently presented and discussed in numerous case studies and theoretical contributions, which established Goldstein's and his collaborators' reputation as early representatives of neuropsychology. Goldstein's main collaborator and coauthor was Adhémar Gelb.

In 1918 Goldstein was appointed as successor of Edinger, and he was promoted in 1929 to full professor of neurology at Frankfurt. In 1930 he moved to Berlin as head of a newly founded division of neurology at the Moabit Hospital and as full professor at the Faculty of Medicine. Denounced as a Jew as well as a political activist for the social-democratic party, he was forced to resign; he emigrated to the Netherlands in 1933, where he joined the University of Amsterdam, and then he finally settled in the United States in 1935. He taught at Columbia University, served as clinical professor of neurology at Tufts Medical School in Boston (1940–45), and then returned to New York City and engaged in private psychotherapeutic practice until he suffered a stroke that resulted in hemiplegia and aphasia.

Goldstein is considered to have been a fervent antilocalizationist. This assessment, however, needs specification. On neo-Kantian grounds, he rejected from the outset the hypothesis that the notions of space and time were materially embodied *in* the brain like memory traces or sensory impressions. By consequence, the possibility of a strict localization of each and every mental function and of its variable contents was also excluded. In addition, clinical data relating to the spontaneous restoration of impaired functions (whether central like speech or peripheral like the retinal sensitivity to light) indicated that the organism's single capacities could not be conceived of as elementary modules with clear-cut functional competences. Both theoretical and clinical considerations led Goldstein to adopt an organismic approach partly cast in terms of the Berlin school of psychology of Wolfgang Köhler. Thus, anything happening to some part of the organism affects the whole organism, the part being defined as figure, the whole organism as ground. In terms of cerebral localization, this meant that mental functions, though being confined within more or less narrow boundaries, are fully operant if, and only if, the whole cortex within the whole brain within the whole organism is working. Rather than anitlocalizationism, the term 'equipotentialism' would certainly be preferable for the characterization of Goldstein's neuropsychological approach. As he put it, 'The individual speech performance is understandable only from the aspect of its relation to the function of the total organism in its endeavor to realize itself as much as possible in the given situation.'

Bibliography

Primary: 1915. *Die transkortikalen Aphasien* (Jena); 1920. (with Gelb, Adhémar) *Psychologische Analysen hirnpathologischer Fälle* (Leipzig); 1934. *Der Aufbau des Organismus* (the Hague); 1940. *Human Nature in the Light of Psychopathology*, (Cambridge, MA); 1948. *Language and Language Disturbances* (New York); 1963. *The Organism: A Holistic Approach to Biology* (New York).

Secondary: Harrington, Anne, 1996. *Reenchanted Science: Holism in German Culture from Wilhelm II to Hitler* (Princeton); Geschwind, Norman, 1974. 'The Paradoxical Position of Kurt Goldstein in the History of Aphasia' in Geschwind, Norman, *Selected Papers on Language and the Brain* (Dordrecht); Simmel, Marianne L., ed., 1968. *The Reach of Mind: Essays in Memory of Kurt Goldstein* (New York).

Alexandre Métraux

GOLGI, CAMILLO   (b. Corteno, Italy, 7 July 1843; d. Pavia, Italy, 21 January 1926), *medicine, physiology, anatomy, parasitology.*

Son of the physician Alessandro, Golgi studied medicine at the University of Pavia, graduating in 1865, at age twenty-two. As an undergraduate, he was a student in the Institute of Psychiatry directed by Cesare Lombroso (1835–1909). After his MD, he entered the Hospital of St Matteo, performing scientific research on neurology and the lymphatic system of the brain in the Institute of General Pathology, directed by Guilio Bizzozero (1846–1901), who introduced Golgi to experimental research and histological techniques.

Golgi's first publication, in 1868, reported studies carried out on pellagra under the direction of Lombroso. Then he analyzed forty-five cases of smallpox, resulting in the first major publication on the pathology of bone marrow. Influenced by Lombroso's theories and by Rudolf Virchow's epoch-making work *Cellular Pathology* (1858), Golgi assumed that mental diseases could be due to organic lesions in the neural centers, and he concentrated on the experimental study of the structure of the nervous system.

For financial reasons, in 1872 Golgi accepted the post of chief physician at the Hospital for the Chronically Sick at Abbiategrasso, a small town near Pavia. He arranged a small laboratory in a kitchen, continuing his investigations into the nervous system, and according to his memoirs, he discovered in 1873 the silver chromate method for staining nerve tissue. This method, called 'reazione nera' [black reaction], made possible the observations of the subtle structure of the nervous system. In 1875 Golgi published an article on the olfactory bulbs containing the first drawings of neural structures as visualized by this technique.

In 1875, at the age of thirty-two, Golgi was invited to Siena as a full professor of anatomy, but he preferred to return to the University of Pavia, as extraordinary professor of histology. The following year he married Lina Aletti, Bizzozero's niece. They had no children, but adopted Golgi's niece Carolina. Golgi remained in Pavia for the remainder of his career and life.

In 1881 he was appointed to the chair of General Pathology at the University of Pavia, but continued his histology teaching. He established a very active laboratory, where he trained many students and foreign guests. He also served as Rector of the university and was made a Senator of the Kingdom of Italy.

With his very productive histological tools Golgi was able to observe the cells that bear his name—the multipolar motor and sensory nerve cells in the cerebral cortex and posterior horns of spinal cord—and suggested the existence of a system of membranes in the cytoplasm of the cell (now named Golgi's apparatus), making up a functional unit concerned with intracellular transport of molecules, the existence of which was confirmed in the 1950s by electron microscopy.

In 1891 Golgi's discoveries on nerve cells led Waldeyer-Hartz (1836–1921) to define the nerve cell or 'neuron' as the basic structural and functional unit of the nervous system, a central point fully developed by Santiago Ramón y Cajal (1852–1934). In 1887 Wilhelm His (1831–1904) showed that the neuron is an embryological unit, because the axons are outgrowths from primitive nerve cells, and by 1889 he suggested the individuality of the nerve cells. The ensemble of these results was called the neuron theory of the nervous system.

Golgi always remained opposed to this theory, although acknowledging that its starting point was to be found in his own work. He attached more importance to the unitary action of the nervous system produced by networks of nervous cells, which instead of working individually act together as a 'diffuse nerve network'. Golgi shared the 1906 Nobel Prize for medicine or physiology with Ramón y Cajal for their work on the structure of the nervous system.

While working at the Hospital of St Matteo, Golgi had studied the causes of malaria, and in a series of seminal papers published between 1885 and 1893, combining clinical observations with laboratory experiments, he was able to show that malaria was produced by three different species of *Plasmodia* (a fourth was subsequently discovered), producing the three clinically differentiated types of intermittent fevers, in which each febrile episode coincided with the reproduction of the parasites in the blood. He also showed that quinine destroyed parasites in the blood, explaining its therapeutic value. In 1890 Golgi also produced beautiful photographs of the characteristic developmental phases of the parasites.

Bibliography

Primary: 1903. *Opera omnia* 3 vols. (Milan); 1885. 'Sulla infezione malarica.' *Giornale della R. Accademica di Medicina di Torino* 33: 734–758; 1892. 'Azione della chinina sui parasiti malarici e sui corrispondenti accessi febbrili.' *Rendiconti del R. Istituto Lombardo* (serie II) 25:163–184, 335–361; 1899. 'Sul ciclo evolutivo dei parassiti malarici nella febbre terzana; diagnosi differenziale tra i parassiti endoglobulari malarici della terzana e quelli della quartana.' *Archivio delle Scienze Mediche* 13: 173; 1929. *Gli studi di Camillo Golgi sulla malaria*, raccolti e ordinati da a cura di A. Perroncito (Rome).

Secondary: Cimino, G., 1999. 'Reticular Theory versus Neuron Theory in the Work of Camillo Golgi.' *Physis* 36: 431–472; Mazzarello, Paolo, 1996, *La struttura nascosta: La vita di Camillo Golgi* (Bologna) [English trans., 1999. *The Hidden Structure. A Scientific Biography of Camillo Golgi* (Oxford)]; *DSB*.

Bernardino Fantini

GORDON, DORIS CLIFTON

GORDON, DORIS CLIFTON (b. Melbourne, Australia, 10 July 1891; d. Stratford, New Zealand, 9 July 1956), *general practice, obstetrics, maternal health.*

Gordon (née Clifton Jolly) was the daughter of Lucy Clifton Couch and Alfred Jolly, a clergyman. Her family emigrated from Australia to New Zealand in 1894, first to Wellington and then, in 1905, to Tapanui, Otago, where her father managed a branch of the National Bank of New Zealand. Gordon graduated MB ChB from the Otago Medical School in 1916, having topped the lists in both the medical and the surgical examinations in 1915. The year after graduation, she married a fellow medical graduate, William (Bill) Gordon, in Palmerston North, and they eventually had four children. After Bill's return from overseas service in 1918, they set up in joint general practice in Stratford, with a small private hospital, called 'Marire'. This was their base for the rest of their working lives, and Doris was probably accurate in her assessment that the two of them became as much a part of the Stratford landscape as Mt Taranaki. Dr Doris, as she was known locally, later described 'back-block' practice as 'bog, bush and candlelight' medicine. She took pride in her practice and specialized in the health of women and children.

While still a medical student, Gordon decided to devote herself to midwifery and specifically to searching for 'a safe, universally applicable method of pain relief' in childbirth. She pioneered the use in New Zealand of 'twilight sleep' in childbirth and was a great supporter of pain relief in childbirth generally. Her 1924 MD thesis was on 'Scopolamine Morphine Narcosis in Childbirth'. Like many of her female contemporaries, she regarded the right to pain relief as a feminist issue and argued that her male colleagues did not know what they were talking about when they promoted natural childbirth and claimed that even stitches after birth 'do not hurt much'. She wanted the same facilities to be available for all women, and she believed that the best services would be provided by doctors rather than midwives. With those goals in mind, she helped found the New Zealand Obstetrical Society in 1927 (later the Obstetrical and Gynaecological Society). She claimed, 'Our aim was the genuine welfare of every mother, irrespective of colour or complexion, and her inviolable right to be treated with the same consideration as would be extended to a Prime Minister's daughter.'

She inspired women's groups to work for improved maternity services and mobilized them into a successful public fund-raising campaign for establishing a chair in obstetrics at the Otago Medical School in 1931 and for the new Queen Mary Maternity Hospital in Dunedin (1938). She was made an MBE in 1935. During World War II, she inspired the women's organizations that led a campaign to fund a postgraduate chair in obstetrics and gynecology in Auckland. The school, with its own hospital, was established in 1947 and later became the National Women's Hospital. From 1946 to 1948, she was Director of Maternal Welfare in the New Zealand Department of Health. In 1925 Gordon was the first woman in Australasia to be appointed a fellow of the Royal College of Surgeons of Edinburgh. She became a member of the British (later Royal) College of Obstetricians and Gynaecologists in 1936 and a fellow in 1954. At that time only twenty leading obstetricians in the world had been made fellows of the College. She was the only woman outside royalty to be so honored and the only recipient in the southern hemisphere. Doris Gordon wrote lively accounts of her life in a two-volume autobiography, the second volume of which appeared in 1957, the year after she died in her own 'Marire' hospital.

Bibliography

Primary: 1955. *Backblocks Baby-Doctor* (London); 1957. *Doctor Down Under* (London).

Secondary: *DNZB*.

Linda Bryder

GORGAS, WILLIAM CRAWFORD (b. Mobile, Alabama, USA, 3 October 1854; d. London, England, 4 July 1920), *public health, military medicine.*

Gorgas was the son of Josiah, an army officer from Pennsylvania, and Amelia Gayle, daughter of a former Alabama governor. The young Gorgas family moved frequently, following the typical trajectory of an army career. In April 1861, however, Josiah took charge of his next assignment. In the country's rapidly changing political landscape, he found his wife's Southern loyalties more compelling than his own Northern ties. Resigning from the army, he moved his family to Charleston, South Carolina, and then traveled to meet with Jefferson Davis. Davis, impressed with his skills, made him Chief of Ordnance. Young 'Willie' was in Charleston with his mother on 12 April, when shots were fired on Fort Sumter. The two spent most of the Civil War in Richmond, Virginia, while Brigadier General Josiah Gorgas oversaw the Confederate Army's munitions needs.

After the war ended, the Gorgases moved to Brierfield, Alabama. There Josiah embarked on an unsuccessful career

as an iron manufacturer. Willie (who became 'W.C.' to all but his family) set his sights on a West Point education and a military career. Educational opportunities were few in Brierfield, so he was sent off to Greensboro, Alabama, and then to New Orleans for his schooling. The opening of the University of the South (1868) proved a fortunate event for the Gorgas family: Josiah was named headmaster of the Junior Department, thereby securing both the family's finances and Willie's education. William Gorgas enrolled in the preparatory school the following summer. He only excelled in his studies after realizing that his poor early performance dismayed his beloved mother and his respected father. It was also during this period that he encountered yellow fever. The disease struck New Orleans, and Gorgas was one of four students who volunteered to provide assistance. Two of his fellow students contracted yellow fever and died. Gorgas never forgot this experience.

After six years, Gorgas graduated AB (August 1875) and—overcoming his father's arguments against the choice—attempted to gain entry to West Point. His several applications were rejected. His path apparently blocked, Gorgas decided to take another route to his desired goal. The army needed doctors. Despite financial constraints, Gorgas moved to New York (1876), attending Bellevue Medical College and eventually winning the admiration of William H. Welch, future dean of medicine at the Johns Hopkins Medical School. He graduated MD in 1879. After a year's internship at Bellevue Hospital, Gorgas entered the Army Medical Department as first lieutenant; like his father, he moved frequently between posts.

It was at Fort Brown, Texas (1882), that he had his next memorable encounter with yellow fever. He had previously experienced the disease's effects, but at one remove: he had not contracted yellow fever and thus was not immune to it. Ignoring this reality during the Texas outbreak, he treated yellow fever patients regularly. One of his patients, Mary Doughty, was the sister-in-law of the post commander. Her condition was so dire that her grave had been dug, and Gorgas had agreed to read her burial service. Surprisingly, she survived. Gorgas, however, finally fell ill, and the pair convalesced from yellow fever together. They were married in 1885.

When the U.S. Army sought a medical officer to lead a sanitary campaign in yellow fever–ridden Havana in the wake of the Spanish-American war (1898), the now-immune and organizationally gifted Gorgas was an obvious choice. At the time, it was widely believed that yellow fever was transmitted by 'fomites': disease-causing materials carried on the soiled bedding and clothing of patients. If 'filth' was the cause, cleanliness would be the cure. Gorgas and his team cleaned Havana, and Havana grew far healthier. Typhoid and dysentery numbers declined; overall mortality rates dropped dramatically. Yet, yellow fever deaths *increased*. Surgeon General George Miller Sternberg sent a special commission, headed by Walter Reed, to study the disease (1900). Gorgas quickly befriended Reed, as he did Cuban doctor Carlos Finlay, who suggested the unlikely theory of mosquito transmission to his American colleagues. Gorgas followed Reed's work closely, but continued his campaign against filth. Reed and his commission soon published their eloquent demonstration that the mosquito—specifically, the *Aedes aegypti* mosquito—was responsible for transmitting yellow fever. Gorgas tailored his sanitary strategies to the life cycle of his newly discovered enemy.

Mosquito species have distinctive preferences for living and breeding. *Aedes aegypti*, he learned, were uncommonly attached to human dwelling spaces. Indeed, areas free of humans were also free of the mosquitoes; however, soon after humans arrived, the mosquitoes followed. Though they did not require human blood to survive, female *Aedes aegypti* did require it to lay eggs, which they laid not in swamps or puddles, but in water-filled artificial containers. Larvae required a water-based incubation period of eight to nine days, during which time they occasionally needed to surface for air. Gorgas used the knowledge to control his enemy. He divided Havana into districts, with a Sanitary Department representative in charge of each. District officers conducted monthly inspections of houses. Where they found mosquito larvae, they fined residents. To enhance cooperation and preserve esprit-de-corps, Gorgas—who often used his Southern charm to great persuasive and even therapeutic effect—ensured that fines were remitted after residents cleaned offending receptacles. Additionally, sanitary workers fumigated buildings and coated rainwater containers with a thin layer of kerosene, to suffocate surfacing larvae. On the other side of the transmission equation, they screened yellow fever patients to keep mosquitoes from feeding on them. By September 1901, Havana was freed of yellow fever.

Malaria, however, persisted. Though less deadly than yellow fever, malaria was a profound problem in its own right, striking and incapacitating large numbers of people, while conferring little if any immunity to future attacks. The same year that Gorgas arrived in Havana, British malariologist Ronald Ross demonstrated that malaria was transmitted by the mosquito. The mosquito-culprit, in this case, was the *Anopheles*. Malaria's mosquito, like the disease itself, was quite different from that of yellow fever.

Gorgas adapted his techniques to the *Anopheles'* life cycle. Though he could not eradicate malaria (an elusive goal, even today), he did successfully contain it.

A similar convergence of American interest and tropical disease concern took Gorgas on his next sanitary campaign. In November 1903 Panama won its independence from Colombia. The Americans, long blocked by Colombia from constructing a canal through Panama that would allow sea access to California, took advantage of the situation. By February 1904 the Panama Canal Convention was formally approved, and plans to construct the canal were soon in place.

History, however, offered a cautionary tale: the French, successful in their Suez Canal–building project, had failed spectacularly in their efforts to build a Panama canal in the 1880s. The chief cause of their failure was disease: specifically, malaria and yellow fever. Though the French did not publicize their health statistics, Gorgas later estimated that yellow fever killed about a third of the white labor force annually (Gibson, p. 96). The lesson for the Americans was clear. Unfortunately, they did not much heed it.

Gorgas knew the lesson well: the United States would not succeed in Panama if they ignored its sanitary challenges. The American Medical Association, still seeking to achieve the political clout it would later enjoy, lobbied unsuccessfully for Gorgas to be named to the Panama Canal Commission. Gorgas was indeed sent to Panama to head up sanitary efforts, but not as a member of the Commission. Consequently, he was forced to appeal to commissioners for all his material and personnel needs. More unfortunately still, the commissioners, who were largely engineers, were hostile to sanitation in general and to the mosquito theory in particular. Gorgas was thus forced to battle not only local mosquitoes, but also the resistance of his superiors. The commissioners, baffled by Gorgas's tendency to ignore filth and bad smells, resented his suggestions that money be 'wasted' on fumigation, water drainage, and sanitary inspections. In June 1905 the Commission recommended to then-Secretary of War William H. Taft that Gorgas be replaced with a more conventional, filth-oriented sanitary officer. President Theodore Roosevelt took matters into his own hands. Consulting with top doctors—including Gorgas's old teacher, Welch—Roosevelt was eventually persuaded that the mosquito theory reflected the best scientific knowledge and that Gorgas was the best American for the job of ensuring Panama's health. Not only did Roosevelt reject the Commission's request; he directed the commissioners to assist Gorgas in his sanitary efforts by approving his requests in a regular and timely fashion. Gorgas was further aided by the appointment of John F. Stevens, a supporter of the mosquito theory, as chief engineer.

Finally enjoying administrative cooperation, Gorgas soon saw the success of his sanitary plans. As in Havana, he divided the area into sanitary districts, employed inspectors, and oversaw drainage, fumigation, and screening projects. In 1906 yellow fever stopped taking victims in the canal zone. Malaria continued, but in a diminished capacity. To control it, Gorgas established a system of dispensaries for quinine distribution. Finally, in 1907 he was named to an overhauled Canal Commission. Though he continued to face opposition to his mosquito control efforts—particularly by the Commission's new leader, Lieutenant Colonel George Washington Goethals—Gorgas had made sufficient sanitary progress that such bureaucratic resistance had little impact. He remained in Panama until late 1913, to guarantee the ultimate success of his methods.

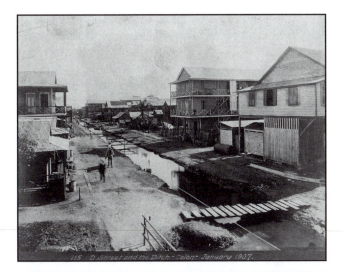

Colón, Panama, during the building of the Panama Canal. A ditch runs down the middle of the unpaved street, January 1907. Photograph, Iconographic Collection, Wellcome Library, London.

His work in Havana and Panama made Gorgas a coveted consultant for other projects of disease containment. It earned him honors, awards, and elected positions in numerous medical societies, including a term as president of the American Medical Association. When the position of Surgeon General opened (1914), Gorgas was the Army's widely praised choice. He was soon promoted to the rank of major general. As the United States prepared for its probable entry into World War I, Gorgas employed his organizational skills on the medical committee of the Council of National Defense. When America went to war, he oversaw an extensive hospital-building project, helped recruit top civilian doctors, and formed the Division of Military Orthopedic Surgery. Moreover, his sanitary experience helped him ensure that the number of American military deaths from disease would be far fewer than from wounds. Regulations required his retirement on his sixty-fourth birthday, which, fortunately, came as the war was ending.

Even in retirement, Gorgas continued his international sanitary efforts. The Rockefeller Foundation's International Health Division sent him to South America as a yellow fever consultant, and in 1920 he was slated to participate in a similar expedition to West Africa. En route, he visited London, where he was to receive the insigne of the Most Distinguished Order of St Michael and St George. When a stroke prevented him from receiving his award at Buckingham Palace, King George V personally presented it to him in his hospital room. Gorgas died on 4 July 1920. The British gave him an official state funeral at St Paul's Cathedral. He was buried at Arlington Cemetery in Virginia.

Bibliography

Primary: 1903. 'A Short Account of the Results of Mosquito Work in Havana, Cuba.' *Journal of the Association of Military Surgeons of the United States* 12: 133–139; 1904. 'Health Conditions on the Isthmus of Panama.' *Scientific American* 57: 238–256; 1909. 'Sanitation of the Tropics with Special Reference to Malaria and Yellow Fever.' *Journal of the American Medical Association* 52: 1075–1077; 1915. *Sanitation in Panama* (London).

Secondary: Litsios, Socrates, 2001. 'William Crawford Gorgas, 1854–1920.' *Perspectives in Biology and Medicine* 44: 368–378; Gibson, John M., 1950. *Physician to the World: The Life of General William C. Gorgas* (Tuscaloosa, AL); Lampson, Robin, 1939. *Death Loses a Pair of Wings* [biographical novel] (New York); Gorgas, Marie D., and Burton J. Hendrick, 1924. *William Crawford Gorgas: His Life and Work* (Philadelphia); Martin, Franklin H., 1924. *Major General William Crawford Gorgas, M.D., USA* (Chicago); *DAMB*.

Kim Pelis

GOTŌ, KONZAN (aka GONZAN) (b. Edo [now Tokyo], Japan, 4 June 1659; d. Kyoto, Japan, 25 October 1733), *Japanese medicine, clinical medicine reform, founder of Kohōha (Ancient Method School).*

Gotō Konzan was born in Edo, the capital of the Tokugawa Shōgun, receiving his early education at the city's Hayashi School of Confucian Studies. He also studied Goseiha, literally the 'Later Generation School' medicine, but following a major fire in which his father's house burned to the ground and the family's assets were destroyed, he moved at age twenty-seven to Kyoto with his family. There, he attempted to enter the school of Nagoya Gen'i (1628–96) but was refused admission because of his inability to pay the entry fee.

Nagoya Gen'i was himself a major figure in the history of Japanese medicine as the first substantial challenger to the Goseiha medical orthodoxy. Gen'i, who had trained in the Goseiha, later read the *Shanghan shanglun*, a Ming dynasty (1368–1644) commentary on the Chinese medical classic, the *Shanghanlun* by Zhang Zhongjing (Jp. *Shōkanron* by Chō Chūkei [196–220]). In addition, Gen'i was stimulated by a new school of Confucian thought called the Kogakuha, or School of Ancient Learning, that challenged the theories of Song Confucianism by emphasizing close readings of the original Confucian classics. Similarly, Gen'i sidestepped the ideas of Manase Dōsan and the Goseiha by emphasizing close readings of ancient Chinese medical classics, especially the *Shanghanlun*, and basing his therapies on interpretations of those classics. As a result, Gen'i is remembered as the father of the Kohōha, or Ancient Method School of medicine. Nevertheless, his refusal to admit Konzan to his school resulted in a major rupture in the genealogy of this approach to medical practice.

Konzan's response to Nagoya Gen'i's refusal to teach him was to study the ancient Chinese medical classics on his own. By dint of his efforts, Konzan far surpassed Gen'i in his own day and established the Kohōha as an important school of Japanese medical theory and practice. Konzan despised the then-current practice whereby physicians shaved their heads and assumed the dress of Buddhist priests. Instead, he allowed his hair to grow and wore ordinary clothes. Thereafter, it was possible to distinguish his followers by their hairstyle and dress. Over two hundred students studied under him, including Kagawa Shūan (1683–1755) and Yamawaki Tōyō (1705–62) and many others who went on to become leading practitioners not only in Kyoto but also throughout the country. Konzan urged his students to integrate their studies of Confucian classics through the Kogakuha, or School of Ancient Learning, with their study of medicine through the Kohōha.

Konzan developed a theory that postulated that all diseases were the result of the stagnation of *qi*. Different symptoms and manifestations of disease simply reflected different locations and manners of this stagnation. For therapy, he emphasized moxibustion, but he also made use of pills that contained the gall bladder of bears and recommended bathing in hot springs. By the time of his death, the Kohōha had entered the mainstream of Japanese medicine.

Bibliography

Primary: 1971. *Nihon shisō taikei* [Works in Japanese Thought] vol. 63 (Tokyo); 1979. Yoshinori, Ōtsuka, and Yakazu Dōmei, eds. *Kinsen Kanpō igakusho shūsei* [Collected works of early modern Kanpō medicine] vol.13 (Tokyo); 1990. *Rinshō shinkyū koten zensho* [Classic works of clinical acupuncture] vol. 20 (Osaka).

Secondary: Fujikawa Yū,1972. *Nihon igaku shi* [Medical history of Japan] (Tokyo).

William Johnston

GOTŌ, SHINPEI

GOTŌ, SHINPEI (b. Shiogama, Mutsu domain [Iwate Prefecture], Japan, 24 July 1857; d. Kyoto, Japan, 13 April 1929), *public health, medical administration.*

Gotō was a public health official-turned-politician who demonstrated his versatile talent beyond the sphere of health and medicine.

Born as a son of a samurai in the northeastern region of Japan, Gotō chose to become a medical man to make his way. After leaving a medical school in the Fukushima Prefecture (1876), he served as a physician to the Aichi Prefectural Hospital in Nagoya and rose to become its director at the age of twenty-four (1881). His proposals for sanitary inspection in Aichi attracted the attention of Sensai Nagayo, the director of the Sanitary Bureau of the Home Ministry. Gotō was called into the Bureau to serve as its medical officer in 1883.

Gotō studied hygiene in Germany (1890–92) and received his MD from the University of Munich. After his return to Japan, he was appointed director of the Sanitary Bureau (1892). He lost the post once, in 1893, because of his involvement in a scandal, but he made a comeback in 1895, having demonstrated his distinguished organizational talent in special quarantine work during and after the Sino-Japanese War. The Infectious Diseases Prevention Act of 1897, a comprehensive statute effective until 1999, was introduced during his tenure. Being aware of the ineffectiveness of one-sided enforcement of laws and regulations, Gotō bent his mind to establish an administrative system in which the state and people would act in cooperation for public health through the medium of local communal agencies.

In 1898 Gotō was singled out to serve as the chief civil administrator to the Colonial Government of Taiwan. Here again, he acknowledged the demerits of the one-sided coercion of Japanese rule. His administration in Taiwan (1898–1906) was characterized especially by the promotion of local people's cooperation through indigenous administrative machineries, of statistics and surveying work, and of social infrastructure such as sewerage systems, which can all be viewed as embodiments of his public health ideas. He pursued a 'biological approach' to colonial management, by which he meant policymaking that was adaptive to the natural, economic, social, and cultural climates of Taiwan, based on 'scientific' investigations and planning.

From a colonialist point of view, his management of Taiwan was successful, and the Japanese government sent him to Manchuria as the first president of the South Manchurian Railway Company, a quasi-official agency of Japanese expansion in the region (1906–08). His high motivation, rational thinking, and active personality, now with distinguished records as an administrator, made Gotō invaluable for Japan's central leadership. He entered the cabinet as the Minister of State for Communications (1908–11, 1912–13), for Home Affairs (1916–18), and for Foreign Affairs (1918).

In his later career, Tokyo became the main field for his 'biological approach'. As the mayor of Tokyo (1920–23), Gotō proposed a comprehensive scheme for urban planning, covering roads and streets, water supply and sewerage systems, waste disposal, open spaces, etc. For investigations, the Tokyo Institute for Municipal Research was established. The scheme, however, came to a dead end, mainly for financial reasons.

In September 1923, four months after his retirement from the mayorship of Tokyo, the city was devastated by the Great Kantō Earthquake. Gotō was restored as Home Minister a day after the earthquake and assigned the reconstruction of the metropolis. He envisaged not just a reconstruction, but a drastic urban restructuring, along the lines of the scheme he had proposed as the mayor. Once again, finance became an obstacle. After his resignation in February 1924, his scheme for the metropolis's reconstruction was reduced in scale and carried out. Some traces of his plans can still be found in Tokyo today.

Bibliography

Primary: 1889. *Kokka Eisei Genri* [Principles of state hygiene] (Tokyo); 1898. 'Shi-chō-son jichi-tai to densenbyō yobō jimu.' [Local government of cities, towns, and villages and prevention of infectious diseases] *Dai-Nihon Shiritsu Eiseikai Zasshi* 16: 675–704.

Secondary: Tsurumi, Yusuke, 1938. *Gotō Shinpei* (Tokyo).

Takeshi Nagashima

GOUDAS, ANASTASIOS   (b. Grammeno Ioanninon, Ottoman Empire, 1816; d. Athens, Greece, 1882), *medicine.*

Born to Nikolaos and Giannoula Goudas, Goudas and his three sisters lost their mother at an early age. Following the outbreak of the Hellenic revolution in 1821, his family, along with others, took refuge in Kerkyra (Corfu), where they were inhumanly persecuted by the British, prompting them to seek asylum in Souli, Epirus. After the revolution, Goudas completed his high school studies in Ioannina, and after the establishment of Athens University in 1837, Goudas went to Athens to become one of the top students in the Medical School. On 9 July 1843, he became the first student of Athens University to be awarded a first-class doctoral degree, for his thesis *On the Illnesses that Appear Frequently in the Royal Sugar Factory in Kainourio.* The factory at issue in his thesis was near the town of Lamia, in central Greece.

After furthering his studies in Paris, Goudas returned to Athens to take up medical practice. Acutely aware of the nascent state of Hellenic medical literature during his day, he began to translate and publish distinguished essays of lauded foreign professors. Goudas personally published two journals, *The Bee of Medicine* (1853–58) and *Bee of Athens* (1864–66), in which appeared several articles on his own unique medical work: 'Studies on the Medical Chorography and Climate of Athens' (*The Bee of Medicine*, 1858, 6: 9), 'On Cholera in Piraeus', and 'Remarks on the Periodic Epidemic Fevers' (*The Bee of Medicine*, 1853, 1: 9). Many of his works were published separately in Greek and French pamphlets. Goudas's contribution through the medical journals was of decisive significance for the support of the formation and domination of 'scientific' knowledge for the benefit of Hellenic society in the nineteenth century.

Beside his involvement in medical science and bibliography, Goudas published articles and headlines of varied content in newspapers and periodicals of that era. In 1860 one of his political articles, appearing in the newspaper *Independence*, prompted charges of blasphemy against King Othon, and Goudas was sentenced to a period of imprisonment. Upon release, he went to Smyrna and later to London, returning to Athens in 1862 following the expulsion of King Othon.

Goudas wrote numerous political articles, among the most important of which were 'Advice to the Future King of Greece' (1863, also in French), 'Memoranda to the Protective Powers of Greece and to the Entire Civilized World' (Athens, 1863; also published in French, Paris 1863), 'The Present Situation in the East Particularly in Greece' (Zakynthos, 1864), 'East and West' (in two periodicals, 1867–68; also in French and English), and 'The Past, the Present and the Future in the East' (1878). His work *Distinguished Men of the Hellenic Revolution*, spanning eight volumes (1869–76), is considered a great contribution to modern Hellenic history. It contains biographies of important actors in various fields of Hellenic life before the fight for independence, based on material offered by their families. Goudas's collection of biographies remained unfinished, probably because of his serious illness, cancer of the larynx, of which he passed away.

Bibliography

Secondary: 1929. *The Great Hellenic Encyclopedia* vol. 8; 1985, 1996. *The Papyros Larousse Britannica* vol. 19.

Maria Korasidou

GOWERS, WILLIAM RICHARD   (b. Hackney, London, England, 20 March 1845; d. London, 4 May 1915), *hematology, neurology.*

Born in the east end of London, the son of William Gowers, a cobbler, and his wife, Ann Venables, the younger William Gowers attended Hackney Free and Parochial Schools in Chatham Place. His father died when he was eleven years old and, his mother sold the cobbler's shop and moved back to her family home in Headington, Oxfordshire. Gowers excelled enough to win a four-year scholarship to Christ Church School, Oxford.

Medical Training

He decided on medicine and in 1861, with the payment of £150 raised by his relatives, he was apprenticed for two years to a country doctor, Thomas Simpson of Coggeshall, Essex. He continued to read widely while learning the practical aspects of medicine, and he entered University College Hospital, London, in 1863, achieving his MRCS in 1867. He graduated MB from the University of London in 1869 and the next year received his MD and the Gold Medal in Medicine. Gowers impressed Sir William Jenner (1815–98), RCP president and physician to the Queen, and asked him to be his house physician and later secretary-assistant. In 1870 he was appointed the first registrar at the National Hospital for the Paralyzed and Epileptic, Queen Square, London, becoming assistant physician (1873) and then full physician (1880). In 1879 he was elected FRCP and gave the Goulstonian Lecturer on epilepsy, published in 1881 with a landmark second edition in 1901 based on his experience with 3,000 cases. He was elected FRS in 1887.

Personal Life

Gowers courted Mary Baines, daughter of a prominent Yorkshire publisher and businessman, married in 1875, and had four children. They lived at 50 Queen Anne Street, London, where he had consulting rooms to see private patients. Not a very sociable man, he was comfortable with his four children, encouraging their activities and sports and taking them on outings and explorations of historic buildings as well as writing and illustrating children's stories for them.

He was a talented artist—his paintings were shown at the Royal Academy of Arts—illustrating his own books with clean drawings and paintings that were superior to those in contemporary textbooks. A slight angular man with an awkward gait, a dignified and distant carriage, steely eyes, and humorless expression, he was admired rather than liked, an 'unclubable' person who seldom attended medical meetings except when he was presenting. Although he had some friends and correspondents, he could be very critical and caustic in his remarks.

Clinical Activities

Gowers became increasingly famous for his clear clinical writings. He could also be very inventive, creating a hemoglobinometer and improving the hemocytometer, which were in wide use for decades. His first paper was on a safety hypodermic syringe. He encouraged use of the ophthalmoscope and wrote a very influential book on the subject (1879), beautifully illustrated with his own paintings of the retina, which were regarded as much superior to the later photographic illustrations. In the book he mentioned that his instrument was one of his own design and outlined how a student could make his own for a few pence.

His writings were based on clinical observation, with clear explanations and his own illustrations. He did no experiments and relied on his own experiences rather than the published work of others. He was a close observer of his patients, making copious shorthand notes. An advocate of shorthand writing, he admonished others to learn the skill, telling one young man on the street that he would never amount to anything for he did not know shorthand. He was admired as an outstanding clinician and teacher, and his lectures were packed with students and visiting physicians.

In 1879 he wrote of the significance of the patellar reflex, which he called the 'knee-jerk', and advised clinicians to use a percussion hammer rather than hand tapping. He participated in an important clinical event when he diagnosed a spinal tumor in an army officer and suggested it could be surgically removed, which was successfully carried out by Victor Horsley (1857–1916) in 1887, the first such operation. His descriptions of myasthenia gravis, post-diphtheritic bulbar palsy, dystrophica myotonica, geniculate herpes, encephalitis periaxilis diffusa, ataxia paraplegia, vasovagal attacks, musicogenic epilepsy, paramyotonia multiplex, sleep paralysis, Wilson's disease, and Foster Kennedy syndrome all came before those who are credited with these descriptions. 'Gowers's sign' refers to the method used by persons with myopathy to rise from the floor, putting their hands on their knees and moving them up their legs until standing. Macdonald Critchley (1900–97) noted his influence on clinical neurology by counting the number of references (132, many more than any other neurologist) to Gowers's contributions mentioned in S. A. Kinnier Wilson's *Neurology* (1940). Sir William Osler (1849–1919) called him 'that brilliant ornament of British medicine' and dedicated his book on chorea to him. Osler visited him often when in London and seemed to be able to develop a friendship with the reserved Gowers, but Osler could be friendly with anyone. Although Gowers's various books and papers were influential and made him one of the best-known English physicians of his age, the greatest work was *A Manual of Diseases of the Nervous System*, which was the most widely used neurology text for decades.

The *Manual* was a landmark book that brought together the personal observations of an astute and experienced clinician with the developing neurosciences of the age. It was profusely illustrated (with Gowers's own drawings), and in typical Gowers style, he did not rely on or refer to many previous authors, but wrote of his experiences and gave his clear explanations for what he had observed. Published in two volumes in England (1886–88) and in one volume in the United States (1888), there were new editions over the next decade, and James Taylor assisted him with the 1899 edition. He had planned a further English one-volume edition by the elimination of much of the anatomy and physiology previously included, but this never appeared—Critchley had in his library the draft papers for a new edition of Volume 2.

Later Life

Gowers was knighted at age forty-two during Queen Victoria's Diamond Jubilee (1897). The next year, he surprised his colleagues by resigning his chair of medicine and his appointment as physician at University College Hospital, stating he could not do justice to his academic activities as well as his increasing private practice. Never in robust health, he was described as prematurely aging, but he pursued interests in painting, archeology, botany, painting and engraving, and antiquarian research of churches. He retired from practice in 1902 at age sixty-two. In his last years, when his health was failing, he was visited a number of times by Osler, who thought he was suffering from a condition Gowers had described, ataxia paraplegia.

His Legacy

His writings were widely influential and clarified the developing field of clinical neurology at a time that it was said to be in chaos. Although it was a period of 'the flowering of neurology', it took someone like Gowers to bring structure and sense to all the new science, coupled with his practical observations on patients. Kennedy (1970) said, 'we should be better doctors, better teachers, better writers, if we from time to time read Gowers'.

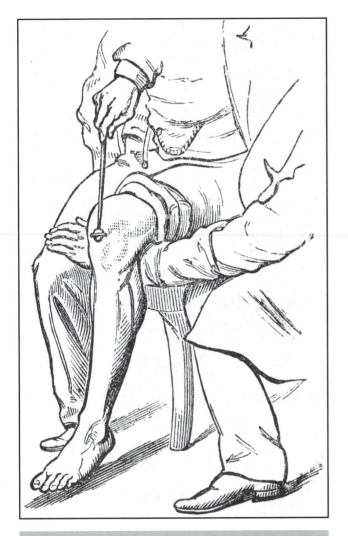

Gowers's method of obtaining the knee-jerk. Lithograph from *A Manual of Diseases of the Nervous System*, London, 1886–1888. Wellcome Library, London.

The *Manual* is a classic text, called a masterpiece and the 'Bible of neurology'. Spillane pondered who first used that phrase, which was widely quoted, and concluded that it 'may not have amounted to a Bible, but it was certainly a New Testament'. Many neurologists use the adage to young colleagues, 'If you think you have discovered something new, first look it up in Gowers.'

Bibliography

Primary: 1879. *A Manual and Atlas of Medical Ophthalmoscopy* (London; 2nd edn., 1882; 3rd edn., 1890; 4th edn., 1904); 1886–1888. *A Manual of Diseases of the Nervous System* 2 vols. (London; 2nd edn., 1892–1893; 3rd edn., 1899); 1895. *Clinical Lectures on Diseases of the Nervous System* (London).

Secondary: Spillane, J. D., 1981. *Doctrine of the Nerves: Chapters in the History of Neurology* (New York); Kennedy, F., 1970. 'William Gowers (1845–1915)' in Haymaker, W., and Francis Schiller, eds., *The Founders of Neurology* (Springfield, IL); Critchley, M., 1949.

Sir William Gowers 1845–1915: A Biographical Appreciation [contains a complete bibliography of Gowers's writings] (London); *Oxford DNB.*

Jock Murray

GOYANES CAPDEVILLA, JOSÉ

GOYANES CAPDEVILLA, JOSÉ (b. Monforte, Lugo, Spain, 16 June 1876; d. Santa Cruz de Tenerife, Spain, 16 May 1964), *cancer surgery, medical history.*

Goyanes Capdevilla was a prestigious Spanish surgeon who led the fight against cancer in Spain before the Spanish Civil War. As a student of medicine (Madrid School of Medicine, 1893–1900) he trained at the department of surgery of the San Carlos University Hospital and worked as assistant at the anatomical museum, earning his PhD in 1901. He soon thereafter became consulting surgeon at Madrid General Hospital (1905–18), where he specialized in cancer surgery. He was one of the founders of the Spanish Committee against Cancer (1909), which was affiliated with the International Association against Cancer and which remained active until World War I. Besides his clinical responsibilities and active role in the campaign against cancer, Goyanes was president of the Spanish Medical-Surgical Academy (1911 and 1912) and a member of the Royal Academy of Medicine at Madrid (1918). He was also dean of the physicians' corps in charge of the Madrid Beneficencia, the public provincial charities (1934). As a leading figure in surgery, he became involved in the founding of the Madrid Society for Surgery (1931) and its aftermath, the Spanish Association of Surgeons, whose members designated him as their first president (1935–49).

In 1918 he replaced surgeon Eulogio Cervera y Ruiz (1855–1917) as Director of the incipient National Cancer Institute (NCI) in Madrid. The Institute was set up after a visit to Spain by Marie Curie in 1919, although it was not officially inaugurated until 1922. It was designed as a center for research and treatment (surgery and radiotherapy), funded by charitable donations and to a lesser degree by the state, at least until the Republican period. Goyanes was director of the NCI until 1931, when his conservative, republican political sympathies led to his dismissal by Marcelino Pascua (1897–1977), Director-General of Health in the recently established Republic.

Goyanes Capdevilla's interest in cancer is reflected in several publications and lectures, such as those given in 1924 at the Royal Academy of Medicine at the founding of the Spanish League against Cancer, similar to other European associations. Its members, before the Second Spanish Republic (1931), were largely female members of the aristocracy. Goyanes became President of the League in 1928 with the main goal of attracting financial support for the NCI. He promoted the study of cancer by all biomedical disciplines on the grounds that it was the 'most terrible plague of the social body' and that it would soon overtake tuberculosis in importance. Goyanes believed that the fight should include prophylaxis against substances linked to cancer as well as the treatment of the diagnosed disease. The NCI achieved developments in both research and treatment under his leadership.

His scientific work received international recognition, and he was named Knight of the Portuguese Order of Santiago, Doctor *honoris causa* by the University of Bordeaux, *Officier de la Légion d'honneur*, and Honorary Fellow of the American College of Surgeons.

Goyanes developed the intra-arterial regional anesthesia approach and various surgical techniques for the treatment of laryngeal cancer. He also published on the statistics, etiology, and pathogenesis of cancer. In addition to his clinical studies, he was a prolific writer of literature. He also published texts on the history of medicine, such as his publications on Miguel Servet [Michael Servetus] (1511–53) and Maimonides [Rabí Mosheh ben Maimon] (1135–1204), and on the portrayal of physicians in the works of the writer Francisco Quevedo (1580–1645).

Bibliography

Primary: 1924. 'La lucha contra el cáncer.' *El Siglo Médico* 73: 268–271.

Secondary: Fraga Vázquez, Xosé A., and Alfonso Mato Domínguez, 1993. *Diccionario histórico das ciencias e das técnicas do Galicia. Autores (1868–1936)* (Galicia); Medina-Doménech, Rosa María, 1996. *¿Curar el cáncer? Los orígenes de la Radioterapia en el primer tercio del siglo XX* (Granada).

Rosa María Medina-Doménech

GRAAF, REINIER DE   (b. Schoonhoven, the Netherlands, 30 July 1641; d. Delft, the Netherlands, 17 August 1673), *anatomy, physiology.*

As a son of Catholic parents—Catharina van Breenen and Cornelis de Graaf—de Graaf went to study in Louvain in the Spanish Netherlands. In 1663 he exchanged Louvain for Utrecht, where he studied medicine with Ysbrand van Diemerbroek, but soon he set out for Leiden, matriculating at Leiden University on 5 April 1663. It was there that de Graaf befriended Jan Swammerdam and Niels Steno, with whom he studied anatomy under Johannes van Horne and Franciscus de le Boë, Sylvius. In 1664 de Graaf published an account of the famous experiment that enabled him to drain some juice from the pancreas of a living dog using a fistula. He performed this experiment for audiences elsewhere and graduated while in Angers (France) on 23 July 1665. In 1666 he set up practice in Delft, where, on 14 June 1672, he married Maria van Dyck. Their firstborn son died in April 1673, only seven weeks old. Shortly after, de Graaf himself expired at the age of thirty-two.

In Delft, de Graaf continued his innovative research. He experimented with the use of the needle and invented a flexible tube that made it possible to apply enemas in private. It was from Delft, too, that de Graaf introduced his fellow citizen Antonie van Leeuwenhoek to the Royal Society in a letter of 28 April 1673. De Graaf, however, had by then become entangled in painful disputes with Jan Swammerdam over questions of priority relating to his research on the male and female genital organs.

A surgeon and anatomist of unusual skill, de Graaf acquired lasting fame for his description of the female reproductive organs, in particular for the idea that mammalian eggs are formed in what we now know as the 'Graafian follicles'. De Graaf examined successive stages of pregnancy in rabbits and studied human ovaries as well as those of cows, sheep, and pigs. He described the process of ovulation without being able to observe the egg itself (it was found only much later, in 1827, by Karl Ernst von Baer). Others, including Niels Steno, had already suggested that the 'female testicles' were in fact ovaries, but de Graaf's *De mulierum organis* of 1672 lent the idea scientific credibility.

De Graaf's experimental way of settling questions through observation and experiment—a method that had become popular among a group of Sylvius's Leiden students—marked a new development in scientific inquiry. The method was not devised in opposition to any medical theory or school. Indeed, the pancreas experiment was supposed to confirm one of Sylvius's iatrochemical views. The pancreatic juice was thought to be the acid factor in a mixture of juices (the *humor triumviratus*) that supposedly caused a process of effervescence in the duodenum.

Gradually improving his methods and discussing his research findings with local colleagues who checked and reexamined them, de Graaf developed into a much-appreciated experimentalist. Already renowned in his own time, his fame has stuck with later generations. Today, the main hospital in his hometown of Delft carries his name.

Bibliography

Primary: 1677. *Opera omnia* (Leiden); 1664. *De succi pancreatici natura et usu* (Leiden); 1668. *De virorum organis generationi inservientibus, de clysteribus et de usu syphonis in anatomia* (Leiden); 1672. *De mulierum organis generationi inservientibus* (Leiden).

Secondary: Houtzager, H. L., ed., 1991. *Reinier de Graaf 1641–1673* (Rotterdam); Lindeboom, G. A., 1975. 'Dog and Frog. Physiological Experiments at Leiden During the Seventeenth Century' in Lunsingh Scheurleer, Th. H., and G. H. M. Posthumus Meyjes, eds., *Leiden University in the Seventeenth Century. An Exchange of Learning* (Leiden) pp. 278–293; *DSB*.

Han van Ruler

GRAEFE, FRIEDRICH WILHELM ERNST ALBRECHT VON   (b. Berlin, Germany, 22 May 1828; d. Berlin, 20 July 1870), *ophthalmology, surgery.*

Graefe was born in the Prussian capital of Berlin in Villa Finkenheerd as the son of Carl Ferdinand von Graefe into a moderate noble family, which had established social relations with many intellectuals and artists of the time, including the writer Karl Immermann and the architect

Friedrich Schinkel. His father was a rather famous surgeon who directed the Clinisch-chirurgisch-augenärztliches Institut in the Surgical Clinic of Berlin University, from 1818. Carl Ferdinand persuaded his son to study medicine.

Medical Training

After going to the elitist French high school in his hometown, Albrecht Graefe graduated with his 'matura' at the early age of fifteen. Graefe took up his medical studies in 1843, at the Friedrich-Wilhelms-University of Berlin, and lived in a small flat next to Oranienburger Tor and Chausseestrasse. At the University Hospital, he was trained in the most up-to-date methods in experimental medicine and was the student of the anatomist and physiologist Johannes Mueller, the physiologist Emil Du Bois-Reymond, and the pathological anatomist Rudolf Virchow. Yet Graefe was also greatly influenced by the clinical approaches of Ludwig Schoenlein, the surgeon Johann Friedrich Dieffenbach, and a representative of the younger generation of university teachers, Johann Christian Juengken, who mutually introduced the novices to the recently introduced type of bedside-teaching and the 'rational' classification of internal diseases. In 1847 Graefe graduated MD in Berlin with a dissertation *De bromo ejusque praesipuis praeparatis*. His thesis was part of the research program of Juengken, who wanted to introduce a new kind of narcosis into surgery. Unfortunately, while working in his private laboratory at Finkenheerd, the experimental apparatus exploded, and Graefe sustained serious lung injury from the bromine vapor. One year later, however, he passed the state examinations and was given the doctor's certificate to practice medicine. In his case, this also included the right to perform general surgery and surgical obstetrics. Just made a young medical doctor, he helped to stem the outbreak of a cholera epidemic in Berlin. This is also reflected in his work: *Über Tannin als Choleramittel* (1848).

In autumn of the revolutionary year 1848, Graefe, who was an antiroyalist, commenced a scientific peregrination that brought him in close contact with Ferdinand Arlt, the famous eye-surgeon at the Allgemeine Krankenhaus of Prague, where Graefe finally decided to become an ophthalmologist. He then went to visit Louis-Auguste Desmarres and Julius Sichel at the Medical Faculty of Paris. The latter had emigrated from Frankfurt am Main to the French capital for political reasons. When Graefe crossed the channel for his residency in London, he met the histologist William Bowman, the ophthalmologist Franciscus Cornelis Donders, and George Critchett. In Donders, who had originally come from Utrecht, Graefe found an ingenious colleague who, like him, was very much occupied with medical research. Later, Donders and Graefe stayed in close contact. On his return to Berlin, Graefe had met many of the key figures of his field and was provided with various innovative concepts and methods. Yet Graefe felt compelled to open a private ophthalmologic practice on 1 November 1851, a practice that was to become the mecca for many young ophthalmologists who came to practice with Graefe. In 1852 he was given the *venia legendi* for surgery and ophthalmology at the Friedrich-Wilhelms-University of Berlin. His Habilitations thesis, *Über die Wirkung der Augenmuskeln*, was on the physiology of eye movement. Being a Privatdozent at the clinic for surgery, Graefe was made the first full professor for ophthalmology in Germany in 1866. His university chair *ad personam* was immediately withdrawn, however, after his death, because of the perpetual financial crisis of the Charité Hospital during the nineteenth century. In addition, Graefe had stated in his will that his private clinic should only be continued if the state would take over the funding of its ongoing costs. This the Prussian administration refused.

Ophthalmology and Ophthalmologic Surgery

The surgeon Johann Christian Juengken, who was also in charge of minor ophthalmologic surgery and the ophthalmologic diseases in the outpatient department of the Charité Hospital, stepped down from his professorship in 1868. Graefe, who was already seriously ill at the time, was given the directorship of the Charité Hospital's ophthalmologic clinic. Graefe died two years later from the effects of lung tuberculosis, which he had contracted at the age of thirty, and his death was marked with a small funeral service at his place of birth. However, he left a wide legacy and had many pupils who were appointed to chairs in ophthalmology all over Germany and even in Switzerland. Typical is the case of Paul Heinrich Braunschweig, who worked as assistant to Graefe until his academic teacher was given emeritus status. Braunschweig went on to receive his *venia legendi* with an exclusively ophthalmologic topic: *Über die Geschwülste des Sehnerven* (1893). In 1902 he was offered a position as a professor of ophthalmology at the University of Halle. There, he committed himself to the early differentiation of the field and advocated the construction of a comparatively large clinic, with forty-five beds for his eye patients and another fifteen for the ear patients.

Together with Donders, Graefe was among the first ophthalmologists who regularly used the ophthalmoscope of Hermann von Helmholtz for the diagnosis of the fundus oculi when going on their ward rounds. After many years of experimental tinkering at his Institute for Physiology at Königsberg, East Prussia, Helmholtz had come up with this new diagnostic instrument in 1850, independently of the work of Charles Babbage in Great Britain. Numerous are Graefe's students' solemn accounts of his diagnostic skills. For example, the ophthalmologist Richard Liebreich, a pupil of Helmholtz who was born in Königsberg and later moved to London, served as assistant to Graefe and learned accurate diagnostic techniques in Graefe's Berlin clinic. When he later moved to London, he proved to be an important popularizer of his mentor's ideas and spread the art of ophthalmoscopy among many physicians of the English capital. Also, Liebreich's delicate and artistic illustrations of the diseases of the eye, as they were displayed in his *Atlas der Ophthalmologie* (1863), made him well known outside the Prussian borders. The art of drawing and the scientific representation of ophthalmic diseases were also pet occupations of Graefe, together with his care for what is now one of the most important collections on ophthalmology, which is housed at the Museum for Medical History in Berlin. This collection also contains many glasses and spectacles; Graefe had been deeply interested in the investigation and cure of weak-sightedness. Already in 1848, he had been engaged with Donders to work on the physiology of sight. They both scrutinized whether the application of specific spectacles would illuminate the relation of accommodation and convergence of the eye. Additionally, the heritage of Graefe is passed on to present generations by the Graefe Museum, established through the Deutsche Ophthalmologische Gesellschaft at the Ruprecht-Karls-University of Heidelberg.

Another landmark of Graefe's achievements was his introduction of a surgical therapy for glaucoma, what he called an 'iridectomy', as a release operation for the increase of intraocular pressure. His method consisted of a surgical intervention into the iris of the eye. He furthermore introduced surgical treatments for squint disorders and modified the cataract operation. Very important for him was the exchange with his clinical colleagues, as Graefe defended the position that many diseases of the eye could only be understood etiologically, when also focusing on internal and neurological diseases. His work even touched on various internal pathologies—for example diabetes, nephritis, and tumors of the brain—and he described the congested papilla as a curvature of the retina, which could be seen in his fundoscopy. He also realized that inflammations of the optic nerve could be a cause for amblyopia. Yet Graefe's main research interest remained weak-sightedness without organic lesion of the eye.

Medical Societies and Specialist Publications

As already noted, Graefe created a wide school of ophthalmologists and was a key figure in the establishment of this 'small discipline' at German universities. Many later *ordinarii* in ophthalmology went through his clinic. Yet in order to connect the small and disseminated scientific community, Graefe was deeply engaged in setting up various medical societies and specialist publications. Among these was the *Archiv fuer Ophthalmologie*, which he founded together with Donders in 1854 and which is still in existence, under its new title *Albrecht von Graefes Archiv für Ophthalmologie*. It is likewise one of the oldest scientific journals among the small clinical disciplines.

In 1857 Graefe initiated the first congress on ophthalmology in Germany, what was later (in 1920) called the Deutsche Ophthalmologische Gesellschaft. This initial congress took place at the University of Heidelberg, as did the following ones during

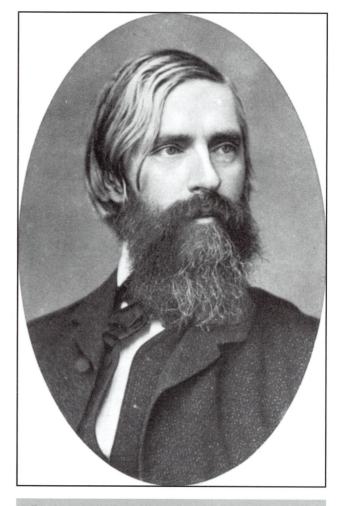

Albrecht von Graefe. Halftone reproduction from *Münchener medizinische Wochenschrift*, 1928. Wellcome Library, London.

Graefe's lifetime. Here, Graefe made use of a wide platform to discuss his innovative ideas and to present patient histories from his private clinic in Berlin. Many of these early presentations were later published in his *Archiv für Ophthalmologie*.

In his day Graefe was very popular, and his methods were often seen as if they stemmed from another world. Graefe was thus also the subject of many local writers, such as Felix Philippi or Eugenie John, who praised his ingenuity and his engagement in the medical treatment of the Berlin poor. Nowadays, the name of Albrecht von Graefe is still associated with the Graefe sign because he realized that in hyperthyroidism and some tumors, the upper eyelid does not follow downward movements of the eye bulb. This pathogenic process causes the white sclera to be rendered visible and continues to be a proper diagnostic sign. Yet Graefe was also an inventor, a passion he shared with his friend Donders, and a surgical instrument, the 'Graefe knife' for cataract operations, is named after him. Acknowledging his wide contributions to the science of ophthalmology, the Deutsche Ophthalmologische Gesellschaft created a Graefe Medal in 1885.

Bibliography

Primary: 1847. *De bromo ejusque praesipuis praeparatis* (Berlin); 1848. *Über Tannin als Choleramittel* (Berlin); 1852. *Über die Wirkungen der Augenmuskeln* (Berlin); 1866. *Stauungspapille bei Hirnerkrankungen* (Berlin).

Secondary: Winau, Rolf, 1987. *Medizin in Berlin* (Berlin and New York) pp. 203–206; Muenchow, Wolfgang, 1978. *Albrecht von Graefe* (Leipzig); Heynold von Graefe, Blida, 1969. *Albrecht von Graefe, ein Leben für das Licht* (Munich).

Frank W. Stahnisch

GRAHAM, EVARTS AMBROSE   (b. Chicago, Illinois, USA, 19 March 1883; d. St Louis, Missouri, USA, 4 March 1957), *surgery.*

Graham was the son of a community surgeon. He received his Baccalaureate degree from Princeton in 1904 (first in his class) and his MD from Rush Medical College in Chicago in 1907. His surgical training was at Rush and Presbyterian Hospital in Chicago. Graham was also a special student in chemistry at the University of Chicago. He had a brief stint as a solo practicing surgeon in Mason City, Iowa, and served in the U.S. Army Medical Corps near the end of World War I. From 1919 to 1951, he was the Bixby Professor of Surgery at Washington University School of Medicine in St Louis and Surgeon-in-Chief at Barnes Hospital and St Louis Children's Hospital. He became Bixby Professor Emeritus in 1951.

Graham was one of the most prominent American surgeons during the middle third of the twentieth century. His research altered the management of empyema, and he was one of the pioneers of the then-new specialty of thoracic surgery. Together with one of his surgical residents, he developed the radiologic method of visualizing the gall bladder (cholecystography, the Graham-Cole test). Graham performed the first successful one-stage pneumonectomy for lung cancer in 1933. His studies carried out with a medical student, Ernst Wynder, were instrumental in establishing the relationship between cigarette smoking and lung cancer. He had major leadership roles in the American College of Surgeons, the American Board of Surgery, and the Joint Commission on Accreditation of Hospitals. He was responsible for training hundreds of surgical residents at Barnes Hospital.

Graham had great integrity and strong convictions, vigorously advocating his objectives and always welcoming a good fight. He strongly opposed fee-splitting, which he had encountered during his brief experience as a practicing surgeon in Iowa. A tall, imposing figure, Graham had a rather abrupt, somewhat reserved demeanor. He was known for his intellectual acuity and dignified manner. He was quiet, polite, and incapable of small talk. He and his wife, Helen, had three sons, one of whom was stillborn.

Graham received a multitude of honors, including fourteen honorary degrees and numerous medals and prizes. Ironically,

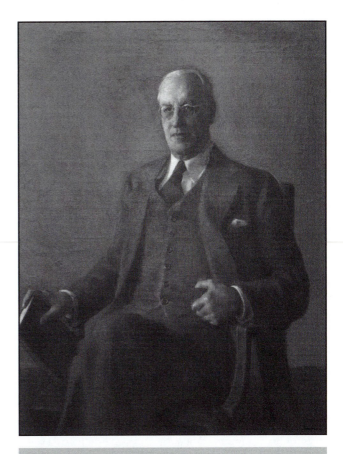

Evarts Graham. Oil Portrait by Robert Brachman, 1952. Becker Medical Library, Washington University School of Medicine.

he continued to be a heavy cigarette smoker despite his groundbreaking work pointing out the association between smoking and lung cancer. He died of that malignancy after a brief illness. Twenty of Graham's protégés became department chairmen at medical schools around the world. Graham's biographer termed him the 'Surgical Spirit of St. Louis'.

Bibliography

Primary: 1920. 'Some Principles Involved in the Treatment of Empyema.' *Surgery, Gynecology & Obstetrics* 31: 60–71; 1924. (with Cole, W. H.) 'Roentgenologic Examination of the Gall Bladder.' *Journal of the American Medical Association* 82: 613–614; 1933. (with Singer, J. J.) 'Successful Removal of an Entire Lung for Carcinoma of the Bronchus.' *Journal of the American Medical Association* 101: 1371–1374; 1950. (with Wynder, Ernst L.). 'Tobacco Smoking as a Possible Etiologic Factor in Bronchogenic Carcinoma.' *Journal of the American Medical Association* 143: 329–336.

Secondary: Mueller, C. Barber, 2002. *Evarts A. Graham: The Life, Lives, and Times of the Surgical Spirit of St. Louis* (Hamilton, Ontario); Olch, Peter D., 1989. 'Evarts A. Graham in World War I: The Empyema Commission and Service in the American Expeditionary Forces.' *Journal of the History of Medicine and Allied Sciences* 44: 430–446; *DAMB*.

Marvin J. Stone

GRAHAM, SYLVESTER (b. West Suffield, Connecticut, USA, 5 July 1794; d. Northampton, Massachusetts, USA, 11 September 1851), *health reform.*

The son of John Graham, a clergyman, and Ruth Graham, Sylvester was reared by a succession of relatives after the death of his father and mental breakdown of his mother. His unsettled childhood was plagued by poor health as well, yet in 1823 he entered Amherst Academy, only to be dismissed within a year on dubious charges of misbehavior. During the episode of illness that followed expulsion, Sarah Earl, whom he married in 1824, nursed him back to health.

Graham was ordained a Presbyterian minister in 1826 and preached for several years in New Jersey. In 1830 he moved to Philadelphia to work as an agent for the Pennsylvania Temperance Society, lecturing on the physical as well as moral harm done by strong drink. He soon expanded his subject matter, attacking other forms of immorality and arguing that any behavior that damaged morals necessarily damaged the body too. Graham's test for immorality was stimulation: any activity that was pleasurable or exciting led to loss of control of carnal appetites, he maintained, resulting in spiritual degradation and bodily injury. On that basis, he condemned coffee, tea, white bread, meat, and sexual indulgence.

Graham was the first prominent vegetarian in America, and the first in the Western world to promote vegetable diet primarily for reasons of health instead of morality. Nevertheless, the basis for his assumption that meat damaged health was a spiritual one, an Old Testament passage stating that the diet originally assigned to humankind by God included only vegetable foods. His physiological rationale for vegetarianism consisted of arguments drawn from moral principles and had little scientific basis.

In the area of sexual hygiene as well, conclusions of physical damage were dictated by moral considerations. Graham warned that much poor health derived from 'marital excess', or engaging in sexual intercourse more than once monthly. Sex outside marriage was condemned as even more injurious than marital intercourse, and he was particularly concerned about the effects of the 'solitary vice', or masturbation. Convinced that the erotic fantasizing that accompanied that act inflamed the brain and that the inflammation could spread through the nervous system, he warned of a host of afflictions culminating in insanity as the outcome of solitary sexual stimulation. Graham was a major catalyst for the formation of Victorian anxieties over pathological effects from sexual activity.

Graham did offer much good hygienic advice, such as his recommendations of daily exercise and bathing and his condemnation of tight-laced corsets and overreliance on medication. He is best known for his promotion of whole-grain bread, made from coarse-ground Graham flour, and Graham crackers, which were regarded as a health food until the early twentieth century. From 1837 to 1839, he produced the *Graham Journal of Health and Longevity* and published several books advocating his health reform principles. Grahamite beliefs would play an influential role in radical health reform programs down to the early twentieth century.

Graham anticipated that adoption of his recommendations would generate increased vigor and lengthened life and that as physical health improved, so would the moral health of individuals and society, until the long-awaited Christian millennium would be brought about by vegetable diet and sexual restraint. Over many generations, he believed, the human race would be restored to the natural lifespan of 900-plus years enjoyed by the biblical patriarchs. Graham died at the age of fifty-seven, after several years of semi-invalidism.

Bibliography

Primary: 1834. *A Lecture to Young Men on Chastity* (Providence); 1837. *A Treatise on Bread and Bread-making* (Boston); 1839. *The Science of Human Life* 2 vols. (Boston).

Secondary: Whorton, James, 1982. *Crusaders for Fitness: The History of American Health Reformers* (Princeton) pp. 13–131; Nissenbaum, Stephen, 1980. *Sex, Diet, and Debility in Jacksonian America: Sylvester Graham and Health Reform* (Westport, CT); Naylor, Mildred, 1942. 'Sylvester Graham, 1794–1851.' *Annals of Medical History* (3rd series) 4: 236–240; *DAMB*.

James Whorton

GRAM, HANS CHRISTIAN JOACHIM (b. Copenhagen, Denmark, 13 September 1853; d. Copenhagen, 14 November 1949), *bacteriology, pharmacology.*

As the oldest son of Frederik Terkel Julius Gram, a professor of law, and Louise Christiane Roulund, Gram initially pursued an interest in botany and began studies in this field in 1872. He was quickly drawn toward medicine through bacteriology, and he received his medical degree from the University of Copenhagen in 1878. He then worked as an assistant at various Copenhagen hospitals and also refined his skills in microscopy. In 1882 he received the gold medal from the University of Copenhagen for an essay on the number and size of red blood corpuscles in chlorotics, and he defended his thesis on the size of red blood corpuscles the following year.

Gram was part of the circle of young researchers in bacteriology that gathered around Carl Julius Salomonsen in the early 1880s. From 1883 to 1885 Gram studied bacteriology and pharmacology in laboratories across Europe, and upon the recommendation of Salomonsen, Gram first visited the pathologist Carl Friedländer in Berlin. Gram became involved in Friedländer's experiments on pneumococci and quickly developed a simple and effective staining method for identifying and differentiating bacteria in tissue samples. Gram found that some bacteria retained the color from aniline gentian violet when first prepared with iodine and then treated with alcohol (gram-positive), whereas others bleached (gram-negative). This method made Gram famous on an international scale and also allowed him to determine that the bacteria grown by Friedländer were different from the bacteria observed in the lungs of pneumonia patients. Perhaps out of consideration for Friedländer, Gram did not pay too much attention to this aspect of his results, but his staining method was employed by Friedländer's main critic, Albert Fraenkel, who went on to identify the pneumococcus.

After 1884 Gram never worked on his staining method again, and upon his return to Copenhagen (1885), he abandoned bacteriology and concentrated on pharmacology and clinical medicine. After serving as an assistant at Kommunehospitalet (1885–89), where he was active in testing new pharmacological products, and as district medical officer (1889–91), he became a professor of pharmacology (1891–1900). During his earlier travels, Gram had worked at Oswald Schmiedeberg's pioneering pharmacological institute in Strasbourg, and though he did not himself take much interest in experimental pharmacology, his contacts were valuable to young Danish researchers in this field. Gram increasingly focused on clinical practice, partly through his position as chief physician in internal medicine at Frederiks Hospital, later Rigshospitalet (1892–1923), and from 1900 as professor of internal medicine. He retired from the university in 1924, but continued his private practice until 1934.

The Gram staining method remains a central diagnostic tool. Counterstaining for gram-negative bacteria quickly became standard, but an explanation for why bacteria are colored differently was not supplied until the 1960s.

Bibliography

Primary: 1883. *Undersøgelser over de røde Blodlegemers Tal og Størrelse hos Mennesket* (Copenhagen); 1884. 'Über die isolierte Färbung der Schizomyceten in Schnitt- und Trockenpräparaten.' *Fortschritte der Medizin* 2: 185–189.

Secondary: Lautrop, Hans, 1982. 'Christian Gram og hans farvemetode med hidtil utrykte breve fra Gram til Salomonsen 1883–84.' *Bibliotek for Læger* 174: 1–30; Jarløv, Ejnar, 1938. 'Chr. Gram.' *Hospitalstidende* 47: 1113–1115; Heiberg, K. A., 1938. 'Chr. Gram.' *Ugeskrift for Læger* 100: 1357.

Søren Bak-Jensen

GRANCHER, JACQUES-JOSEPH (b. Felletin, France, 29 September 1843; d. Paris, France, 13 July 1907), *tuberculosis, pediatrics.*

Grancher's early career illustrates both his talents and his struggles as a medical student of unusually humble origins (his father was a tailor). He began study at the Paris Faculty of Medicine in 1862 and then delayed the degree in order to begin earning a salary as an intern at various Paris hospitals while studying histology with Ranvier and Cornil. In 1869 he began a ten-year stint as the director of a pathology laboratory for the Paris hospital administration. After a brief attachment to the military surgical service in the Franco-Prussian War (1870–71), he finally received his degree in 1873, quickly obtained the coveted post of hospital doctor, and opened a private practice, all the while continuing research in pathology. In 1885 he was appointed to the post of clinical professor of pediatric diseases at the Paris Faculty of Medicine. He was a member of the Academy of Medicine (elected 1892), and he served on the national public health council and the national antituberculosis commission.

Grancher's thesis, *De l'unité de la phthisie* (1873), marked a lifelong dedication to the etiological study and eradication of tuberculosis. He used his skills in cellular anatomy to argue for the *uniciste* understanding of pulmonary tuberculosis as one essential disease with multiple manifestations, publishing a notable article on this subject in the *Archives de Physiologie* in 1872. Grancher's study on the relative importance of contagion as opposed to heredity in the etiology of tuberculosis placed him in the vanguard of the germ theory of disease and led him into a public controversy. In 1902 he created a foundation, later known as the *Ouevre Grancher*, to prevent the development of tuberculosis in urban children at risk because of exposure within the family. One program—inspired by a tangle of altruism and experimentalism—placed such children with rural families and was subjected to the critical scrutiny of the press. Grancher followed his preventive medicine into electoral office: as a city councilor and, later, mayor of Cambo-les-Bains (1900–05), he advocated open-air schools and sanatoriums to prevent childhood tuberculosis.

Grancher's second involvement in controversy arose from his work with the antirabies program developed by Louis Pasteur. One of the early clinicians to join Pasteur's team, Grancher studied microbiology in Pasteur's laboratory in the early 1880s and quickly became his intimate friend, personal physician, and essential colleague. In 1885 Pasteur turned to him to administer inoculations and supervise care for his first patients, Joseph Meister and Jean-Baptiste Jupille, and then to take charge of the antirabies clinic on the rue Vauquelin. When the program was attacked at the Academy of Medicine in January 1887 by Michel Peter, a faculty professor of clinical medicine, Grancher played the central role in orchestrating the defense. His advocacy of Pasteur was further carried out in medical journals that he cofounded or edited: *Bulletin médical,* the *Archives de médecine expérimentale,* and the *Revue de la tuberculose.* Grancher developed new protocols for antiseptic care in his pediatric wards and published results showing a dramatic reduction in mortality (1900). He was one of the organizers of the Pasteur Institute (Paris) and later its vice-president (1900) and president (1905).

Bibliography

Primary: 1873. *De l'unité de la phthisie* (Paris); 1897–98. *Traité des maladies de l'enfance* 5 vols. (Paris); 1900. *Un service antiseptique de médecine; statistique de dix années* (Paris).

Secondary: Gelfand, Toby, 2002. '11 January 1887, the Day Medicine Changed: Joseph Grancher's Defense of Pasteur's Treatment for Rabies.' *Bulletin of the History of Medicine* 76: 698–718; Debré, Patrice, 1998. *Louis Pasteur* [trans. Forster, Elborg] (Baltimore); Roussillat, Jacques, 1989. *Un patron des hôpitaux de Paris à la Belle Époque: la vie de Joseph Grancher* (Guérat); Archives de l'Institut Pasteur, http:www.Pasteur.fr./infosci/archives/grc0.html.

Martha Hildreth

GRASSI, GIOVANNI BATTISTA (b. Rovellasca, Como, Italy, 27 March 1854; d. Rome, Italy, 4 May 1925), *medicine, parasitology, zoology, hygiene, epidemiology.*

The son of Luigi, a public official, and Costanza Mazzucchetti, of peasant origin, Grassi first studied at Saronno, and then in 1872 he moved to the University of Pavia, where he studied under Camillo Golgi (1843–1926) and Giulio Bizzozero (1846–1901), receiving his MD in 1878.

While still a student, he carried out scientific observations on parasitic helminths in animals and man. After earning his degree, he decided to become a zoologist rather than a clinician. Financed by a scholarship, he began to work at Messina and at the Zoological Station at Naples, publishing a monograph on the *Chetognaths* (1882). Then he decided to complete his training as a zoologist and spent a period (1879–80) in the laboratories of Gegenbaur and Bütschli in Heidelberg, where he also met Maria Koenen, who became his wife. In 1882 he published a monograph on the development of the vertebral column in fish.

In 1883, at the early age of twenty-nine, Grassi won a contest and was appointed professor of Comparative Zoology at the University of Catania, where he returned to his studies on parasitic helminths. He discovered that, unusually, the life cycle of *Hymenolepis nana* does not require an intermediate host. At the same time in collaboration with Sauveur Calandruccio, Grassi studied the life cycle of eels, demonstrating in the field and in the laboratory the metamorphosis of the larval eels or leptocephali, previously considered a different species. Together with Calandruccio, he continued to study various parasites of man and animals.

In Catania, Grassi also started to study entomology, discovering a new species and studying the determination of the castes among the termites, demonstrating the role of parasitic protozoans in the maturation of sex organs during development.

In 1888 he began to investigate malaria transmission in birds, in collaboration with the clinician Raimondo Feletti, describing two of the parasites, *Laverania danilevski* and *Haemamoeba pracox.* He and Feletti proposed names for the malarial parasites of man, two of which (*vivax* and *malariae*) remained in use. In 1895 Grassi was appointed at the University of Rome as professor of anatomy and comparative physiology.

After Ross's preliminary results in India in 1897 on human malaria and his experimental demonstration (1898) of the transmission of bird malaria by *Culex,* Grassi in July 1898 undertook an extensive biogeographical study, correlating the presence of malaria with the presence of a special genre of mosquitoes, *Anopheles.* Collaborating with the clinicians Amico Bignami and Guiseppe Bastianelli, Grassi studied the life cycle of the *Plasmodium* in man and in mosquitoes, and in November 1898 they experimentally produced the transmission of malaria in a healthy person through the bites of *Anopheles* collected in malarious areas. The following year Grassi was able to show that *Anopheles* are born uninfected

and are able to transmit malaria only after biting an infected human. He therefore announced what has been called the 'Grassi's law': malaria = *Anopheles* + infected humans.

In 1900 Grassi published a monograph on malaria, with beautiful microscopical illustrations of the life cycle of the *Plasmodia.* Between 1900 and 1902 Grassi, in collaboration with Pittaluga and Noè, made a series of studies in areas endemic for malaria near Rome and on the plain of Capaccio, near Paestum, where he successfully demonstrated mechanical protection against malaria.

In 1902 Ross was awarded the Nobel Price for discovering the mode of malaria transmission. Grassi could not accept that his contribution to the discovery of the transmission of human malaria had been dismissed, and for the following two decades a bitter dispute ensued. Ross continued to insist that the 'Italians' had just filled in a few details, whereas Grassi repeatedly stressed that Ross's discovery in birds was not conclusive for human malaria and that he had been the first to identify its specific vector of human malaria, the mosquitoes of the genus *Anopheles.*

Because of this disaffection, Grassi abandoned the study of malaria and devoted his research mainly to the life cycle of the parasite of the grape vine (*Phylloxera vastatrix*), which at the turn of the century brought incalculable damage to wine production in Europe, showing the differences between the European and America strains and suggesting appropriate control measures. In this same period, Grassi became interested in industrial hygiene and in particular phosphonecrosis, a disease common among workers in the match industry. He also conducted experimental studies of goiter, endemic in Alpine valleys.

At the end of World War I, which produced a severe recrudescence of malaria, Grassi decided to go back to the subject and in 1918 established a 'malaria observatory' at Fiumicino, in the Tiber Delta, studying mosquito flight habits. He also made a wide epidemiological study of the incidence of malaria in the area and suggested various methods of malaria control. Up to his death, he continued to study malaria and was correcting a manuscript of his study of the biology of *Anopheles superpictus* when he died in Rome. According to his last will, he was buried in the small cemetery of Fiumicino.

Grassi was elected a member of twenty-four scientific academies. He received the Royal Society of London's Darwin Medal (1896) for his zoological work on termites and eels, the University of Leipzig's doctoral degree *honoris causa* (1909), the Turin academy's Vallauri prize (1904), and the Accademia dei Lincei's Royal Prize. In 1908 he was made a member of the Italian Senate for his scientific achievements.

Bibliography

Primary: 1893. (with Saudias, A.) *Costituzione e sviluppo della società dei Termitidi* (Catania); 1896. 'The Reproduction and Metamorphosis of the Common Eel (*Anguilla vulgaris*).' *Proc. R. Soc. London* 60: 260–271; 1898. 'Rapporti tra la malaria e peculiari insetti (Zanzaroni e zanzare palustri).' *Rendiconti della Reale Acca-*

demia dei Lincei 7: 163–172; 1900. *Studi di uno zoologo sulla malaria* (Rome; 2nd enlarged edn., 1901).

Secondary: Snowden, Frank, M., 2006. *The Conquest of Malaria: Italy, 1900–1962* (New Haven and London); Capanna, Ernesto, ed., 1996. *Battista Grassi, uno zoologo per la malaria* (Rome); Neghme, A., 1964. 'An Appraisal of Giovan Battista Grassi: His Work in Biology and Parasitology.' *Experimental Parasitology* 15: 260–278; Corti, A., 1961. *Battista Grassi e la trasmissione della malaria* (Pavia); Janicki, Constantin, 1928, 'Giovan Battista Grassi. Ein grosser Zoologe und Parasitologe Italiens.' *Naturwissenschaft* 14: 225–231; *DSB*.

Bernardino Fantini

GRAVES, ROBERT JAMES (b. Dublin, Ireland, 28 March 1796; d. Banagher, King's County, Ireland, 20 March 1853), *medicine, physiology, medical education.*

Graves belonged to a distinguished Anglo-Irish intellectual dynasty. He was the youngest son of Richard Graves (1763–1829), Church of Ireland Dean of Ardagh and regius professor of divinity in Trinity College Dublin. His namesake, the poet Robert Graves (1895–1985) was his grandnephew. He excelled as an undergraduate at Trinity in both classics BA (1815) and medicine MB (1818). He extended his medical studies in London, Edinburgh, Berlin, and other clinical centers on the continent, returning to Dublin in 1821. In 1824 Graves helped found the Park Street medical school and became physician to the Meath Hospital.

He and William Stokes (1804–78) were responsible for first introducing into the British Isles the central European practice he had encountered in Berlin, practice in which clinical teaching was focused on the patient's bedside rather than on the lecture theater. Students were taught the virtues of careful observation and the taking of a case history with notes directly from the patient. The core tools of diagnosis were percussion as advocated by Leopold Auenbrugger (1722–1809) and auscultation, most particularly with the use of the stethoscope to diagnose valvular disease. Detailed discussion of symptoms, pathology, and therapy all happened at the bedside. Teaching at Park Street was similarly pioneering in its foregrounding of the primacy of hospital experience. Graves was also unusual in following the German practice of addressing poor patients sympathetically and informatively rather than abusively and dismissively, as was the Dublin tradition.

The methods of Graves and Stokes were given wider circulation through the 1843 publication of Graves's *Clinical lectures*. Subsequently translated into French, German, and Italian, the *Clinical lectures* transformed Dublin medicine from an outhouse of Edinburgh University into an international center of clinical excellence and a major influence on research, teaching, and practice throughout Europe, America, and the British Empire. At the request of its founder, John Cheyne (1777–1836), Graves edited the fifth and final volume of the journal *Dublin Hospital Reports*. In 1832 he cofounded with Robert Kane (1809–90) the *Dublin*, later *Irish Journal of Medical Science*, and was a prolific contributor to the *London Medical and Surgical Journal* and the *London Medical Gazette*. An accomplished linguist, his *Edinburgh Medical and Surgical Journal* column was a conduit for the dissemination of German research into English from the 1820s.

In the *Clinical Lectures* Graves gave so comprehensive a description to exophthalmic goiter that Armand Trousseau (1801–67) gave it the name 'Graves' disease'. He effected a paradigmatic shift in the treatment of fevers, replacing the traditional regime of starving, bleeding, and purging with one based on feeding, and he suggested 'He fed fevers' for his epitaph. During the Great Famine of the 1840s, he highlighted the role of contagion in the spread of typhus and cholera. He was a vociferous critic of overcrowding at centers of famine relief and of the paltry fees authorized by the Board of Health for the payment of famine doctors.

In 1827 Graves became King's Professor of the Institutes of Medicine (physiology, pathology, and therapeutics) at Trinity College. He was president of the King and Queen's (later Royal) College of Physicians of Ireland in 1843–44 and FRS from 1849.

Bibliography

Primary: 1835. 'Newly Observed Affection of the Thyroid Gland in Females.' *London Medical and Surgical Journal* 8: 2516–2517, repr. in Major, R. H., 1945. *Classic Descriptions of Disease* (Springfield, IL) pp. 280–281; 1843. *Clinical Lectures on the Practice of Medicine* (Dublin); 1863. (Stokes, William, ed.) *Studies in Physiology and Medicine* (London).

Secondary: O'Brien, Eoin, 1975. 'Dublin Masters of Clinical Expression: V. Robert Graves (1796–1853).' *Journal of the Irish Colleges of Physicians and Surgeons* 4: 4; Widdess, J. D. H., 1963. *A History of the Royal College of Physicians of Ireland, 1654–1963* (Dublin); Ormsby, Lambert H., 1888. *Medical History of the Meath Hospital and County Dublin Infirmary* (Dublin); *Oxford DNB*.

James McGeachie

GREENWOOD, MAJOR (b. Shoreditch, London, England, 9 August 1880; d. London, 5 October 1949), *medical statistics, epidemiology.*

Born into a long line of doctors (his father, both grandfathers, and several near relatives were physicians), Greenwood grew up in London's East End. At the age of eighteen, he entered the London Hospital Medical School and read *The Grammar of Science* (1892) by the statistical pioneer Karl Pearson (1857–1936). In 1904 Greenwood received his license to practice medicine and spent the 1904–05 academic year studying under Pearson at University College London. In 1905 Greenwood was given a research scholarship by the British Medical Association, and he became the demonstrator in the physiological laboratory of Leonard Hill (1866–1952) in the London Hospital Medical School. In 1910 Charles James Martin (1866–1955), director of the Lister Institute of Preventive Medicine, created the position of medical statistician for Greenwood. At the time, this was the only post in Britain that had been designed to deal with medical data using Pearsonian methods, and its creation signaled that Greenwood's career had been launched. In 1920 Greenwood left the Lister Institute to become the first senior Statistical Officer at the Ministry of Health; in 1927 he became the first professor of epidemiology and medical statistics at the London School of Hygiene and Tropical Medicine and the head of the Statistical Research Unit at the Medical Research Council (MRC); in 1928 he was elected FRS. While at the MRC, Greenwood collaborated with the bacteriologist W. W. C. Topley (1886–1944) in research that studied the rise and fall of epidemic diseases within populations of laboratory mice. In their studies, Greenwood and Topley focused on mouse typhoid to illustrate the relative importance of environment, host, and agent factors in disease occurrence. Greenwood retired in 1945.

Reflecting the views of Pearson, Greenwood held that, because science involved demonstrating the association between the same antecedents and consequents (on multiple occasions), scientific reasoning was fundamentally statistical. Eventually, Greenwood's views drew him into a public controversy with Sir Almroth Wright (1861–1947), a prominent bacteriologist in early twentieth-century Britain. Although the debate was ignited by Greenwood's statistical criticism of Wright's diagnostic technique called an opsonic index (named for the blood serum substance opsonin), the debate actually reflected fundamentally differing views on the nature of science. For Wright, statistical results could, at most, illustrate a *possible* connection between two events, but an underlying *causal* connection could only be established by a well-designed 'crucial experiment' in the controlled environment of a laboratory setting. For Greenwood, by contrast, 'crucial experiments' did not exist; as he would observe in *Epidemiology: Historical and Experimental*, 'In the biological experimentation … there can be no crucial experiments, reasoning must be stochastic, inferences no more than probable' (Greenwood, 1932, p. 80).

As the first medical student to be trained in the mathematical statistical techniques that Pearson had pioneered, Greenwood could be characterized as the first professionally trained medical statistician of the twentieth century. Through the positions that he held and the students that he taught, Greenwood laid the foundation for the emergence of a statistically based epidemiology, which would come to maturity in the second half of the twentieth century in the work of his colleague and successor Sir Austin Bradford Hill (1897–1991).

Bibliography

Primary: 1932. *Epidemiology: Historical and Experimental* (Baltimore); 1935. *Epidemics and Crowd-Diseases: An Introduction to the Study of Epidemiology* (New York); 1936. *The Medical Dictator and Other Biographical Studies* (London).

Secondary: Magnello, Eileen, 2002. 'The Introduction of Mathematical Statistics into Medical Research: The Roles of Karl Pearson, Major Greenwood, and Austin Bradford Hill' in Magnello, Eileen, and Anne Hardy, eds., *The Road to Medical Statistics* (Amsterdam) pp. 95–123; Matthews, J. Rosser, 2002. 'Almroth Wright, Vaccine Therapy, and British Biometrics: Disciplinary Expertise versus Statistical Objectivity' in Magnello, Eileen, and Anne Hardy, eds., *The Road to Medical Statistics* (Amsterdam) pp. 125–147; Hogben, Lancelot, 1950. 'Major Greenwood, 1880–1949.' *Obituary Notices of Fellows of the Royal Society* 7: 139–154; *Oxford DNB*.

J. Rosser Matthews

GREGG, NORMAN McALISTER (b. Sydney, Australia, 7 March 1892; d. Sydney, 27 July 1966), *ophthalmology, teratology.*

Gregg, the youngest of the six children of James and Mary Gregg, was educated at Homebush Grammar School and Sydney Grammar School where, from an early age, he was a brilliant all-rounder. During medical studies at the University of Sydney, he gained many academic distinctions and graduated with first-class honors in 1915. He was president of the Undergraduates Association and a director of the University Union. Excelling in many sports, he represented his state in cricket and tennis and was on the university's swimming and baseball teams. He later became captain, and then President, of the Royal Sydney Golf Club. While serving with the Royal Army Medical Corps in France during World War I, Gregg was awarded the Military Cross 'for conspicuous gallantry and devotion to duty during a raid'.

Like many antipodean medical graduates of his era, Gregg traveled to England for postgraduate training and experience at London's Moorfields Eye Hospital and the Royal Westminster Ophthalmic Hospital, and also at the Birmingham and Midland Eye Hospital.

Back in Sydney, he became an ophthalmic surgeon at Royal Prince Alfred Hospital and the Royal Alexandra Hospital for Children and commenced private practice. In 1923 he married Haidee Margaret Carson; they had two daughters.

Consideration had occasionally been given in the early 1940s to the possibility that maternal infection during pregnancy could cause birth defects and other serious consequences, but this hypothesis lacked evidence. Following a widespread epidemic of rubella in eastern Australia in 1940–41, exacerbated by a susceptible population and wartime conditions, Gregg gathered evidence from his own practice and from other ophthalmologists that maternal rubella infection caused atypical congenital cataracts, other eye abnormalities, and heart and other birth defects. Three years later, he identified deafness in young children as another feature of maternal rubella. The astuteness of Gregg's clinical observations in his classic paper in 1941 was confirmed when the expanded congenital rubella syndrome was described after the major epidemic in the United States in the mid-1960s.

Already a prominent clinician in Sydney, Gregg was regarded as an inspiring teacher and mentor. He became

President of the Board of Management at the Royal Alexandra Hospital for Children and an active member of many professional and community committees, while continuing his busy private practice. Among many honors, Gregg was awarded the prestigious Charles Mickle Fellowship by the University of Toronto (1951) and honorary doctorates by three Australian universities. He was knighted in 1953.

Gregg's findings had major implications for clinical medicine, scientific research, and public health. His studies showed that rubella, previously regarded as a mild infectious disease, could cause cataracts and other significant birth defects if susceptible pregnant women became infected in the first few months of pregnancy. His work stimulated laboratory research scientists to eventually isolate the rubella virus two decades after his initial observations. Primary prevention of birth defects resulting from rubella later became possible when a vaccine was developed. Gregg's discovery also stimulated rapid development of the fledgling field of teratology, the study of birth defects and their causes.

Bibliography

Primary: 1941. 'Congenital Cataract Following German Measles in the Mother.' *Transactions of the Ophthalmological Society of Australia* 3: 35–46; 1944. 'Further Observations on Congenital Defects in Infants Following Maternal Rubella.' *Transactions of the Ophthalmological Society of Australia* 4: 119–131.

Secondary: Heagney, Brenda, comp., 1992. *Rubella: Essays in Honour of the Birth of Sir Norman McAlister Gregg, 1892–1966* (Sydney); Burgess, Margaret A., 1991. 'Gregg's Rubella Legacy.' *The Medical Journal of Australia* 155: 355–357; Cooper, L. Z., 1975. 'Congenital Rubella in the United States' in Krugman, S., and A. A. Gershon, eds., *Infections of the Fetus and Newborn Infant. Progress in Clinical and Biological Research* (New York); Obituary, 1966. 'Norman McAlister Gregg.' *The Medical Journal of Australia* 2: 1166–1169.

Paul A. L. Lancaster

GREGORY, ALFRED JOHN (b. England, *c.* 1851; d. Richmond Hill, Surrey, England, 14 July 1927), *medicine, bacteriology.*

Little is known of Gregory's early years other than that he completed his medical training at Durham, where he also received his Diploma in Public Health in 1891. Later that year, he emigrated to the Cape Colony. Two years later, he became the first officially appointed medical adviser to the Cape Government and rose to become the colony's leading medical figure until the Union of South Africa was created in 1910.

Gregory almost single-handedly built the medical department in the Cape Colony and was the prime mover of public health reform legislation in 1897. His rise was controversial and earned him the resentment especially of South African–born Cape Town practitioners. Efficient but authoritarian, progressive yet intolerant, Gregory possessed a sanitarian's approach to infectious diseases and a contempt for all behavior that did not conform to late Victorian bourgeois norms. Typical of his time and place in South Africa, Gregory showed neither sympathy nor understanding for the structural causes of overcrowded and squalid housing, and he was a firm believer in residential segregation by race and even by ethnicity.

Gregory was acting Medical Officer of Health for Cape Colony when bubonic plague broke out late in 1900. Together with the leading British expert on plague at the time, William J. R. Simpson, Gregory launched an intensive public health campaign, which also had strong political overtones, namely the forced removal of black Africans from Cape Town to a new residential location later to be called Ndabeni.

Gregory became Medical Officer of Health for Cape Colony in 1901 and served as adviser on the preparation of a new Native Reserve Locations bill the following year. He quarreled with the Native Affairs Department because he felt they were reluctant to coerce Africans and because they opposed a comprehensive pass system, which he favored. He was also influential in other social legislation, such as the Aliens Immigration Act of 1902, designed to exclude Indian laborers primarily, but directed also against poor Eastern European immigrants, especially Jews.

Gregory was disappointed not to be named Medical Officer of Health when the Cape joined the new Union of South Africa in 1910. He took retirement on a pension the next year and in 1912 became chairman of a special commission on tuberculosis. The commission's report was poorly received by parliament, especially its steep cost, which included Gregory's large honorarium. He left South Africa for England in May 1914, settling in Bournemouth. During World War I, he served as civil surgeon at the South African Military Hospital at Richmond.

Although his social attitudes were offensive, Gregory's success in establishing a centralized and efficient public health department deserves recognition. Gregory's energy and single-minded faith in the importance of the state's role in building modern public health infrastructure cannot be denied, and in this he had much in common with the new generation of sanitarians all over the world. On the other hand, Gregory's prejudices blinded him to the structural causes of poverty and disease in his city and contributed to the facile political decisions to invest in separate and unequal African locations rather than in better housing and wages.

Bibliography

Primary: 1899. 'Notes on Some Recent Cases of Plague in South Africa.' *South African Medical Journal* 7: 81–85.

Secondary: van Heyningen, Elizabeth, 1989. 'Agents of Empire: The Medical Profession in the Cape Colony, 1880-1910.' *Medical History* 33: 450–471; van Heyningen, Elizabeth, 1981. 'Cape Town and the Plague of 1901' in Saunders, C., H. Phillips, and E. B. van

Heyningen, eds., *Studies in the History of Cape Town* vol. 4 (Cape Town) pp. 66–107.

Myron Echenberg

GREGORY, JOHN (b. Aberdeen, Scotland, 3 June 1724; d. Edinburgh, Scotland, 9 February 1773), *medicine, medical education, medical ethics.*

Gregory, son of James Gregorie, professor of medicine, King's College Aberdeen, and Anna Chalmers, began his studies at Aberdeen grammar school and King's College Aberdeen. In 1742 he went to Edinburgh University to study medicine and took courses with Alexander Monro *primus* (1697–1767), Andrew Sinclair, and John Rutherford (1695–1779). He also joined the student society, the Royal Medical Society. In 1745 Gregory went to Leiden and studied under Hieronymus Gaubius (1705–80) and Bernard Albinus (1697–1770). He received his MD from King's College Aberdeen in 1746.

In the same year Gregory returned to Aberdeen. He had received an education suitable for an aspiring professor, and his family had been closely associated with King's College for several generations. In the eighteenth century, professorial positions were often treated as a kind of family property, and Gregory's half-brother, James, had taken over the professorship of medicine on the death of their father. John, who had been greatly influenced by the ethical ideas of his cousin, the philosopher Thomas Reid (1710–96), became professor of philosophy in 1746. He also started a medical practice, which grew rapidly enough for him to resign his position as professor in 1749. In 1752 he married Elizabeth Forbes, and the couple had six children, one of whom, James Gregory, also became a physician and professor. When his half-brother died in 1755, John Gregory was appointed to the chair of medicine at King's College. He was elected FRS in 1756.

In Aberdeen, Gregory was a founding member, with Reid, of the Aberdeen Philosophical Society, also known as the Wise Club. Papers he read to the Society were subsequently collected and published as *A Comparative View of the State and Faculties of Man, with Those of the Animal World* (1765). In 1764 Gregory moved to Edinburgh to take up the professorship of the practice of medicine. His continued interest in ethical issues led to his writing *Observations on the Duties and Offices of a Physician, and on the Method of Prosecuting Enquiries in Philosophy* (1770) (subsequently published as *Lectures on the Duties and Qualifications of a Physician*). Along with Thomas Percival's *Medical Ethics* (1803), this forms a link between Scottish Common Sense philosophy and the codes of ethics that became an integral part of nineteenth-century British and American medical professionalization.

Courses in the practice of medicine, or pathology, together with those in anatomy and surgery, formed the core of the eighteenth-century medical curriculum. Gregory's most lasting contribution as a medical educator, however, was in his clinical teaching. Starting in the late seventeenth century, hospitals attached to medical schools were gradually supplanting apprenticeship as the venue for medical students to gain clinical experience. Gregory's clinical lectures wholeheartedly promoted the value of bedside teaching as the basis for medical practice. 'A gentleman can declaim on the causes of diseases', he began his lectures, 'but [if] he was never conversant with the sick, he is embarrassed with his erudition, and deceived in cases, in which an apothecary's apprentice would find no difficulty' (*Lectures*, 1771). As is often the case with clinical textbooks, the lecture in which he stated this was copied and recopied by students in preference to actual hospital experience.

After the death of his wife in 1761, Gregory wrote *A Father's Legacy to his Daughters*, which was published by his son in 1774. Though later condemned by feminist writers such as Mary Wollstonecraft (1759–97), it is noteworthy for promoting vigorous outdoor exercise for women, including walking and horseback riding. It was probably the mostly widely read of all his published works.

Bibliography

Primary: 1765. *A Comparative View of the State and Faculties of Man, with Those of the Animal World* (London); 1770. *Observations on the Duties and Offices of a Physician, and on the Method of Prosecuting Enquiries in Philosophy* (London); 1771. 'Notes from Dr. Gregory's Clinical Lectures in the Royal Infirmary 1771.' Royal Medical Society Library (Edinburgh); 1774. *A Father's Legacy to His Daughters* (London).

Secondary: McCullough, L. B., 1998. *John Gregory and the Invention of Professional Medical Ethics and the Profession of Medicine* (Dordrecht); Smellie, William, 1800. *Literary and Characteristical Lives of John Gregory and Others* (Edinburgh); *Oxford DNB*.

Lisa Rosner

GRENFELL, WILFRED THOMASON (b. Parkgate, England, 28 February 1865; d. Charlotte, Vermont, USA, 9 October 1940), *medical philanthropy, missionary medicine.*

Grenfell was born at Parkgate, near Chester, to Jane Georgina Hutchinson and the Reverend Algernon Sidney Grenfell, schoolmaster at Mostyn School. A good athlete but a lackluster student at Marlborough School, he considered the army or clergy, but settled on medicine, entering the London Hospital Medical College. Coincidentally, his father, periodically mentally unstable and despondent about his failure as a schoolmaster, was appointed chaplain to the London Hospital, serving only a year before he was admitted to an asylum where he hanged himself.

Grenfell's medical school career was also undistinguished, with a rating of 'very poor' in his clinical clerkship. He was uninterested in his classes, but impressed by Sir Arthur Clark's diagnostic skill and antialcohol campaigns and by Frederick Treves's talents as a teacher, surgeon, social reformer, athlete, and self-promoter, an 'all round man' with strong Christian beliefs. In the summers Grenfell organized country camping for East End London apprentices and factory workers, learning that he could express his Christian ideals through the organization of people for their own good and that publicity could advance this work.

A visit to an evangelical tent meeting set him on a course toward missionary work, and after graduation he was encouraged by Treves to become involved with the Mission to Deep Sea Fishermen as they were looking for a strong teetotaler physician who would preach Christianity. During the arduous two-month winter voyage on the North Atlantic, he found the fishermen unresponsive to his preaching, but he gained attention from a reporter who came on board and found the young doctor a handsome figure to feature in his stories. When some administrators were dismissed for financial irregularities, Grenfell, age twenty-four, was appointed superintendent of the Mission fleet. He exercised his organizational skills by providing facilities for recreation, reading, and education for the fishermen, as well as soup kitchens, libraries, and a series of public lectures. An effective writer, he began a regular series of stories of the hardship and heroism of the fishermen in the Mission monthly magazine, *Toilers of the Deep*.

Grenfell sailed in a hospital ship to Newfoundland, entering St John's harbor as the city was being destroyed by fire. Visiting the fishing ships, he treated 693 patients in one month, recognizing that more could be done with proper ships and resources. He convinced fish plant owners and the government to build and support two small hospitals. Back in England, he increased public attention for the Mission with his writings and lantern slide lectures. The Mission leaders valued his fundraising, but felt he was now neglecting his other duties.

He returned to the Labrador coast in 1893 with a hospital ship and a refurbished steamer, accompanied by two additional nurses and two other physicians. He combined medical and missionary work with his heroic and sometimes reckless adventures, and stories about the brave Christian missionary doctor caught the attention of the public and also powerful and rich supporters. The story of his remarkable survival on an ice floe that was drifting out into the ocean added to his public aura. He survived many days of freezing weather on the ice by sacrificing his dogs to make protective clothing. He lectured over North America and Britain, and although not a great orator, his handsome appearance, public image, and straightforward manner enthralled his audiences.

Increasingly on his own path, he worked tirelessly for his vision of social and political change for the people of Labrador, often stepping on the toes of the local church, the government, the Mission, and the fishery owners. Even the local people he served sometimes felt embarrassed by his public discussion of their poverty and passivity. He often came under criticism as a self-publicist who was an effective fund-raiser but financially inept, capable of grand vision but bored with detail. Despite this, increasingly the work of all Mission personnel was becoming identified with Grenfell, and in 1913 a separate International Grenfell Association was established for fundraising.

After serving as a major in the Royal Army Medical Corps during World War I, he returned to missionary work to find the Mission with few staff and his own financial situation insecure. His spiritual autobiography, *A Labrador Doctor*, was successful, and although it was more about the Mission than about him, it advanced his international standing. His fame was having unexpected repercussions, as an increasing number of books about him began to decrease his own book sales.

In 1920 he became independent of the Mission, and the Grenfell Foundation of Great Britain and Ireland was formed. He worked diligently for the organization, which had new staff and physicians to carry on the work as he lectured and raised funds. He began to accumulate honors, with a knighthood in 1927 and nine honorary degrees. His last few years were of increasing infirmity and depression following the death of his wife, Anne, who was his only confidant and who contributed significantly to his writings. He had a final heart attack after a dinner at his summer home in Charlotte, Vermont. His ashes were buried at St Anthony.

At the time of his death, he had authored thirty books and had founded six hospitals, seven nursing stations, fourteen industrial centers, three agricultural stations, twelve clothing distribution centers, orphanage–boarding schools, cooperative stores, and a cooperative sawmill. The Grenfell Mission continues to provide medical care to the people of northern Newfoundland and Labrador.

Bibliography

Primary: 1895. *Vikings of Today, or, Life and Medical Work among the Fishermen of Labrador* (London); 1919. *A Labrador Doctor: The Autobiography of Wilfred Thomason Grenfell MD (Oxon) C.M.G.* (Boston and New York).

Secondary: Rompkey, R., 1991. *Grenfell of Labrador: A Biography* (Toronto).

Jock Murray

GRIERSON, CECILIA   (b. Buenos Aires, Argentina, 22 November 1859; d. Buenos Aires, 10 April 1934), *obstetrics, kinesiology.*

Most widely known in Argentina as the first female physician to graduate from a South American university, Grierson made many concrete contributions to the practice of medicine in a wide variety of fields. Daughter of upper-class families of Scottish and Irish descent, Grierson acquired an early education in Buenos Aires's best schools. At the age of twenty-three, she enrolled at the medical school of the University of Buenos Aires. While still a medical student, she helped to organize the first school of nursing in Argentina in

1885; she directed it until 1913 (it was named for her in 1935). After graduation from medical school in 1889, with a specialization in obstetrics and gynecology, she took on a series of posts in city hospitals, beginning with a clinical practice in gynecology at the Hospital Ramos Mejìa. She played a leadership role in that field, founding both the National Obstetric Association in 1901 and the medical journal *Revista Obstètrica*. She taught obstetrics at the medical school, but within a few years began clinical work in kinesiology and emergency medicine at a number of Buenos Aires hospitals. She published numerous books and articles in all of her fields of practice, including pioneering works in Argentina on physical therapy.

Though Grierson took on the health and well-being of women and children as her primary concern, she did not limit herself to the treatment of them, as was commonly expected of female practitioners. Rather, she pioneered new techniques and practices in emergency medicine, kinesiology, and nursing. In emergency medicine, she promoted the teaching of novel techniques for treating accident victims, and in 1892 she founded the Argentine First Aid Society (Sociedad Argentina de Primeros Auxilios). She simultaneously engaged in teaching and research on physical therapy, resulting in her appointment to teach the first courses in kinesiology and physical therapy at the University of Buenos Aires medical school.

Grierson was active in the first generation of physicians who imported the French approach to pediatrics, related to eugenics and known as puericulture, at the turn of the century. Along with other physicians in this new field, she suggested more widespread efforts to train women in their early childbearing years in the latest scientific approaches to child care. Her particular emphasis in the field of puericulture was in improved nursing and training of women in modern medical techniques related to child health.

An active member of the Argentine socialist and feminist movements, she also pursued her lifelong interests in education of women and children, especially children with disabilities. Building on her early, premedical career in education, she founded the School for Home Economics in 1902 and taught the subject in girls' schools in Buenos Aires, simultaneously with her medical work. A leader in the struggle for basic women's rights in her country, Grierson presided over the First International Feminist Congress of Argentina, held in Buenos Aires in 1910, and contributed to efforts to reform the civil code to grant women the right to divorce and political rights. Later in life, she became a patron of the arts in Argentina, donating part of her considerable wealth to cultural and educational institutions. A collection of Grierson's papers are held at the Universidad de San Andrès in Buenos Aires.

Bibliography

Primary: 1889. *Histero-ovariotomías efectuadas en el hospital de mujeres desde 1883 a 1889* (Buenos Aires); 1897. *Masaje práctico con los ejercicios activos complementarios y un atlas de anatomía descriptiva y topográfica para enfermeras y masajistas* (Buenos Aires); 1909. *Primeros Auxilios en casos de accidentes y prevención contra las enfermedades infecciosas* (Buenos Aires); 1910. *Enseñanza de enfermeras y masajistas* (Buenos Aires).

Secondary: Taboada, Asunción, 1983. *Vida y obra de Cecilia Grierson* (Buenos Aires); Kohn Loncarica, Alfredo Guillermo, 1976. *Cecilia Grierson. Vida y obra de la primera médica argentina* (Buenos Aires).

Julia Rodriguez

GRIESINGER, WILHELM (b. Stuttgart, Germany, 29 July 1817; d. Berlin, Germany, 26 October 1869), *neurology, psychiatry, internal medicine.*

Born in Stuttgart, Griesinger was a leading figure of nineteenth-century neurology and psychiatry. Together with close friends of his youth, Carl Reinhold August Wunderlich und Wilhelm Roser, he shared many programmatic concepts for modern medical practice, based on the approaches of the natural sciences. Griesinger attended his first medical courses at the Eberhard-Karls-University of Tübingen (1834–37), where he was actively engaged in a students' fraternity. After some fraternity pranks, he was hauled before the university's rector and expelled from his 'alma mater'. He then registered at the University of Zurich (1837–38), where he studied with Johann Lukas Schönlein, whose clinical demonstrations Griesinger admired. He was later allowed to return to Tübingen, graduating MD in 1838.

Having completed his medical examination, Griesinger practiced medicine in Friedrichshafen, Lake Constance, and began an internship at the mental asylum of Winnenthal, where he wrote his famous handbook *Pathologie und Therapie der psychischen Krankheiten* (1845). After a journey to Vienna and Paris, Griesinger served as university assistant to Wunderlich. When he was made 'Privatdozent' at Tübingen, he collaborated with Wunderlich on the editorial board of *Archiv für physiologische Heilkunde* (1847–49). With this organ he could propagate his revolutionary ideas on modern psychiatry, based on pathological anatomy, experimental physiology, and 'rational' critique of clinical practice. In 1847 Griesinger was made 'Extraordinarius' for general pathology, material medica, and history of medicine. Although he was stimulated by the political ideals of the revolution of 1848 in his home country Wurttemberg, he left Tübingen on receiving a call for the chair in medical pathology and therapy at the Christian-Albrechts-University of Kiel.

Shortly after, the Vice-King of Egypt invited Griesinger to be his personal physician as well as director of the Cairo School of Medicine, where he stayed until 1852. On his return from Egypt, he was made director of the medical clinic at Tübingen (1854), before accepting the directorship of the Canton Hospital and mental asylum at Zurich (1860–64). Already in the second edition of his *Handbook* (1861),

Griesinger sided with the 'non-restraint-movement'. His overall achievements made him the choice for the 'Ordinarius' in psychiatry at Berlin Charité, when Karl August von Solbrig declined it. When Griesinger accepted the call, his patients were housed either in the wards of the medical clinic or, together with the syphilitics and sick prisoners, in a closed asylum. However, the board of directors offered Griesinger a neurological ward with the outpatients department at his disposal. During his stay in the Prussian capital (1865–68), Griesinger changed Berlin's psychiatric landscape. Following on from his dictum that mental illness is caused by pathological processes of the brain, he founded two major scientific platforms in Berlin, a society (the 'Berliner medicinisch-psychologische Gesellschaft', 1867) and a journal (the *Archiv für Psychiatrie und Nervenkrankheiten*, 1868). When Griesinger conceptualized his approach for psychiatric care, he focused on separated wards for neurological and psychiatric pathologies. This was an insult to traditional Charité politics, which had placed the neurology patients in the medical clinic—under the directorship of Friedrich Theodor Frerichs. A long struggle over the 'nerve material' ended in Griesinger's favor, mainly because of ministerial interference. He was also successful in implementing hospital care, in the middle of the capital, for acute patients in the Charité wards, while he established an 'agrarian colony' for chronic patients in the city's outskirts. Thus, Griesinger was a major driving force with regard to the institutionalization of distinct neurological and psychiatric clinics and the distribution of new concepts for home-based and community-oriented psychiatric care.

Bibliography

Primary: 1845. (English trans. of 2nd edn., 1867). *Die Pathologie und Therapie der psychischen Krankheiten* (Stuttgart); 1860. 'Diagnostische Bemerkungen über Hirnkrankheiten.' *Archiv für Heilkunde* 1: 51–85; 1872. *Gesammelte Abhandlungen* 2 vols. (Berlin).

Secondary: Hess, Volker, and Eric Engstrom, 2000. 'Neurologie an der Charité zwischen medizinischer und psychiatrischer Klinik' in Holdorff, Bernd, and Rolf Winau, eds., *Geschichte der Neurologie in Berlin* (Berlin and New York) pp. 99–110; Schmiedebach, Heinz-Peter, 1986. *Psychiatrie und Psychologie im Widerstreit. Die Auseinandersetzung in der Berliner medicinisch-psychologischen Gesellschaft (1867–1899)* (Husum); Wahrig-Schmidt, Bettina, 1985. *Der junge Griesinger im Spannungsfeld zwischen Philosophie und Physiologie* (Tübingen).

Frank W. Stahnisch

GRINKER, ROY RICHARD (b. Chicago, Illinois, USA, 2 August 1900; d. Chicago, 9 May 1993), *neurology, psychiatry.*

Grinker, son of Julius Grinker, a neurologist at the Postgraduate Hospital in Chicago, graduated from the University of Chicago in 1919 and received his MD from Rush Medical College in the same city in 1921. After a number of internships and further study at the universities of Vienna,

Zurich, Hamburg, and London, he was appointed in 1924 as instructor at the Northwestern University Medical School and in 1929 as assistant professor in neurology at the University of Chicago. With Percival Bailey, he combined neurology and neurosurgery in one division. Grinker was encouraged to establish a division of psychiatry, and from 1933 to 1935, he was on a two-year study-leave for further training, supported by a fellowship from the Rockefeller Foundation. Part of this time he spent in Vienna, where he was in psychoanalysis with Sigmund Freud. He also studied at the Maudsley Hospital in London and the Phipps Clinic at Johns Hopkins University. Upon his return, Grinker found conditions at the University of Chicago unfavorable to the development of psychiatry. In 1937 he returned to Michael Reese Hospital, where he became the head of the Division of Neurology and Psychiatry.

In 1942 Grinker enlisted in the U.S. Army Air Corps. With his former resident John P. Spiegel, he experimented in Tunisia with methods of short-term abreactive psychotherapy to treat soldiers suffering from war neurosis or shell shock. With the aid of a sodium pentothal injection, a dream-state was induced that aided the recovery and abreaction of traumatic memories (this treatment was called narcosynthesis). The experiences in North Africa are reflected in Grinker's two most influential books (coauthored with Spiegel), which investigate the reactions of normal individuals to extraordinary stresses, such as those of warfare. In 1943 he became the head of the Don Cesar Convalescent Hospital for the Air Corps in St Petersburg, Florida, where ex-servicemen suffering from war neuroses were treated and psychiatric training for army medical officers was provided.

Upon his return to Michael Reese Hospital, Grinker intended to organize a training program for psychiatrists. In 1951 the Institute for Psychosomatic and Psychiatric Research and Training was founded; Grinker was its director until his retirement in 1976, and he continued teaching there until 1989. Despite the fact that Grinker's institute was not affiliated with a university, it conducted influential research and trained a number of influential psychiatrists. It organized interdisciplinary research into psychosomatic medicine, schizophrenia, anxiety and stress, and borderline states. Grinker expanded the realm of psychoanalysis with his studies in dynamic psychiatry and his analysis of transactional processes in psychoanalysis and psychotherapy. In his later years, he aimed to develop a general theory of human behavior, integrating previous work in psychiatry and psychoanalysis with the findings of psychology, sociology, and anthropology.

In 1946, upon the founding of the National Institute of Mental Health, Grinker became a member of its Research Study Group. He was active in the Group for the Advancement of Psychiatry, which was founded in 1946 by a number of military psychiatrists with a broad psychoanalytic orientation intent on reforming the discipline. From 1956 to 1969, Grinker was chief editor of *AMA Archives of General*

Psychiatry. In 1972 he received the Distinguished Service Award of the American Psychiatric Association.

Bibliography

Primary: 1934. *Neurology* (Springfield, IL; several subsequent edns.); 1945. (with Spiegel, John P.) *War Neuroses* (Philadelphia); 1945. (with Spiegel, John P.) *Men under Stress* (Philadelphia); 1979. *Fifty Years in Psychiatry: A Living History* (Springfield, IL).

Secondary: Offer, Daniel, and Daniel X. Freedman, eds., 1972. *Modern Psychiatry and Clinical Research: Essays in Honor of Roy R. Grinker, Sr.* (New York); Weinberg, Jack, 1980. 'Roy R. Grinker, Sr: Some Biographical Notes.' *Journal of the American Academy of Psychoanalysis* 8(3): 441–449.

Hans Pols

GROSS, SAMUEL DAVID (b. Easton, Pennsylvania, USA, 8 July 1805; d. Philadelphia, Pennsylvania, USA, 14 February 1884), *urology, medical history, pathology, surgery.*

Gross, son of Philip and Juliana Gross, was the fifth of six children born to this farming family, which lived on a 200-acre farm, four miles from Easton, Pennsylvania. His great-grandfather had emigrated from the Lower Palatinate of Germany in the 1600s. The family would have been considered Pennsylvania Dutch (*Deutch* until World War I) and spoke a dialect of German. Although this was Mennonite country, his mother was a strict Lutheran, as was he, along with his two sisters and three brothers.

His early education was obtained in the fabled one-room schoolhouse, where he first learned English at the age of twelve. By the age of six, he had already decided upon a career in medicine, as he later recalled in his autobiography. Recognizing the limitations of his education, he read everything he could obtain, studying English, Latin, and German. He spent several months at an academy in nearby Wilkes-Barre and then at Lawrenceville Academy, New Jersey. In 1824 he started a medical apprenticeship, but he was disappointed in the two local physicians he met. The third was Joseph K. Swift, a University of Pennsylvania graduate, to whom he paid $300 in advance for a three-year period. Still not pleased with his education, he prevailed upon Swift in 1826 to give him a letter of introduction to the University. Once in Philadelphia, he found George McClellan, who was one of the founders of Jefferson Medical College in 1824, and Gross became his private pupil for eighteen months, before enrolling at Jefferson and graduating with the Class of 1828. His thesis was 'The Nature and Treatment of Cataract'.

Gross entered private practice in Philadelphia near Jefferson and supported himself by translating foreign textbooks such as Bayle and Holland's *Manual of Practical Obstetrics* and Tavernier's *Operative Surgery* into English. Not only did this give him a good grounding in the medical literature, but it also stimulated his writing ability, which enabled him to publish numerous textbooks and many papers. After two years in practice, Gross still could not make enough to sup-

port his new wife and stepson, so he returned to Easton. His practice grew rapidly, but he wanted more intellectual pursuits. He turned a small shed near his home into an anatomy laboratory and gathered material for a textbook of descriptive anatomy, using English rather than Latin, but this project never reached fruition. During this time, he did publish *The Anatomy, Physiology, and Diseases of Bones and Joints* (1830).

In 1833 he moved his family to Cincinnati, Ohio, to become demonstrator in anatomy in the Medical College of Ohio. Two years later, this school closed, and he was appointed professor of pathological anatomy in the medical department of Cincinnati College. He conducted innumerable postmortems, making extensive notes about his findings. This culminated in his producing *Elements of Pathological Anatomy* (1839), the first significant American book on the subject. The text went through two more editions (1845, 1857), the third edition containing histopathologic descriptions by Jacob Mendes Da Costa. The work made Gross an international celebrity. He also undertook studies in experimental and forensic pathology. When he could not offer a good explanation about a strangulation case, he devised several experiments using rabbits in order to understand the physiology involved. From this experience, he published guidelines for medical examiners relating to strangulation (1836).

When this medical school closed in 1839, Gross was offered positions in New Orleans and in Charlottesville, Virginia. The next year, he accepted the professorship of surgery at the Louisville (Kentucky) Institute of Medicine, which became a part of the University of Louisville. He remained in this city until 1856, save for 1850, when he served as professor of surgery at the University of New York. He developed a successful practice in Louisville and continued his experimental studies. These included determining the maximum size an intestinal wound can be in dogs before the development of peritonitis (less than one-half inch) and culminated in the book *Wounds of the Intestines* (1843).

The University of Pennsylvania offered him a professorship in 1855, but he declined. The next year, upon the death of Thomas Dent Mutter, Jefferson invited Gross to become professor of surgery. Gross accepted and had the distinction of being the first alumnus to achieve a professorship at Jefferson.

Gross became the most prominent American surgeon during his twenty-six years in Philadelphia. His reputation grew enormously, and his operating room was memorialized in the famous painting by Thomas Eakins. In 1859 he published *A System of Surgery; Pathological, Diagnostic, Therapeutic and Operative,* a two-volume work of 2,360 pages. He incorporated histopathologic studies here, also, as well as discussions about malignancies and tuberculosis.

'The Nestor of Surgery' distinguished himself as a urologist with his text *Practical Treatise on the Diseases, Injuries, and Malformations of the Urinary Bladder, the Prostate Gland and the Urethra* (1851). Gross also became the first American trauma surgeon and was well-known as a military surgeon for his work during the American Civil War (1861–65). His *A Manual of Military Surgery* appeared in Philadelphia in 1862 and was pirated by a Confederate publisher the same year. This book also was translated into German and Japanese.

How could one man be so productive and so prolific? 'I generally spent from 5 to 8 hours per day upon my manuscript, subject of course to frequent and sometimes annoying interruptions by patients', he wrote in his autobiography. He found time to write *A Century of American Medicine* for the American Centennial celebration in 1876 and *A Memoir of John Hunter and his Pupils* for the First Annual Oration for the Philadelphia Academy of Surgery, which he founded (1881).

Gross was founder and president of the Kentucky Medical Society, Philadelphia Pathological Society, Jefferson Medical Alumni Association, the Philadelphia Academy of Surgery, and the American Surgical Association. He served as president of the American Philosophical Society and the American Academy of Sciences. His membership in foreign societies and his honorary degrees make for a lengthy list, including honors from the universities of Pennsylvania, Oxford, Cambridge, and Edinburgh. He was an avid book collector and donated his extant library to the College of Physicians of Philadelphia; two thousand of his books had been destroyed by fire at the University of Louisville.

Bibliography

Primary: 1857. *Elements of Pathological Anatomy* (Philadelphia); 1861. *A Manual of Military Surgery; or Hints on the Emergencies of Field, Camp and Hospital Practice. Illustrated with Wood Cuts* (Philadelphia); 1887. (with Gross, S. W., et al.) *Autobiography of Samuel D. Gross, M.D. Emeritus Professor of Surgery in the Jefferson Medical College of Philadelphia* (Philadelphia).

Secondary: Malkin, H. M., 2001. 'Samuel David Gross—America's First Pathologist.' *Ann. Diagn. Pathol.* 5(2): 121–127; Mullins, R. J., and D. D. Trunkey, 1990. 'Samuel D. Gross: Pioneer Academic Trauma Surgeon of 19th Century America.' *J. Trauma* 30(5): 528–538; Wagner, F. B., 1989. *Thomas Jefferson University: Tradition and Heritage.* (Philadelphia); Wagner, F. B., 1988. *Eakins's Gross Clinic: The Acme of Medicine in Art.* (Düsseldorf); Wagner, F. B., Jr., 1981. 'Revisit of Samuel D. Gross, M.D.' *Surg. Gynecol. Obstet.* 152(5): 663–674; Da Costa, J. M., 1884. *Biographical Sketch of Professor Samuel D. Gross.* (Philadelphia); *DAMB.*

Lawrence Charles Parish

GROTJAHN, ALFRED (b. Schladen, Germany, 25 November 1869; d. Berlin, Germany, 4 September 1931), *social hygiene.*

Grotjahn's father was a rural medical practitioner, whose morphine addiction and violent temper, along with the early death of Grotjahn's mother and the manic depression of his stepmother, made Grotjahn's childhood difficult. He attended a succession of schools, and while at *Gymnasium* in

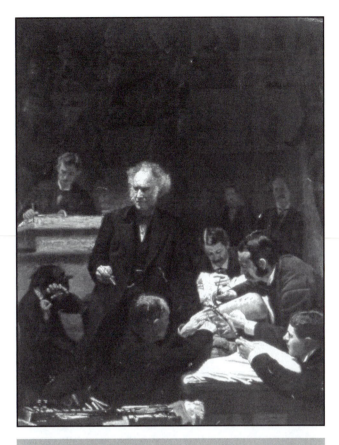

Gross pauses, scalpel in hand, to address his students during an anatomical dissection. Photomechanical reproduction of a painting by Thomas Eakins entitled *The Gross Clinic, 1875.* Courtesy of the National Library of Medicine.

Wolfenbüttel, he met Albert Südekum (1871–1944), later member of parliament for the Social Democratic Party (SPD) and minister of finance in Prussia, a lifelong friend. Together they started to attend political meetings. Grotjahn would have liked to study economics or become a journalist, but his father disapproved. In 1890 he enrolled in medicine at Greifswald and continued his studies at Leipzig, Kiel, and finally Berlin. In Leipzig, in addition to preclinical courses, he attended lectures in economics. In Kiel he combined studies in the clinical subjects with seminars held by the sociologist Ferdinand Tönnies (1855–1936). Inspired by Tönnies, Südekum and Grotjahn sought contact with the local labor movement. In Berlin, Grotjahn intensified his extracurricular activities, joining both a circle of socialist students, which could have led to exclusion from the university, and an association of social science students, which brought him into contact with the professor of economics Gustav Schmoller (1838–1917). A plan to study the statistical relationship between social class and venereal disease failed. Instead, in 1893 Grotjahn gained his MD with a more conventional dissertation. He passed his state exam in 1895–96.

Grotjahn (like other pioneers of social hygiene) worked as a general practitioner in Berlin for almost twenty years, during which time his political outlook became less radical and he sympathized with Naumann's liberals. Meanwhile he studied economics with Schmoller, graduating in 1903. Grotjahn developed his concepts in opposition to what he characterized as 'physical-biological hygiene'. He looked at nutrition and alcoholism, but was also concerned about the declining birthrate and the inheritance of mental and physical problems. Especially in his later writings, it was difficult to demarcate social from racial hygiene. He published prolifically and cofounded and edited several journals. He was also active in a number of associations that dominated debates over medicine and health in early twentieth-century Germany, such as the Society for Social Medicine, Hygiene, and Medical Statistics and the Society to Combat Venereal Disease, as well as the Society for Racial Hygiene and the *Leipziger Verband*. In 1912 he published his textbook, *Soziale Pathologie*, and with Ignaz Kaup (1870–1944), a *Handbook of Social Hygiene*. In 1914, finally, supported by Schmoller and the Berlin professor of hygiene Carl Flügge (1847–1923), and against the resistance of other members of the medical faculty, he attained his Habilitation.

In 1915 an appointment as head of the new municipal department of social hygiene allowed Grotjahn to retire from his practice. In 1921, as a replacement candidate for the SPD, he won a seat in the German parliament. Until the end of his mandate in 1924, he contributed to a number of health and social policy initiatives. He is credited with codesigning the SPD health program of 1922, which called for a socialization of medical services. In the final years of his life, Grotjahn came to sympathize with the lifestyle reform movement. In 1920, after much controversy between medical faculty and Prussian government, Grotjahn was appointed professor of social hygiene at Berlin University, but without funds to run an institute. However, his influence was considerable. Grotjahn taught both at the university and at academies for medical officers of health, and whereas some of his students came to hold influential positions during the Nazi dictatorship, many others emigrated and implemented some of his ideas abroad. After World War II, while social hygienists in the GDR claimed Grotjahn's heritage, Grotjahn students also continued to exert influence in the Federal Republic.

Bibliography

Primary: 1912. *Soziale Pathologie* (Berlin); 1932. *Erlebtes und Erstrebtes* (Berlin).

Secondary: Hubenstorf, Michael, 1987. 'Alfred Grotjahn' in Treue, Wilhelm, and Rolf Winau, eds., *Berlinische Lebensbilder: Ärzte* (Berlin); Weindling, Paul, 1987. 'Medical Practice in Imperial Berlin: The Casebook of Alfred Grotjahn.' *Bulletin of the History of Medicine* 61: 397–410; Tutzke, Dietrich, 1979. *Alfred Grotjahn* (Leipzig).

Carsten Timmermann

GUIDO DA VIGEVANO (b. Pavia, Italy, *c.* 1280; d. Paris, France, 1349), *anatomy*.

Guido was born in Pavia to a noble family from nearby Vigevano, and he probably studied medicine at the University of Bologna. He became a member of the retinue of the Holy Roman Emperor Henry VII in 1310 when the latter visited Italy to firm up support. The emperor's untimely death in 1313 curtailed Guido's appointment, and he returned to Pavia to practice medicine for a time. Sometime after 1323, Guido joined the French royal court, first as physician to Marie of Luxemburg, a relative of Emperor Henry VII and wife of King Charles IV of France. Still later, he became physician to another French queen, Jeanne of Burgundy, wife of King Phillip VI (r. 1328–50).

While serving at court, Guido was swept up in a project for a new crusade, and in 1335 he wrote a treatise titled *Texaurus Regis Francie*, the *Treasury of the King of France for the acquisition of the Holy Land from beyond the sea, and also for the health of his body and the prolongation of his life, together with care against poison*. Guido advised his king on siegecraft and included a regimen for the king's health while on campaign, as well as a small treatise outlining his original experiments on aconite (monkshood) poisoning.

The siegecraft portion of the treatise is illustrated and ranges from extremely practical suggestions (ladders and towers made of prefabricated, interchangeable parts) to the fantastic (windmill-powered assault 'tanks'). Modern commentators have frequently praised Guido's detailed knowledge of mechanical technologies such as wagons and mills, even as they have criticized his fantasies.

Guido's regimen of health was based on the Galenic 'nonnaturals', six elements that make up the daily regimen of the patient. Taken together, they represented a counsel of moderation and balance, adapted in this case to the special needs of an 'old man' (King Phillip was in his forties!) on a military campaign. The additional medical material concerned cramps and aconite poisoning, for which Guido provided his own—self-tested—remedy.

The crusade never got past the planning stage, and ten years later, Guido produced a second, longer treatise, *Liber notabilium*. Again, it is divided into three parts, a book of extracts from the Latin Galen as known to the middle ages; another regimen of health very similar to the 1335 treatise, but without the emphasis on military campaigns; and an illustrated *Anatomia*.

The last was modeled on the famous anatomy of Mondino de' Liuzzi (*c.* 1270–1326), and like his predecessor's work, Guido's work seems to have been based at least in part on dissections of human cadavers. Commentators have noted that Guido's anatomy displays a certain independence of spirit. Italian physicians were the only persons who practiced human dissection in the fourteenth century, and Guido may have introduced the practice to France. He certainly insisted on the value of anatomy in the training of physicians. Guido's drawings are considerably improved over those of his

French contemporary, the surgeon Henry of Mondeville (d. c. 1320). One innovation in representation is that several of Guido's drawings have parchment flaps that fold; closed, they present the surface of the cadaver's skin; open, they reveal the organs beneath the surface.

Guido da Vigevano disappeared from court records in 1349. It has been speculated that he died in the plague epidemic that ravaged Paris between 1348 and 1350.

Bibliography

Primary: 1926. (Wickersheimer, E., ed.) *Anatomies de Mondino dei Luzzi et de Guido de Vigevano* (Paris); 1993. (Ostuni, G., ed.) *Le Macchine del Re: Il Texaurus Regis Francie di Guido da Vigenvano* (Vigevano).

Secondary: Hall, B. S., 1982. 'Guido da Vigevano's *Texaurus Regis Francie*, 1335' in Eamon, W., ed., *Studies on Medieval Fachliteratur* (Brussels); Hall, A. R., 1976. 'Guido's *Texaurus*, 1335' in Hall, B. S., and D. C. West, eds., *On Pre-Modern Technology and Science: Essays in Honor of Lynn White, Jr.* (Los Angeles); Gille, B., 1966. *Renaissance Engineers* (London).

Bert Hall

GUILERA MOLAS, LLUÍS GONZAGA   (b. El Prat de Llobregat, Barcelona, Spain, 10 September 1896; d. Barcelona, Spain, 5 June 1969), *radiotherapy, oncology.*

Guilera—histologist, radiotherapist, and gynecologist—made a major contribution to the development of oncology in Catalonia (Spain) as director of the Cancer Pavilion at the Santa Cruz y San Pablo Hospital (SCSPH), an important hospital in the Catalan network of charitable medical care. He studied Medicine in Barcelona and obtained his PhD in Madrid (1919) with a focus on histology.

In 1917, in collaboration with Enrique Ribas Ribas, Guilera managed to buy one mg of radium in order to create a radiotherapy dispensary as part of the Gynecology Service headed by Adolfo Pujol Brull in the SCSPH. This dispensary was the seedbed of the SCSPH Cancer Pavilion.

At this time, he was funded by the official Board for Advanced Studies and Scientific Research to travel to Swiss clinics to investigate radium and the effects of x-rays on ovaries and gynecological cancer. He was also visiting researcher at radiology clinics in Berlin, Munich, Erlangen, and Vienna.

From 1921 to 1929, he was in charge of the Radiotherapy Section at the Gynecology Department at the SCSPH, where he was able to increase the amount of radium available for therapeutic purposes thanks to charitable donations. In 1929 he obtained the chair of histology at the University of Granada although he never took up the position. In his private laboratory he researched on experimental cancer, publishing his studies and presenting papers at scientific meetings, such as those of the Catalonian Society of Biology.

In 1930 the radiotherapy section of the gynecology department became the cancer department of the SCSPH.

The establishment of this Department within a dedicated Cancer Pavilion was an organizational innovation in Spanish hospitals and led to the full recognition of oncology as a medical specialty, also encouraging collaborative work between surgeons and radiotherapists. The building and opening of the Cancer Pavilion was financed by charitable donations—originally intended for a cancer hospice—and by the Catalan Provincial Government. Guilera was head of the oncology department at the SCSPH and professor of histology and pathology at the University of Barcelona. In 1936 he was secretary of the charitable organization the Catalan League against Cancer. He also edited various medical journals such as the *Radiología Cancerológica-Revista Ibérica de Ciencias Médicas*, which became the journal of the Spanish Society of Medical Radiology and Electrology in 1946. Soon after the Spanish Civil War, Guilera moved to the University of Seville as professor of histology (1941–43), although he returned to Barcelona to his former position at the SCSPH until retirement in 1966.

Among Guilera's publications, his papers on radiotherapy outcomes in cancer patients deserve special mention. His studies reveal a more rigorous scientific approach to cancer therapy than was usual in Spain at that time. In the debate on cancer campaign policy in 1934, during the Second Spanish Republic, Guilera called for the state to support a wide clinical program to treat cancer patients rather than only fund research on the causes of the disease. As a result of his experience with continental European clinics, he placed special emphasis on the use of radiotherapy and promoted the consolidation of oncology as a medical specialty.

Bibliography

Primary: 1928. *Diagnòstic i tractament del càncer de l'uter* (Barcelona); 1935. *La lluita contra el càncer à Catalunya* (Barcelona).

Secondary: Medina-Doménech, Rosa María, 1996. *¿Curar el cáncer? Los orígenes de la Radioterapia en el primer tercio del siglo XX* (Granada); Calbet i Camarasa, Josep Maria, and Jacint Corbella i Corbella, 1981. *Diccionari Biogràfic de Metges Catalans* vol. 2 (Barcelona) p. 69.

Rosa Maria Medina-Doménech

GUILLAIN, GEORGES   (b. Rouen, France, 3 March 1876; d. Paris, France, 29 June 1961), *neurology.*

Of high bourgeoisie origins, Guillain studied first in Rouen. He then came to Paris, where he ascended the ranks of the university medical faculty and hospital hierarchy with distinction. He was placed first in the competition for internship (1898), and he served as chief resident (1902–05), hospital physician (1906), and assistant professor (1910). A student of Pierre Marie, Guillain's early work combined the anatomical-clinical tradition with a physiological approach in studies on the ventral cortico-spinal tract, Turck's tract, the internal capsule, the red nucleus, and the olivary nucleus.

During World War I, Guillain was chief of an army neurological unit. His *Travaux Neurologiques de Guerre* (1920) collected studies published in collaboration with his assistant, J-A. Barré, who had studied under Babinski. Outstanding among these was a 1916 study identifying an acute peripheral polyneuropathy with characteristic findings in the cerebro-spinal fluid, later to be named Guillain-Barré syndrome. In 1936 Guillain's definitive study of the syndrome surveyed a vast literature. In 1953 he published a synthesis including nineteen unpublished cases from his own practice. Here he identified forms of the disease affecting the cranial nerves and higher centers that could lead to death.

After the war Guillain pursued research begun with Barré into neurological diagnosis and described the nasopalpebral and pubic reflexes. His work on the cerebro-spinal fluid dominated this phase of his career, especially the colloidal-benzoin reaction (1920), which remained of primary diagnostic significance in multiple sclerosis and other diseases until the appearance of electrophoresis of proteins in the 1960s.

In 1923 Guillain succeeded Pierre Marie to the chair of neurology at the Salpêtrière, a position he would hold until 1947. Although he faithfully followed the traditions and practices put in place by Charcot, he made institutional renovations, adding an Institute of Neurobiology, then a laboratory of electroencephalography, and in 1942 a neurosurgical unit under his direction. With an entourage of distinguished colleagues—Ivan Bertrand, Alajouanine, Garcin, Mollaret, and many others—constituting a leading center of neurology, Guillain's research covered the entire field of organic disorders, leaving aside psychopathology, without neglecting his teaching responsibilities. His eight volumes of *Etudes Neurologiques* (1924–39) united his most important current and older studies. Two examples drawn from this huge work illustrate its rigorous methodology. In a series of publications on *palatal myoclonus* (1930–33), Guillain elaborated the specific symptomatology and, by means of analysis of the neuropathological lesions, was able to elucidate the physiopathological mechanism of this disorder.

Another example was Guillain's synthesis under the designation *spino-cerebellar hereditary degeneration* (1936, vol. 7) of three neurological entities (Friedrich's ataxia, cerebellar hereditary ataxia, and Stumpell-Lorrain familial spastic paraplegia) previously considered to be separate and distinct diseases. He proved that all displayed a pyramidal syndrome either alone or associated with other features.

Then, when he had managed to re-establish the supremacy of the Salpêtrière school without offending such powerful personalities as André-Thomas and Jean Lhermitte, World War II once again dispersed Guillain's colleagues. During the Occupation, he was able to return to work in progress and reorganize his teaching and research. Despite being cut off from the rest of the world, Guillain succeeded in maintaining the international stature of French neurology.

In 1947 Guillain's student Théophile Alajouanine succeeded to his chair of neurology. Guillain's reception into the Academy of Sciences in 1951 marked official recognition of his reputation as an extraordinary scientific personage. After revising his analysis of the Guillain-Barré syndrome in 1951, Guillain turned to the project of a biography of Charcot, which became the first book-length study of the founder of French neurology, whose students had been Guillain's own mentors and whose tradition he carried on.

Bibliography

Primary: 1920. *Travaux neurologiques de guerre* (Paris); 1924–39. *Etudes neurologiques* 8 vols. (Paris); 1955. *Charcot* (Paris and New York).

Secondary: Bonduelle, Michel, 1997. 'Georges Guillain.' *Revue Neurologique* 153: 163–171.

Michel Bonduelle

GUISLAIN, JOSEPH (b. Ghent, Belgium, 2 February 1797; d. Ghent, 1 April 1860), *psychiatry*.

Guislain, who was born into a wealthy family, took his MD degree in 1819 at Ghent University. Having familiarized himself early on with the ideas of the famous French reformer Philippe Pinel, he made his name with the prize-winning essay *Traité sur l'aliénation mentale et sur les hospices des aliénés*, published in 1826. Two years later, he was appointed chief physician of the two mental asylums of Ghent on the intercession of the canon Petrus-Joseph Triest (1760–1836). Together, they transformed the mental health system of Ghent, which was to become a model for all Belgium. In 1835 Guislain was appointed professor of physiology at Ghent University. In 1841 he became a member of a governmental committee that was expected to report on the living conditions in the Belgian lunatic asylums. It took until 1850 before the recommendations of the committee (made in 1842) were transformed into legislation. In 1852 the town council of Ghent—to which Guislain was elected—decided to build a model institution for the mentally ill.

When Guislain was appointed chief physician of the asylums of Ghent, the mentally disturbed were generally in a dire condition. Guislain had set his mind to improving the situation. He wanted to humanize mental health care by medicalizing it. He was convinced that improvement and even cure of the mentally disturbed was possible, and he did everything to realize the preconditions for it. Following such people as Tuke, Pinel, Esquirol, Heinroth, Reil, and Schroeder van der Kolk, he propagated the principles of 'moral treatment'. According to Guislain—who founded his psychiatric system on vitalistic principles—mental illness is essentially a disturbed frame of mind. This is not to say, however, that he disregarded somatic factors. He was a follower of Brown, to whom the concepts of sthenia and asthenia were of crucial importance. Hence, in therapeutics, Guislain advocated either calming down (comfort, visits, leave) or stimulation (physical exercise such as working, walking, or horseback riding; stimulation of the mental capacities by painting, reading, or making music). He agreed with Conolly that there was to be no—or at least very limited—restraint. When the etiology was thought to be a physical one, therapeutics included medicaments such as opium, digitalis, or quinine sulfate; purgatives such as hellebore, rhubarb, or aloe; hot and cold baths; cauterium actuale; and, finally, surgical intervention (such as castration or extirpation of the ovaries).

With regard to institutional care, Guislain established the fact that the Belgian asylums were lacking in organization. In the regulation he drafted in 1829, he stressed the need for a humane treatment of the mentally ill, taking good care of food and hygiene. Guards and caretakers were expected to observe their patients rather than constraining them. He tried to generalize what he had accomplished locally by putting pressure on the national government to enforce legislation for all Belgium. The law of 1850 that settled the legal position of the mentally disturbed was to a great extent his doing. A next step was to bring housing in line with modern ideas and legislation. Guislain's views found an architectonic expression in the 1850s, when a new asylum was built in Ghent, designed by Adolphe Pauli. The Ghent asylum—completed in 1857—was generally considered a model institution, attracting interested visitors from all over the world.

Bibliography

Primary: 1826. *Traité sur l'aliénation mentale et sur les hospices des aliénés* 2 vols. (Amsterdam); 1833. *Traité sur les phrénopathies ou doctrine nouvelle des maladies mentales* (Brussels); 1846. *La nature considérée comme force instinctive des organes* (Brussels); 1852. *Leçons orales sur les phrénopathies ou traité théorique et pratique des maladies mentales* 3 vols. (Ghent).

Secondary: Staeyen, E. A. van, 1993. 'Oorzaken van krankzinnigheid volgens J. Guislain (1797–1860).' *Psychiatrie en verpleging* 69: 184–192; Staeyen, E. A. van, 1987. 'Dr. Joseph Guislain (1797–1860), Vitalist.' *Psychiatrie en verpleging* 63: 120–129, 175–182; Schmidt, F. J. M., 1985. *Die Entwicklung der Irrenpflege in den Niederlanden. Vom Tollhaus bis zur gesetzlich anerkannten Irrenanstalt* (Herzogenrath).

Eduard A. van Staeyen

GUITERAS GENER, JUAN (b. Matanzas, Cuba, 4 January 1852; d. Matanzas, Cuba, 28 October 1925), *tropical medicine, public health.*

Guiteras was born into a family of accomplished writers and educators. His father, Eusebio, was a teacher, novelist, and poet, and his brother Pedro José was a historian of Cuba. Two other brothers, Antonio and Eusebio Jr., were writers and educators, and a final brother, Gregorio, took up the medical profession along with Juan. In 1869, one year after the beginning of Cuba's Ten Years' War, the family left for Philadelphia. Juan had completed one year of medical school at the University of Havana, and upon his arrival in the United States, he enrolled in the University of Pennsylvania's medical school, where he received his degree in 1873.

After working as an intern at the Philadelphia Hospital for six years (1873–79), Guiteras joined the Marine Hospital Service as a researcher of yellow fever epidemics in the United States, thus beginning a long engagement with both the U.S. military and epidemiology. That same year, Guiteras was named to a commission to study yellow fever in Cuba, with specific instructions to study sanitation conditions in the ports of Matanzas and Havana in the interest of preventing the spread of yellow fever and other contagious diseases. During this period he also published a number of studies on yellow fever and other diseases, in both Cuban and American journals, including the *Therapeutic Gazette*, the *Medical News of Philadelphia*, and the *Annals of the Academy of Science in Havana*.

In 1900, after serving as professor of medicine at the University of Charleston (1885–89) and as professor of pathology at the University of Pennsylvania (1889–1900), Guiteras went to Santiago, Cuba, to join the United States Provisional Government as yellow fever specialist and commander of the Medical Corps of the U.S. Army. After several months in Santiago, he was named professor at the University of Havana, where he taught general pathology and intertropical pathology. This latter subject, created by Guiteras, was the first of its kind in the Americas. In 1901 he was named director of Las Animas Hospital, a post he held for twenty years. During this period he also served in the Cuban government, as president of the Commission on Infectious Diseases and Director of Sanitation. He left the directorship of Las Animas Hospital in 1921 when President Alfredo Zayas named him Secretary of Health and Sanitation. This appointment did not last long, ending as it did with his departure in 1922. Guiteras died in his native city of Matanzas three years later.

Guiteras collaborated with and supported Carlos Finlay in his efforts to eradicate yellow fever and to demonstrate Finlay's theory of transmission through the mosquito. Soon after joining the provisional government, he participated in the research and subsequent eradication campaign, led by Finlay and U.S. Army Surgeon General William Gorgas, which definitively eliminated yellow fever in Cuba in late 1901.

As an epidemiologist, Guiteras was involved in controlling a brief outbreak of bubonic plague in Cuba in 1912. His work was noted by the Rockefeller Foundation, which invited him in 1916 to join William Gorgas and other physicians on a tour of the Caribbean, including Panama, Ecuador, Peru, Colombia, Venezuela, Brazil, Curacao, Puerto Rico, Trinidad, and Barbados, for the purpose of definitively eradicating yellow fever. Four years later, in 1920, he was again commissioned by the Rockefeller Foundation, along with Gorgas, on a yellow fever campaign to Africa, which included visits to Nigeria, Dahomey, the Congo (French and Belgian), Senegal, and Canary Islands.

Bibliography

Primary: 1904. *Prophylaxis against Yellow Fever* (Washington, DC); 1911. *Contra el cólera asiático: Instrucciones populares* (Havana); 1914. *La peste bubónica en Cuba* (Havana).

Secondary: Roig de Leuchsenring, Emilio, 1965. *Médicos y medicina en Cuba: Historia, biografía, costumbrismo* (Havana); Ministerio de Salubridad y Asistencia Social, 1951. *Centenario del nacimiento del Dr. Juan Guiteras Gener* (Havana); Rodríguez Expósito, César, 1947. *Dr. Juan Guiteras, apunte biográfico* (Havana).

Alejandra Bronfman

GULL, WILLIAM WITHEY (b. Colchester, Essex, England, 31 December 1816; d. London, England, 29 January 1890), *medicine.*

The youngest of six children of John Gull, barge owner and wharfinger, Gull was brought up by his mother from the age of ten after his father died of cholera. He started as a schoolmaster's assistant in Lewes, Sussex, but in 1837 William Harrison, the treasurer at Guy's Hospital, London, offered him an apprenticeship there. Thus, he was able to attend lectures for medical students and graduate in 1841, one of the first graduates from the then-new University of London. Gull was appointed a lecturer at the medical school in 1843, became assistant physician to Guy's hospital in 1851, and rose to full physician five years later.

Gull was noted for his unhurried thoroughness, diagnostic flair, and interest in his patients: 'his manner was the same in a hospital ward as in a palace.' Skeptical about the indiscriminate use of drugs of unproven worth, he stated that 'medicine acts best when there is a tendency to get well' and wrote a paper on acute rheumatism treated by mint water. With a deep interest in the training of nurses, he maintained that, though nursing was sometimes a trade and sometimes a profession, it ought to be a religion. He was the first to describe several important conditions: paroxysmal hemoglobinuria, thrombosis of the mesenteric artery, and myxedema. The last condition he documented was a cretinoid state in five women that was associated with obesity and sluggishness, and though he could not identify its cause, when Charles Hilton Fagge (1838–83) showed that it was due to thyroid disease, Gull generously paid tribute to his colleague.

Gull is also claimed to have been the first to describe anorexia nervosa. In 1868, in an address to the British Medical Association, he briefly mentioned 'young women emaciated to the last degree through hysterical apepsia'. Five years later, a French psychiatrist, Charles Lasègue (1816–83), published 'De l'anorexie hysterique' (1873), a major article describing eight women studied during the siege of Paris in the Franco-Prussian war. Rapidly translated into English and published a month before Gull gave two lectures on the condition, Gull referred to Lasègue's work as 'confirmatory'. Nevertheless, any dispute about priority soon fizzled out, and the condition itself became firmly labeled as anorexia nervosa.

Though he never published a book, Gull wrote extensively—including about rheumatic fever, paraplegia, tabes dorsalis, nephritis, brain abscess, and cholera (drawing up a report on the last for the RCP in 1854). He held every office at the RCP except that of President, and in 1871, after attending the Prince of Wales, who was seriously ill with typhoid fever at Sandringham, he was created a baronet. This connection with the court was to surface many years later, when the extraordinary claim was made that Gull had had a major role in the Jack the Ripper murders of prostitutes in the East End of London—given that the Royal family had had to remove any evidence of Prince Albert Victor (the future Edward VII) consorting with streetwalkers.

Gull acquired a large practice, leaving over £344,000 at his death. His career showed that several virtues could be combined in one person: a smiling public persona with a keen interest in all classes of people, together with broad outside interests (he was an expert linguist and a keen naturalist). He represented the best of observational medicine in the Victorian era, combining this with an open mind and humility: 'However clever you are', he maintained, 'you are sure to overlook phthisis, syphilis, and itch.'

Bibliography

Primary: 1894–1896. (Acland, Theodore Dyke, ed. and arr.) *A collection of the published writings of William Withey Gull* (London).

Secondary: Vandereycken, W., and R. Van Deth, 1994. *From Fasting Saints to Anorexic Girls* (London); *Munk's Roll; Oxford DNB.*

Stephen Lock

GULLSTRAND, ALLVAR (b. Landskrona, Sweden, 5 June 1862; d. Stockholm, Sweden, 28 July 1930), *physiological optics, ophthalmology.*

Gullstrand was born in the town of Landskrona in the south of Sweden, where his father, Pehr Alfred Gullstrand, married to Sofia Mathilda Korsell, worked as a medical officer. The family moved to Jönköping, where Gullstrand graduated from high school in 1880. He showed a particular bent for mathematics and dedicated his spare time to analytical geometry and differential and integral calculus. Pehr Gullstrand, who was familiar with the use of the ophthalmoscope, recognized the mathematical talent of his son and advised him to study to become an oculist. Gullstrand fulfilled his father's wish. After graduating in medicine in Uppsala 1884, he went to Vienna, accompanied by his wife Signe Christina Breitholtz, to study the elements of ophthalmology.

Back in Sweden, Gullstrand pursued his scientific path with remarkable consequence. He became licentiat in medicine (1888) in Stockholm, worked as an amanuensis in the eye clinic at the Serafimer hospital, and practiced as an eye specialist at the polyclinic for eye diseases. He defended his doctoral thesis in Uppsala in 1890 and was appointed lecturer in ophthalmology at the Karolinska Institute in Stockholm in 1891. In 1894 he returned to Uppsala, where he was appointed the first professor of ophthalmology. Gullstrand crowned his career with the Nobel Prize in Physiology or Medicine in 1911 and with a personal professorship in physical and physiological optics at Uppsala University in 1914.

Gullstrand's research concerned the geometry of optics, a subject that required a profound knowledge of mathematics and physics. Already in his dissertation on the problems of astigmatism, Gullstrand had demonstrated his exceptional mental acumen. His analysis of the nature of the pencil of rays that forms the image on the retina was grounded on derivations from equations that were obtained from the laws of the refraction of light. Through these equations, Gullstrand was able to estimate the degree of asymmetry with which light enters the eye. He pursued his dioptrical research throughout the 1890s. In a number of studies published in the early 1900s, Gullstrand delivered a definitive theory on the refraction in the eye. His investigations gave rise to a new understanding of the optical representation. Gullstrand showed that the lens of the eye during accommodation not only deforms on the surface, but also changes in the layer. Gullstrand's work contributed considerably to the knowledge of the eye's accommodation.

Although he mainly was occupied with problems of a high level of mathematical abstraction, Gullstrand also took interest in the practical side of optics. He contributed to the improvement of glasses and designed a number of optical instruments, such as the slit lamp, which enabled examinations of the living eye without disturbing light reflections. His reflex-free ophthalmoscope should also be mentioned. With the aid of this instrument, eye doctors could make far better examinations of the bottom of the eye. Combined with proper lenses, these techniques could also be used in order to study the inner structures of the living eye in microscopic magnitude.

Gullstrand embodied the spirit of scientific medicine, with its firm belief in the importance of specialization, its valuation of physics, and its technical inventiveness. Physiological optics, the subject that Gullstrand came to master, developed rapidly in the latter half of the nineteenth century. As a ramification of laboratory physiology, it appropriated an experimental ideal. Its theories, methods, and instruments, however, soon spread from the laboratories to eye clinics. At the turn of the century, ophthalmology had become a discipline of its own. Gullstrand's career mirrored this development.

Bibliography

Primary: 1890. *Bidrag till astigmatismens teori* (Stockholm); 1900. *Allgemeine Theorie des monochromatischen Aberrationen und ihre nächsten Ergebnisse für die Ophtalmologie* (Uppsala); 1908. *Die optische Abbildung in heterogenen Medien und die Dioptrik der Kristallinse des Menschen* (Uppsala and Stockholm).

Secondary: Tengroth, Björn, 1997. 'Allvar Gullstrand: Sveriges första nobelpristagare i fysiologi eller medicin.' *Förhandlingar från XVI Nordiska medicinhistoriska kongressen i Stockholm, Svensk medicinhistorisk tidskrift* (Supplement 1) 1: 77–84; Nilsson, Gunnar, 1945. *Berömda svenska läkare* (Uppsala); *DSB.*

Jan Eric Olsén

GULLY, JAMES MANBY (b. Kingston, Jamaica, 14 March 1808; d. London, England, 27 March 1883), *hydropathy.*

Gully was the son of Daniel Gully, a Jamaican coffee planter. When the family moved to England just before the end of the Napoleonic wars, James began a medical education that would take him to Paris and Edinburgh, gaining his MD at the latter in 1829. Any brief sense of security stemming from this was abruptly halted the following year: both Gully's parents died, the woman he had hoped to marry died, and the legal freedom granted to slaves led to the collapse of the family's plantation-based fortune. Under severe pressures, Gully went to work in London, combining a medical practice with medical journalism and the translation of continental medical texts. In 1831 he also married Fanny Court, with whom he had four children before her death from smallpox in 1838. Gully kept writing medical treatises as well as practicing but seemed dogged by misfortune until the early 1840s.

It was then that an old friend, James Wilson, returned from the Continent with the news that the hydropathic water cure system of Vincent Priessnitz was established as a proper alternative to medical orthodoxy and that they should combine forces and become medical hydropaths. They (rather astutely) chose the spa town of Malvern in Worcestershire as their center of operations, set up separate practices, and with remarkable rapidity attracted a very affluent clientele. This famously included the naturalist Charles Darwin (1809–82) and the poet Alfred, Lord Tennyson (1809–92). Gully both wrote a book on the water cure and from the mid-1850s became heavily involved in building up Malvern's amenities, including a newspaper, a good hotel, a new school, and a new railway station. He had long supported the practices of mesmerism and homeopathy and in the latter case urged some of its methods of treatments on his Malvern patients: by the 1860s, spiritualism was added, Gully becoming a fervent believer. But as in earlier periods of his life, a strange mix of bad luck and theatricality visited again. In retirement, which began in the early 1870s, Gully's name was romantically linked with a woman who was accused of murdering her husband. An inquiry into the case tainted Gully's name thereafter.

Critical of medical orthodoxy throughout his life, Gully found the perfect commercial solution in hydropathy, with its appeal to nervously exhausted eminent Victorians. Their often protracted visits to Malvern were almost always followed up by their returning home to continue to there follow a daily routine firmly based on the one followed while resident in Malvern itself. The respectability, indeed fame, of much of Gully's patient population and the (often locally disliked) way that he put Malvern on their medical map sat in odd contrast with the vicissitudes, agonies, and scandals of his private life.

Bibliography

Primary: 1846. *The Water Cure in Chronic Disease* (London); 1863. *A Guide to Domestic Hydrotherapeia* (London).

Secondary: Browne, Janet, 1990. 'Spas and Sensibilities: Darwin at Malvern' in Porter, Roy, ed., *The Medical History of Waters and Spas* (London); *Oxford DNB*.

Michael Neve

GUTHRIE, GEORGE JAMES (b. London, England, 1 May 1785; d. London, 1 May 1856), *surgery*.

Descended from an old Forfarshire family, whose members settled in Wexford, Guthrie's father, Andrew, was manager of a business that sold lead plaister. At age thirteen, Guthrie was apprenticed to Dr Phillips, a surgeon in Pall Mall, London, and also attended the Windmill Street School of Medicine. From June 1800 to March 1801, he served as a hospital mate at York Hospital, Chelsea, but was not then medically qualified. Shortly afterward, an order was issued that obliged all hospital mates to be a Member of the College of Surgeons. He entered the army as an assistant surgeon to the 29th Regiment of Foot at the age of sixteen, having passed the MRCS examination on 5 February 1801, shortly after the order was issued. He served in Canada for five years with the 29th Regiment and was then transferred to the Peninsula. He served there, except for a brief period in 1810, from 1808 to 1814. He saw much service and was especially commended by the Duke of Wellington.

In 1811 he was promoted staff surgeon, and in 1812 to deputy inspector of hospitals, but the Medical Board in London refused to confirm this appointment because of his youth. In the Peninsula he acted in this capacity in various battles, including Albuera, where he was in charge of over 3,000 wounded. Unlike John Hunter (1728–93), he particularly favored primary amputations on the battlefield rather than secondary amputations in the treatment of gunshot injuries requiring amputation. He was placed on half-pay in 1814 and then practiced privately in London. At this time, he attended the Windmill Street School and listened to the lectures of Charles Bell (1774–1842) and Benjamin Brodie (1783–1862) and those of John Abernethy (1764–1831) at St Bartholomew's.

James McGrigor (1771–1858) invited him to rejoin the Army Medical Department, but he declined. After the Battle of Waterloo, he journeyed to Brussels and advised on the management of a number of cases. His services were well received there, and he carried out major surgery on a number of individuals, including a successful case of amputation through the hip joint. On retiring to London, he took charge of two wards at the York Hospital for two years. When offered a knighthood by the Duke of York, he declined it on the grounds that he could not afford to accept this honor.

He also lectured *gratis* for twenty years to medical officers in all of the public services. These lectures were extremely popular and were often interspersed with anecdotes from his own military career in the Peninsular War. In 1816 he founded the Royal Westminster Ophthalmic Hospital at Charing Cross and from 1823 served as an assistant surgeon. From 1823 to 1843, he was also a full surgeon at the Westminster Hospital. He served from 1824 to 1856 as a Member of Council and from 1828 to 1856 as a Member of the Court of Examiners, and he was elected Vice-President of the RCS on five occasions. He was elected its President three times (1833, 1841, and 1854). He was also the RCS Hunterian professor of anatomy, physiology, and surgery from 1828 to 1832 and was elected FRS in 1827.

Bibliography

Primary: 1815. *On Gun-Shot Wounds of the Extremities, Requiring the Different Operations of Amputation* (London); 1853. *Commentaries on the Surgery of the War in Portugal, Spain, France, and the Netherlands ... Showing the Improvements made during and since that period in the great art and science of surgery on all the subjects to which they relate*, 5th edn. (London).

Secondary: Anon., 1850. 'Biographical Sketch of G.J. Guthrie, esq., F.R.S.' *Lancet* i: 726–736; Pettigrew, T. J., 1839. 'George James Guthrie, F.R.S., &c., &c., &c' in Pettigrew, T. J., *Medical Portrait Gallery* vol. 4 (pt. 5) (London) pp. 1–22; *Oxford DNB*.

Matthew Howard Kaufman